T0191794

Contributions to Statistics

More information about this series at http://www.springer.com/series/2912

S. Ejaz Ahmed
Editor

Big and Complex Data Analysis

Methodologies and Applications

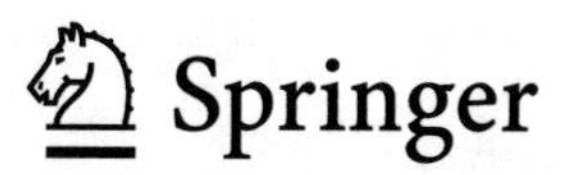

Editor
S. Ejaz Ahmed
Department of Mathematics & Statistics
Brock University
St. Catherines, Ontario
Canada

ISSN 1431-1968
Contributions to Statistics
ISBN 978-3-319-82387-4 ISBN 978-3-319-41573-4 (eBook)
DOI 10.1007/978-3-319-41573-4

© Springer International Publishing AG 2017
Softcover reprint of the hardcover 1st edition 2017
This work is subject to copyright. All rights are reserved by the Publisher, whether the whole or part of the material is concerned, specifically the rights of translation, reprinting, reuse of illustrations, recitation, broadcasting, reproduction on microfilms or in any other physical way, and transmission or information storage and retrieval, electronic adaptation, computer software, or by similar or dissimilar methodology now known or hereafter developed.
The use of general descriptive names, registered names, trademarks, service marks, etc. in this publication does not imply, even in the absence of a specific statement, that such names are exempt from the relevant protective laws and regulations and therefore free for general use.
The publisher, the authors and the editors are safe to assume that the advice and information in this book are believed to be true and accurate at the date of publication. Neither the publisher nor the authors or the editors give a warranty, express or implied, with respect to the material contained herein or for any errors or omissions that may have been made. The publisher remains neutral with regard to jurisdictional claims in published maps and institutional affiliations.

Printed on acid-free paper

This Springer imprint is published by Springer Nature
The registered company is Springer International Publishing AG
The registered company address is: Gewerbestrasse 11, 6330 Cham, Switzerland

Preface

This book comprises a collection of research contributions toward high-dimensional data analysis. In this data-centric world, we are often challenged with data sets containing many predictors in the model at hand. In a host of situations, the number of predictors may very well exceed the sample size. Truly, many modern scientific investigations require the analysis of such data. There are a host of buzzwords in today's data-centric world, especially in digital and print media. We encounter data in every walk of life, and for analytically and objectively minded people, data is everything. However, making sense of the data and extracting meaningful information from it may not be an easy task. Sometimes, we come across buzzwords such as big data, high-dimensional data, data visualization, data science, and open data without a proper definition of such words. The rapid growth in the size and scope of data sets in a host of disciplines has created a need for innovative statistical and computational strategies for analyzing such data. A variety of statistical and computational tools are needed to deal with such type of data and to reveal the data story.

This book focuses on variable selection, parameters estimation, and prediction based on high-dimensional data (HDD). In classical regression context, we define HDD where a number of predictors (d) are larger than the sample size (n). There are situations when the number of predictors is in millions and sample size maybe in hundreds. The modeling of HDD, where the sample size is much smaller than the size of the data element associated with each observation, is an important feature in a host of research fields such as social media, bioinformatics, medical, environmental, engineering, and financial studies, among others. A number of the classical techniques are available when $d < n$ to tell the data story. However, the existing classical strategies are not capable of yielding solutions for HDD. On the other hand, the term "big data" is not very well defined, but its problems are real and statisticians need to play a vital role in this data world. Generally speaking, big data relates when data is very large and may not even be stored at one place. However, the relationship between n and d may not be as crucial when comparing with HDD. Further, in some cases, users are not able to make the distinction between population and sampled data when dealing with big data. In any event, the big data or data science is an emerging field stemming equally from research enterprise and public and private sectors. Undoubtedly, big data is the future of research in a host of research fields, and transdisciplinary programs are required to develop the skills for data scientists. For example, many private and public agencies are using sophisticated number-crunching, data mining, or big data analytics to reveal patterns based on collected information. Clearly, there is an increasing demand for efficient prediction strategies for analyzing such data. Some examples of big data that have prompted demand are gene expression arrays; social network modeling; clinical, genetics, and phenotypic spatiotemporal data; and many others.

In the context of regression models, due to the trade-off between model prediction and model complexity, the model selection is an extremely important and challenging problem in the big data arena. Over the past two decades, many penalized regularization approaches have been developed to perform variable selection and estimation simultaneously. This book makes a seminal contribution in the arena of big data analysis including HDD. For a smooth reading and understanding of the contributions made in this book, it is divided in three parts as follows:

General High-dimensional theory and methods (chapters "Regularization After Marginal Learning for Ultra-High Dimensional Regression Models"–"Bias-Reduced Moment Estimators of Population Spectral Distribution and Their Applications")

Network analysis and big data (chapters "Statistical Process Control Charts as a Tool for Analyzing Big Data"–"Nonparametric Testing for Heterogeneous Correlation")

Statistics learning and applications (chapters "Optimal Shrinkage Estimation in Heteroscedastic Hierarchical Linear Models"–"A Mixture of Variance-Gamma Factor Analyzers")

We anticipate that the chapters published in this book will represent a meaningful contribution to the development of new ideas in big data analysis and will showcase interesting applications. In a sense, each chapter is self-contained. A brief description of the contents of each of the eighteen chapters in this book is provided.

Chapter "Regularization After Marginal Learning for Ultra-High Dimensional Regression Models" (Feng) introduces a general framework for variable selection in ultrahigh-dimensional regression models. By combining the idea of marginal screening and retention, the framework can achieve sign consistency and is extremely fast to implement.

In chapter "Empirical Likelihood Test for High Dimensional Generalized Linear Models" (Zang et al.), the estimation and model selection aspects of high-dimensional data analysis are considered. It focuses on the inference aspect, which can provide complementary insights to the estimation studies, and has at least two notable contributions. The first is the investigation of both full and partial tests, and the second is the utilization of the empirical likelihood technique under high-dimensional settings.

Abstract random projections are frequently used for dimension reduction in many areas of machine learning as they enable us to do computations on a more succinct representation of the data. Random projections can be applied row-

and column-wise to the data, compressing samples and compressing features, respectively. Chapter “Random Projections For Large-Scale Regression” (Thanei et al.) discusses the properties of the latter column-wise compression, which turn out to be very similar to the properties of ridge regression. It is pointed out that further improvements in accuracy can be achieved by averaging over least squares estimates generated by independent random projections.

Testing a hypothesis subsequent to model selection leads to test problems in which nuisance parameters are present. Chapter “Testing in the Presence of Nuisance Parameters: Some Comments on Tests Post-Model-Selection and Random Critical Values” (Leeb and Pötscher) reviews and critically evaluates proposals that have been suggested in the literature to deal with such problems. In particular, the chapter reviews a procedure based on the worst-case critical value, a more sophisticated proposal based on earlier work, and recent proposals from the econometrics literature. It is furthermore discussed why intuitively appealing proposals, for example, a parametric bootstrap procedure, as well as another recently suggested procedure, do not lead to valid tests, not even asymptotically.

As opposed to extensive research of covariate measurement error, error in response has received much less attention. In particular, systematic studies on general clustered/longitudinal data with response error do not seem to be available. Chapter “Analysis of Correlated Data with Error-Prone Response Under Generalized Linear Mixed Models” (Yi et al.) considers this important problem and investigates the asymptotic bias induced by the error in response. Valid inference procedures are developed to account for response error effects under different situations, and asymptotic results are appropriately established.

Statistical inference on large covariance matrices has become a fast growing research area due to the wide availability of high-dimensional data, and spectral distributions of large covariance matrices play an important role. Chapter “Bias-Reduced Moment Estimators of Population Spectral Distribution and Their Applications” (Qin and Li) derives bias-reduced moment estimators for the population spectral distribution of large covariance matrices and presents consistency and asymptotic normality of these estimators.

Big data often take the form of data streams with observations of a related process being collected sequentially over time. Statistical process control (SPC) charts provide a major statistical tool for monitoring the longitudinal performance of the process by online detecting any distributional changes in the sequential process observations. So, SPC charts could be a major statistical tool for analyzing big data. Chapter “Statistical Process Control Charts as a Tool for Analyzing Big Data” (Qiu) introduces some basic SPC concepts and methods and demonstrates the use of SPC charts for analyzing certain real big data sets. This chapter also describes some recent SPC methodologies that have a great potential for handling different big data applications. These methods include disease dynamic screening system and some recent profile monitoring methods for online monitoring of profile/image data that is commonly used in modern manufacturing industries.

Chapter “Fast Community Detection in Complex Networks with a K-Depths Classifier” (Tian and Gel) introduces a notion of data depth for recovery of community structures in large complex networks. The authors propose a new data-driven algorithm, K-depths, for community detection using the L_1 depth in an unsupervised setting. Further, they evaluate finite sample properties of the K-depths method using synthetic networks and illustrate its performance for tracking communities in online social media platform Flickr. The new method significantly outperforms the classical K-means and yields comparable results to the regularized K-means. Being robust to low-degree vertices, the new K-depths method is computationally efficient, requiring up to 400 times less CPU time than the currently adopted regularization procedures based on optimizing the Davis-Kahan bound.

Chapter "How Different are Estimated Genetic Networks of Cancer Subtypes?" (Shojaie and Sedaghat) presents a comprehensive comparison of estimated networks of cancer subtypes. Specifically, the networks estimated using six estimation methods were compared based on various network descriptors characterizing both local network structures, that is, edges, and global properties, such as energy and symmetry. This investigation revealed two particularly interesting properties of estimated gene networks across different cancer subtypes. First, the estimates from the six network reconstruction methods can be grouped into two seemingly unrelated clusters, with clusters that include methods based on linear and nonlinear associations, as well as methods based on marginal and conditional associations. Further, while the local structures of estimated networks are significantly different across cancer subtypes, global properties of estimated networks are less distinct. These findings can guide future research in computational and statistical methods for differential network analysis.

Statistical analysis of big clustered time-to-event data presents daunting statistical challenges as well as exciting opportunities. One of the challenges in working with big biomedical data is detecting the associations between disease outcomes and risk factors that involve complex functional forms. Many existing statistical methods fail in large-scale settings because of lack of computational power, as, for example, the computation and inversion of the Hessian matrix of the log-partial likelihood is very expensive and may exceed computation memory. Chapter "A Computationally Efficient Approach for Modeling Complex and Big Survival Data" (He et al.) handles problems with a large number of parameters and propose a novel algorithm, which combines the strength of quasi-Newton, MM algorithm, and coordinate descent. The proposed algorithm improves upon the traditional semiparametric frailty models in several aspects. For instance, the proposed algorithms avoid calculation of high-dimensional second derivatives of the log-partial likelihood and, hence, are competitive in term of computation speed and memory usage. Simplicity is obtained by separating the variables of the optimization problem. The proposed methods also provide a useful tool for modeling complex data structures such as time-varying effects.

Asymptotic inference for the concentration of directional data has attracted much attention in the past decades. Most of the asymptotic results related to concentration parameters have been obtained in the traditional large sample size and fixed dimension case. Chapter "Tests of Concentration for Low-Dimensional and High-Dimensional Directional Data" (Cutting et al.) considers the extension of existing testing procedures for concentration to the large n and large d case. In this high-dimensional setup, the authors provide tests that remain valid in the sense that they reach the correct asymptotic level within the class of rotationally symmetric distributions.

"Nonparametric testing for heterogeneous correlation" covers the big data problem of determining whether a weak overall monotone association between two variables persists throughout the population or is driven by a strong association that is limited to a subpopulation. The idea of homogeneous association rests on the underlying copula of the distribution. In chapter "Nonparametric Testing for Heterogeneous Correlation" (Bamattre et al.), two copulas are considered, the Gaussian and the Frank, under which components of two respective ranking measures, Spearman's footrule and Kendall's tau, are shown to have tractable distributions that lead to practical tests.

Shrinkage estimators have profound impacts in statistics and in scientific and engineering applications. Chapter "Optimal Shrinkage Estimation in Heteroscedastic Hierarchical Linear Models" (Kou and Yang) considers shrinkage estimation in the presence of linear predictors. Two heteroscedastic hierarchical regression models are formulated, and the study of optimal shrinkage estimators in each model is thoroughly presented. A class of shrinkage estimators, both parametric and semiparametric, based on unbiased risk estimate is proposed and is shown to be (asymptotically) optimal under mean squared error loss in each model. A simulation study is conducted to compare the performance of the proposed methods with existing shrinkage estimators. The authors also apply the method to real data and obtain encouraging and interesting results.

Chapter "High Dimensional Data Analysis: Integrating Submodels" (Ahmed and Yuzbasi) considers efficient prediction strategies in sparse high-dimensional model. In high-dimensional data settings, many penalized regularization strategies are suggested for simultaneous variable selection and estimation. However, different strategies yield a different submodel with different predictors and number of predictors. Some procedures may select a submodel with a relatively larger number of predictors than others. Due to the trade-off between model complexity and model prediction accuracy, the statistical inference of model selection is extremely important and a challenging problem in high-dimensional data analysis. For this reason, we suggest shrinkage and pretest post estimation strategies to improve the prediction performance of two selected submodels. Such a pretest and shrinkage strategy is constructed by shrinking an overfitted model estimator in the direction of an underfitted model estimator. The numerical studies indicate that post selection pretest and shrinkage strategies improved the prediction performance of selected submodels. This chapter reveals many interesting results and opens doors for further research in a host of research investigations.

Chapter "High-Dimensional Classification for Brain Decoding" (Croteau et al.) discusses high-dimensional classification within the context of brain decoding where spatiotemporal neuroimaging data are used to decode latent cognitive states. The authors discuss several approaches for feature selection including persistent homology, robust functional principal components analysis, and mutual information networks. These features are incorporated into a multinomial logistic classifier, and model estimation is based on penalized likelihood using the elastic net penalty. The approaches are illustrated in an application where the task is to infer, from brain activity measured with magnetoencephalography (MEG), the type of video stimulus shown to a subject.

Principal components analysis is a widely used technique for dimension reduction and characterization of variability in multivariate populations. In chapter "Unsupervised Bump Hunting Using Principal Components" (A. D'ıaz-Pach'on et al.), the authors interest lies in studying when and why the rotation to principal components can be used effectively within a response-predictor set relationship in the context of mode hunting. Specifically focusing on the Patient Rule Induction Method (PRIM), the authors first develop a fast version of this algorithm (fastPRIM) under normality which facilitates the theoretical studies to follow. Using basic geometrical arguments, they then demonstrate how the principal components rotation of the predictor space alone can in fact generate improved mode estimators. Simulation results are used to illustrate findings.

The analysis of high-dimensional data is challenging in multiple aspects. One aspect is interaction analysis, which is critical in biomedical and other studies. Chapter "Identifying Gene-Environment Interactions Associated with Prognosis Using Penalized Quantile Regression" (Wang et al.) studies high-dimensional interactions using a robust approach. The effectiveness demonstrated in this study opens doors for other robust methods under high-dimensional settings. This study will also be practically useful by introducing a new way of analyzing genetic data.

In chapter "A Mixture of Variance-Gamma Factor Analyzers" (McNicholas et al.), a mixture modeling approach for clustering high-dimensional data is developed. This approach is based on a mixture of variance-gamma distributions, which is interesting because the variance-gamma distribution has been underutilized in multivariate statistics—certainly, it has received far less attention than the skew-t distribution, which also parameterizes location, scale, concentration, and skewness. Clustering is carried out using a mixture of variance-gamma factor analyzers (MVGFA) model, which is an extension of the well-known mixture of factor analyzers model that can accommodate clusters that are asymmetric and/or heavy tailed. The formulation of the variance-gamma distribution used can be represented as a normal mean variance mixture, a fact that is exploited in the development of the associated factor analyzers.

In summary, several directions for innovative research in big data analysis were highlighted in this book. I remain confident that this book conveys some of the surprises, puzzles, and success stories in the arena of big data analysis. The research in this arena is ongoing for a foreseeable future.

As an ending thought, I would like to thank all the authors who submitted their papers for possible publication in this book as well as all the reviewers for their valuable input and constructive comments on all submitted manuscripts. I would like to express my special thanks to Veronika Rosteck at Springer for the encouragement and generous support on this project and helping me to arrive at the finishing line.

My special thanks go to Ulrike Stricker-Komba at Springer for outstanding technical support for the production of this book. Last but not least, I am thankful to my family for their support for the completion of this book.

Niagara-On-The-Lake, Ontario, Canada S. Ejaz Ahmed
August 2016

Contents

Part I
General High-Dimensional Theory and Methods

Regularization After Marginal Learning for Ultra-High Dimensional Regression Models

Yang Feng and Mengjia Yu

Abstract Regularization is a popular variable selection technique for high dimensional regression models. However, under the ultra-high dimensional setting, a direct application of the regularization methods tends to fail in terms of model selection consistency due to the possible spurious correlations among predictors. Motivated by the ideas of screening (Fan and Lv, J R Stat Soc Ser B Stat Methodol 70:849–911, 2008) and retention (Weng et al, Manuscript, 2013), we propose a new two-step framework for variable selection, where in the first step, marginal learning techniques are utilized to partition variables into different categories, and the regularization methods can be applied afterwards. The technical conditions of model selection consistency for this broad framework relax those for the one-step regularization methods. Extensive simulations show the competitive performance of the new method.

Keywords Independence screening • Lasso • Marginal learning • Retention • Selection • Sign consistency

1 Introduction

With the booming of information and vast improvement for computation speed, we are able to collect large amount of data in terms of a large collections of n observations and p predictors, where $p \gg n$. Recently, model selection gains increasing attention especially for ultra-high dimensional regression problems. Theoretically, the accuracy and interpretability of selected model are crucial in variable selection. Practically, algorithm feasibility and efficiency are vital in applications.

A great variety of penalized methods have been proposed in recent years. The regularization techniques for simultaneous variable selection and estimation are particularly useful to obtain sparse models compared to simply apply traditional criteria such as Akaike's information criterion [1] and Bayesian information

Y. Feng (✉) • M. Yu
Department of Statistics, Columbia University, New York, NY 10027, USA
e-mail: yangfeng@stat.columbia.edu

© Springer International Publishing AG 2017

S.E. Ahmed (ed.), *Big and Complex Data Analysis*, Contributions to Statistics,
DOI 10.1007/978-3-319-41573-4_1

criterion [18]. The least absolute shrinkage and selection operator (Lasso) [19] have been widely used as the l_1 penalty shrinks most coefficients to 0 and fulfills the task of variable selection. Many other regularization methods have been developed; including bridge regression [13], the smoothly clipped absolute deviation method [5], the elastic net [26], adaptive Lasso [25], LAMP [11], among others. Asymptotic analysis for the sign consistency in model selection [20, 24] has been introduced to provide theoretical support for various methods. Some other results such as parameter estimation [17], prediction [15], and oracle properties [5] have been introduced under different model contexts.

However, in ultra-high dimensional space where the dimension $p = \exp(n^a)$ (where $a > 0$), the conditions for sign consistency are easily violated as a consequence of large correlations among variables. To deal with such challenges, Fan and Lv [6] proposed the sure independence screening (SIS) method which is based on correlation learning to screen out irrelevant variables efficiently. Further analysis and generalization can be found in Fan and Song [7] and Fan et al. [8]. From the idea of retaining important variables rather than screening out irrelevant variables, Weng et al. [21] proposed the regularization after retention (RAR) method. The major differences between SIS and RAR can be summarized as follows. SIS makes use of marginal correlations between variables and response to screen noises out, while RAR tries to retain signals after acquiring these coefficients. Both of them relax the irrepresentable-type conditions [20] and achieve sign consistency.

In this paper, we would like to introduce a general multi-step estimation framework that integrates the idea of screening and retention in the first step to learn the importance of the features using the marginal information during the first step, and then impose regularization using corresponding weights. The main contribution of the paper is two-fold. First, the new framework is able to utilize the marginal information adaptively in two different directions, which will relax the conditions for sign consistency. Second, the idea of the framework is very general and covers the one-step regularization methods, the regularization after screening method, and the regularization after retention method as special cases.

The rest of this paper is organized as follows. In Sect. 2, we introduce the model setup and the relevant techniques. The new variable selection framework is elaborated in Sect. 3 with connections to existing methods explained. Section 4 develops the sign consistency result for the proposed estimators. Extensive simulations are conducted in Sect. 5 to compare the performance of the new method with the existing approaches. We conclude with a short discussion in Sect. 6. All the technical proofs are relegated to the appendix.

2 Model Setup and Several Methods in Variable Selection

2.1 Model Setup and Notations

Let (X_i, Y_i) be i.i.d. random pairs following the linear regression model:

$$Y_i = X_i\beta + \varepsilon_i, \quad i = 1, \ldots, n,$$

where $X_i = (X_i^1, \ldots, X_i^p)^T$ is p_n-dimensional vector distributed as $N(0, \Sigma)$, $\beta = (\beta_1, \ldots, \beta_p)^T$ is the true coefficient vector, $\varepsilon_1, \ldots, \varepsilon_n \overset{i.i.d.}{\sim} N(0, \sigma^2)$, and $\{X_i\}_{i=1}^n$ are independent of $\{\varepsilon_i\}_{i=1}^n$. Note here, we sometimes use p_n to emphasize the dimension p is diverging with the sample size n. Denote the support index set of β by $S = \{j : \beta_j \neq 0\}$ and the cardinality of S by s_n, and $\Sigma_{S^c|S} = \Sigma_{S^cS^c} - \Sigma_{S^cS}(\Sigma_{SS})^{-1}\Sigma_{SS^c}$. Both p_n and s_n are allowed to increase as n increases. For conciseness, we sometimes use signals and noises to represent relevant predictors S and irrelevant predictors S^c (or their corresponding coefficients) respectively.

For any set A, let A^c be its complement set. For any k dimensional vector w and any subset $K \subseteq \{1, \ldots, k\}$, w_K denotes the subvector of w indexed by K, and let $\|w\|_1 = \sum_{i=1}^k |w_i|$, $\|w\|_2 = (\sum_{i=1}^k w_i^2)^{1/2}$, $\|w\|_\infty = \max_{i=1,\ldots,k} |w_i|$. For any $k_1 \times k_2$ matrix M, any subsets $K_1 \subseteq \{1, \ldots, k_1\}$, $K_2 \subseteq \{1, \ldots, k_2\}$, $M_{K_1K_2}$ represents the submatrix of M consisting of entries indexed by the Cartesian product $K_1 \times K_2$. Let M_{K_2} be the columns of M indexed by K_2 and M^j be the j-th column of M. Denote $\|M\|_2 = \{\Lambda_{\max}(M^TM)\}^{1/2}$ and $\|M\|_\infty = \max_{i=1,\ldots,k} \sum_{j=1}^k |M_{ij}|$. When $k_1 = k_2 = k$, let $\rho(M) = \max_{i=1,\ldots,k} M_{ii}$, $\Lambda_{\min}(M)$ and $\Lambda_{\max}(M)$ be the minimum and maximum eigenvalues of M, respectively.

2.2 Regularization Techniques

The Lasso [19] defined as

$$\hat{\beta} = \arg\min_{\beta} \left\{ (2n)^{-1} \sum_{i=1}^{n} (Y_i - X_i^T\beta)^2 + \lambda_n \sum_{j=1}^{p_n} |\beta_j| \right\}, \quad \lambda_n \geq 0 \tag{1}$$

is a popular variable selection method. Thanks to the invention of efficient algorithms including LARS [4] and the coordinate descent algorithm [14], Lasso and its variants are applied to a wide range of different scenarios in this big data era. There is a large amount of research related to the theoretical properties of Lasso. Zhao and Yu [24] proposed almost necessary and sufficient conditions for the sign consistency for Lasso to select true model in the large p_n setting as n increases. Considering the sensitivity of tuning parameter λ_n and consistency for model selection, Wainwright

[20] has identified precise conditions of achieving sparsity recovery with a family of regularization parameters λ_n under deterministic design.

Another effective approach to the penalization problem is adaptive Lasso (AdaLasso) [25], which uses an adaptively weighted l_1-penalty term, defined as

$$\hat{\beta} = \arg\min_{\beta} \left\{ (2n)^{-1} \sum_{i=1}^{n} (Y_i - X_i^T \beta)^2 + \lambda_n \sum_{j=1}^{p_n} \omega_j |\beta_j| \right\}, \quad \lambda_n \geq 0. \tag{2}$$

where $\omega_j = 1/|\hat{\beta}_{\text{init}}|^{\gamma}$ for some $\gamma \geq 0$, in which $\hat{\beta}_{\text{init}}$ is some initial estimator. When signals are weakly correlated to noises, Huang et al. [16] proved AdaLasso is sign consistent with $\omega_j = 1/|\hat{\beta}_j^M| \equiv 1/|(\tilde{X^j})^T Y|$, where $\tilde{X}$ is the centered and scaled data matrix. One potential issue of this weighting choice is that when the correlations between some signals and response are too small, those signals would be severely penalized and may be estimated as noises. We will use numeric examples to demonstrate this point in the simulation section.

2.3 *Sure Independence Screening*

To reduce dimension from ultra-high to a moderate level, Fan and Lv [6] proposed a sure independence screening (SIS) method, which makes use of marginal correlations as a measure of importance in first step and then utilizes other operators such as Lasso to fulfill the target of variable selection. In particular, first we calculate the component-wise regression coefficients for each variable, i.e., $\hat{\beta}_j^M = (\tilde{X^j})^T \tilde{Y}$, $j = 1, \ldots, p_n$, where $\tilde{X^j}$ is the standardized j-th column of data X and $\tilde{Y}$ is the standardized response. Second, we define a sub-model with respect to the largest coefficients

$$\mathcal{M}_\gamma = \{1 \leq j \leq p_n : |\hat{\beta}_j^M| \text{ is among the first } \lfloor \gamma n \rfloor \text{ of all}\}.$$

Predictors that are not in $\mathcal{M}_\gamma$ are regarded as noise and therefore discarded for further analysis. SIS reduces the number of candidate covariates to a moderate level for the subsequent analysis. Combining SIS and Lasso, Fan and Lv [6] introduced SIS-Lasso estimator,

$$\begin{aligned} \hat{\beta} &= \arg\min_{\beta \in \mathcal{M}_\gamma} \left\{ (2n)^{-1} \sum_{i=1}^{n} (Y_i - X_i^T \beta)^2 + \lambda_n \sum_{j \in \mathcal{M}_\gamma} |\beta_j| \right\} \\ &= \arg\min_{\beta} \left\{ (2n)^{-1} \sum_{i=1}^{n} (Y_i - X_i^T \beta)^2 + \lambda_n \sum_{j \in \mathcal{M}_\gamma} |\beta_j| + \infty \sum_{j \in \mathcal{M}_\gamma^c} |\beta_j| \right\}. \end{aligned} \tag{3}$$

Clearly, γ should be chosen carefully to avoid screening out signals. To deal with the issue that signals may be marginally uncorrelated with the response in some cases, iterative-SIS was introduced [6] as a practical procedure but without rigorous theoretical support for the sign consistency. As a result, solely relying on marginal information is sometimes a bit too risky, or greedy, for model selection purpose.

3 Regularization After Marginal Learning

3.1 Algorithm

From Sect. 2, one potential drawback shared between AdaLasso and SIS-Lasso is that they may miss important covariates that are marginally weakly correlated with the response.

Now, we introduce a new algorithm, regularization after marginal (RAM) learning, to solve the issue. It utilizes marginal correlation to divide all variables into three candidate sets: a retention set, a noise set, and an undetermined set. Then regularization is imposed to find signals in the uncertainty set as well as to identify falsely retention signals and falsely screened noises.

A detailed description of the algorithm is as follows:

Step 0 (Marginal Learning) *Calculate the marginal regression coefficients after standardizing each predictor, i.e.,*

$$\hat{\beta}_j^{\mathcal{M}} = \sum_{i=1}^{n} \frac{(X_i^j - \bar{X}^j)}{\hat{\sigma}_j} Y_i, \quad 1 \le j \le p_n, \tag{4}$$

where $\bar{X}^j = \frac{1}{n}\sum_{i=1}^n X_i^j$ *and* $\hat{\sigma}_j^2 = \sqrt{\frac{\sum_{i=1}^n (X_i^j - \bar{X}^j)^2}{n-1}}$.

Define a retention set by $\hat{\mathcal{R}} = \{1 \le j \le p : |\hat{\beta}_j^{\mathcal{M}}| \ge \gamma_n\}$, *for a positive constant* γ_n; *a noise set by* $\hat{\mathcal{N}} = \{1 \le j \le p : |\hat{\beta}_j^{\mathcal{M}}| \le \tilde{\gamma}_n\}$, *for a positive constant* $\tilde{\gamma}_n < \gamma_n$; *and an undetermined set by* $\hat{\mathcal{U}} = (\hat{\mathcal{R}} \cup \hat{\mathcal{N}})^c$.

Step 1 (Regularization After Screening Noises Out) *Search for signals in* $\hat{\mathcal{U}}$ *by solving*

$$\hat{\beta}_{\hat{\mathcal{R}},\hat{\mathcal{U}}_1} = \arg\min_{\beta_{\hat{\mathcal{N}}}=0} \left\{ (2n)^{-1} \sum_{i=1}^{n} \Big(Y_i - \sum_{j \in \hat{\mathcal{U}}} X_{ij}\beta_j - \sum_{k \in \hat{\mathcal{R}}} X_{ik}\beta_k \Big)^2 + \lambda_n \sum_{j \in \hat{\mathcal{U}}} |\beta_j| \right\}, \tag{5}$$

where the index $\hat{\mathcal{U}}_1$ *is denoted as the set of variables that are estimated as signals in* $\hat{\mathcal{U}}$, *namely* $\hat{\mathcal{U}}_1 = \{j \in \hat{\mathcal{U}} | (\hat{\beta}_{\hat{\mathcal{R}},\hat{\mathcal{U}}_1})_j \ne 0\}$. *After Step 1, the selected variable set is* $\hat{\mathcal{R}} \cup \hat{\mathcal{U}}_1$.

Step 2 (Retrieve Falsely Discarded Signals) *Reevaluate the set* $\hat{\mathcal{N}}$ *to check whether it contains any signals. Solve*

$$\hat{\beta}_{\hat{\mathcal{R}},\hat{\mathcal{U}}_1,\hat{\mathcal{N}}_1} = \underset{\beta_{\hat{\mathcal{U}}_2}=0}{\arg\min} \left\{ (2n)^{-1} \sum_{i=1}^{n} \Big(Y_i - \sum_{j\in\hat{\mathcal{N}}} X_{ij}\beta_j - \sum_{k\in\hat{\mathcal{R}}\cup\hat{\mathcal{U}}_1} X_{ik}\beta_k \Big)^2 + \lambda_n^{\star} \sum_{j\in\hat{\mathcal{N}}} |\beta_j| \right\}, \tag{6}$$

where $\hat{\mathcal{U}}_2 = \hat{\mathcal{U}} \backslash \hat{\mathcal{U}}_1$.

This step is used to retrieve important variables which are weakly correlated to response marginally. This step can be omitted if we are sure about the noise set $\hat{\mathcal{N}}$. The selected variable set is now $\hat{\mathcal{R}} \cup \hat{\mathcal{U}}_1 \cup \hat{\mathcal{N}}_1$.

Step 3 (Remove Falsely Retained Signals) *Inspect the retention set* $\hat{\mathcal{R}}$ *to check whether it contains any noises. Solve*

$$\hat{\beta}_{\hat{\mathcal{R}}_1,\hat{\mathcal{U}}_1,\hat{\mathcal{N}}_1} = \underset{\beta_{\hat{\mathcal{U}}_2\cup\hat{\mathcal{N}}_2}=0}{\arg\min} \left\{ (2n)^{-1} \sum_{i=1}^{n} \Big(Y_i - \sum_{j\in\hat{\mathcal{R}}} X_{ij}\beta_j - \sum_{k\in\hat{\mathcal{U}}_1\cup\hat{\mathcal{N}}_1} X_{ik}\beta_k \Big)^2 + \lambda_n^{\star\star} \sum_{j\in\hat{\mathcal{R}}} |\beta_j| \right\}, \tag{7}$$

where $\hat{\mathcal{N}}_2 = \hat{\mathcal{N}} \backslash \hat{\mathcal{N}}_1$.

This step is used to remove noises which are highly correlated with the response marginally. This step can be omitted if we are sure about the retention set $\hat{\mathcal{R}}$. The final selected variable set is $\hat{\mathcal{R}}_1 \cup \hat{\mathcal{U}}_1 \cup \hat{\mathcal{N}}_1$.

The final estimator $\hat{\beta}_{\hat{\mathcal{R}}_1,\hat{\mathcal{U}}_1,\hat{\mathcal{N}}_1}$ is called the regularization after marginal (RAM) learning estimator. Note that the optimization problem described Step 2 in the RAM algorithm is of the same complexity as the original Lasso problem. A more efficient version of the algorithm where we remove Step 2 is called RAM-2. The corresponding selected variable set of RAM-2 is $\hat{\mathcal{R}}_1 \cup \hat{\mathcal{U}}_1$ as $\hat{\mathcal{N}}_1 = \emptyset$.

3.2 Connections to SIS and RAR

In the preparation Step 0 of RAM, marginal correlation provides us with a first evaluation of the importance for all variables. Usually, we expect that the variables with high marginal correlations are likely to be signals, while noises tend to have low marginal correlations. The choice of the thresholds γ_n and $\tilde{\gamma}_n$ are critical to ensure the accuracy of the retention set and the noise set. We follow Weng et al. [21] to select γ_n using a permutation-based approach. In particular, denote $Y_{(1)}, \ldots, Y_{(n)}$ as randomly permuted responses. Let γ_n be the largest marginal regression coefficient between permuted response and original data, i.e.,

$$\gamma_n = \max_{1\le j\le p_n} \left\{ |D_j| \,\Big|\, D_j = \sum_{i=1}^{n} \frac{(X_i^j - \bar{X}^j)}{\hat{\sigma}_j} Y_{(i)} \right\}. \tag{8}$$

In practice, we may adjust the threshold to ensure at most $\lceil n^{1/2} \rceil$ variables are included in the retention set, considering the root n consistency of classical least square estimators as well as SIS-based models. For $\tilde{\gamma}_n$, we can set it as the n-th largest coefficient in magnitude so that the cardinality of $\hat{\mathcal{R}} \cup \hat{\mathcal{U}}$ is $n-1$.

RAM-2 is closely connected to SIS. Technically, it utilizes marginal information to remove as many noises as possible. In addition, RAM-2 can be viewed as a greedy implementation of RAR+ [21], which is summarized in the following.

- (Retention) Define a retention set $\hat{R}$ which represents the coefficients strongly correlated to response marginally.
- (Regularization) Apply penalization on $\hat{R}^c$ to recover signals

$$\breve{\beta} = \arg\min_{\beta} \left\{ (2n)^{-1} \sum_{i=1}^{n} (Y_i - X_i^T \beta)^2 + 0 \sum_{j \in \hat{R}} |\beta_j| + \lambda_n \sum_{j \in \hat{R}^c} |\beta_j| \right\}. \tag{9}$$

- (Redemption) Denote $Q = \{j \in \hat{R}^c : \breve{\beta}_j \neq 0\}$, additional signals detected from the second step. Calculate the following penalized least square problem:

$$\tilde{\beta} = \arg\min_{\beta_{(\hat{R} \cup Q)^c} = 0} \left\{ (2n)^{-1} \sum_{i=1}^{n} \Big(Y_i - \sum_{j \in \hat{R}} X_{ij} \beta_j - \sum_{k \in Q} X_{ik} \beta_k \Big)^2 + \lambda_n^* \sum_{j \in \hat{R}} |\beta_j| \right\}, \tag{10}$$

  where λ_n^* is the penalty parameter and is in general different from λ_n in the previous step.

The regularization step only imposes penalty to variables that are not in $\hat{R}$. When all covariates in $\hat{R}$ are signals, we need only to recover the sparsity in $\hat{R}^c$. Although RAR performs well when the retention set $\hat{R} \subseteq S$, it could fail to recover the true sparsity pattern when $\hat{R}$ contains noises. Hence, the redemption step is necessary to rule out falsely selected noises.

As the intrinsic idea for RAR is retention, RAR+ can be regarded as a bidirectional and self-corrected version of RAR. Motivated by SIS-Lasso (3) and RAR+ (10), RAM first explores data by dividing variables into three sets in which one contains signal-like variables, one contains noise-like variables, and one contains the remaining undetermined variables. In Steps 1 and 3, RAM-2 combines advantages of SIS and RAR: on one hand, in terms of computational efficiency, like SIS, it is very efficient, thanks to the many noises screened out in the first step; on the other hand, RAM-2 could relax the regularity condition for sign consistency due to the retention set.

3.3 From RAM-2 to RAM

Though RAM-2 takes advantages of both SIS and RAR+, it shares the same drawback as SIS since signals that are marginally uncorrelated with the response could be removed during Step 1. To avoid fully replying on marginal correlation, RAM adds Step 2 to recover such signals.

Instead of re-examining $\hat{\mathcal{R}}$ immediately, the optional Step 2 is designed to reexamine the "noise" set $\hat{\mathcal{N}}$ and find signals in it. Intuitively, the retention of signals in $\hat{\mathcal{U}}_1 \cup \hat{\mathcal{R}}$ gives "weak" signals in $\hat{\mathcal{N}}_1$ an opportunity to show their significance in regression. Furthermore, noises in $\hat{\mathcal{R}}$ will also be weakly correlated with the residues $Y - X_{\mathcal{U}_1 \cup \mathcal{N}_1} \beta_{\mathcal{U}_1 \cup \mathcal{N}_1}$ in Step 3. Thus, we do not start to eliminate unnecessary variables in $\hat{\mathcal{R}}$ until all the other signals have been identified. Step 2 in RAM reduces the risk of signal losses, and increases the reliability of the model selection process.

We provide a brief comparison in Table 1 to show the similarities as well as differences among SIS-Lasso, RAR/RAR+, and RAM-2/RAM. The last row of Table 1 shows the final variable selection result. Note that, though some of the notations for different methods are same in Table 1, they are not necessarily identical since different procedures may lead to different results. Among these methods, RAM-2 and SIS-Lasso remove the variables in the noise set detected via marginal learning; RAR retains all variables in $\mathcal{R}$; RAM and RAR+ perform a recheck on all the candidate sets.

Table 1 Differences among 5 regularization methods using marginal information

<table>
<tr><th>RAM-2</th><th>RAM</th><th>SIS-Lasso</th><th>RAR</th><th>RAR+</th></tr>
<tr><td colspan="2" rowspan="2">$\mathcal{R}$: Retention set
$\mathcal{U}$: Undetermined set
$\mathcal{N}$: Noise set</td><td>$\mathcal{N}^c$: Candidates</td><td colspan="2">$\mathcal{R}$: Retention set
$\mathcal{R}^c$: Candidates</td></tr>
<tr><td>$\mathcal{N}$: Noise set</td><td colspan="2"></td></tr>
<tr><td>Retain $\mathcal{R}$</td><td>Retain $\mathcal{R}$</td><td>Check $\mathcal{N}^c$</td><td colspan="2"></td></tr>
<tr><td>Check $\mathcal{U}$</td><td>Check $\mathcal{U}$</td><td>Remove $\mathcal{N}$</td><td colspan="2"></td></tr>
<tr><td>Remove $\mathcal{N}$</td><td></td><td></td><td colspan="2"></td></tr>
<tr><td></td><td>Retain $\mathcal{R} \cup \mathcal{U}_1$</td><td></td><td colspan="2">Retain $\mathcal{R}$</td></tr>
<tr><td></td><td>Check $\mathcal{N}$</td><td></td><td colspan="2">Check $\mathcal{R}^c$</td></tr>
<tr><td colspan="2">Retain $\mathcal{U}_1 \cup \mathcal{N}_1$</td><td></td><td></td><td>Retain $(\mathcal{R}^c)_1$</td></tr>
<tr><td colspan="2">Check $\mathcal{R}$</td><td></td><td></td><td>Check $\mathcal{R}$</td></tr>
<tr><td>$\mathcal{R}_1 \cup \mathcal{U}_1$</td><td>$\mathcal{R}_1 \cup \mathcal{U}_1 \cup \mathcal{N}_1$</td><td>$(\mathcal{N}^c)_1$</td><td>$\mathcal{R} \cup (\mathcal{R}^c)_1$</td><td>$\mathcal{R}_1 \cup (\mathcal{R}^c)_1$</td></tr>
</table>

The subscript 1 for each set denotes the signals recovered from the corresponding sets

4 Asymptotic Analysis

4.1 Sure Independence Screening Property

Considering the linear regression model under the scaling $\log p_n = O(n^{a_1})$, $s_n = O(n^{a_2}), a_1 > 0, a_2 > 0, a_1 + 2a_2 < 1$, which is also required for achieving Strong Irrepresentable Condition in Zhao and Yu [24]. Under the conditions below, Fan and Lv [6] showed that SIS asymptotically achieves to screen only noises out. This result is necessary for the consistency in SIS-Lasso (3) as well as in RAM-2.

Condition 1 $var(Y_1) = \beta_S^T \Sigma_{SS} \beta_S = O(1)$.

Condition 2 $\Lambda_{max}(\Sigma) \le Cn^{\tau}$ *for a sufficiently large* $C, \tau \ge 0$.

Condition 3 $min_{j \in S} |cov(\beta_j^{-1} Y_1, X_1^j)| \ge c$ *for some positive constant c.*

Corollary 1 *Under Conditions 1–3, if* $min_{j \in S} |\beta_j| \ge Cn^{-a_3/2}$ *for some* $a_3 \in (0, 1 - a_1)$, *then there exists some* $\theta < 1 - a_1 - a_3$ *such that when* $\gamma \asymp n^{-\theta}$, *we have*

$$pr(S \subset \mathcal{M}_{\gamma}) \to 1 \quad as\ n \to \infty.$$

Condition 1 implies that there cannot be too many variables that have marginal regression coefficients exceeding certain thresholding level as in Fan and Song [7]. When Condition 2 fails, there is heavy collinearity in X, which leads to difficulty for differentiating signals from linearly correlated noises. Condition 3 rules out the situation that signals are jointly correlated with Y but their marginal correlations are relatively weak.

4.2 Sign Consistency for RAM-2

Given the success of screening in the first step, the following conditions are necessary to achieve sign consistency for RAM-2.

Condition 4 $\|\Sigma\beta\|_{\infty} = O(n^{(1-2\kappa)/8})$, *where* $0 < \kappa < \frac{1}{2}$ *is a constant.*

Condition 5 $min_{j \in S} |\beta_j| \ge Cn^{-\delta + a_2/2}$ *for a sufficiently large C, where* $0 < \delta < \{1 - max(a_1, a_2)\}/2$.

Condition 6 $\Lambda_{min}(\Sigma_{S \cup Z, S \cup Z}) \ge C_{min} > 0$, *where the strong noise set is defined as* $Z = \{j \in S^c : |\beta_j^M| \ge \gamma_n - c_1 n^{-\kappa}\}$ *with cardinality* z_n.

Condition 7 $\|\Sigma_{ZS} \Sigma_{SS}^{-1}\|_{\infty} \le 1 - \alpha$, *where* $\alpha > 0$.

Condition 8 $max_{S \subset Q \subset S \cup Z} \|\{\Sigma_{Q^c Q}(\Sigma_{QQ})^{-1}\}_{S \cap R^c}\|_{\infty} \le 1 - \gamma_1$, *where the strong signal set is defined as* $R = \{j \in S : |\beta_j^{\mathcal{M}}| > \gamma_n + c_1 n^{-\kappa}\}$ *and* $\gamma_1 > 0$.

Theorem 1 *If Conditions 1–8 are satisfied and* $\gamma = \tilde{\gamma}_n$ *holds for Corollary 1, then when* $z_n/s_n \to 0, s_n \to \infty$ *and* $\lambda_n \asymp n^{-\delta}, \lambda_n^{**} \asymp n^{-\delta}$, *RAM-2 achieves sign consistency*

$$pr(\hat{\beta}_{\hat{\mathcal{R}}_1,\hat{\mathcal{U}}_1,\hat{\mathcal{N}}_1} \text{ is unique and } sign(\hat{\beta}_{\hat{\mathcal{R}}_1,\hat{\mathcal{U}}_1,\hat{\mathcal{N}}_1}) = sign(\beta)) \to 1, \text{ as } n \to \infty.$$

Under the scaling conditions described in Theorem 1, Conditions 1 and 4 are required for establishing the uniform deviation results for marginal regression coefficients. Condition 5, which is a similar condition as that in Corollary 1, imposed a lower bound for magnitudes of the marginal regression coefficients. When strong noises in Z are not highly correlated to the signals, the probability of sign consistency converges to 1 as $n \to \infty$. In fact, when Z is an empty set, Conditions 6–8 are generalizations of some key conditions in Wainwright [20]. They relax the irrepresentable condition in Zhao and Yu [24] and give a toleration level on Z.

4.3 Sign Consistency for RAM

The key point for achieving sign consistency is the restriction for $\hat{\mathcal{U}}_1$ in Condition 8. In Step 2, we require similar restrictions on $\hat{\mathcal{N}}_1$ to guarantee the sign consistency of RAM. Different with RAM-2, we will take a second look on $\hat{\mathcal{N}}$ so that the success of RAM does not heavily depend on the screening step. We still control the scale as $\log p_n = O(n^{a_1}), s_n = O(n^{a_2}), a_1 > 0, a_2 > 0, a_1 + 2a_2 < 1$.

Theorem 2 *Under Conditions 4–8, when* $z_n/s_n \to 0, s_n \to \infty$ *and* $\lambda_n, \lambda_n^*, \lambda_n^{**} \asymp n^{-\delta}$, *RAM achieves sign consistency*

$$pr(\hat{\beta}_{\hat{\mathcal{R}}_1,\hat{\mathcal{U}}_1,\hat{\mathcal{N}}_1} \text{ is unique and } sign(\hat{\beta}_{\hat{\mathcal{R}}_1,\hat{\mathcal{U}}_1,\hat{\mathcal{N}}_1}) = sign(\beta)) \to 1, \text{ as } n \to \infty.$$

5 Numerical Study

5.1 Tuning Parameter Selection

In Weng et al. [21], the reports of successes are with respect to the oracle performance, namely the existence of an estimator that recovers the true model on the solution path. When comes to practice, it is necessary to choose an effective criterion for assessment of models under different tuning parameters λ_n. Chen and Chen [3] proposed an extended Bayesian information criterion (EBIC),

$$\text{BIC}_\gamma = \text{BIC} + 2\gamma \log \tau(\mathcal{S}_k), \quad 0 \le \gamma \le 1, \tag{11}$$

where $\mathcal{S}_k$ is the collection of all models with k covariates, and $\tau(\mathcal{S}_k)$ is the size of $\mathcal{S}_k$. Clearly, in our linear model, $\tau(\mathcal{S}_k) = \binom{p_n}{k}$. EBIC ($\text{BIC}_\gamma$) usually leads to a model with smaller size than BIC, since the additional term penalizes heavily on the model size. Therefore it is suitable for the ultra-high dimensional scenario we are considering. Chen and Chen [3] also established EBIC's consistency property. For all the penalize solution path calculation in the numeric studies, we apply EBIC for choosing the penalty parameter. Note that beside using a criterion function to select tuning parameter, another popular way is to use cross-validation-based approaches including Friedman et al. [14], Feng and Yu [12], and Yu and Feng [23].

5.2 *Simulations*

Note that in the RAM algorithm, we can replace the Lasso penalty with the adaptive Lasso penalty for all regularization steps. We implement both versions and call the corresponding estimators RAM-2-Lasso, RAM-2-AdaLasso, RAM-Lasso, and RAM-AdaLasso.

We compare the performances of model selection and parameter estimation under various ultra-high dimensional linear regression settings. The methods included for comparison are Lasso, AdaLasso, SIS-Lasso, RAR, RAR+, RAM-2-Lasso, RAM-2-AdaLasso, RAM-Lasso, and RAM-AdaLasso. We set $n =$ 100, 200, 300, 400, 500, and $p_n = \lfloor 100\exp(n^{0.2})\rfloor$, where $\lfloor k\rfloor$ is the largest integer not exceeding k. The number of repetitions is 200 for each triplet (n, s_n, p_n). We calculate the proportion of exact sign recovery and compare the MSE of the coefficient estimates, i.e., $\|\hat{\beta} - \beta\|_2^2$. All the penalization steps are implemented by using the R package glmnet [14] with corresponding weights. Note that other solution path calculation methods can also be used, including LARS [4] and APPLE [22]. The following scenarios are considered.

(1) The covariance matrix Σ is

$$\Sigma = \begin{bmatrix} \Sigma_{11} & 0 \\ 0 & I \end{bmatrix}, \text{ where } \Sigma_{11} = \begin{bmatrix} 1 & \dots & r \\ \vdots & \ddots & \vdots \\ r & \dots & 1 \end{bmatrix}_{2s_n \times 2s_n}.$$

Set $r = 0.6, \sigma = 3.5, s_n = 4, \beta_S = (3, -2, 2, -2)^T, \beta = (\beta_S^T, 0^T)^T$. After calculation, the absolute value of correlations between response and predictors are $(0.390, 0.043, 0.304, 0.043, 0.130, 0.130, 0.130, 0.130, 0, 0, \dots)^T$.

(2) The covariance matrix Σ is

$$\Sigma = \begin{bmatrix} \Sigma_{11} & 0 \\ 0 & I \end{bmatrix}, \text{ where } \Sigma_{11} = \begin{bmatrix} 1 & \dots & r & 0 \\ \vdots & \ddots & \vdots & \vdots \\ r & \dots & 1 & 0 \\ 0 & \dots & 0 & 1 \end{bmatrix}_{(2s_n-1)\times(2s_n-1)}.$$

(2a) Set $r = 0.5, \sigma = 2.5, s_n = 5, \beta_S = (3, 2, 1, -1, 0.75)^T, \beta = (0, 0, 0, 0, \beta_S^T, 0^T)^T$. After calculation, the absolute value of correlations between response and predictors are (0.483, 0.483, 0.483, 0.483, 0.772, 0.676, $0.579, 0.386, 0.145, 0, 0, \dots)^T$.

(2b) Set $r = 0.5, \sigma = 2, s_n = 5, \beta_S = (2.5, 2, 1, -1, 0.5)^T, \beta = (0, 0, 0, 0, \beta_S^T, 0^T)^T$. After calculation, the absolute value of correlations between response and predictors are (0.497, 0.497, 0.497, 0.497, 0.773, 0.718, $0.607, 0.387, 0.110, 0, 0, \dots)^T$.

For SIS-Lasso, we select the top $n - 1$ variables with largest absolute value of marginal correlations for fair comparison with RAMs. For AdaLasso, the weights are $\omega_j = 1/|\hat{\beta}_j^{\mathcal{M}}|$ as shown in (4). According to Weng et al. [21], the threshold γ_n for RAR/RAR+ is determined by one time permuted data,

$$\gamma_n = \max_{1\leq j\leq p} \left\{ |D_j^*| \middle| D_j^* = \sum_{i=1}^n \frac{(X_i^j - \bar{X}^j)}{\sum_{i=1}^n (X_i^j - \bar{X}^j)^2} Y_{(i)} \right\}.$$

For all penalized estimators, EBIC is used to select the tuning parameter. Tables 2 and 3 show the sign recovery proportion and MSE for each method.

In Scenario 1, only RAR+ and RAM-Lasso perform well especially when the dimension p_n becomes large. As the consequence of small marginal correlation coefficients β_2 and β_4, the two corresponding signals are screened out at the beginning, leading to the failure of SIS-Lasso and RAM-2. Their weak marginal correlations also lead to heavy penalties in regularization, which leads to the low sign recovery proportion and large MSE of AdaLasso as well as RAM-AdaLasso. In this scenario, RAR+ and RAM-Lasso perform the best in terms of both sign recovery proportion and the MSE.

In Scenario 2, an independent signal is included in both Scenario 2a and Scenario 2b, which leads to some interesting findings. For Scenario 2a, RAM-2-AdaLasso has impressive high success rates as RAM-AdaLasso does. This emphasizes the important role of marginal learning (RAM-AdaLasso v.s. AdaLasso) and the advantage from screening (RAM-2-AdaLasso v.s. AdaLasso). Noteworthy, RAM-2-Lasso is also comparable to RAR+ and RAM-Lasso, so it indicates that the more efficient version RAM-2 is a worthwhile alternative for variable selection. In Scenario 2b, with respect to the sign recovery proportion and the MSE criteria, RAR+ takes the lead while RAM-Lasso and RAM-2-Lasso follow closely.

Table 2 Sign recovery proportion over 200 simulation rounds of each method

n	100	200	300	400	500
Scenario 1					
Lasso	0.000	0.000	0.045	0.235	0.450
SIS-Lasso	0.000	0.000	0.015	0.065	0.095
AdaLasso	0.000	0.000	0.010	0.025	0.035
RAR	0.015	0.245	0.370	0.320	0.360
RAR+	**0.025**	**0.515**	**0.870**	**0.900**	**0.935**
RAM-2-Lasso	0.000	0.040	0.125	0.130	0.145
RAM-Lasso	**0.090**	**0.630**	**0.890**	**0.880**	**0.870**
RAM-2-AdaLasso	0.000	0.015	0.050	0.065	0.090
RAM-AdaLasso	0.000	0.050	0.190	0.290	0.330
Scenario 2a					
Lasso	0.000	0.000	0.005	0.010	0.035
SIS-Lasso	0.000	0.000	0.000	0.005	0.030
AdaLasso	0.000	0.125	0.380	0.625	0.675
RAR	0.000	0.000	0.000	0.000	0.000
RAR+	0.000	0.095	0.295	0.550	0.665
RAM-2-Lasso	0.000	0.080	0.300	0.530	0.675
RAM-Lasso	0.000	0.100	0.300	0.505	0.645
RAM-2-AdaLasso	**0.000**	**0.105**	**0.420**	**0.680**	**0.835**
RAM-AdaLasso	**0.000**	**0.125**	**0.425**	**0.710**	**0.850**
Scenario 2b					
Lasso	0.000	0.000	0.005	0.105	0.300
SIS-Lasso	0.000	0.000	0.005	0.090	0.255
AdaLasso	0.000	0.075	0.200	0.335	0.390
RAR	0.000	0.000	0.000	0.000	0.000
RAR+	**0.000**	**0.160**	**0.330**	**0.560**	**0.720**
RAM-2-Lasso	**0.000**	**0.110**	**0.315**	**0.495**	**0.630**
RAM-Lasso	**0.005**	**0.125**	**0.350**	**0.535**	**0.680**
RAM-2-AdaLasso	0.000	0.100	0.300	0.445	0.575
RAM-AdaLasso	0.000	0.120	0.315	0.470	0.645

Note: By setting $p_n = \lfloor 100 \exp(n^{0.2}) \rfloor$, the number of variables are 1232, 1791, 2285, 2750, and 3199, respectively. The bold values represent the best performing methods under each scenario

6 Discussion

In this work, we propose a general framework for variable selection in ultra-high dimensional linear regression model by incorporating marginal information before regularization. It is shown to have sign consistency under a weaker condition compared with the one-step procedure if the marginal information is helpful.

The framework is quite general and can be easily extended to the case of generalized linear models as well as any other penalty form. Another important

Table 3 Mean square error $\|\hat{\beta} - \beta\|_2^2$ over 200 simulation rounds of each method

n	100	200	300	400	500
Scenario 1					
Lasso	4.0218	3.5174	2.3559	1.3320	0.8017
SIS-Lasso	4.0606	3.5962	3.1029	2.9109	2.7388
AdaLasso	3.9857	3.6522	3.2897	3.0739	2.7821
RAR	3.3556	1.6786	0.9485	0.7303	0.6733
RAR+	**3.4226**	**1.5673**	**0.7130**	**0.5413**	**0.4585**
RAM-2-Lasso	3.9420	3.3433	2.9404	2.8482	2.7078
RAM-Lasso	**3.0516**	**1.3942**	**0.7336**	**0.6030**	**0.5093**
RAM-2-AdaLasso	3.9469	3.4311	3.0538	2.9292	2.7711
RAM-AdaLasso	3.7514	2.9639	2.0931	1.7351	1.5575
Scenario 2a					
Lasso	1.7728	1.5525	1.3311	1.1789	1.0086
SIS-Lasso	1.7684	1.5488	1.3385	1.1724	0.9764
AdaLasso	1.7296	1.3663	0.8032	0.5767	0.4101
RAR	1.6421	0.9908	0.7189	0.6048	0.5104
RAR+	1.8041	1.3893	0.9026	0.6154	0.4390
RAM-2-Lasso	1.8471	1.4442	1.0207	0.6850	0.5125
RAM-Lasso	1.8900	1.4271	1.0111	0.6608	0.4937
RAM-2-AdaLasso	**1.8362**	**1.4144**	**0.8883**	**0.5946**	**0.4340**
RAM-AdaLasso	**1.8279**	**1.4105**	**0.8534**	**0.5873**	**0.4351**
Scenario 2b					
Lasso	1.5437	1.4189	1.2009	0.8720	0.5943
SIS-Lasso	1.5344	1.4152	1.1709	0.8118	0.5503
AdaLasso	1.5372	0.8574	0.5612	0.4743	0.4279
RAR	1.2475	0.7910	0.6334	0.5047	0.4399
RAR+	**1.5458**	**0.9677**	**0.6210**	**0.4027**	**0.3242**
RAM-2-Lasso	**1.5932**	**1.0729**	**0.6631**	**0.4806**	**0.4106**
RAM-Lasso	**1.6032**	**1.0598**	**0.6585**	**0.4759**	**0.3867**
RAM-2-AdaLasso	1.5786	0.9240	0.5973	0.4957	0.4237
RAM-AdaLasso	1.5781	0.9262	0.5999	0.4880	0.4026

The bold values represent the best performing methods under each scenario

extension would be the high dimensional classification [9, 10]. How to develop the parallel theory for those extensions would be an interesting future work.

Acknowledgements This work was partially supported by NSF grant DMS-1308566. The authors would like to thank the Editor and the referee for constructive comments which greatly improved the paper. The majority of the work was done when Mengjia Yu was an M.A. student at Columbia University.

Appendix

Proof of Theorem 1 Denote the design matrix by X, response vector by Y, and error vector by ε. The scale condition is $\log p_n = O(n^{a_1})$, $s_n = O(n^{a_2}), a_1 > 0, a_2 > 0, a_1 + 2a_2 < 1$.

Step I: Recall the index of variables with large coefficients

$$\mathcal{M}_{\tilde{\gamma}_n} = \{1 \leq j \leq p : |\hat{\beta}_j^M| \text{ is among the first} \lfloor \tilde{\gamma}_n \rfloor \text{ of all } \} = \mathcal{N}^c.$$

Under Corollary 1,

$$\text{pr}(S \subset \mathcal{M}_{\tilde{\gamma}_n} = \mathcal{N}^c = \mathcal{R} \cup \mathcal{U}) \to 1 \quad \text{as } n \to \infty.$$

Hence with high probability the set $\hat{\mathcal{N}}$ contains only noises.

Step II: Next we will show that RAM-2 succeeds in detecting signals in $\hat{\mathcal{N}}^c$. Let $S = \{1 \leq j \leq p : \beta_j \neq 0\}$. Denote the compositions $S = \hat{\mathcal{R}}_1 \cup \hat{\mathcal{U}}_1$ and define the set of noises left in $\hat{\mathcal{N}}^c$ as $(\hat{\mathcal{R}} \setminus \hat{\mathcal{R}}_1) \cup (\hat{\mathcal{U}} \setminus \hat{\mathcal{U}}_1) \doteq \hat{\mathcal{R}}_2 \cup \hat{\mathcal{U}}_2$, where $\hat{\mathcal{R}}_1$ and $\hat{\mathcal{U}}_1$ are signals from $\hat{\mathcal{R}}$ and $\hat{\mathcal{U}}$, respectively.

Firstly, we would like to introduce an important technique in RAR+. Define the set of true signals as S, and in an arbitrary regularization, define the set that is hold without penalty as H while the set that needs to be checked with penalty as C. Let

$$\check{\beta} = \arg\min_{\beta} \left\{ (2n)^{-1} \|Y - X\beta\|_2^2 + \lambda_n \|\beta_C\|_1 \right\}, \tag{12}$$

$$\bar{\beta} = \arg\min_{\beta_{(S\cup H)^c}=0} \left\{ (2n)^{-1} \|Y - X\beta\|_2^2 + \lambda_n \|\beta_{C\cap S}\|_1 \right\}. \tag{13}$$

Now we define $Q = S \cup H$ which are the variables we would like to retain, and then the variables that are supposed to be discarded are $Q^c = C \setminus S$.

By optimality conditions of convex problems [2], $\check{\beta}$ is a solution to (12) if and only if

$$n^{-1} X^T (Y - X\check{\beta}) = \lambda_n \partial \|\check{\beta}_C\|, \tag{14}$$

where $\partial \|\check{\beta}_C\|$ is the subgradient of $\|\beta_C\|_1$ at $\beta = \check{\beta}$. Namely, the ith $(1 \leq i \leq p_n)$ element of $\partial \|\check{\beta}_C\|$ is

$$(\partial \|\check{\beta}_C\|)_i = \begin{cases} 0 & \text{if } i \in C; \\ \text{sign}(\check{\beta}_i) & \text{if } i \in C^c \text{ and } \check{\beta}_i \neq 0; \\ t & \text{otherwise,} \end{cases}$$

where t can be any real number with $|t| \leq 1$. Similarly, $\bar{\beta}$ is the unique solution to (13) if and only if

$$\bar{\beta}_{Q^c} = 0, \quad n^{-1}X_Q^T(Y - X_Q\bar{\beta}_Q) = \lambda_n \mathrm{sig}(\bar{\beta}_Q), \tag{15}$$

where $\mathrm{sig}(\bar{\beta}_Q)$, a vector of length card(Q), is the subgradient of $\|\beta_{\bar{Q}^c}\|_1$ at $\beta_Q = \bar{\beta}_Q$. Then it is not hard to see that the unique solution $\bar{\beta}$ is also a solution for (13) if

$$\|n^{-1}X_{Q^c}^T(Y - X_Q\bar{\beta}_Q)\|_\infty < \lambda_n, \tag{16}$$

simply because (15) and (16) imply $\bar{\beta}$ satisfies (14). Solving the equation in (15) gives

$$\bar{\beta}_Q = (X_Q^TX_Q)^{-1}\left[X_Q^TY - n\lambda_n \mathrm{sig}(\bar{\beta}_Q)\right]. \tag{17}$$

Using (17) and $Y = X_S\beta_S + \varepsilon$, (16) is equivalent to

$$\begin{aligned}&\|X_{Q^c}^TX_Q(X_Q^TX_Q)^{-1}\mathrm{sig}(\bar{\beta}_Q)\\&\quad + (n\lambda_n)^{-1}X_{Q^c}^T(I - X_Q(X_Q^TX_Q)^{-1}X_Q^T)(X_S\beta_S + \varepsilon)\|_\infty < 1\end{aligned} \tag{18}$$

Since $(I - X_Q(X_Q^TX_Q)^{-1}X_Q^T)X_Q = 0$, (18) can be simplified as

$$\|X_{Q^c}^TX_Q(X_Q^TX_Q)^{-1}\mathrm{sig}(\bar{\beta}_Q) + (n\lambda_n)^{-1}X_{Q^c}^T(I - X_Q(X_Q^TX_Q)^{-1}X_Q^T)\varepsilon\|_\infty < 1. \tag{19}$$

Note that, if there is a unique solution for (12), say $\check{\beta}$, and $\bar{\beta}$ satisfies (19), then $\bar{\beta}$ is indeed the unique solution for (12). This is equivalent to $\check{\beta}_{Q^c} = 0$. Furthermore, if $\min_{j\in Q}|\beta_j| > \|\beta_j - \bar{\beta}_j\|_\infty$ also holds, we can conclude $\check{\beta}_Q \neq 0$. Thus (12) achieves sign recovery. In the following, we will make use of this idea repeatedly.

Secondly, consider the Step 1 (5),

$$\begin{aligned}\hat{\beta}_{\hat{\mathcal{R}},\hat{\mathcal{U}}_1} &= \underset{\beta_{\hat{\mathcal{N}}}=0}{\arg\min}\left\{(2n)^{-1}\sum_{i=1}^n\left(Y_i - \sum_{j\in\hat{\mathcal{U}}}X_{ij}\beta_j - \sum_{k\in\hat{\mathcal{R}}}X_{ik}\beta_k\right)^2 + \lambda_n\sum_{j\in\hat{\mathcal{U}}}|\beta_j|\right\},\\&= \underset{\beta_{\hat{\mathcal{N}}}=0}{\arg\min}\left\{(2n)^{-1}\|Y - X\beta\|_2^2 + \lambda_n\|\beta_{\hat{\mathcal{U}}}\|_1\right\}.\end{aligned} \tag{20}$$

Here, denote $\check{\beta} = \hat{\beta}_{\hat{\mathcal{R}},\hat{\mathcal{U}}_1}$. After this step, the ideal result is that with high probability,

$$\check{\beta}_{\hat{\mathcal{U}}_1} \neq 0 \text{ and } \check{\beta}_{\hat{\mathcal{U}}\setminus\hat{\mathcal{U}}_1} = 0. \tag{21}$$

Therefore, define an oracle estimator of (20),

$$\bar{\beta} = \underset{\beta_{(\hat{\mathcal{R}}\cup\hat{\mathcal{U}}_1)^c}=0}{\arg\min} \left\{ (2n)^{-1}\|Y - X_{\hat{Q}}\beta_{\hat{Q}}\|_2^2 + \lambda_n\|\beta_{\hat{\mathcal{U}}_1}\|_1 \right\}, \tag{22}$$

where $\hat{Q} = \hat{\mathcal{R}} \cup \hat{\mathcal{U}}_1 = S \cup \hat{\mathcal{R}}_2$. Now, we plug $\breve{\beta}, \bar{\beta}$, and $\hat{Q}$ back to (12), (13), and (19), then it is sufficient to prove (20) has a unique solution and it achieves sign consistency with $Q = \hat{Q}$.

Let

$$\begin{aligned} F &= X_{\hat{Q}^c}^T - \Sigma_{\hat{Q}^c\hat{Q}}\Sigma_{\hat{Q}\hat{Q}}^{-1}X_{\hat{Q}}^T, \\ K_1 &= \Sigma_{\hat{Q}^c\hat{Q}}\Sigma_{\hat{Q}\hat{Q}}^{-1}\text{sig}(\bar{\beta}_{\hat{Q}}), \\ K_2 &= FX_{\hat{Q}}(X_{\hat{Q}}^TX_{\hat{Q}})^{-1}\text{sig}(\bar{\beta}_{\hat{Q}}) + (n\lambda_n)^{-1}F\{I - X_{\hat{Q}}(X_{\hat{Q}}^TX_{\hat{Q}})^{-1}X_{\hat{Q}}^T\}\varepsilon. \end{aligned}$$

Then, (19) is equivalent to

$$\|K_1 + K_2\|_\infty < 1.$$

To be more clear that, since we have already screen $\hat{\mathcal{N}}$ out, $\hat{Q}^c$ is in fact the complement of $\hat{Q}$ under the "universe" $\hat{\mathcal{R}}\cup\hat{\mathcal{U}}$. We write $\hat{Q}^c$ instead of $(\hat{\mathcal{R}}\cup\hat{\mathcal{U}})\backslash\hat{Q} = \hat{\mathcal{U}}_2$ to show a close connection with the analysis in first part above.

Now let

$$\begin{aligned} A &= \{R \subset \hat{\mathcal{R}}_1 \subset S, S \subset \hat{Q} \subset S \cup Z\}, \\ B &= \{S \subset \hat{Q} \subset S \cup Z\}, \\ \mathcal{T}_A &= \{(\mathcal{R}_1, Q) | R \subset \mathcal{R}_1 \subset S, S \subset Q \subset S \cup Z\}. \end{aligned}$$

From Conditions 1 and 4, $P(A) \to 1$ as a direct result of Proposition 2 in Weng et al. [21]. Since Condition 8 implies

$$\text{pr}(\|K_1\|_\infty \leq 1 - \gamma_1) \geq \text{pr}(\{\|K_1\|_\infty \leq 1 - \gamma_1\} \cap A) = \text{pr}(A) \to 1 \tag{23}$$

as given A

$$\|K_1\|_\infty = \|\Sigma_{\hat{Q}^c\hat{Q}}\Sigma_{\hat{Q}\hat{Q}}^{-1}\text{sig}(\bar{\beta}_{\hat{Q}})\|_\infty \leq \|\{\Sigma_{\hat{Q}^c\hat{Q}}\Sigma_{\hat{Q}\hat{Q}}^{-1}\}_{\hat{\mathcal{U}}_1}\|_\infty$$

is always less than $1 - \gamma_1$.

Denote $K_2(\mathcal{R}_1, Q)$ as the analogy of K_2 and $\bar{\beta}_Q$ as the analogy of $\bar{\beta}_{\hat{Q}}$ by replacing $\hat{\mathcal{R}}_1$ and $\hat{Q}$ in (22) with $\mathcal{R}_1$ and Q. Since given X_Q and ε, the j-th element of $K_2(\mathcal{R}_1, Q)$, namely

$$F(j)X_Q(X_Q^TX_Q)^{-1}\text{sig}(\bar{\beta}_Q) + (n\lambda_n)^{-1}F(j)\{I - X_Q(X_Q^TX_Q)^{-1}X_Q^T\}\varepsilon, \tag{24}$$

is normally distributed with mean 0 and variance V_j, where

$$V_j \le (\Sigma_{Q^c|Q})_{jj}\Big[\mathrm{sig}(\bar{\beta}_Q)^T(X_Q^TX_Q)^{-1}\mathrm{sig}(\bar{\beta}_Q) + (n\lambda_n)^{-2}\varepsilon^T\{I - X_Q(X_Q^TX_Q)^{-1}X_Q^T\}\varepsilon\Big]$$
$$\le \mathrm{sig}(\bar{\beta}_Q)^T(X_Q^TX_Q)^{-1}\mathrm{sig}(\bar{\beta}_Q) + (n\lambda_n)^{-2}\|\varepsilon\|_2^2.$$

Hence, we let

$$H = \bigcup_{(\mathcal{R}_1,Q)\subset\mathcal{T}_A}\Big\{\mathrm{sig}(\bar{\beta}_Q)^T(X_Q^TX_Q)^{-1}\mathrm{sig}(\bar{\beta}_Q) + (n\lambda_n)^{-2}\|\varepsilon\|_2^2$$
$$> \frac{s_n + z_n}{nC_{\min}}(8(s_n + z_n)^{1/2}n^{-1/2} + 1) + (1 + s_n^{1/2}n^{-1/2})/(n\lambda_n^2)\Big\}.$$

Next, we want to show

$$\mathrm{pr}\Big(\|K_2\|_\infty > \frac{\gamma_1}{2}\Big) \le \mathrm{pr}\Big(\Big\{\|K_2\|_\infty > \frac{\gamma_1}{2}\Big\} \cap A\Big) + \mathrm{pr}(A^c)$$
$$\le \mathrm{pr}\Big(\Big\{\bigcup_{(\mathcal{R}_1,Q)\subset\mathcal{T}_A}\|K_2(\mathcal{R}_1,Q)\|_\infty > \frac{\gamma_1}{2}\Big\} \cap A\Big) + \mathrm{pr}(A^c)$$
$$\le \mathrm{pr}\Big(\bigcup_{(\mathcal{R}_1,Q)\subset\mathcal{T}_A}\|K_2(\mathcal{R}_1,Q)\|_\infty > \frac{\gamma_1}{2} \mid H^c\Big) + \mathrm{pr}(H) + \mathrm{pr}(A^c)$$
$$\longrightarrow 0. \tag{25}$$

By the tail probability inequality of Gaussian distribution (inequality (48) in Wainwright [20]), it is not hard to see that

$$\mathrm{pr}\Big(\bigcup_{(\mathcal{R}_1,Q)\subset\mathcal{T}_A}\|K_2(\mathcal{R}_1,Q)\|_\infty > \frac{\gamma_1}{2} \mid H^c\Big)$$
$$\le \sum_{(\mathcal{R}_1,Q)\subset\mathcal{T}_A}\mathrm{pr}(\|K_2(\mathcal{R}_1,Q)\|_\infty > \frac{\gamma_1}{2} \mid H^c)$$
$$\le 2^{s_n+z_n}\cdot \max_{(\mathcal{R}_1,Q)\subset\mathcal{T}_A}\mathrm{pr}(\|K_2(\mathcal{R}_1,Q)\|_\infty > \frac{\gamma_1}{2} \mid H^c)$$
$$\le 2^{s_n+z_n}\cdot 2(p_n - s_n)\exp(-\gamma_1^2/8V), \tag{26}$$

where $V = (1 + s_n^{1/2}n^{-1/2})/(n\lambda_n^2) + \frac{s_n+z_n}{nC_{\min}}(8(s_n + z_n)^{1/2}n^{-1/2} + 1) \ge V_j$ under condition H^c. Since $\log[2^{s_n+z_n+1}(p_n - s_n)] = o(\gamma_1^2/8V)$ under our scaling, (26) $\to 0$.

To bound pr(H), note that

$$\begin{aligned}\mathrm{pr}(H) \le \mathrm{pr}\Big(\bigcup_{(\mathcal{R}_1,Q)\subset\mathcal{T}_A}\Big\{&\mathrm{sig}(\bar\beta_Q)^T(X_Q^TX_Q)^{-1}\mathrm{sig}(\bar\beta_Q)\\ &> \frac{s_n+z_n}{nC_{\min}}(8(s_n+z_n)^{1/2}n^{-1/2}+1)\Big\}\Big)\\ &+\mathrm{pr}\Big((n\lambda_n)^{-2}\|\varepsilon\|_2^2 > (1+s_n^{1/2}n^{-1/2})/(n\lambda_n^2)\Big)\end{aligned} \tag{27}$$

Since $\|\varepsilon\|_2^2 \sim \chi^2(n)$, using the inequality of (54a) in Wainwright [20], we get

$$\begin{aligned}\mathrm{pr}\Big((n\lambda_n)^{-2}\|\varepsilon\|_2^2 > (1+s_n^{1/2}n^{-1/2})/(n\lambda_n^2)\Big) &\le \mathrm{pr}\Big(\|\varepsilon\|_2^2 \ge (1+s_n^{1/2}n^{-1/2})n\Big)\\ &\le \exp(-\frac{3}{16}s_n),\end{aligned} \tag{28}$$

whenever $s_n/n < 1/2$. For any given Q that satisfying $S\subset Q\subset S\cup Z$,

$$\begin{aligned}\mathrm{sig}(\bar\beta_Q)^T(X_Q^TX_Q)^{-1}\mathrm{sig}(\bar\beta_Q) &\le (s_n+z_n)\|(X_Q^TX_Q)^{-1}\|_2\\ &\le (s_n+z_n)/n\Big(\|(X_Q^TX_Q/n)^{-1}-\Sigma_{QQ}^{-1}\|_2+\|\Sigma_{QQ}^{-1}\|_2\Big)\\ &\le (s_n+z_n)/n\Big(\|(X_Q^TX_Q/n)^{-1}-\Sigma_{QQ}^{-1}\|_2+1/C_{\min}\Big).\end{aligned}$$

holds for any $\mathcal{R}_1$ that satisfying $R\subset\mathcal{R}_1\subset S$. Therefore, by the concentration inequality of (58b) in Wainwright [20],

$$\begin{aligned}&\mathrm{pr}\Big(\bigcup_{(\mathcal{R}_1,Q)\subset\mathcal{T}_A}\Big\{\mathrm{sig}(\bar\beta_Q)^T(X_Q^TX_Q)^{-1}\mathrm{sig}(\bar\beta_Q) > \frac{s_n+z_n}{nC_{\min}}(8(s_n+z_n)^{1/2}n^{-1/2}+1)\Big\}\Big)\\ &\le\sum_{S\subset Q\subset S\cup Z}\mathrm{pr}\Big(\bigcup_{R\subset\mathcal{R}_1\subset S}\Big\{\mathrm{sig}(\bar\beta_Q)^T(X_Q^TX_Q)^{-1}\mathrm{sig}(\bar\beta_Q) > \frac{s_n+z_n}{nC_{\min}}(8(s_n+z_n)^{1/2}n^{-1/2}+1)\Big\}\Big)\\ &\le\sum_{S\subset Q\subset S\cup Z}\mathrm{pr}\Big(\|(X_Q^TX_Q/n)^{-1}-\Sigma_{QQ}^{-1}\|_2\ge\frac{8}{C_{\min}}(s_n+z_n)^{1/2}n^{-1/2}\Big)\\ &\le\sum_{S\subset Q\subset S\cup Z}\mathrm{pr}\Big(\|(X_Q^TX_Q/n)^{-1}-\Sigma_{QQ}^{-1}\|_2\ge\frac{8}{C_{\min}}(\mathrm{Card}(Q))^{1/2}n^{-1/2}\Big)\\ &\le 2^{z_n+1}\exp\Big(-\frac{s_n}{2}\Big).\end{aligned} \tag{29}$$

Hence, (28) and (29) imply pr$(H)\le 2^{z_n+1}\exp(-\frac{s_n}{2})+\exp(-\frac{3}{16}s_n)\to 0$.

Since $P(A^c) = 1 - P(A) \to 0$, the inequalities (26)–(29) imply (25) under the scaling in Theorem 1. Thus $\|K_1 + K_2\|_\infty < 1$ achieves with high probability, which also means $\breve{\beta}_{\hat{\mathcal{U}}\setminus\hat{\mathcal{U}}_1} = 0$ achieves asymptotically.

From our analysis in the first part, the following goal is the uniqueness of (20). If there is another solution, let's call it $\breve{\beta}'$. For any t such that $0 < t < 1$, the linear combination $\breve{\beta}(t) = t\breve{\beta} + (1-t)\breve{\beta}'$ is also a solution to (20) as a consequence of the convexity. Note that, the new solution point $\breve{\beta}(t)$ satisfies (16) and $\breve{\beta}(t)_{Q^c} = 0$, hence it is a solution to (13). From the uniqueness of (13), we conclude that $\breve{\beta} = \breve{\beta}'$.

The last part of this step is to prove $\bar{\beta}_{\mathcal{U}_1} \neq 0$ with high probability. By (17) and $Y = X_S\beta_S + \varepsilon = X_{\hat{Q}}\beta_{\hat{Q}} + \varepsilon$, we have

$$\begin{aligned}
\|\beta_{\hat{Q}} - \bar{\beta}_{\hat{Q}}\|_\infty &= \|\lambda_n(X_{\hat{Q}}^T X_{\hat{Q}}/n)^{-1}\mathrm{sig}(\bar{\beta}_{\hat{Q}}) - (X_{\hat{Q}}^T X_{\hat{Q}})^{-1}X_{\hat{Q}}^T\varepsilon\|_\infty \\
&\leq \lambda_n\|(X_{\hat{Q}}^T X_{\hat{Q}}/n)^{-1}\|_\infty + \|(X_{\hat{Q}}^T X_{\hat{Q}})^{-1}X_{\hat{Q}}^T\varepsilon\|_\infty \\
&\leq \lambda_n(s_n + z_n)^{1/2}\|(X_{\hat{Q}}^T X_{\hat{Q}}/n)^{-1}\|_2 + \|(X_{\hat{Q}}^T X_{\hat{Q}})^{-1}X_{\hat{Q}}^T\varepsilon\|_\infty \\
&\leq \lambda_n(s_n + z_n)^{1/2}(\|(X_{\hat{Q}}^T X_{\hat{Q}}/n)^{-1} - \Sigma_{\hat{Q}\hat{Q}}^{-1}\|_2 + 1/C_{\min}) \\
&\quad + \|(X_{\hat{Q}}^T X_{\hat{Q}})^{-1}X_{\hat{Q}}^T\varepsilon\|_\infty
\end{aligned} \tag{30}$$

for any $\hat{Q}$ satisfying $S \subset \hat{Q} \subset S \cup Z$. In (29), we have already got

$$\mathrm{pr}\Big(\|(X_{\hat{Q}}^T X_{\hat{Q}}/n)^{-1} - \Sigma_{\hat{Q}\hat{Q}}^{-1}\|_2 \geq \frac{8}{C_{\min}}(s_n + z_n)^{1/2}n^{-1/2}\Big) \leq 2\exp(-\frac{s_n}{2}) \tag{31}$$

Let $G = \Big\{\|(X_{\hat{Q}}^T X_{\hat{Q}})^{-1}\|_2 > 9/(nC_{\min})\Big\}$, by the inequality (60) in Wainwright [20],

$$\mathrm{pr}(G) \leq \mathrm{pr}(\|(X^T X)^{-1}\|_2 > 9/(nC_{\min})) \leq 2\exp(-n/2).$$

Since $(X_{\hat{Q}}^T X_{\hat{Q}})^{-1}X_{\hat{Q}}^T\varepsilon \mid X_{\hat{Q}} \sim N(0, (X_{\hat{Q}}^T X_{\hat{Q}})^{-1})$, then when we condition on G and achieve

$$\begin{aligned}
&\mathrm{pr}\Big(\|(X_{\hat{Q}}^T X_{\hat{Q}})^{-1}X_{\hat{Q}}^T\varepsilon\|_\infty > \frac{(s_n + z_n)^{1/2}}{n^{1/2}C_{\min}^{1/2}}\Big) \\
&\leq \mathrm{pr}\Big(\|(X_{\hat{Q}}^T X_{\hat{Q}})^{-1}X_{\hat{Q}}^T\varepsilon\|_\infty > \frac{(s_n + z_n)^{1/2}}{n^{1/2}C_{\min}^{1/2}} \mid G^c\Big) + \mathrm{pr}(G) \\
&\leq 2(s_n + z_n)e^{-(s_n+z_n)/18} + 2e^{-n/2},
\end{aligned} \tag{32}$$

since under G^c, each component of $(X_{\hat{Q}}^T X_{\hat{Q}})^{-1}X_{\hat{Q}}^T\varepsilon \mid X_{\hat{Q}}$ is normally distributed with mean 0 and variance that is less than $9/(nC_{\min})$.

Hence (30)–(32) together imply that,

$$\|\bar{\beta}_{\hat{Q}}-\beta_{\hat{Q}}\|_\infty \leq U_n \doteq \lambda_n(s_n+z_n)^{1/2}\Big(\frac{8}{C_{\min}}(s_n+z_n)^{1/2}n^{-1/2}+1/C_{\min}\Big)+\frac{(s_n+z_n)^{1/2}}{n^{1/2}C_{\min}^{1/2}}$$

holds with probability larger than $2(s_n + z_n)e^{-(s_n+z_n)/18} + 2e^{-n/2} + 2\exp^{-s_n/2}$. Therefore,

$$\begin{aligned}
&\mathrm{pr}(\|\bar{\beta}_{\hat{Q}} - \beta_{\hat{Q}}\|_\infty \geq U_n) \\
&\leq \mathrm{pr}\Big(\bigcup_{S\subset Q \subset S\cup Z} \{\|\bar{\beta}_Q - \beta_Q\|_\infty \geq U_n\} \cap B\Big) + \mathrm{pr}(B^c) \\
&\leq 2^{z_n}\Big(2(s_n + z_n)e^{-(s_n+z_n)/18} + 2e^{-n/2} + 2\exp^{-s_n/2}\Big) + \mathrm{pr}(B^c) \qquad (33)
\end{aligned}$$

Under the scaling of Theorem 1, we have $\mathrm{pr}(B) \geq \mathrm{pr}(A) \to 1$ and $2^{z_n}(2(s_n + z_n)e^{-(s_n+z_n)/18} + 2e^{-n/2} + 2\exp^{-s_n/2}) \to 0$. From Condition 5, it is easy to verify that

$$\min_{j\in S} |\beta_j| > U_n,$$

for sufficiently large n. Thus with high probability $\min_{j\in S} |\beta_j| > \|\bar{\beta}_{\hat{Q}} - \beta_{\hat{Q}}\|_\infty$ as n increases, which also implies $\check{\beta}_{\hat{Q}} \neq 0$ with high probability.

Finally, $\hat{\beta}_{\hat{\mathcal{R}},\hat{\mathcal{U}}_1}$ exactly recover signals with high probability as $n \to \infty$.

Step III: We need to prove that RAM-2 succeeds in detecting signals via Step 3. Similar to Step II, we need to define proper $\check{\beta}$ in (12) and $\bar{\beta}$ in (13). Since the main idea is the same as the procedure above, we only describe the key steps in the following proof. Recall the estimator (7),

$$\begin{aligned}
\hat{\beta}_{\hat{\mathcal{R}}_1,\hat{\mathcal{U}}_1,\hat{\mathcal{N}}_1} &= \underset{\beta_{\hat{\mathcal{U}}_2\cup\hat{\mathcal{N}}_2}=0}{\arg\min} \Big\{(2n)^{-1}\sum_{i=1}^{n}\Big(Y_i - \sum_{j\in\hat{\mathcal{R}}} X_{ij}\beta_j - \sum_{k\in\hat{\mathcal{U}}_1\cup\hat{\mathcal{N}}_1} X_{ik}\beta_k\Big)^2 + \lambda_n^{\star\star}\sum_{j\in\hat{\mathcal{R}}}|\beta_j|\Big\} \\
&= \underset{\beta_{\hat{\mathcal{N}}\cup\hat{\mathcal{U}}\setminus\hat{\mathcal{U}}_1}=0}{\arg\min} \Big\{(2n)^{-1}\|Y - X\beta\|_2^2 + \lambda_n^{\star\star}\|\beta_{\hat{\mathcal{R}}}\|_1\Big\}. \qquad (34)
\end{aligned}$$

This is a new "$\check{\beta}$" in (12), and we denote it as $\tilde{\beta}$. After this step, the ideal result is that with high probability,

$$\tilde{\beta}_{\hat{\mathcal{R}}_1} \neq 0 \text{ and } \tilde{\beta}_{\hat{\mathcal{R}}\setminus\hat{\mathcal{R}}_1} = 0. \qquad (35)$$

Therefore, define an oracle estimator of (34),

$$\mathring{\beta} = \arg\min_{\beta_{S^c}=0} \left\{ (2n)^{-1}\|Y - X_S\beta_S\|_2^2 + \lambda_n^{\star\star}\|\beta_{\hat{\mathcal{R}}_1}\|_1 \right\}. \tag{36}$$

Now, we plug $\tilde{\beta}$ and $\mathring{\beta}$ back to (12), (13), and (18), then it is sufficient to prove (34) has a unique solution and it achieves sign consistency with $Q = S$. Let

$$\begin{aligned}
F' &= X_{\hat{\mathcal{R}}_2}^T - \Sigma_{\hat{\mathcal{R}}_2 S}\Sigma_S^{-1}X_S^T,\\
K_1' &= \Sigma_{\hat{\mathcal{R}}_2 S}\Sigma_{SS}^{-1}\mathrm{sig}(\mathring{\beta}_S),\\
K_2' &= F'X_S(X_S^TX_S)^{-1}\mathrm{sig}(\mathring{\beta}_S) + (n\lambda_n^{\star\star})^{-1}F'\{I - X_S(X_S^TX_S)^{-1}X_S^T\}\varepsilon.
\end{aligned}$$

Similarly,

$$\mathrm{pr}\Big(\|K_1'\|_\infty \le 1-\alpha\Big) \ge \mathrm{pr}\Big(\{\|K_1'\|_\infty \le 1-\alpha\} \cap D\Big) \ge \mathrm{pr}(D) \ge \mathrm{pr}(A) \to 1, \tag{37}$$

where $D = \{\hat{\mathcal{R}}_2 \subset Z\}$ and it implies $\|K_1'\|_\infty \le 1-\alpha$ under Condition 7. Let

$$\begin{aligned}
H' = \bigcup_{R\subset\mathcal{R}_2\subset S} \Big\{ &\mathrm{sig}(\mathring{\beta}_S)^T(X_S^TX_S)^{-1}\mathrm{sig}(\mathring{\beta}_S) + (n\lambda_n^{\star\star})^{-2}\|\varepsilon\|_2^2 > \frac{s_n}{nC_{\min}}\big(8s_n^{1/2}n^{-1/2}+1\big)\\
&+ \big(1+s_n^{1/2}n^{-1/2}\big)/\big(n(\lambda_n^{\star\star})^2\big)\Big\}.
\end{aligned}$$

Then,

$$\begin{aligned}
\mathrm{pr}\Big(\|K_2'\|_\infty > \frac{\alpha}{2}\Big) &\le \mathrm{pr}\Big(\{\|K_2'\|_\infty > \frac{\alpha}{2}\} \cap A\Big) + \mathrm{pr}(A^c)\\
&\le \mathrm{pr}\Big(\bigcup_{\substack{(\mathcal{R}_2,\mathcal{R}_1)\\ \mathcal{R}_2\subset Z\\ R\subset\mathcal{R}_1\subset S}} \Big\{\|\tilde{K}_2(\mathcal{R}_2,\mathcal{R}_1)\|_\infty > \frac{\alpha}{2}\Big\}\Big) + \mathrm{pr}(A^c)\\
&\le \mathrm{pr}\Big(\bigcup_{\substack{(\mathcal{R}_2,\mathcal{R}_1)\\ \mathcal{R}_2\subset Z\\ R\subset\mathcal{R}_1\subset S}} \Big\{\|\tilde{K}_2(\mathcal{R}_2,\mathcal{R}_1)\|_\infty > \frac{\alpha}{2}\Big\} \mid \tilde{H}^c\Big) + \mathrm{pr}(\tilde{H}) + \mathrm{pr}(A^c)\\
&\le 2^{z_n+s_n+1}z_n e^{-\alpha^2/8V'} + 2e^{-\frac{s_n}{2}} + e^{-\frac{3}{16}s_n} + \mathrm{pr}(A^c)\\
&\longrightarrow 0,
\end{aligned} \tag{38}$$

where the last step of (38) follows from (26), (28), and (29) in the proof of Step II, and $V' = \frac{s_n}{nC_{\min}}(8s_n^{1/2}n^{-1/2}+1)+(1+s_n^{1/2}n^{-1/2})/(n(\lambda_n^{\star\star})^2)$.

Equations (37) and (38) indicate $\tilde{\beta}_{\hat{\mathcal{R}}\setminus\hat{\mathcal{R}}_1} = 0$. We skip the proof of uniqueness and move to the next step of proving $\tilde{\beta}_{\hat{\mathcal{R}}_1} \neq 0$.

$$\|\mathring{\beta}_S - \beta_S\|_\infty = \|(X_S^TX_S)^{-1}(X_S^TY - n\lambda_n^{\star\star}\text{sig}(\mathring{\beta}_S)) - \beta_S\|_\infty$$
$$\leq \|(X_S^TX_S)^{-1}X_S^T\varepsilon\|_\infty + \|\lambda_n^{\star\star}(X_S^TX_S/n)^{-1}\|_\infty.$$

Let $W_n = \lambda_n^{\star\star}s_n^{1/2}\big(\frac{8}{C_{\min}}s_n^{1/2}n^{-\frac{1}{2}}+\frac{1}{C_{\min}}\big)+\frac{s_n^{1/2}}{n^{1/2}C_{\min}^{1/2}} = o(n^{a_2/2-\delta})$. In the same way, we can show that as $n\to\infty$

$$\text{pr}(\|\mathring{\beta}_S - \beta_S\|_\infty \leq W_n) \to 0$$

Hence, Condition 5 ensures that as $n\to\infty$,

$$\text{pr}\big(\min_{j\in S}|\beta_j| > \|\mathring{\beta}_S - \beta_S\|_\infty\big) \to 1, \tag{39}$$

which is equivalent to $\tilde{\beta}_{\hat{\mathcal{R}}_1} \neq 0$.

Finally, combining Step I, Step II, and Step III, we conclude that

$$P(\hat{\beta}_{\hat{\mathcal{R}}_1,\hat{\mathcal{U}}_1,\hat{\mathcal{N}}_1} \text{ is unique and } \text{sign}(\hat{\beta}_{\hat{\mathcal{R}}_1,\hat{\mathcal{U}}_1,\hat{\mathcal{N}}_1}) = \text{sign}(\beta)) \to 1, \quad \text{as } n\to\infty.$$

□

Proof of Theorem 2 Denote the compositions $S = \hat{\mathcal{R}}_1 \cup \hat{\mathcal{U}}_1 \cup \hat{\mathcal{N}}_1$ and define the set of noises left in $\hat{\mathcal{U}}^c$ as $(\hat{\mathcal{R}}\setminus\hat{\mathcal{R}}_1)\cup(\hat{\mathcal{N}}\setminus\hat{\mathcal{N}}_1)\doteq\hat{\mathcal{R}}_2\cup\hat{\mathcal{N}}_2$, where $\hat{\mathcal{R}}_1$, $\hat{\mathcal{U}}_1$, and $\hat{\mathcal{N}}_1$ are signals from $\hat{\mathcal{R}}$, $\hat{\mathcal{U}}$, and $\hat{\mathcal{N}}$, respectively.

Step I: Consider the Step 1 in (5), which is exactly the same as (20). Since there is no difference from the Step II in the proof of Theorem 1, we skip the details here.

Step II: Let's consider the Step 2 in (6).

$$\hat{\beta}_{\hat{\mathcal{R}},\hat{\mathcal{U}}_1,\hat{\mathcal{N}}_1} = \mathop{\arg\min}_{\beta_{\hat{\mathcal{U}}\setminus\hat{\mathcal{U}}_1}=0}\left\{(2n)^{-1}\sum_{i=1}^n\Big(Y_i - \sum_{j\in\hat{\mathcal{N}}}X_{ij}\beta_j - \sum_{k\in\hat{\mathcal{R}}\cup\hat{\mathcal{U}}_1}X_{ik}\beta_k\Big)^2 + \lambda_n^\star\sum_{j\in\hat{\mathcal{N}}}|\beta_j|\right\}$$
$$= \mathop{\arg\min}_{\beta_{\hat{\mathcal{U}}\setminus\hat{\mathcal{U}}_1}=0}\left\{(2n)^{-1}\|Y - X\beta\|_2^2 + \lambda_n^\star\|\beta_{\hat{\mathcal{N}}}\|_1\right\}. \tag{40}$$

Here, denote $\check{\beta} = \hat{\beta}_{\hat{\mathcal{R}},\hat{\mathcal{U}}_1,\hat{\mathcal{N}}_1}$. After this step, the ideal result is that with high probability,

$$\check{\beta}_{\hat{\mathcal{N}}_1} \neq 0 \text{ and } \check{\beta}_{\hat{\mathcal{N}}\setminus\hat{\mathcal{N}}_1} = 0. \tag{41}$$

Then, define an oracle estimator of (20),

$$\bar{\beta} = \underset{\beta_{(\hat{\mathcal{R}}\cup\hat{\mathcal{U}}_1\cup\hat{\mathcal{N}}_1)^c}=0}{\arg\min} \left\{ (2n)^{-1}\|Y - X_{\hat{Q}}\beta_{\hat{Q}}\|_2^2 + \lambda_n^\star \|\beta_{\hat{\mathcal{N}}_1}\|_1 \right\}, \tag{42}$$

where $\hat{Q} = (\hat{\mathcal{R}} \cup \hat{\mathcal{U}}_1) \cup \hat{\mathcal{N}}_1 = S \cup \hat{\mathcal{R}}_2$. Similar to Step II in proof of Theorem 1, let

$$\begin{aligned}
F &= X_{\hat{\mathcal{N}}_2}^T - \Sigma_{\hat{Q}^c\hat{Q}}\Sigma_{\hat{Q}\hat{Q}}^{-1}X_{\hat{Q}}^T,\\
K_1 &= \Sigma_{\hat{\mathcal{N}}_2\hat{Q}}\Sigma_{\hat{Q}\hat{Q}}^{-1}\mathrm{sig}(\bar{\beta}_{\hat{Q}}),\\
K_2 &= FX_{\hat{Q}}(X_{\hat{Q}}^T X_{\hat{Q}})^{-1}\mathrm{sig}(\bar{\beta}_{\hat{Q}}) + (n\lambda_n)^{-1}F\{I - X_{\hat{Q}}(X_{\hat{Q}}^T X_{\hat{Q}})^{-1}X_{\hat{Q}}^T\}\varepsilon,
\end{aligned}$$

and

$$\begin{aligned}
A &= \{R \subset \hat{\mathcal{L}}_1 \doteq \hat{\mathcal{R}}_1 \cup \hat{\mathcal{U}}_1 \subset S, S \subset \hat{Q} \subset S \cup Z\},\\
B &= \{S \subset \hat{Q} \subset S \cup Z\},\\
\mathcal{T}_A &= \{(\mathcal{L}_1, Q) | R \subset \mathcal{L}_1 \subset S, S \subset Q \subset S \cup Z\}.
\end{aligned}$$

Similarly, we get

$$\mathrm{pr}(\|K_1\|_\infty \leq 1 - \gamma_1) \geq \mathrm{pr}(\{\|K_1\|_\infty \leq 1 - \gamma_1\} \cap A) \geq \mathrm{pr}(A) \to 1. \tag{43}$$

To obtain $\mathrm{pr}(\|K_2\|_\infty > \frac{\gamma_1}{2}) \to 0$, we define event H as

$$\begin{aligned}
H = \bigcup_{(\mathcal{L}_1, Q)\subset\mathcal{T}_A} &\Big\{\mathrm{sig}(\bar{\beta}_Q)^T(X_Q^T X_Q)^{-1}\mathrm{sig}(\bar{\beta}_Q) + (n\lambda_n)^{-2}\|\varepsilon\|_2^2\\
&> \frac{s_n + z_n}{nC_{\min}}\big(8(s_n + z_n)^{1/2}n^{-1/2} + 1\big) + \big(1 + s_n^{1/2}n^{-1/2}\big)/(n\lambda_n^2)\Big\}.
\end{aligned}$$

Then, following (25)–(29),

$$\begin{aligned}
\mathrm{pr}\Big(\|K_2\|_\infty > \frac{\gamma_1}{2}\Big) &\leq \mathrm{pr}\Big(\Big\{\|K_2\|_\infty > \frac{\gamma_1}{2}\Big\} \cap A\Big) + \mathrm{pr}(A^c)\\
&\leq \mathrm{pr}\Big(\bigcup_{(\mathcal{L}_1, Q)\subset\mathcal{T}_A} \|K_2(\mathcal{L}_1, Q)\|_\infty > \frac{\gamma_1}{2} \mid H^c\Big) + \mathrm{pr}(H) + \mathrm{pr}(A^c)\\
&\leq 2^{s_n+z_n} \cdot 2(p_n - s_n)\exp(-\gamma_1^2/8V) + 2^{z_n+1}\exp\Big(-\frac{s_n}{2}\Big)\\
&\quad + \exp\Big(-\frac{3}{16}s_n\Big)\\
&\longrightarrow 0,
\end{aligned} \tag{44}$$

where $V = (1 + s_n^{1/2}n^{-1/2})/(n(\lambda_n^\star)^2) + s_n n^{-1}C_{\min}^{-1}(8s_n^{1/2}n^{-1/2} + 1)$.

Again, we skip the uniqueness of $\check{\beta}$ and move to bound $\|\bar{\beta}_{\hat{Q}} - \beta_{\hat{Q}}\|_\infty$. By (30)–(32) in the proof of Theorem 1, we have

$$\begin{aligned}
&\mathrm{pr}\big(\|\bar{\beta}_{\hat{Q}} - \beta_{\hat{Q}}\|_\infty \geq U_n\big) \\
&\quad \leq 2^{z_n}\big(2(s_n + z_n)e^{-(s_n+z_n)/18} + 2e^{-n/2} + 2\exp^{-s_n/2}\big) + \mathrm{pr}(B^c) \to 0,
\end{aligned}$$

where $U_n = \lambda_n(s_n + z_n)^{1/2}\Big(\frac{8}{C_{\min}}(s_n + z_n)^{1/2}n^{-1/2} + 1/C_{\min}\Big) + \frac{(s_n+z_n)^{1/2}}{n^{1/2}C_{\min}^{1/2}}$. As $\min_{j\in S}|\beta_j| \gg U_n$ with sufficiently large n, we conclude that with high probability $\min_{j\in S}|\beta_j| > \|\bar{\beta}_{\hat{Q}} - \beta_{\hat{Q}}\|_\infty$ as n increases, which also implies $\check{\beta}_{\hat{Q}} \neq 0$ with high probability.

Therefore, $\hat{\beta}_{\hat{\mathcal{R}},\hat{\mathcal{U}}_1,\hat{\mathcal{N}}_1}$ successfully recover signals from $\hat{\mathcal{N}}$ with high probability when n is large enough.

Step III: Following the same steps as in Step III in the proof of Theorem 1, we have

$$P\big(\hat{\beta}_{\hat{\mathcal{R}}_1,\hat{\mathcal{U}}_1,\hat{\mathcal{N}}_1} \text{ is unique and } \mathrm{sign}(\hat{\beta}_{\hat{\mathcal{R}}_1,\hat{\mathcal{U}}_1,\hat{\mathcal{N}}_1}) = \mathrm{sign}(\beta)\big) \to 1, \quad \text{as } n \to \infty.$$

□

References

1. Akaike, H.: A new look at the statistical model identification. IEEE Trans. Autom. Control **19**, 716–723 (1974)
2. Bach, F., Jenatton, R., Mairal, J., Obozinski, G.: Optimization with sparsity-inducing penalties. arXiv preprint arXiv:1108.0775 (2011)
3. Chen, J., Chen, Z.: Extended bayesian information criteria for model selection with large model spaces. Biometrika **95**, 759–771 (2008)
4. Efron, B., Hastie, T., Johnstone, I., Tibshirani, R.: Least angle regression. Ann. Stat. **32**, 407–499 (2004)
5. Fan, J., Li, R.: Variable selection via nonconcave penalized likelihood and its oracle properties. J. Am. Stat. Assoc. **96**, 1348–1360 (2001)
6. Fan, J., Lv, J.: Sure independence screening for ultrahigh dimensional feature space. J. R. Stat. Soc. Ser. B Stat. Methodol. **70**, 849–911 (2008)
7. Fan, J., Song, R.: Sure independence screening in generalized linear models with np-dimensionality. Ann. Stat. **38**, 3567–3604 (2010)
8. Fan, J., Feng, Y., Song, R.: Nonparametric independence screening in sparse ultra-high dimensional additive models. J. Am. Stat. Assoc. **106**, 544–557 (2011)
9. Fan, J., Feng, Y., Tong, X.: A road to classification in high dimensional space: the regularized optimal affine discriminant. J. R. Stat. Soc. Ser. B. **74**, 745–771 (2012)
10. Fan, J., Feng, Y., Jiang, J., Tong, X.: Feature augmentation via nonparametrics and selection (fans) in high dimensional classification. J. Am. Stat. Assoc. (2014, to appear)
11. Feng, Y., Li, T., Ying, Z.: Likelihood adaptively modified penalties. arXiv preprint arXiv:1308.5036 (2013)

12. Feng, Y., Yu, Y.: Consistent cross-validation for tuning parameter selection in high-dimensional variable selection. arXiv preprint arXiv:1308.5390 (2013)
13. Frank, I.E., Friedman, J.H.: A statistical view of some chemometrics regression tools. Technometrics **35**, 109–135 (1993)
14. Friedman, J., Hastie, T., Tibshirani, R.: Regularization paths for generalized linear models via coordinate descent. J. Stat. Softw. **33**, 1–22 (2010)
15. Greenshtein, E., Ritov, Y.: Persistence in high-dimensional linear predictor selection and the virtue of overparametrization. Bernoulli **10**, 971–988 (2004)
16. Huang, J., Ma, S., Zhang, C.-H.: Adaptive lasso for sparse high-dimensional regression models. Stat. Sin. **18**, 1603 (2008)
17. Knight, K., Fu, W.: Asymptotics for lasso-type estimators. Ann. Stat. **28**, 1356–1378 (2000)
18. Schwarz, G.: Estimating the dimension of a model. Ann. Stat. **6**, 461–464 (1978)
19. Tibshirani, R.: Regression shrinkage and selection via the lasso. J. R. Stat. Soc. Ser. B Methodol. **58**, 267–288 (1996)
20. Wainwright, M.J.: Sharp thresholds for high-dimensional and noisy sparsity recovery. IEEE Trans. Inf. Theory **55**, 2183–2202 (2009)
21. Weng, H., Feng, Y., Qiao, X.: Regularization after retention in ultrahigh dimensional linear regression models. Manuscript (2013). Preprint, arXiv:1311.5625
22. Yu, Y., Feng, Y.: Apple: approximate path for penalized likelihood estimators. Stat. Comput. **24**, 803–819 (2014)
23. Yu, Y., Feng, Y.: Modified cross-validation for lasso penalized high-dimensional linear models. J. Comput. Graph. Stat. **23**, 1009–1027 (2014)
24. Zhao, P., Yu, B.: On model selection consistency of lasso. J. Mach. Learn. Res. **7**, 2541–2563 (2006)
25. Zou, H.: The adaptive lasso and its oracle properties. J. Am. Stat. Assoc. **101**, 1418–1429 (2006)
26. Zou, H., Hastie, T.: Regularization and variable selection via the elastic net. J. R. Stat. Soc. Ser. B Stat. Methodol. **67**, 301–320 (2005)

Empirical Likelihood Test for High Dimensional Generalized Linear Models

Yangguang Zang, Qingzhao Zhang, Sanguo Zhang, Qizhai Li, and Shuangge Ma

Abstract Technological advances allow scientists to collect high dimensional data sets in which the number of variables is much larger than the sample size. A representative example is genomics. Consequently, due to their loss of accuracy or power, many classic statistical methods are being challenged when analyzing such data. In this chapter, we propose an empirical likelihood (EL) method to test regression coefficients in high dimensional generalized linear models. The EL test has an asymptotic chi-squared distribution with two degrees of freedom under the null hypothesis, and this result is independent of the number of covariates. Moreover, we extend the proposed method to test a part of the regression coefficients in the presence of nuisance parameters. Simulation studies show that the EL tests have a good control of the type-I error rate under moderate sample sizes and are more powerful than the direct competitor under the alternative hypothesis under most scenarios. The proposed tests are employed to analyze the association between rheumatoid arthritis (RA) and single nucleotide polymorphisms (SNPs) on chromosome 6. The resulted p-value is 0.019, indicating that chromosome 6 has an influence on RA. With the partial test and logistic modeling, we also find that the SNPs eliminated by the sure independence screening and Lasso methods have no significant influence on RA.

Y. Zang • Q. Zhang • S. Zhang
School of Mathematical Sciences, University of Chinese Academy of Sciences, Beijing, China

Key Laboratory of Big Data Mining and Knowledge Management, Chinese Academy of Sciences, Beijing, China
e-mail: zangyangguang@mails.ucas.ac.cn; qzzhang@ucas.ac.cn; sgzhang@ucas.ac.cn

Q. Li
Key Laboratory of Systems and Control, Academy of Mathematics and Systems Science, Chinese Academy of Sciences, Beijing, China
e-mail: liqz@amss.ac.cn

S. Ma (✉)
Department of Statistics, Taiyuan University of Technology, Taiyuan, China

Department of Biostatistics, School of Public Health, Yale University, New Haven, CT, USA
e-mail: shuangge.ma@yale.edu

© Springer International Publishing AG 2017

S.E. Ahmed (ed.), *Big and Complex Data Analysis*, Contributions to Statistics,
DOI 10.1007/978-3-319-41573-4_2

1 Introduction

High dimensional data are now routinely encountered in many scientific fields such as genome-wide association studies (GWAS), DNA microarray analysis, and brain imaging studies. With, for example, GWAS data, the number of SNPs (p) is in the order of tens of thousands, whereas the sample size (n) is much smaller, usually at most in the order of hundreds. This is the so-called large p, small n paradigm. The analysis of high dimensional data poses many challenges for statisticians and calls for new statistical methodologies and theories [10].

Generalized linear models (GLM), including the logistic, Poisson, and Negative Binomial regression models, are widely employed statistical models in various applications. In this chapter, we consider the problem of testing regression coefficients for GLM under the "large p, small n" paradigm. Although the proposed method has broad applicability, it has been partly motivated by the analysis of a rheumatoid arthritis (RA) data with SNP measurements. See Sect. 5 for more details. In this RA study, we are interested in testing whether a large number of SNPs on chromosome 6 are associated with RA. Or equivalently, whether their regression coefficients in a GLM are simultaneously equal to zero.

When p is fixed, there exist two popular multivariate tests: the likelihood ratio test and the Wald test. However, when the dimension p becomes larger than the sample size n, these two tests become invalid. That is because the two tests involve the estimator of the inverse sample covariance matrix, which becomes problematic for large p. To solve this problem, Geoman et al. [13] pioneered a score test statistic that has a quadratic form of the residuals of the null model and derived the asymptotic distribution in GLM with canonical link functions. Chen et al. [5] investigated the test of [13] and discovered that the high dimensionality can adversely impact the power of the test when the inverse of the link function in GLM is unbounded, for instance, the log link in the Poisson or Negative Binomial regression. They then proposed a U-statistic test which can avoid the adverse impact of the high dimensionality. Zhong and Chen [28] proposed simultaneous tests for coefficients in high dimensional linear regression models with factorial designs.

On the other hand, it is well known that the empirical likelihood (EL) ratio test is a powerful nonparametric likelihood approach [19]. Many advantages of the empirical likelihood method have been shown in the literature. In particular, the empirical likelihood method does not involve any variance estimation, which saves a lot of effort. For more details on empirical likelihood methods, we refer to [7, 21]. There are some publications on empirical likelihood tests for high dimensional data. Wang et al. [26] proposed a jackknife empirical likelihood test method for testing equality of two high dimensional means. Some empirical likelihood tests for testing whether a covariance matrix equals a given one or has a banded structure were investigated in [27]. Peng et al. [22] considered an empirical likelihood test for coefficients in high dimensional linear models.

Motivated by the empirical likelihood tests [22] and U-statistic tests [5], we develop an empirical likelihood test for testing regression coefficients in GLM. We show that the empirical likelihood test has an asymptotic chi-squared distribution with two degrees of freedom under the null hypothesis, and this result is independent of the number of covariates. The computational time of our proposed method is shown to be much lower than that of the competing alternative. In addition, we consider the partial test problem which is more useful in practice. Simulation results show that the proposed test statistic has a good control of the type-I error rate under moderate sample sizes, and that the proposed method is more powerful than those in [5] under the alternative hypothesis.

The paper is organized as follows. Section 2 presents a new methodology to the GLM's global test, and Sect. 3 considers the situation with nuisance parameters. In Sect. 4, we conduct simulations to evaluate the performance of proposed method. Section 5 provides a real data example, and Sect. 6 gives some discussions. Some technical details are provided in Appendix.

2 The Proposed Test

For $i = 1, \ldots, n$, Y_i is a scalar response variable, which can be binary, categorical, or continuous in the framework of GLM. $X_i = (X_{i1}, \ldots, X_{ip})^\top$ is a p-dimensional random vector with $\Sigma = E(X_i X_i^\top)$. X_i can be seen as a group of predictors of interest, such as p SNPs from a candidate gene or region. Consider the GLM

$$E(Y|X) = g(X^\top \beta) \text{ and } \mathrm{var}(Y|X) = V\{g(X^\top \beta)\}, \tag{1}$$

where $g(\cdot)$ is a given function, β is the vector of regression coefficients, and $V(\cdot)$ is a non-negative function. Note that $g^{-1}(\cdot)$ is called the link function, and "$\top$" denotes the matrix transpose. Our first aim is to test the significance of the regression coefficients, that is,

$$H_0 : \beta = \beta_0 \ \text{ vs } \ H_1 : \beta \neq \beta_0 \tag{2}$$

for a specific $\beta_0 \in R^p$ under $n < p$.

Remark 1 In the existing high dimensional studies, much attention has been paid to the estimation problem. To cope with the high dimensionality, usually special data/model structures need to be assumed. A popular assumption is sparsity, which has led to the family of penalization methods and others. For references, we refer to [2, 12, 17]. Without making strong assumptions on, for example, the sparsity structure, hypothesis testing provides an alternative way of analyzing high dimensional data.

Write $\psi(X_i, \beta_0) = g'(X_i^\top \beta_0)/V\{g(X_i^\top \beta_0)\}$, where $g'(\cdot)$ is the first-order derivative of $g(t)$ with respect to t. To test (2), the statistic in [13] is

$$S_n = \frac{[\sum_{i=1}^n (Y_i - \mu_{0i})\psi(X_i, \beta_0)X_i]^\top [\sum_{i=1}^n (Y_i - \mu_{0i})\psi(X_i, \beta_0)X_i]}{\sum_{i=1}^n (Y_i - \mu_{0i})^2 \psi^2(X_i, \beta_0)X_i^\top X_i},$$

where $\mu_{0i} = g(X_i^\top \beta_0)$. Chen and Guo [5] noticed that S_n can be written in the form $S_n = 1 + U_n/A_n$, where

$$A_n = \frac{1}{n}\sum_{i=1}^n (Y_i - \mu_{0i})^2 \psi^2(X_i, \beta_0)X_i^\top X_i$$

and

$$U_n = \frac{1}{n}\sum_{i \neq j}^n (Y_i - \mu_{0i})(Y_j - \mu_{0j})\psi(X_i, \beta_0)\psi(X_j, \beta_0)X_i^\top X_j.$$

They also pointed out that the term A_n is redundant since it increases the variance and decreases the power. Therefore, they only considered the term U_n as the statistic which can also avoid the adverse impact of high dimensionality. Notice that U_n is the estimate of $(n-1)\Delta_{\beta_0,\beta}^\top \Delta_{\beta_0,\beta}$, where

$$\Delta_{\beta_0,\beta} = E\left\{[g(X_i^\top \beta) - g(X_i^\top \beta_0)]\psi(X_i, \beta_0)X_i\right\}.$$

Motivated by this work, we build the statistic as

$$T_i = (Y_i - \mu_{0i})(Y_{i+m} - \mu_{0i+m})\psi(X_i, \beta_0)\psi(X_{i+m}, \beta_0)X_i^\top X_{i+m}, \tag{3}$$

where $i = 1, \ldots, m$, $m = \lfloor n/2 \rfloor$, the maximal integer less than $n/2$. The sample splitting method has also been used in [22, 26, 27]. It is easy to see that the expectation of T_i equals $\Delta_{\beta_0,\beta}^\top \Delta_{\beta_0,\beta}$. Since $\Delta_{\beta_0,\beta}^\top \Delta_{\beta_0,\beta}$ is $O(||\beta - \beta_0||_2^2)$, if we assume that $g'(\cdot)$ and $\psi(\cdot, \cdot)$ are finite, the power may decrease when $||\beta - \beta_0||_2$ is smaller than 1, where $||\cdot||_2$ denotes the L_2 norm. Therefore another statistic S_i with the order of $O(||\beta - \beta_0||_2)$ is considered:

$$S_i = (Y_i - \mu_{0i})\psi(X_i, \beta_0)X_i^\top \alpha + (Y_{i+m} - \mu_{0i+m})\psi(X_{i+m}, \beta_0)X_{i+m}^\top \alpha, \tag{4}$$

where the vector $\alpha \in R^p$ can be chosen based on prior information or just simply set as $\mathbf{1}_p = (1, \ldots, 1)^\top \in R^p$.

The EL technique has been applied to linear models [20], GLMs [15, 18], confidential interval construction [19], quantiles [6], and others. Here we use it for high dimensional testing. Set $Z_i = (T_i, S_i)^\top$. Based on [24], the EL test statistic is

$l_m = -2\log L_m$, where L_m is defined as

$$L_m = \sup\left\{\prod_{i=1}^{m}(mw_i)\,\middle|\, w_i \geq 0, \sum_{i=1}^{m} w_i = 1, \sum_{i=1}^{m} w_i Z_i = \mathbf{0}\right\}.$$

Using the Lagrange multiplier technique, we can obtain

$$l_m = -2\sum_{i=1}^{m}\log(1+\lambda^{\top}Z_i),$$

where λ satisfies

$$\frac{1}{m}\sum_{i=1}^{m}\frac{Z_i}{1+\lambda^{\top}Z_i} = \mathbf{0}.$$

Let $\varepsilon = Y - g(X^{\top}\beta)$. To establish the asymptotic properties of the empirical likelihood test, we first make the following assumptions:

Condition 1. Let Ω be the support of X. There exist positive constants δ and K such that $E\left(|\varepsilon|^{2+\delta}\,|X = x\right) \leq K$ for any $x \in \Omega$.

Condition 2. $g(\cdot)$ is continuously differentiable, $V(\cdot) > 0$ and is finite, and there exist positive constants c_1 and c_2 such that $c_1 \leq \psi^2(x, \beta_0) \leq c_2$ for any $x \in \Omega$.

Remark 2 Condition 1 postulates that the error term has a finite $(2+\delta)$th moment, which is common in the analysis of GLM [5].

The following theorem establishes the asymptotic properties of the EL test:

Theorem 1 *Suppose that* $n \to \infty$, $\alpha^{\top}\Sigma\alpha > 0$, *Conditions 1–2 hold, and*

$$\frac{E|X_i^{\top}X_{i+m}|^{2+\delta}}{[tr\{\Sigma^2\}]^{(2+\delta)/2}} = o(m^{\frac{\delta}{2}}), \tag{5}$$

and

$$\frac{E|X_i^{\top}\alpha + X_{i+m}^{\top}\alpha|^{2+\delta}}{[\alpha^{\top}\Sigma\alpha]^{(2+\delta)/2}} = o(m^{\frac{\delta}{2}}). \tag{6}$$

Then, under H_0, l_m converges in distribution to a chi-squared distribution with two degrees of freedom.

Based on this theorem, we reject H_0 when $l_m > \chi^2_{2,b}$, where $\chi^2_{2,b}$ is the $(1-b)$-quantile of a chi-squared distribution with two degrees of freedom and b is the significance level. Since conditions (5) and (6) are abstract, we introduce two intuitive examples which satisfy these conditions, and we can see that p can be very large in the two examples.

Example 1 Let X be a Gaussian random vector with mean 0 and covariance matrix Σ where Σ is an arbitrary p by p positive definite matrix. Then (5) and (6) hold.

Example 2 Consider the factor model, which is illustrated in [1, 9, 26]. There exists a s-variate random vector $F_i = (F_{i1}, \ldots, F_{is})^\top$ for some $s \geq p$ so that $X_i = \Gamma F_i$, where Γ is a $p \times s$ matrix such that $\Gamma \Gamma^\top = \Sigma$, $E(F_i) = \mathbf{0}$, and $\text{var}(F_i) = I_s$, where I_s is the $s \times s$ identity matrix. Each F_{ij} has a finite 8th moment and $E(F_{ij}^4) = 3 + \Delta$ for some constant Δ. For any integer $l_v \geq 0$ with $\sum_{v=1}^{q} l_v = 8$ and distinct $j_1, \ldots, j_q$, $E(F_{ij_1}^{l_1} F_{ij_2}^{l_2} \ldots F_{ij_q}^{l_q}) = E(F_{ij_1}^{l_1}) E(F_{ij_2}^{l_2}) \ldots E(F_{ij_q}^{l_q})$. Then (5) and (6) hold.

Theorem 2 *Assume that $n \to \infty$, and $\alpha^\top \Sigma \alpha$ is positive. Under Example 1 or Example 2 and Conditions 1–2, l_m converges in distribution to a chi-squared distribution with two degrees of freedom under H_0.*

Remark 3 The effects of data dimensionality on empirical likelihood have been investigated [8]. The empirical likelihood ratio statistic does not asymptotically converge to chi-squared distribution with p degrees of freedom under the null hypothesis. We project the p-dimensional data onto a two-dimensional space. Therefore, the EL test still enjoys the Wilks' phenomenon.

3 The Partial Test with Nuisance Parameters

In this section, we extend the method developed in Sect. 2 to test part of the regression coefficients with the presence of nuisance parameters. Such a test has practical importance. For example, in a GWAS, we are also interested in a specific region or specific genes, with the presence of other SNPs.

Without loss of generality, we partition $X_i = (X_i^{(1)\top}, X_i^{(2)\top})^\top$, where the dimensions of $X_i^{(1)}$ and $X_i^{(2)}$ are p_1 and p_2, respectively. Accordingly, the regression coefficient vector can be partitioned as $\beta = (\beta^{(1)\top}, \beta^{(2)\top})^\top$. Consider the test

$$\tilde{H}_0 : \beta^{(2)} = \beta_0^{(2)} \text{ vs } \tilde{H}_1 : \beta^{(2)} \neq \beta_0^{(2)}. \tag{7}$$

To test (7), we need to estimate $\beta_0^{(1)}$ first. The quasi-likelihood score of $\beta^{(1)}$ is

$$q(\beta^{(1)}, \beta^{(2)}) = \frac{\partial Q_n(\beta)}{\partial \beta^{(1)}} = \sum_{i=1}^{n} \{Y_i - \mu_i(\beta)\} \psi(X_i, \beta) X_i^{(1)},$$

where $\mu_i(\beta) = g(X_i^\top \beta)$ and $Q_n(\beta) = \sum_{i=1}^{n} \int_{Y_i}^{\mu_i(\beta)} \frac{Y_i - t}{V(t)} dt$. The maximum quasi-likelihood estimator $\beta^{(1)}$ can be obtained by solving the equation $q(\beta^{(1)}, \beta_0^{(2)}) = 0$, which is denoted as $\hat{\beta}_0^{(1)}$.

Set $\hat{\beta}_0 = (\hat{\beta}_0^{(1)\top}, \beta_0^{(2)\top})^\top$ and $\hat{\mu}_{0i} = \mu_i(\hat{\beta}_0)$. Similar to Sect. 2, we consider the statistic $\tilde{Z}_i = (\tilde{T}_i, \tilde{S}_i)^\top$, where

$$\tilde{T}_i = (Y_i - \hat{\mu}_{0i})(Y_{i+m} - \hat{\mu}_{0i+m})\psi(X_i, \hat{\beta}_0)\psi(X_{i+m}, \hat{\beta}_0)X_i^{(2)\top}X_{i+m}^{(2)}, \tag{8}$$

$$\tilde{S}_i = (Y_i - \hat{\mu}_{0i})\psi(X_i, \hat{\beta}_0)X_i^{(2)\top}\tilde{\alpha} + (Y_{i+m} - \hat{\mu}_{0i+m})\psi(X_{i+m}, \hat{\beta}_0)X_{i+m}^{(2)\top}\tilde{\alpha}, \tag{9}$$

and $\tilde{\alpha} \in R^{p_2}$. By applying the empirical likelihood method, we have

$$\tilde{l}_m = -2\sum_{i=1}^{m} \log(1 + \tilde{\lambda}^\top \tilde{Z}_i),$$

where $\tilde{\lambda}$ satisfies

$$\frac{1}{m}\sum_{i=1}^{m} \frac{\tilde{Z}_i}{1 + \tilde{\lambda}^\top \tilde{Z}_i} = \mathbf{0}.$$

Denote $\Sigma_{X^{(j)}}, j = 1, 2$ as the covariance matrices of $X^{(1)}$ and $X^{(2)}$, respectively. To establish the asymptotic properties of $\tilde{l}_m$, we need the following conditions:

Condition 3. As $n \to \infty$, $p_1 n^{-1/4} \to 0$, and there exists a $\beta^{*(1)} \in R^{p_1}$ such that $||\hat{\beta}_0^{(1)} - \beta^{*(1)}||_2 = O_p(p_1 n^{-1/2})$. In particular under $\tilde{H}_0$, we have $\beta^{*(1)} = \beta_0^{(1)}$, where $\beta = (\beta_0^{(1)\top}, \beta_0^{(2)\top})^\top$ is the true parameter.

Condition 4. $\Sigma_{X^{(1)}}$ is a positive definite matrix, and its eigenvalues are bounded away from zero and infinity.

Condition 5. $g(\cdot)$ is first-order continuously differentiable. Define $\beta_0^* = (\beta_0^{*(1)\top}, \beta_0^{(2)\top})^\top$, where $\beta_0^{*(1)}$ is defined in Condition 3. There exist positive constants c_1 and c_2 such that $c_1 \le \psi^2(x, \beta_0^*) \le c_2$, $[\partial\psi(x, \beta_0^*)/\partial(x^\top\beta_0^*)]^2 \le c_2$ for any $x \in \Omega$.

The main properties of the test can be summarized as follows:

Theorem 3 *Suppose that* $n \to \infty$, $\tilde{\alpha}^\top \Sigma_{X^{(2)}}\tilde{\alpha} > 0$, *and Conditions 1, 3–5 hold. Then if*

$$\frac{E|X_i^{(2)\top}X_{i+m}^{(2)}|^{2+\delta}}{[tr\{\Sigma_{X^{(2)}}^2\}]^{(2+\delta)/2}} = o(m^{\frac{\delta}{2}}) \;\; and \;\; \frac{E|X_i^{(2)\top}\tilde{\alpha} + X_{i+m}^{(2)\top}\tilde{\alpha}|^{2+\delta}}{[\tilde{\alpha}^\top \Sigma_{X^{(2)}}\tilde{\alpha}]^{(2+\delta)/2}} = o(m^{\frac{\delta}{2}})$$

are satisfied, then under $\tilde{H}_0$, $\tilde{l}_m$ *converges in distribution to a chi-squared distribution with two degrees of freedom.*

4 Simulation Study

In a published study [3], five popular methods have been compared, including the multivariate score test [4], the Fisher's method for combining p-values, the minimum p-value approach, a Fourier transform method [25], and a Bayesian score statistic [13]. It is found that the minimum p-value method and the Bayesian score method outperform the others. Chen et al. [5] further showed that their method performs better than the Bayesian score method. Thus in this section, we focus on comparing the proposed method against that in [5] (denoted as CG).

SIMULATION I. The $p \times 1$ iid vectors $\{X_i\}_{i=1}^n$ are generated from a moving average model,

$$X_{ij} = Z_{ij} + \rho Z_{i(j+1)} \quad (i = 1, \ldots, n,\ j = 1, \ldots, p), \tag{10}$$

where for each i, $\{Z_{ij}\}_{j=1}^{p+1}$ are independently generated from a $(p+1)$ standard normal distribution $N(0, I_{p+1})$.

Following [5], we consider three GLMs: logistic, Poisson, and Negative Binomial. In the logistic model, $Y_i \sim$ Bernoulli$\{1, g(X_i^\top \beta)\}$ conditioning on X_i. In the Poisson model, $Y_i \sim$ Poisson$\{g(X_i^\top \beta)\}$. In the Negative Binomial model, the conditional distribution of Y given X is NB$\{\exp(X^\top \beta), 1/2\}$. We set ρ in (10) to be 1 in the logistic model and 0.5 in the Poisson and Negative Binomial models.

To examine performance under both the $p < n$ and $p > n$ situations, we set the sample size $n = 500$ and the dimension $p = 100, 300, 500, 800, 1000$. For the coefficient vector $\beta = (\beta_1, \ldots, \beta_p)^\top$, β_i equals c_1 if $i \leq [c_2 p]$, otherwise β_i equals zero. The parameter c_2 controls the sparsity level of β. We select $c_2 = 0.75$ for the dense case and 0.25 for the sparse case. In order to have a reasonable range for the response variables, we restrict the value of $\exp\{X^\top \beta\}$ between $\exp(-4)$ and $\exp(4)$ in the Logistic model and between $\exp(0) = 1$ and $\exp(4) = 55$ in the Poisson and Negative Binomial models. The power is calculated by choosing $c_1 = 0.01$, and the type-I error rate is obtained with $c_1 = 0$. We set $\alpha = (1, \ldots, 1)^\top$ in the proposed test.

Summary statistics based on 1000 replicates are shown in Table 1. We can see that both methods have a good control of the type-I error rate. For example, under the Logistic model with $n = 500, p = 1000$, and dense data, the sizes of the EL and CG tests are 0.051 and 0.054, respectively. The EL test is more powerful than CG in most cases. For example, under the same setting, the power of the EL and CG tests are 0.998 and 0.318, respectively.

SIMULATION II. Here we consider different α values. The data generating models are the same as Simulation I. Notice that we set the first c_2 proportion of β to be c_1. Therefore we consider two cases of α: first, set $\alpha_i = 1$ if $i \leq \lfloor c_3 d \rfloor$; second, set $\alpha_i = 1$ if $i \geq p - \lfloor c_3 d \rfloor$. We choose c_3 from $\{0.25, 0.5, 0.75, 1\}$. Here we provide results for the logistic model. Performance under the other two models is similar.

Table 1 Empirical type-I error rates and power of EL and CG at significance level 5 % under Simulation I

	Logistic				Poisson				Negative Binomial			
	$c_1 = 0$		$c_1 = 0.01$		$c_1 = 0$		$c_1 = 0.01$		$c_1 = 0$		$c_1 = 0.01$	
(n, p)	EL	CG	EL	CG	EL	CG	EL	CG	EL	CG	EL	CG
Dense												
(500, 100)	0.058	0.056	0.297	0.118	0.053	0.053	0.620	0.262	0.063	0.058	0.382	0.136
(500, 300)	0.052	0.065	0.760	0.208	0.060	0.054	0.982	0.463	0.063	0.052	0.801	0.200
(500, 500)	0.044	0.052	0.921	0.238	0.050	0.060	0.997	0.595	0.060	0.050	0.950	0.270
(500, 800)	0.044	0.064	0.982	0.298	0.062	0.056	1.000	0.728	0.063	0.052	0.999	0.382
(500, 1000)	0.051	0.054	0.998	0.318	0.065	0.056	1.000	0.796	0.065	0.059	1.000	0.415
Sparse												
(500, 100)	0.056	0.061	0.079	0.085	0.067	0.060	0.112	0.102	0.059	0.059	0.108	0.086
(500, 300)	0.051	0.057	0.115	0.087	0.063	0.055	0.250	0.130	0.065	0.065	0.167	0.098
(500, 500)	0.050	0.054	0.186	0.102	0.066	0.062	0.388	0.164	0.060	0.059	0.218	0.109
(500, 800)	0.057	0.059	0.273	0.105	0.059	0.045	0.575	0.229	0.067	0.057	0.326	0.114
(500, 1000)	0.059	0.051	0.322	0.137	0.060	0.057	0.661	0.259	0.060	0.056	0.435	0.159

Table 2 Power of EL with different α values at significance level 5 % under Simulation II

(n, p)	$c_3 = 0.25$	$c_3 = 0.5$	$c_3 = 0.75$	$c_3 = 1$
$\alpha_i = 1$ if $i \leq \lfloor c_3 d \rfloor$; $(c_1 = 0.01, c_2 = 0.25)$				
(500, 100)	0.103	0.090	0.063	0.075
(500, 300)	0.225	0.143	0.111	0.093
(500, 500)	0.372	0.185	0.156	0.118
(500, 800)	0.546	0.292	0.220	0.153
(500, 1000)	0.669	0.380	0.255	0.176
$\alpha_i = 1$ if $i \geq p - \lfloor c_3 d \rfloor$; $(c_1 = 0.01, c_2 = 0.25)$				
(500, 100)	0.044	0.050	0.049	0.075
(500, 300)	0.058	0.057	0.054	0.093
(500, 500)	0.064	0.056	0.057	0.118
(500, 800)	0.049	0.050	0.058	0.153
(500, 1000)	0.042	0.055	0.061	0.176

Table 2 suggests that the power can increase if the data structure is known beforehand. For example, under the Logistic model with $n = 500, p = 1000$, and sparse data, we obtain the highest power by choosing the α that represents the same sparsity structure.

SIMULATION III. We conduct simulation for testing (7) in the presence of nuisance parameters. Specifically, $\beta^{(1)}$ has $p_1 = 10$ and is generated randomly from $U(0, 1)$ in the Logistic model and from $U(-0.5, 0.5)$ in the Poisson and Negative Binomial models. $\{X_i\}_{i=1}^n$ are generated from a moving average model

$$X_{ij} = \rho_1 Z_{ij} + \rho_2 Z_{i(j+1)} \quad (i = 1, \ldots, n, \ j = 1, \ldots, p), \tag{11}$$

where for each i, $\{Z_{ij}\}_{j=1}^{p+1}$ are independently generated from a $(p + p_1 + 1)$ standard normal distribution $N(0, I_{p+p_1+1})$. We choose ρ_1 and ρ_2 randomly from $U(0, 1)$. The other settings are similar to Simulation I. The results are shown in Table 3.

In addition, in order to show that the proposed method behaves independently of p and has a good control of type-I error when n is large, we also consider $n = 1000$, $p = 1000, 2000, 5000$. The results are listed in Table 4. Note that as the CG method encounters computational difficulty, we only apply the proposed method.

The observations in Table 3 are similar to those in the previous tables. That is, both methods have a good control of the type-I error, and the proposed method is more powerful under most simulation settings. Table 4 further suggests that, when n is reasonably large, performance of the proposed method is insensitive to the value of p.

In Figs. 1 and 2, we plot the cumulative distributions of EL test statistics under the null in a logistic model for the tests developed in Sects. 2 and 3, respectively. Comparing against the cumulative distribution of the chi-squared distribution with

Table 3 Empirical type-I error rate and power of EL and CG at significance level 5 % under Simulation III

	Logistic				Poisson				Negative Binomial			
	$c_1 = 0$		$c_1 = 0.1$		$c_1 = 0$		$c_1 = 0.1$		$c_1 = 0$		$c_1 = 0.1$	
(n, p)	EL	CG	EL	CG	EL	CG	EL	CG	EL	CG	EL	CG
Dense												
(500, 100)	0.056	0.058	0.174	0.170	0.060	0.056	0.373	0.291	0.071	0.048	0.769	0.702
(500, 300)	0.056	0.061	0.432	0.342	0.062	0.062	0.740	0.524	0.068	0.064	0.914	0.858
(500, 500)	0.057	0.057	0.551	0.505	0.062	0.062	0.866	0.717	0.072	0.052	0.964	0.903
(500, 800)	0.058	0.055	0.647	0.536	0.061	0.058	0.908	0.811	0.064	0.061	0.974	0.806
(500, 1000)	0.055	0.053	0.690	0.513	0.063	0.057	0.930	0.742	0.072	0.057	0.980	0.759
Sparse												
(500, 100)	0.055	0.048	0.073	0.063	0.062	0.049	0.089	0.071	0.073	0.048	0.275	0.282
(500, 300)	0.054	0.049	0.126	0.115	0.061	0.054	0.237	0.152	0.071	0.063	0.668	0.604
(500, 500)	0.047	0.048	0.151	0.151	0.056	0.056	0.410	0.321	0.068	0.062	0.792	0.726
(500, 800)	0.053	0.050	0.243	0.267	0.061	0.057	0.607	0.445	0.072	0.052	0.0887	0.827
(500, 1000)	0.051	0.049	0.259	0.282	0.060	0.055	0.659	0.532	0.073	0.063	0.882	0.813

Table 4 Empirical type-I error rate and power of EL and CG at significance level 5 % under Simulation III

(n, p)	Logistic	Poisson	Negative Binomial
(1000, 1000)	0.052	0.057	0.057
(1000, 2000)	0.048	0.050	0.058
(1000, 5000)	0.050	0.055	0.056

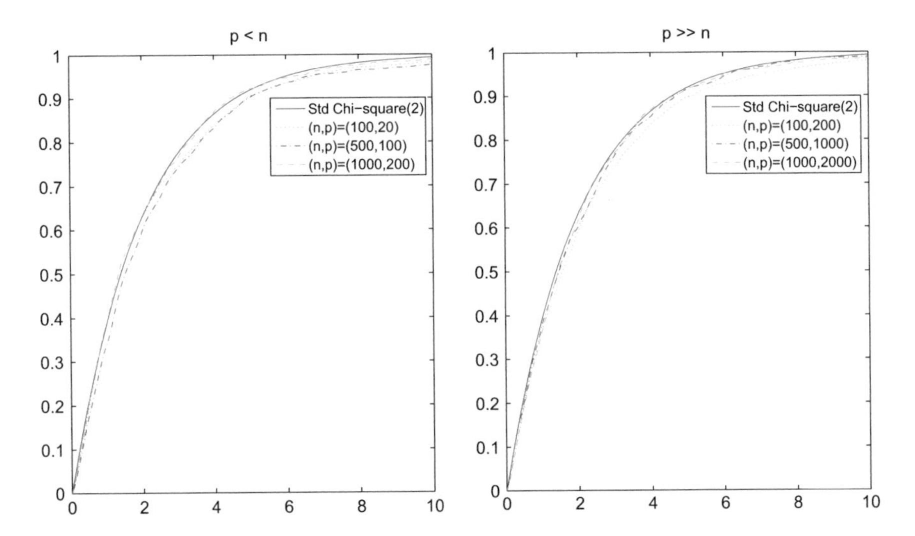

Fig. 1 The EL test statistics under the null hypothesis without the presence of nuisance parameters

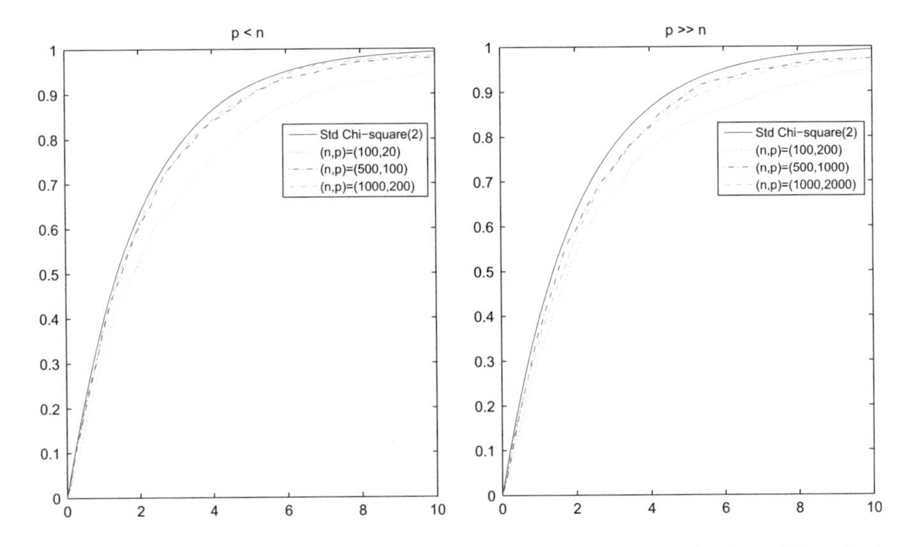

Fig. 2 The EL test statistics in the partial test with nuisance parameters under the null hypothesis

two degrees of freedom suggests the validity of the asymptotic distribution results under various settings.

5 Data Analysis

We analyze data from the North American Rheumatoid Arthritis Consortium (NARAC) provided by the GAW16. The initial batch consisted of 868 cases and 1194 controls genotyped with the 500k Illumina chip (545,080 SNPs). Detailed descriptions of the data can be found in [23]. In the literature, it has been suggested that RA is associated with genetic changes on chromosome 6 [11, 16]. We analyze data to prove this.

Consider the logistic model

$$E(Y_i|X_i) = \frac{\exp(X_i^\top \beta)}{1 + \exp(X_i^\top \beta)},$$

where $Y_i = 0$ or 1 indicates whether subject i is a control or a case, and X_i represents the SNP measurements on chromosome 6 of the ith subject. There are a total of 35,574 SNPs measured. The genotype of each SNP is classified as aa, Aa, and AA and denoted as 0, 1, and 2. We conduct the following processing: (1) remove SNPs with a high missing rate; (2) remove SNPs that have a low minor allele frequency. Specifically, set $a = \frac{2x+y}{2z}$ and $b = \frac{z}{2062}$, where x, y represent the frequencies of genotype 0 and 1, respectively, and z is the frequency of missing value. We select 35,429 SNPs with conditions $0.1 < \min(a, 1-a) < 0.5$ and $b > 0.15$. After this processing, we impute the remaining missing values with sample medians. Applying the proposed method, we obtain a p-value of 0.019, which suggests that SNPs on chromosome 6 are associated with RA.

Multiple methods are applicable to identify important SNPs that are associated with response. Two popular examples are the sure independence screening [12] and the iterated lasso [14]. It is of interest to ask, after the important SNPs have been identified by these methods, whether the remaining still have influence on the response. To answer such a question, we first split the data into two parts randomly: one part is used to identify the important SNPs and the other one is used to test. Then we apply the sure independence screening method to reduce dimensionality. Let $\beta^* = (\beta_1^*, \ldots, \beta_p^*)^\top$ be a p-vector where β_j^* denotes the estimation of β_j in the model

$$E(Y_i|X_{ij}) = \frac{\exp(a + X_{ij}^\top \beta_j)}{1 + \exp(a + X_{ij}^\top \beta_j)},$$

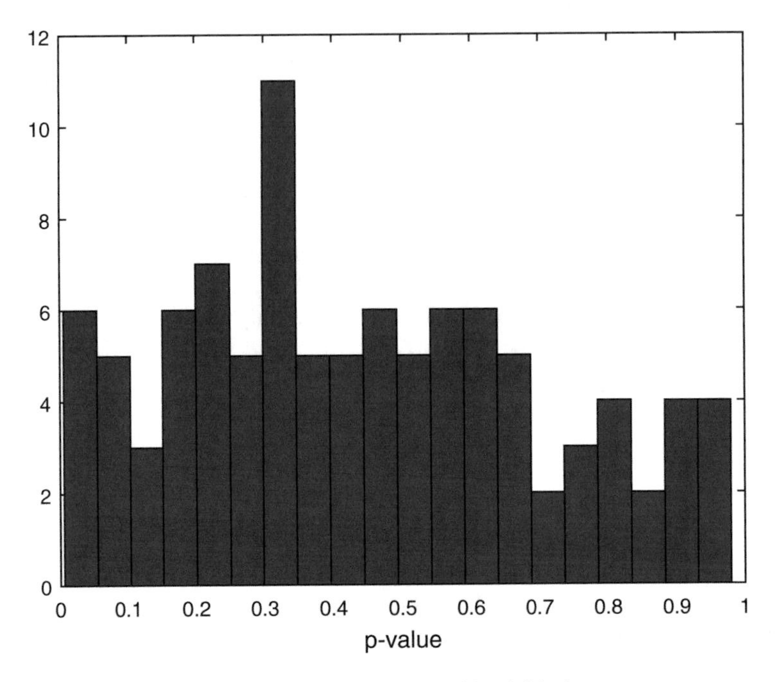

Fig. 3 The p-values of the partial test with the rheumatoid arthritis data

and a is the intercept term. Define

$$M = \left\{ 1 \le j \le p : |\beta_j^*| \text{ is among the first } \left\lfloor \frac{n}{\log(n)} \right\rfloor \text{ largest of all} \right\}.$$

With this method, the resulted M has a size of 263. Further, we apply the iterated lasso method with the tuning parameter chosen using fivefold cross validation. Finally, based on our proposed empirical likelihood test method, we can test whether the remaining SNPs have an effect on RA. We repeat this process 100 times and the histogram of the p-values is showed in Fig. 3. From Fig. 3 we can see that most of the p-values are larger than 0.05, which implies that the remaining SNPs likely have no association with the response.

6 Discussion

High dimensional data are now commonly encountered in multiple scientific fields. GLMs have been extensively used to model such data. The existing studies have been mostly focused on the estimation aspect. In this article, we have considered inference with the whole set of regression coefficients as well as a subset of coefficients. We have rigorously established the asymptotic properties of the proposed tests. In simulation, it is found that the proposed method has a similar control of the type-I error as the alternative but can have better power. The analysis of a GWAS dataset demonstrates the applicability of proposed method. In addition, it is also shown that the proposed method can be coupled with the existing estimation methods and make the results more conclusive.

A limitation of the proposed method is that the statistics converge slower to the limiting distribution compared to that in [5], since we split the data into two parts. Therefore to control the type-I error rate, we usually need more samples. In our limited numerical studies, we have found that usually the proposed method behaves well when there are at least a few hundred samples. For computational feasibility, the number of variables cannot be too large. The proposed method may have problematic performance when there are $\sim$10 samples. Another practical limitation is that β_0 may not be easy to specify. The "default" null with $\beta_0 = 0$ usually does not hold. With high dimensional data, our knowledge is often very limited, and it is not easy to have an informative β_0. However, as shown in data analysis, the proposed method can be coupled with the existing estimation methods to pin down the unimportant variable set.

Acknowledgements We thank the organizers and participants of "The Fourth International Workshop on the Perspectives on High-dimensional Data Analysis." Q. Zhang was partly supported by the China Postdoctoral Science Foundation (Grant No. 2014M550799) and the National Science Foundation of China (11401561). Q. Li was supported in part by the National Science Foundation of China (11371353, 61134013) and the Strategic Priority Research Program of the Chinese Academy of Sciences. S. Ma was supported by the National Social Science Foundation of China (13CTJ001, 13&ZD148).

Appendix

Recall that $\mu_{0i} = g(X_i^\top \beta_0), \psi(X_i, \beta_0) = g'(X_i^\top \beta_0)/V\{g(X_i^\top \beta_0)\}$, $\varepsilon_i = Y_i - g(X_i^\top \beta_0)$,

$$T_i = (Y_i - \mu_{0i})(Y_{i+m} - \mu_{0i+m})\psi(X_i, \beta_0)\psi(X_{i+m}, \beta_0)X_i^\top X_{i+m}$$

and

$$S_i = (Y_i - \mu_{0i})\psi(X_i, \beta_0)X_i^\top \alpha + (Y_{i+m} - \mu_{0i+m})\psi(X_{i+m}, \beta_0)X_{i+m}^\top \alpha.$$

Without loss of generality, we assume $\mu_{0i} = 0$. Now we prove Theorem 1.

Proof According to Theorem 3.2 in [21], it suffices to prove that under the assumptions of Theorem 1, Conditions 1–2, and the null hypothesis, we have that as $n \to \infty$,

$$\frac{1}{\sqrt{m}}\left(\sum_{i=1}^{m} T_i/\sigma_1,\ \sum_{i=1}^{m} S_i/\sigma_2\right)^{\top} \xrightarrow{d} N(0, I_2), \tag{12}$$

and

$$\frac{\sum_{i=1}^{m} T_i^2}{m\sigma_1^2} \xrightarrow{p} 1, \frac{\sum_{i=1}^{m} S_i^2}{m\sigma_2^2} \xrightarrow{p} 1, \frac{\sum_{i=1}^{m} T_i S_i}{m\sigma_1\sigma_2} \xrightarrow{p} 0, \tag{13}$$

where

$$\sigma_1^2 = \mathrm{tr}\left\{[E(V(g(X_1^{\top}\beta_0))\psi^2(X_1, \beta_0)X_1X_1^{\top})]^2\right\}$$

and

$$\sigma_2^2 = 2E\left(V(g(X_1^{\top}\beta_0))\psi^2(X_1, \beta_0)\alpha^{\top}X_1X_1^{\top}\alpha\right).$$

Notice that

$$\begin{aligned}
&\frac{E\left|X_i^{\top}X_{i+m}\psi(X_i, \beta_0)\psi(X_{i+m}, \beta_0)\varepsilon_i\varepsilon_{i+m}\right|^{2+\delta}}{\sigma_1^{(2+\delta)}}\\
&= \frac{E\left\{E\left|X_i^{\top}X_{i+m}\psi(X_i, \beta_0)\psi(X_{i+m}, \beta_0)\varepsilon_i\varepsilon_{i+m}\right|^{2+\delta} \mid X_i = x_i, X_{i+m} = x_{i+m}\right\}}{\sigma_1^{(2+\delta)}}\\
&= \frac{E\left\{\left|x_i^{\top}x_{i+m}\psi(x_i, \beta_0)\psi(x_{i+m}, \beta_0)\right|^{2+\delta} E(|\varepsilon_i|^{2+\delta} \mid X_i = x_i)E(|\varepsilon_{i+m}|^{2+\delta} \mid X_{i+m} = x_{i+m})\right\}}{\sigma_1^{(2+\delta)}}.
\end{aligned}$$

According to Conditions 1–2 and (5), we have

$$\frac{E\left|X_i^{\top}X_{i+m}\psi(X_i, \beta_0)\psi(X_{i+m}, \beta_0)\varepsilon_i\varepsilon_{i+m}\right|^{2+\delta}}{\sigma_1^{(2+\delta)}} = o(m^{\frac{\delta}{2}}).$$

Based on the Lyapunov central limit theorem, we can immediately get $\sum_{i=1}^{m} T_i/\sqrt{m}\sigma_1 \xrightarrow{\mathrm{d}} N(0, 1)$. Similarly we can obtain $\sum_{i=1}^{m} S_i/\sqrt{m}\sigma_2 \xrightarrow{\mathrm{d}} N(0, 1)$. To show (12), we still need to prove that for any constants a and b,

$$a\frac{\sum_{i=1}^{m} T_i}{\sqrt{m}\sigma_1} + b\frac{\sum_{i=1}^{m} S_i}{\sqrt{m}\sigma_2} \xrightarrow{\mathrm{d}} N\left(0, a^2 + b^2\right). \tag{14}$$

Notice that under the null hypothesis,

$$
\begin{aligned}
& a\frac{\sum_{i=1}^m T_i}{\sqrt{m}\sigma_1} + b\frac{\sum_{i=1}^m S_i}{\sqrt{m}\sigma_2} \\
&= \frac{a}{\sqrt{m}\sigma_1}\sum_{i=1}^m \psi(X_i,\beta_0)\psi(X_{i+m},\beta_0)X_i^\top X_{i+m}\varepsilon_i\varepsilon_{i+m} \\
&+ \frac{b}{\sqrt{m}\sigma_2}\sum_{i=1}^m [\psi(X_i,\beta_0)X_i^\top \varepsilon_i + \psi(X_{i+m},\beta_0)X_{i+m}^\top \varepsilon_{i+m}].
\end{aligned}
$$

Then it is easy to obtain that

$$
E\left\{a\frac{\sum_{i=1}^m T_i}{\sqrt{m}\sigma_1} + b\frac{\sum_{i=1}^m S_i}{\sqrt{m}\sigma_2}\right\} = 0,\ \mathrm{var}\left\{a\frac{\sum_{i=1}^m T_i}{\sqrt{m}\sigma_1} + b\frac{\sum_{i=1}^m S_i}{\sqrt{m}\sigma_2}\right\} = a^2 + b^2.
$$

By the Lyapunov central limit theorem, we conclude that (14) holds. That is, we prove (12).

To show the first result in (13), it is obviously that

$$
\frac{\sum_{i=1}^m T_i^2}{m} = \frac{1}{m}\sum_{i=1}^m [\psi(X_i,\beta_0)\psi(X_{i+m},\beta_0)X_i^\top X_{i+m}\varepsilon_i\varepsilon_{i+m}]^2 \xrightarrow{\mathrm{p}} \sigma_1^2.
$$

Therefore the first result in (13) holds. Similarly, we can obtain the rest two results in (13). □

To prove Theorem 2, we first establish Lemma 1.

Lemma 1 *For any $\delta > 0$,*

$$
E|X_1^\top X_{1+m}|^{2+\delta} \le p^\delta \left(\sum_{j=1}^p E|X_{1j}|^{2+\delta}\right)^2 \tag{15}
$$

and

$$
E|\alpha^\top (X_1 + X_{1+m})|^{2+\delta} \le 2^{4+\delta}||\alpha||^{2+\delta}p^{\delta/2}\sum_{j=1}^p E|X_{1j}|^{2+\delta}. \tag{16}
$$

Proof The proof of Lemma 1 is similar to that of Lemma 6 in [26]. □

Proof [Proof of Theorem 2] It suffices to verify that (5) and (6) hold in Theorem 1. Consider Example 1. Assume that $Q_1 = O\Sigma^{-1/2}X_1$, and $Q_{1+m} =$

$O\Sigma^{-1/2}X_{1+m}$, where O is an orthogonal matrix satisfying that $O\Sigma O^\top$ is diagonal. Then $X_1^\top X_{1+m} = Q_1^\top O\Sigma O^\top Q_{1+m} = \sum_{j=1}^p \phi_j Q_{1j}Q_{1+m,j}$, where ϕ_j's are the eigenvalues of Σ. Therefore

$$E\left[(X_1^\top X_{1+m})^4\right] = E\left[\left(\sum_{j=1}^p \phi_j Q_{1j}Q_{1+mj}\right)^4\right] \le 9\left(\sum_{j=1}^p \phi_j^2\right)^2 = 9[\mathrm{tr}\{\Sigma^2\}]^2.$$

Thus we obtain that $E[(X_1^\top X_{1+m})]^4/[\mathrm{tr}\{\Sigma^2\}]^2 = O(1)$ is bounded uniformly for any p, i.e., (5) holds. Equation (6) can be verified in the same way.

As for Example 2, we define $\Sigma' = \Gamma^\top\Gamma = (\sigma'_{i,j})_{1\le i,j\le m}$ and $\alpha^\top\Gamma = (a_1,\ldots,a_m)$. Since $X_i = \Gamma F_i$,

$$X_1^\top X_{1+m} = \sum_{j,j'=1}^s \sigma'_{j,j'}F_{1j}F_{(1+m)j'},$$

where $F_{(1+m)j}$ denotes the jth element of F_{1+m}, and

$$\alpha^\top(X_1 + X_{1+m}) = \sum_{j=1}^m a_j(F_{1j} + F_{(1+m)j}).$$

Denote $\delta_{j_1,\ldots,j_8} = E\left(\prod_{k=1}^8 F_{1j_k}\right)$. The other cases of $\sum_{v=1}^d l_v \le 8$ can be proved in the same way. Notice that

$$E(X_1^\top X_{1+m})^8 = \sum_{j_1,\ldots,j_8=1}^s \sum_{j'_1,\ldots,j'_8=1}^s \prod_{k=1}^8 \sigma'_{j_k j'_k}\delta_{j_1,\ldots,j_8}\delta_{j'_1,\ldots,j'_8}.$$

$\delta_{j_1,\ldots,j_8} \ne 0$ only when $\{j_1,\ldots,j_8\}$ form pairs of integers. Denote $\sum^*$ as the summation of the situations that $\delta_{j_1,\ldots,j_8}\delta_{j'_1,\ldots,j'_8} \ne 0$. By Lemma 1 we have

$$\begin{aligned} E(X_1^\top X_{1+m})^8 &= O\left(\sum^* \prod_{k=1}^8 \sigma'_{j_k j'_k}\right) \\ &= O\left(\mathrm{tr}\{\Sigma'^8\}\right) = O\left([\mathrm{tr}\{\Sigma'^2\}]^4\right). \end{aligned}$$

Similarly we have

$$
\begin{aligned}
E(\alpha^T(X_1+X_{1+m}))^8 &\le 2^8 E\left(\sum_{j=1}^{s} a_j F_{1j}\right)^8 \\
&= O\left(\sum_j a_j^8\right) + O\left(\sum_{j,j'} a_j^6 a_{j'}^2\right) + O\left(\sum_{j,j'} a_j^4 a_{j'}^4\right) + O\left(\sum_{j,j',j''} a_j^4 a_{j'}^2 a_{j''}^2\right) \\
&\quad + O\left(\sum_{j,j',j'',j'''} a_j^2 a_{j'}^2 a_{j''}^2 a_{j'''}^2\right) \\
&= O\left(\left(\sum_j a_j^2\right)^4\right) = O\left(\left(\alpha^T \Gamma \Gamma^T \alpha\right)^4\right).
\end{aligned}
$$

Then according to Theorem 1, we can prove Theorem 2. □

Proof [Proof of Theorem 3] Similar to the proof of Theorem 1, we only need to show that under Conditions 1, 3–5, and the null hypothesis, as $n \to \infty$,

$$
\frac{1}{\sqrt{m}}\left(\sum_{i=1}^{m} \tilde{T}_i/\tilde{\sigma}_1, \ \sum_{i=1}^{m} \tilde{S}_i/\tilde{\sigma}_2\right)^{\top} \xrightarrow{d} N(0, I_2) \tag{17}
$$

$$
\frac{\sum_{i=1}^m \tilde{T}_i^2}{m\tilde{\sigma}_1^2} \xrightarrow{p} 1, \ \frac{\sum_{i=1}^m \tilde{S}_i^2}{m\tilde{\sigma}_2^2} \xrightarrow{p} 1, \ \frac{\sum_{i=1}^m \tilde{T}_i\tilde{S}_i}{m\tilde{\sigma}_1\tilde{\sigma}_2} \xrightarrow{p} 0, \tag{18}
$$

where

$$
\tilde{\sigma}_1^2 = \operatorname{tr}\left\{[E(V(g(X_1^\top \beta_0))\psi^2(X_1, \beta_0)X_1^{(2)}X_1^{(2)\top})]^2\right\},
$$

and

$$
\tilde{\sigma}_2^2 = 2E\left(V(g(X_1^\top \beta_0))\psi^2(X_1, \beta_0)\alpha^\top X_1^{(2)}X_1^{(2)\top}\alpha\right).
$$

To prove (17), it suffices to prove the following three asymptotic results:

$$
\begin{aligned}
&\frac{\sum_{i=1}^m \tilde{T}_i}{\sqrt{m}\tilde{\sigma}_1} \xrightarrow{\mathrm{d}} N(0,1), \\
&\frac{\sum_{i=1}^m \tilde{S}_i}{\sqrt{m}\tilde{\sigma}_2} \xrightarrow{\mathrm{d}} N(0,1), \text{ and } a\frac{\sum_{i=1}^m \tilde{T}_i}{\sqrt{m}\tilde{\sigma}_1} + b\frac{\sum_{i=1}^m \tilde{S}_i}{\sqrt{m}\tilde{\sigma}_2} \xrightarrow{\mathrm{d}} N(0, a^2+b^2).
\end{aligned}
$$

Notice that under the null hypothesis $\tilde{H}_0$, we have

$$\frac{\sum_{i=1}^{m}\tilde{T}_i}{\sqrt{m}\tilde{\sigma}_1} = \frac{1}{\sqrt{m}\tilde{\sigma}_1}\sum_{i=1}^{m} h_{1i}(\hat{\beta}_0)$$

$$= \frac{1}{\sqrt{m}\tilde{\sigma}_1}\sum_{i=1}^{m} h_{1i}(\beta_0) + \frac{1}{\sqrt{m}\tilde{\sigma}_1}\sum_{i=1}^{m}(h_{1i}(\hat{\beta}_0) - h_{1i}(\beta_0)),$$

where

$$h_{1i}(\beta) = \psi(X_i, \beta_0)\psi(X_{i+m}, \beta_0)X_i^{(2)\top}X_{i+m}^{(2)}\left(y_i - g(X_i^\top\beta)\right)\left(y_{i+m} - g(X_{i+m}^\top\beta)\right).$$

Through proper calculation and according to Conditions 3–5, we have

$$E\left(\frac{1}{\sqrt{m}\tilde{\sigma}_1}\sum_{i=1}^{m}(h_{1i}(\hat{\beta}_0) - h_{1i}(\beta_0))\right)^2 = o(1).$$

Then by applying the Markov equality, we have

$$\frac{1}{\sqrt{m}\tilde{\sigma}_1}\sum_{i=1}^{m}(h_{1i}(\hat{\beta}_0) - h_{1i}(\beta_0)) = o_p(1).$$

Therefore $\frac{\sum_{i=1}^{m}\tilde{T}_i}{\sqrt{m}\tilde{\sigma}_1}$ can be written as the summation of independent statistics and $o_p(1)$, namely

$$\frac{\sum_{i=1}^{m}\tilde{T}_i}{\sqrt{m}\tilde{\sigma}_1} = \frac{1}{\sqrt{m}\tilde{\sigma}_1}\sum_{i=1}^{m} h_{1i}(\beta_0) + o_p(1).$$

Therefore similar to the proof of (12) in Theorem 1, we can prove (17).

To show the first result in (18), it is obvious that

$$\frac{1}{m\tilde{\sigma}_1^2}\sum_{i=1}^{m}\tilde{T}_i^2 = \frac{1}{m\tilde{\sigma}_1^2}\sum_{i=1}^{m} h_{1i}^2(\hat{\beta}_0) = \frac{1}{m\tilde{\sigma}_1^2}\sum_{i=1}^{m} h_{1i}^2(\beta_0) + \frac{1}{m\tilde{\sigma}_1^2}\sum_{i=1}^{m}(h_{1i}^2(\hat{\beta}_0) - h_{1i}^2(\beta_0)).$$

By applying Conditions 3–5 and with proper computation, we can obtain

$$E\left(\frac{1}{m\tilde{\sigma}_1^2}\sum_{i=1}^{m}(h_{1i}^2(\hat{\beta}_0) - h_{1i}^2(\beta_0))\right)^2 = o(1).$$

According to the Markov equality, we obtain $\frac{1}{m\tilde{\sigma}_1^2}\sum_{i=1}^m(h_{1i}^2(\hat{\beta}_0)-h_{1i}^2(\beta_0))=o_p(1)$. Therefore we have

$$\frac{\sum_{i=1}^m \tilde{T}_i^2}{m\tilde{\sigma}_1^2}=\frac{1}{m\tilde{\sigma}_1^2}\sum_{i=1}^m h_{1i}^2(\beta_0)+o_p(1). \tag{19}$$

By adopting the method similar to the proof of (13) in Theorem 1, we can obtain the first result in (18). Similarly, we can prove the other two results in (18). □

References

1. Bai, Z.D., Saranadasa, H.: Effect of high dimension: by an example of a two sample problem. Stat. Sin. **6**, 311–329 (1996)
2. Bühlmann, P., et al.: Statistical significance in high-dimensional linear models. Bernoulli **19**(4), 1212–1242 (2013)
3. Chapman, J., Whittaker, J.: Analysis of multiple snps in a candidate gene or region. Genet. Epidemiol. **32**, 560–566 (2008)
4. Chapman, J.M., Cooper, J.D., Todd, J.A., Clayton, D.G.: Detecting disease associations due to linkage disequilibrium using haplotype tags: a class of tests and the determinants of statistical power. Hum. Hered. **56**, 18–31 (2003)
5. Chen, S.X., Guo, B.: Tests for high dimensional generalized linear models. arXiv preprint. arXiv:1402.4882 (2014)
6. Chen, S.X., Hall, P.: Smoothed empirical likelihood confidence intervals for quantiles. Ann. Stat. **21**, 1166–1181 (1993)
7. Chen, S.X., Van Keilegom, I.: A review on empirical likelihood methods for regression. Test **18**(3), 415–447 (2009)
8. Chen, S.X., Peng, L., Qin, Y.L.: Effects of data dimension on empirical likelihood. Biometrika **96**, 711–722 (2009)
9. Chen, S.X., Zhang, L.X., Zhong, P.S.: Tests for high-dimensional covariance matrices. J. Am. Stat. Assoc. **106**, 260–274 (2010)
10. Donoho, D.L., et al.: High-dimensional data analysis: the curses and blessings of dimensionality. In: AMS Math Challenges Lecture, pp. 1–32 (2000)
11. Ellinghaus, E., Stuart, P.E., Ellinghaus, D., Nair, R.P., Debrus, S., Raelson, J.V., Belouchi, M., Tejasvi, T., Li, Y., Tsoi, L.C., et al.: Genome-wide meta-analysis of psoriatic arthritis identifies susceptibility locus at REL. J. Invest. Dermatol. **132**, 1133–1140 (2012)
12. Fan, J., Song, R., et al.: Sure independence screening in generalized linear models with NP-dimensionality. The Annals of Statistics **38**, 3567–3604 (2010)
13. Goeman, J.J., Van De Geer, S.A., Van Houwelingen, H.C.: Testing against a high dimensional alternative. J. R. Stat. Soc. Ser. B (Stat Methodol.) **68**, 477–493 (2006)
14. Huang, J., Ma, S., Zhang, C.H.: The iterated lasso for high-dimensional logistic regression. The University of Iowa Department of Statistical and Actuarial Science Technical Report (392) (2008)
15. Kolaczyk, E.D.: Empirical likelihood for generalized linear models. Stat. Sin. **4**, 199–218 (1994)
16. Li, Q., Hu, J., Ding, J., Zheng, G.: Fisher's method of combining dependent statistics using generalizations of the gamma distribution with applications to genetic pleiotropic associations. Biostatistics **15**, 284–295 (2013)

17. Meinshausen, N., Meier, L., Bühlmann, P.: P-values for high-dimensional regression. J. Am. Stat. Assoc. **104**(488), 1671–1681 (2009)
18. Newey, W.K., Smith, R.J.: Higher order properties of gmm and generalized empirical likelihood estimators. Econometrica **72**, 219–255 (2004)
19. Owen, A.B.: Empirical likelihood ratio confidence intervals for a single functional. Biometrika **75**, 237–249 (1988)
20. Owen, A.B.: Empirical likelihood for linear models. Ann. Stat. **11**, 1725–1747 (1991)
21. Owen, A.: Empirical Likelihood. Chapman and Hall/CRC, Boca Raton (2001)
22. Peng, L., Qi, Y., Wang, R.: Empirical likelihood test for high dimensional linear models. Stat. Probab. Lett. **86**, 74–79 (2014)
23. Plenge, R.M., Seielstad, M., Padyukov, L., Lee, A.T., Remmers, E.F., Ding, B., Liew, A., Khalili, H., Chandrasekaran, A., Davies, L.R., et al.: Traf1-c5 as a risk locus for rheumatoid arthritis–a genomewide study. N. Engl. J. Med. **357**(12), 1199–1209 (2007)
24. Qin, J., Lawless, J.: Empirical likelihood and general estimating equations. Ann. Stat. **22**, 300–325 (1994)
25. Wang, T., Elston, R.C.: Improved power by use of a weighted score test for linkage disequilibrium mapping. Am. J. Hum. Genet. **80**, 353–360 (2007)
26. Wang, R., Peng, L., Qi, Y.: Jackknife empirical likelihood test for equality of two high dimensional means. Stat. Sin. **23**, 667–690 (2013)
27. Zhang, R., Peng, L., Wang, R., et al.: Tests for covariance matrix with fixed or divergent dimension. Ann. Stat. **41**, 2075–2096 (2013)
28. Zhong, P.S., Chen, S.X.: Tests for high-dimensional regression coefficients with factorial designs. J. Am. Stat. Assoc. **106**, 260–274 (2011)

Random Projections for Large-Scale Regression

Gian-Andrea Thanei, Christina Heinze, and Nicolai Meinshausen

Abstract Fitting linear regression models can be computationally very expensive in large-scale data analysis tasks if the sample size and the number of variables are very large. Random projections are extensively used as a dimension reduction tool in machine learning and statistics. We discuss the applications of random projections in linear regression problems, developed to decrease computational costs, and give an overview of the theoretical guarantees of the generalization error. It can be shown that the combination of random projections with least squares regression leads to similar recovery as ridge regression and principal component regression. We also discuss possible improvements when averaging over multiple random projections, an approach that lends itself easily to parallel implementation.

1 Introduction

Assume we are given a data matrix $\mathbf{X} \in \mathbb{R}^{n \times p}$ (n samples of a p-dimensional random variable) and a response vector $\mathbf{Y} \in \mathbb{R}^n$. We assume a linear model for the data where $\mathbf{Y} = \mathbf{X}\beta + \varepsilon$ for some regression coefficient $\beta \in \mathbb{R}^p$ and ε i.i.d. mean-zero noise. Fitting a regression model by standard least squares or ridge regression requires $\mathcal{O}(np^2)$ or $\mathcal{O}(p^3)$ flops. In the situation of large-scale (n, p very large) or high dimensional ($p \gg n$) data these algorithms are not applicable without having to pay a huge computational price.

Using a random projection, the data can be "compressed" either row- or column-wise. Row-wise compression was proposed and discussed in [7, 15, 19]. These approaches replace the least-squares estimator

$$\underset{\gamma \in \mathbb{R}^p}{\operatorname{argmin}} \|\mathbf{Y} - \mathbf{X}\gamma\|_2^2 \qquad \text{with the estimator} \qquad \underset{\gamma \in \mathbb{R}^p}{\operatorname{argmin}} \|\boldsymbol{\psi}\mathbf{Y} - \boldsymbol{\psi}\mathbf{X}\gamma\|_2^2, \tag{1}$$

where the matrix $\boldsymbol{\psi} \in \mathbb{R}^{m \times n}$ ($m \ll n$) is a random projection matrix and has, for example, i.i.d. $\mathcal{N}(0, 1)$ entries. Other possibilities for the choice of $\boldsymbol{\psi}$ are

G.-A. Thanei • C. Heinze • N. Meinshausen (✉)
ETH Zürich, Rämistrasse 101, 8092 Zürich, Switzerland
e-mail: thanei@stat.math.ethz.ch; heinze@stat.math.ethz.ch; meinshausen@stat.math.ethz.ch

© Springer International Publishing AG 2017

S.E. Ahmed (ed.), *Big and Complex Data Analysis*, Contributions to Statistics,
DOI 10.1007/978-3-319-41573-4_3

discussed below. The high dimensional setting and ℓ_1-penalized regression are considered in [19], where it is shown that a sparse linear model can be recovered from the projected data under certain conditions. The optimization problem is still p-dimensional, however, and computationally expensive if the number of variables is very large.

Column-wise compression addresses this later issue by reducing the problem to a d-dimensional optimization with $d \ll p$ by replacing the least-squares estimator

$$\underset{\gamma \in \mathbb{R}^p}{\operatorname{argmin}} \|\mathbf{Y} - \mathbf{X}\gamma\|_2^2 \qquad \text{with the estimator} \qquad \boldsymbol{\phi} \underset{\gamma \in \mathbb{R}^d}{\operatorname{argmin}} \|\mathbf{Y} - \mathbf{X}\boldsymbol{\phi}\gamma\|_2^2, \tag{2}$$

where the random projection matrix is now $\boldsymbol{\phi} \in \mathbb{R}^{p \times d}$ (with $d \ll p$). By right multiplication to the data matrix $\mathbf{X}$ we transform the data matrix to $\mathbf{X}\boldsymbol{\phi}$ and thereby reduce the number of variables from p to d and thus reducing computational complexity. The Johnson–Lindenstrauss Lemma [5, 8, 9] guarantees that the distance between two transformed sample points is approximately preserved in the column-wise compression.

Random projections have also been considered under the aspect of preserving privacy [3]. By pre-multiplication with a random projection matrix as in (1) no observation in the resulting matrix can be identified with one of the original data points. Similarly, post-multiplication as in (2) produces new variables that do not reveal the realized values of the original variables.

In many applications the random projection used in practice falls under the class of Fast Johnson–Lindenstrauss Transforms (FJLT) [2]. One instance of such a fast projection is the Subsampled Randomized Hadamard Transform (SRHT) [17]. Due to its recursive definition, the matrix–vector product has a complexity of $\mathcal{O}(p \log(p))$, reducing the cost of the projection to $\mathcal{O}(np \log(p))$. Other proposals that lead to speedups compared to a Gaussian random projection matrix include random sign or sparse random projection matrices [1]. Notably, if the data matrix is sparse, using a sparse random projection can exploit sparse matrix operations. Depending on the number of non-zero elements in $\mathbf{X}$, one might prefer using a sparse random projection over an FJLT that cannot exploit sparsity in the data. Importantly, using $\mathbf{X}\boldsymbol{\phi}$ instead of $\mathbf{X}$ in our regression algorithm of choice can be disadvantageous if $\mathbf{X}$ is extremely sparse and d cannot be chosen to be much smaller than p. (The projection dimension d can be chosen by cross validation.) As the multiplication by $\boldsymbol{\phi}$ "densifies" the design matrix used in the learning algorithm the potential computational benefit of sparse data is not preserved.

For OLS and row-wise compression as in (1), where n is very large and $p < m < n$, the SRHT (and similar FJLTs) can be understood as a subsampling algorithm. It preconditions the design matrix by rotating the observations to a basis where all points have approximately uniform leverage [7]. This justifies uniform subsampling in the projected space which is applied subsequent to the rotation in order to reduce the computational costs of the OLS estimation. Related ideas can be found in the way columns and rows of $\mathbf{X}$ are sampled in a CUR-matrix decomposition [12]. While the approach in [7] focuses on the concept of leverage, McWilliams et al.

[15] propose an alternative scheme that allows for outliers in the data and makes use of the concept of influence [4]. Here, random projections are used to approximate the influence of each observation which is then used in the subsampling scheme to determine which observations to include in the subsample.

Using random projections column-wise as in (2) as a dimensionality reduction technique in conjunction with (ℓ_2 penalized) regression has been considered in [10, 11, 13]. The main advantage of these algorithms is the computational speedup while preserving predictive accuracy. Typically, a variance reduction is traded off against an increase in bias. In general, one disadvantage of reducing the dimensionality of the data is that the coefficients in the projected space are not interpretable in terms of the original variables. Naively, one could reverse the random projection operation by projecting the coefficients estimated in the projected space back into the original space as in (2). For prediction purposes this operation is irrelevant, but it can be shown that this estimator does not approximate the optimal solution in the original p-dimensional coefficient space well [18]. As a remedy, Zhang et al. [18] propose to find the dual solution in the projected space to recover the optimal solution in the original space. The proposed algorithm approximates the solution to the original problem accurately if the design matrix is low-rank or can be sufficiently well approximated by a low-rank matrix.

Lastly, random projections have been used as an auxiliary tool. As an example, the goal of McWilliams et al. [16] is to distribute ridge regression across variables with an algorithm called LOCO. The design matrix is split across variables and the variables are distributed over processing units (workers). Random projections are used to preserve the dependencies between all variables in that each worker uses a randomly projected version of the variables residing on the other workers in addition to the set of variables assigned to itself. It then solves a ridge regression using this local design matrix. The solution is the concatenation of the coefficients found from each worker and the solution vector lies in the original space so that the coefficients are interpretable. Empirically, this scheme achieves large speedups while retaining good predictive accuracy. Using some of the ideas and results outlined in the current manuscript, one can show that the difference between the full solution and the coefficients returned by LOCO is bounded.

Clearly, row- and column-wise compression can also be applied simultaneously or column-wise compression can be used together with subsampling of the data instead of row-wise compression. In the remaining sections, we will focus on the column-wise compression as it poses more difficult challenges in terms of statistical performance guarantees. While row-wise compression just reduces the effective sample size and can be expected to work in general settings as long as the compressed dimension $m < n$ is not too small [19], column-wise compression can only work well if certain conditions on the data are satisfied and we will give an overview of these results. If not mentioned otherwise, we will refer with compressed regression and random projections to the column-wise compression.

The structure of the manuscript is as follows: We will give an overview of bounds on the estimation accuracy in the following Sect. 2, including both known results and new contributions in the form of tighter bounds. In Sect. 3 we will discuss the possibility and properties of variance-reducing averaging schemes, where estimators based on different realized random projections are aggregated. Finally, Sect. 4 concludes the manuscript with a short discussion.

2 Theoretical Results

We will discuss in the following the properties of the column-wise compressed estimator as in (2), which is defined as

$$\hat{\beta}_d^{\boldsymbol{\phi}} = \boldsymbol{\phi} \operatorname*{argmin}_{\gamma \in \mathbb{R}^d} \|\mathbf{Y} - \mathbf{X}\boldsymbol{\phi}\gamma\|_2^2, \tag{3}$$

where we assume that ϕ has i.i.d. $\mathcal{N}(0, 1/d)$ entries. This estimator will be referred to as the compressed least-squares estimator (CLSE) in the following. We will focus on the unpenalized form as in (3) but note that similar results also apply to estimators that put an additional penalty on the coefficients β or γ. Due to the isotropy of the random projection, a ridge-type penalty as in [11, 16] is perhaps a natural choice. An interesting summary of the bounds on random projections is, on the other hand, that the random projection as in (3) already acts as a regularization and the theoretical properties of (3) are very much related to the properties of a ridge-type estimator of the coefficient vector in the absence of random projections.

We will restrict discussion of the properties mostly to the mean-squared error (MSE)

$$\mathbb{E}_{\boldsymbol{\phi}}\left[\mathbb{E}_{\varepsilon}(\|\mathbf{X}\beta - \mathbf{X}\hat{\beta}_d^{\boldsymbol{\phi}}\|_2^2)\right]. \tag{4}$$

First results on compressed least squares have been given in [13] in a random design setting. It was shown that the bias of the estimator (3) is of order $\mathcal{O}(\log(n)/d)$. This proof used a modified version of the Johnson–Lindenstrauss Lemma. A recent result [10] shows that the $\log(n)$-term is not necessary for fixed design settings where $\mathbf{Y} = \mathbf{X}\beta + \varepsilon$ for some $\beta \in \mathbb{R}^p$ and ε is i.i.d. noise, centred $\mathbb{E}_{\varepsilon}[\varepsilon] = 0$ and with the variance $\mathbb{E}_{\varepsilon}[\varepsilon\varepsilon'] = \sigma^2 I_{n\times n}$. We will work with this setting in the following.

The following result of [10] gives a bound on the MSE for fixed design.

Theorem 1 ([10]) *Assume fixed design and* $\text{Rank}(\mathbf{X}) \geq d$. *Then*

$$\mathbb{E}_{\boldsymbol{\phi}}\left[\mathbb{E}_{\varepsilon}(\|\mathbf{X}\beta - \mathbf{X}\hat{\beta}_d^{\boldsymbol{\phi}}\|_2^2)\right] \leq \sigma^2 d + \frac{\|\mathbf{X}\beta\|_2^2}{d} + \text{trace}(\mathbf{X}'\mathbf{X})\frac{\|\beta\|_2^2}{d}. \tag{5}$$

Proof See Appendix.

Compared with [13], the result removes an unnecessary $\mathcal{O}(\log(n))$ term and demonstrates the $\mathcal{O}(1/d)$ behaviour of the bias. The result also illustrates the tradeoffs when choosing a suitable dimension d for the projection. Increasing d

will lead to a $1/d$ reduction in the bias terms but lead to a linear increase in the estimation error (which is proportional to the dimension in which the least-squares estimation is performed). An optimal bound can only be achieved with a value of d that depends on the unknown signal and in practice one would typically use cross validation to make the choice of the dimension of the projection.

One issue with the bound in Theorem 1 is that the bound on the bias term in the noiseless case ($Y = \mathbf{X}\beta$)

$$\mathbb{E}_{\boldsymbol{\phi}}\left[\mathbb{E}_{\varepsilon}(\|\mathbf{X}\beta - \mathbf{X}\hat{\beta}_d^{\boldsymbol{\phi}}\|_2^2)\right] \leq \frac{\|\mathbf{X}\beta\|_2^2}{d} + \mathrm{trace}(\mathbf{X}'\mathbf{X})\frac{\|\beta\|_2^2}{d} \tag{6}$$

is usually weaker than the trivial bound (by setting $\hat{\beta}_d^{\boldsymbol{\phi}} = 0$) of

$$\mathbb{E}_{\boldsymbol{\phi}}\left[\mathbb{E}_{\varepsilon}(\|\mathbf{X}\beta - \mathbf{X}\hat{\beta}_d^{\boldsymbol{\phi}}\|_2^2)\right] \leq \|\mathbf{X}\beta\|_2^2 \tag{7}$$

for most values of $d < p$. By improving the bound, it is also possible to point out the similarities between ridge regression and compressed least squares.

The improvement in the bound rests on a small modification in the original proof in [10]. The idea is to bound the bias term of (4) by optimizing over the upper bound given in the foregoing theorem. Specifically, one can use the inequality

$$\begin{aligned}
&\mathbb{E}_{\boldsymbol{\phi}}[\mathbb{E}_{\varepsilon}[\|\mathbf{X}\beta - \mathbf{X}\boldsymbol{\phi}(\boldsymbol{\phi}'\mathbf{X}'\mathbf{X}\boldsymbol{\phi})^{-1}\boldsymbol{\phi}'\mathbf{X}'\mathbf{X}\beta\|_2^2]] \\
&\leq \min_{\hat{\beta}\in\mathbb{R}^p} \mathbb{E}_{\boldsymbol{\phi}}[\mathbb{E}_{\varepsilon}[\|\mathbf{X}\beta - \mathbf{X}\boldsymbol{\phi}\boldsymbol{\phi}'\hat{\beta}\|_2^2]],
\end{aligned}$$

instead of

$$\begin{aligned}
&\mathbb{E}_{\boldsymbol{\phi}}[\mathbb{E}_{\varepsilon}[\|\mathbf{X}\beta - \mathbf{X}\boldsymbol{\phi}(\boldsymbol{\phi}'\mathbf{X}'\mathbf{X}\boldsymbol{\phi})^{-1}\boldsymbol{\phi}'\mathbf{X}'\mathbf{X}\beta\|_2^2]] \\
&\leq \mathbb{E}_{\boldsymbol{\phi}}[\mathbb{E}_{\varepsilon}[\|\mathbf{X}\beta - \mathbf{X}\boldsymbol{\phi}\boldsymbol{\phi}'\beta\|_2^2]].
\end{aligned}$$

To simplify the exposition we will from now on always assume we have rotated the design matrix to an orthogonal design so that the Gram matrix is diagonal:

$$\Sigma = \mathbf{X}'\mathbf{X} = \mathrm{diag}(\lambda_1, \ldots, \lambda_p). \tag{8}$$

This can always be achieved for any design matrix and is thus not a restriction. It implies, however, that the optimal regression coefficients β are expressed in the basis in which the Gram matrix is orthogonal, this is the basis of principal components. This will turn out to be the natural choice for random projections and allows for easier interpretation of the results.

Furthermore note that in Theorem 1 we have the assumption Rank($\mathbf{X}$) $\geq d$, which tells us that we can apply the CLSE in the high dimensional setting $p \gg n$ as long as we choose d small enough (smaller than Rank($\mathbf{X}$), which is usually equal to n) in order to have uniqueness.

With the foregoing discussion on how to improve the bound in Theorem 1 we get the following theorem:

Theorem 2 *Assume* Rank($\mathbf{X}$) $\geq d$*, then the MSE (4) can be bounded above by*

$$\mathbb{E}_{\phi}[\mathbb{E}_{\varepsilon}[\|\mathbf{X}\beta - \mathbf{X}\hat{\beta}_d^{\phi}\|_2^2]] \leq \sigma^2 d + \sum_{i=1}^{p} \beta_i^2 \lambda_i w_i \tag{9}$$

where

$$w_i = \frac{(1+1/d)\lambda_i^2 + (1+2/d)\lambda_i \operatorname{trace}(\Sigma) + \operatorname{trace}(\Sigma)^2/d}{(d+2+1/d)\lambda_i^2 + 2(1+1/d)\lambda_i \operatorname{trace}(\Sigma) + \operatorname{trace}(\Sigma)^2/d}. \tag{10}$$

Proof See Appendix.

The w_i are shrinkage factors. By defining the proportion of the total variance observed in the direction of the ith principal component as

$$\alpha_i = \frac{\lambda_i}{\operatorname{trace}(\Sigma)}, \tag{11}$$

we can rewrite the shrinkage factors in the foregoing theorem as

$$w_i = \frac{(1+1/d)\alpha_i^2 + (1+2/d)\alpha_i + 1/d}{(d+2+1/d)\alpha_i^2 + 2(1+1/d)\alpha_i + 1/d}. \tag{12}$$

Analyzing this term shows that the shrinkage is stronger in directions of high variance compared to directions of low variance. To explain this relation in a bit more detail we compare it to ridge regression. The MSE of ridge regression with penalty term $\lambda\|\beta\|_2^2$ is given by

$$\mathbb{E}_{\varepsilon}[\|\mathbf{X}\beta - \mathbf{X}\beta^{\text{Ridge}}\|_2^2] = \sigma^2 \sum_{i=1}^{p} \Big(\frac{\lambda_i}{\lambda_i + \lambda}\Big)^2 + \sum_{i=1}^{p} \beta_i^2 \lambda_i \Big(\frac{\lambda}{\lambda + \lambda_i}\Big)^2. \tag{13}$$

Imagine that the signal lives on the space spanned by the first q principal directions, that is $\beta_i = 0$ for $i > q$. The best MSE we could then achieve is $\sigma^2 q$ by running a regression on the first q first principal directions. For random projections, we can see that we can indeed reduce the bias term to nearly zero by forcing $w_i \approx 0$ for $i = 1, \ldots, q$. This requires $d \gg q$ as the bias factors will then vanish like $1/d$. Ridge regression, on the other hand, requires that the penalty λ is smaller than the qth largest eigenvalue λ_q (to reduce the bias on the first q directions) but large enough to render the variance factor $\lambda_i/(\lambda_i + \lambda)$ very small for $i > q$. The tradeoff in choosing the penalty λ in ridge regression and choosing the dimension d for random projections is thus very similar. The number of directions for which the eigenvalue λ_i is larger than the penalty λ in ridge corresponds to the effective dimension and will yield the same variance bound as in random projections. The analogy between the MSE bounds (9) for random projections and (13) for ridge regression illustrates thus a close relationship between compressed least squares and ridge regression or principal component regression, similar to Dhillon et al. [6].

Instead of an upper bound for the MSE of CLSE as in [10, 13], we will in the following try to derive explicit expressions for the MSE, following the ideas in [10, 14] and we give a closed form MSE in the case of orthonormal predictors. The derivation will make use of the following notation:

Definition 1 Let $\boldsymbol{\phi} \in \mathbb{R}^{p \times d}$ be a random projection. We define the following matrices:

$$\boldsymbol{\phi}_d^{\mathbf{X}} = \boldsymbol{\phi}(\boldsymbol{\phi}'\mathbf{X}'\mathbf{X}\boldsymbol{\phi})^{-1}\boldsymbol{\phi}' \in \mathbb{R}^{p \times p} \quad \text{and} \quad T_d^{\boldsymbol{\phi}} = \mathbb{E}_{\boldsymbol{\phi}}[\boldsymbol{\phi}_d^{\mathbf{X}}] = \mathbb{E}_{\boldsymbol{\phi}}[\boldsymbol{\phi}(\boldsymbol{\phi}'\mathbf{X}'\mathbf{X}\boldsymbol{\phi})^{-1}\boldsymbol{\phi}'] \in \mathbb{R}^{p \times p}.$$

The next Lemma [14] summarizes the main properties of $\boldsymbol{\phi}_d^{\mathbf{X}}$ and $T_d^{\boldsymbol{\phi}}$.

Lemma 1 *Let $\boldsymbol{\phi} \in \mathbb{R}^{p \times d}$ be a random projection. Then*

(i) $(\boldsymbol{\phi}_d^{\mathbf{X}})' = \boldsymbol{\phi}_d^{\mathbf{X}}$ *(symmetric),*
(ii) $\boldsymbol{\phi}_d^{\mathbf{X}}\mathbf{X}'\mathbf{X}\boldsymbol{\phi}_d^{\mathbf{X}} = \boldsymbol{\phi}_d^{\mathbf{X}}$ *(projection),*
(iii) if $\Sigma = \mathbf{X}'\mathbf{X}$ *is diagonal* $\Rightarrow T_d^{\boldsymbol{\phi}}$ *is diagonal.*

Proof See Marzetta et al. [14].

The important point of this lemma is that when we assume orthogonal design then $T_d^{\boldsymbol{\phi}}$ is diagonal. We will denote this by

$$T_d^{\boldsymbol{\phi}} = \operatorname{diag}(1/\eta_1, \ldots, 1/\eta_p),$$

where the terms η_i are well defined but without an explicit representation.

A quick calculation reveals the following theorem:

Theorem 3 *Assume* $\operatorname{Rank}(\mathbf{X}) \geq d$*, then the MSE (4) equals*

$$\mathbb{E}_{\boldsymbol{\phi}}[\mathbb{E}_{\varepsilon}[\|\mathbf{X}\beta - \mathbf{X}\hat{\beta}_d^{\boldsymbol{\phi}}\|_2^2]] = \sigma^2 d + \sum_{i=1}^{p} \beta_i^2 \lambda_i \Big(1 - \frac{\lambda_i}{\eta_i}\Big). \tag{14}$$

Furthermore we have

$$\sum_{i=1}^{p} \frac{\lambda_i}{\eta_i} = d. \tag{15}$$

Proof See Appendix.

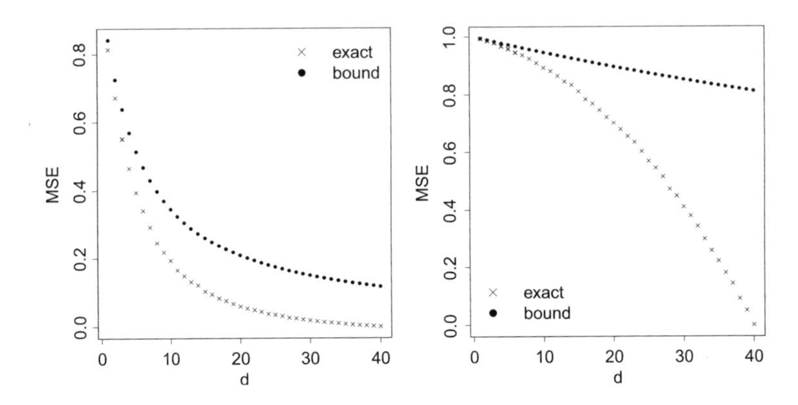

Fig. 1 Numerical simulations of the bounds in Theorems 2 and 3. *Left*: the exact factor $(1-\lambda_1/\eta_1)$ in the MSE is plotted versus the bound w_1 as a function of the projection dimension d. *Right*: the exact factor $(1-\lambda_p/\eta_p)$ in the MSE and the upper bound w_p. Note that the upper bound works especially well for small values of d and for the larger eigenvalues and is always below the trivial bound 1

By comparing coefficients in Theorems 2 and 3, we obtain the following corollary, which is illustrated in Fig 1:

Corollary 1 *Assume* Rank(**X**) $\geq d$*, then*

$$\forall i \in \{1, \ldots, p\}: \ 1 - \frac{\lambda_i}{\eta_i} \leq w_i \tag{16}$$

As already mentioned in general we cannot give a closed form expression for the terms η_i in general. However, for some special cases (26) can help us to get to an exact form of the MSE of CLSE. If we assume orthonormal design ($\Sigma = CI_{p\times p}$), then we have that λ_i/η_i is a constant for all i and and thus, by (26), we have $\eta_i = Cp/d$. This gives

$$\mathbb{E}_{\phi}[\mathbb{E}_{\varepsilon}[\|\mathbf{X}\beta - \mathbf{X}\hat{\beta}_d^{\phi}\|_2^2]] = \sigma^2 d + C\sum_{i=1}^{p} \beta_i^2 \Big(1 - \frac{d}{p}\Big), \tag{17}$$

and thus we end up with a closed form MSE for this special case.

Providing the exact mean-squared errors allows us to quantify the conservativeness of the upper bounds. The upper bound has been shown to give a good approximation for small dimensions d of the projection and for the signal contained in the larger eigenvalues.

3 Averaged Compressed Least Squares

We have so far looked only into compressed least-squares estimator with one single random projection. An issue in practice of the compressed least-squares estimator is its variance due to the random projection as an additional source of randomness. This variance can be reduced by averaging multiple compressed least-squares estimates coming from different random projections. In this section we will show some properties of the averaged compressed least-squares estimator (ACLSE) and discuss its advantage over the CLSE.

Definition 2 (ACLSE) Let $\{\boldsymbol{\phi}_1, \ldots, \boldsymbol{\phi}_K\} \in \mathbb{R}^{p\times d}$ be independent random projections, and let $\hat{\beta}_d^{\boldsymbol{\phi}_i}$ for all $i \in \{1, \ldots, K\}$ be the respective compressed least-squares estimators. We define the averaged compressed least-squares estimator (ACLSE) as

$$\hat{\beta}_d^K := \frac{1}{K}\sum_{i=1}^{K}\hat{\beta}_d^{\boldsymbol{\phi}_i}. \tag{18}$$

One major advantage of this estimator is that it can be calculated in parallel with the minimal number of two communications, one to send the data and one to receive the result. This means that the asymptotic computational cost of $\hat{\beta}_d^K$ is equal to the cost of $\hat{\beta}_d^{\boldsymbol{\phi}}$ if calculations are done on K different processors. To investigate the MSE of $\hat{\beta}_d^K$, we restrict ourselves for simplicity to the limit case

$$\hat{\beta}_d = \lim_{K\to\infty}\hat{\beta}_d^K \tag{19}$$

and instead only investigate $\hat{\beta}_d$. The reasoning being that for large enough values of K (say $K > 100$) the behaviour of $\hat{\beta}_d$ is very similar to $\hat{\beta}_d^K$. The exact form of the MSE in terms of the η_i's is given in [10]. Here we build on these results and give an explicit upper bound for the MSE.

Theorem 4 *Assume* Rank($\mathbf{X}$) $\geq d$. *Define*

$$\tau = \sum_{i=1}^{p}\left(\frac{\lambda_i}{\eta_i}\right)^2.$$

The MSE of $\hat{\beta}_d$ *can be bounded from above by*

$$\mathbb{E}_{\boldsymbol{\phi}}[\mathbb{E}_{\varepsilon}[\|\mathbf{X}\beta - \mathbf{X}\hat{\beta}_d\|_2^2]] \leq \sigma^2\tau + \sum_{i=1}^{p}\beta_i^2\lambda_i w_i^2,$$

where the w_i*'s are given (as in Theorem 1) by*

$$w_i = \frac{(1+1/d)\lambda_i^2 + (1+2/d)\lambda_i \operatorname{trace}(\Sigma) + \operatorname{trace}(\Sigma)^2/d}{(d+2+1/d)\lambda_i^2 + 2(1+1/d)\lambda_i \operatorname{trace}(\Sigma) + \operatorname{trace}(\Sigma)^2/d}.$$

and

$$\tau \in [d^2/p, d].$$

Proof See Appendix.

Comparing averaging to the case where we only have one single estimator we see that there are two differences: First the variance due to the model noise ε turns into $\sigma^2\tau$ with $\tau \in [d^2/p, d]$, thus $\tau \leq d$. Second the shrinkage factors w_i in the bias are now squared, which in total means that the MSE of $\hat{\beta}_d$ is always smaller or equal to the MSE of a single estimator $\hat{\beta}_d^{\phi}$.

We investigate the behaviour of τ as a function of d in three different situations (Fig. 2). We first look at two extreme cases of covariance matrices for which the respective upper and lower bounds $[d^2/p, d]$ for τ are achieved. For the lower bound, let $\Sigma = I_{p\times p}$ be orthonormal. Then $\lambda_i/\eta_i = c$ for all i, as above. From

$$\sum_{i=1}^{p} \lambda_i/\eta_i = d$$

we get $\lambda_i/\eta_i = d/p$. This leads to

$$\tau = \sum_{i=1}^{p} (\lambda_i/\eta_i)^2 = p\frac{d^2}{p^2} = \frac{d^2}{p},$$

which reproduces the lower bound.

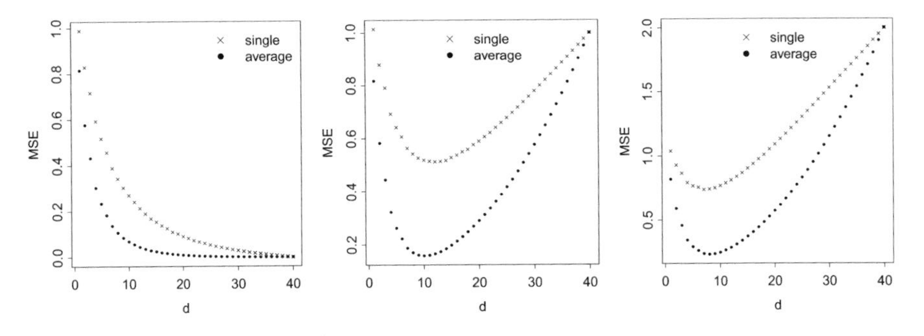

Fig. 2 MSE of averaged compressed least squares (*circle*) versus the MSE of the single estimator (*cross*) with covariance matrix $\Sigma_{i,i} = 1/i$. On the *left* with $\sigma^2 = 0$ (only bias), in the *middle* $\sigma^2 = 1/40$ and on the *right* $\sigma^2 = 1/20$. One can clearly see the quadratic improvement in terms of MSE as predicted by Theorem 4

We will not be able to reproduce the upper bound exactly for all $d \leq p$. But we can show that for any d there exists a covariance matrix Σ, such that the upper bound is reached. The idea is to consider a covariance matrix that has equal variance in the first d direction and almost zero in the remaining $p - d$. Define the diagonal covariance matrix

$$\Sigma_{i,j} = \begin{cases} 1, & \text{if } i = j \text{ and } i \leq d \\ \epsilon, & \text{if } i = j \text{ and } i > d \\ 0, & \text{if } i \neq j \end{cases} . \tag{20}$$

We show $\lim_{\epsilon \to 0} \tau = d$. For this decompose Φ into two matrices $\Phi_d \in \mathbb{R}^{d \times d}$ and $\Phi_r \in \mathbb{R}^{(p-d) \times d}$:

$$\Phi = \begin{pmatrix} \Phi_d \\ \Phi_r \end{pmatrix} .$$

The same way we define β_d, β_r, $\mathbf{X}_d$ and $\mathbf{X}_r$. Now we bound the approximation error of $\hat{\beta}_d^{\Phi}$ to extract information about λ_i/η_i. Assume a squared data matrix ($n = p$) $\mathbf{X} = \sqrt{\Sigma}$, then

$$\begin{aligned}
\mathbb{E}_{\Phi}[\operatorname*{argmin}_{\gamma \in \mathbb{R}^d} \|\mathbf{X}\beta - \mathbf{X}\Phi\gamma\|_2^2] &\leq \mathbb{E}_{\Phi}[\|\mathbf{X}\beta - \mathbf{X}\Phi\Phi_d^{-1}\beta_d\|_2^2] \\
&= \mathbb{E}_{\Phi}[\|\mathbf{X}_r\beta_r - \mathbf{X}_r\Phi_r\Phi_d^{-1}\beta_d\|_2^2] \\
&= \epsilon\mathbb{E}_{\Phi}[\|\beta_r - \Phi_r\Phi_d^{-1}\beta_d\|_2^2] \\
&\leq \epsilon(2\|\beta_r\|_2^2 + 2\|\beta_d\|_2^2\mathbb{E}_{\Phi}[\|\Phi_r\|_2^2]\mathbb{E}_{\Phi}[\|\Phi_d^{-1}\|_2^2]) \\
&\leq \epsilon C,
\end{aligned}$$

where C is independent of ϵ and bounded since the expectation of the smallest and largest singular values of a random projection is bounded. This means that the approximation error decreases to zero as we let $\epsilon \to 0$. Applying this to the closed form for the MSE of $\hat{\beta}_d^{\Phi}$ we have that

$$\sum_{i=1}^{p} \beta_i^2 \lambda_i \Big(1 - \frac{\lambda_i}{\eta_i}\Big) \leq \sum_{i=1}^{d} \beta_i^2 \Big(1 - \frac{\lambda_i}{\eta_i}\Big) + \epsilon \sum_{i=d+1}^{p} \beta_i^2 \Big(1 - \frac{\lambda_i}{\eta_i}\Big)$$

has to go to zero as $\epsilon \to 0$, which in turn implies

$$\lim_{\epsilon \to 0} \sum_{i=1}^{d} \beta_i^2 \Big(1 - \frac{\lambda_i}{\eta_i}\Big) = 0,$$

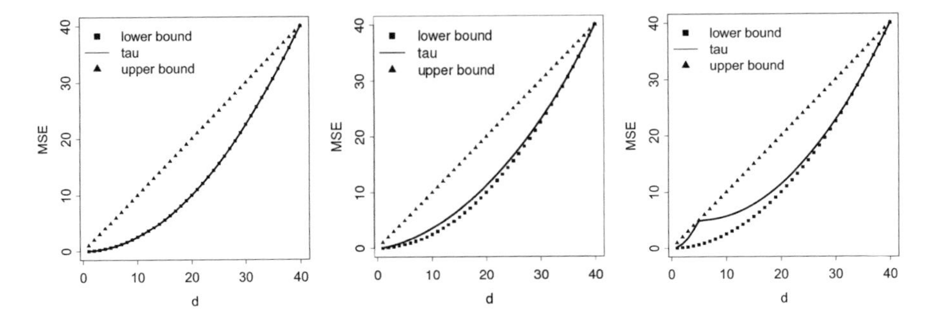

Fig. 3 Simulations of the variance factor τ (*line*) as a function of d for three different covariance matrices and in lower bound (d^2/p) and upper bound (d) (*square, triangle*). On the *left* ($\Sigma = I_{p\times p}$) τ as proven reaches the lower bound. In the *middle* ($\Sigma_{i,i} = 1/i$) τ reaches almost the lower bound, indicating that in most practical examples τ will be very close to the lower bound and thus averaging improves MSE substantially compared to the single estimator. On the *right* the extreme case example from (20) with $d = 5$, where τ reaches the upper bound for $d = 5$

and thus $\lim_{\epsilon\to 0} \lambda_i/\eta_i = 1$ for all $i \in \{1, \ldots, d\}$. This finally yields a limit

$$\lim_{\epsilon\to 0} \sum_{i=1}^{p} \frac{\lambda_i^2}{\eta_i^2} = d.$$

This illustrates that the lower bound d^2/p and upper bound d for the variance factor τ can both be attained. Simulations suggest that τ is usually close to the lower bound, where the variance of the estimator is reduced by a factor d/p compared to a single iteration of a compressed least-squares estimator, which is on top of the reduction in the bias error term. This shows, perhaps unsurprisingly, that averaging over random projection estimators improves the mean-squared error in a Rao–Blackwellization sense. We have quantified the improvement. In practice, one would have to decide whether to run multiple versions of a compressed least-squares regression in parallel or run a single random projection with a perhaps larger embedding dimension. The computational effort and statistical error tradeoffs will depend on the implementation but the bounds above will give a good basis for a decision (Fig. 3).

4 Discussion

We discussed some known results about the properties of compressed least-squares estimation and proposed possible tighter bounds and exact results for the mean-squared error. While the exact results do not have an explicit representation, they allow nevertheless to quantify the conservative nature of the upper bounds on the error. Moreover, the shown results allow to show a strong similarity of the error of compressed least squares, ridge and principal component regression. We also discussed the advantages of a form of Rao–Blackwellization, where multiple compressed least-square estimators are averaged over multiple random projections. The latter averaging procedure also allows to compute the estimator trivially in a distributed way and is thus often better suited for large-scale regression analysis. The averaging methodology also motivates the use of compressed least squares in the high dimensional setting where it performs similar to ridge regression and the use of multiple random projection will reduce the variance and result in a non-random estimator in the limit, which presents a computationally attractive alternative to ridge regression.

Appendix

In this section we give proofs of the statements from the section theoretical results.

Theorem 1 ([10]) *Assume fixed design and* $\mathrm{Rank}(\mathbf{X}) \geq d$*, then the AMSE 4 can be bounded above by*

$$\mathbb{E}_{\boldsymbol{\phi}}[\mathbb{E}_{\varepsilon}[\|\mathbf{X}\beta - \mathbf{X}\hat{\beta}_d^{\boldsymbol{\phi}}\|_2^2]] \leq \sigma^2 d + \frac{\|\mathbf{X}\beta\|_2^2}{d} + \mathrm{trace}(\mathbf{X}'\mathbf{X})\frac{\|\beta\|_2^2}{d}. \tag{21}$$

Proof (Sketch)

$$\begin{aligned}\mathbb{E}_{\boldsymbol{\phi}}[\mathbb{E}_{\varepsilon}[\|\mathbf{X}\beta - \mathbf{X}\hat{\beta}_d^{\boldsymbol{\phi}}\|_2^2]] &= \mathbb{E}_{\boldsymbol{\phi}}[\|\mathbf{X}\beta - \mathbf{X}\boldsymbol{\phi}(\boldsymbol{\phi}'\mathbf{X}'\mathbf{X}\boldsymbol{\phi})^{-1}\boldsymbol{\phi}'\mathbf{X}'\mathbf{X}\beta\|_2^2] + \sigma^2 d \\ &\leq \mathbb{E}_{\boldsymbol{\phi}}[\|\mathbf{X}\beta - \mathbf{X}\boldsymbol{\phi}(\boldsymbol{\phi}'\mathbf{X}'\mathbf{X}\boldsymbol{\phi})^{-1}\boldsymbol{\phi}'\mathbf{X}'\mathbf{X}\boldsymbol{\phi}\boldsymbol{\phi}'\beta\|_2^2] + \sigma^2 d \\ &= \mathbb{E}_{\boldsymbol{\phi}}[\|\mathbf{X}\beta - \mathbf{X}\boldsymbol{\phi}\boldsymbol{\phi}'\beta\|_2^2] + \sigma^2 d.\end{aligned}$$

Finally a rather lengthy but straightforward calculation leads to

$$\mathbb{E}_{\boldsymbol{\phi}}[\|\mathbf{X}\beta - \mathbf{X}\boldsymbol{\phi}\boldsymbol{\phi}'\beta\|_2^2] = \frac{\|\mathbf{X}\beta\|_2^2}{d} + \mathrm{trace}(\mathbf{X}'\mathbf{X})\frac{\|\beta\|_2^2}{d} \tag{22}$$

and thus proving the statement above. □

Theorem 2 *Assume* $\mathrm{Rank}(\mathbf{X}) \geq d$*, then the AMSE (4) can be bounded above by*

$$\mathbb{E}_{\boldsymbol{\phi}}[\mathbb{E}_{\varepsilon}[\|\mathbf{X}\beta - \mathbf{X}\hat{\beta}_d^{\boldsymbol{\phi}}\|_2^2]] \leq \sigma^2 d + \sum_{i=1}^{p} \beta_i^2 \lambda_i w_i \tag{23}$$

where

$$w_i = \frac{(1+1/d)\lambda_i^2 + (1+2/d)\lambda_i \operatorname{trace}(\Sigma) + \operatorname{trace}(\Sigma)^2/d}{(d+2+1/d)\lambda_i^2 + 2(1+1/d)\lambda_i \operatorname{trace}(\Sigma) + \operatorname{trace}(\Sigma)^2/d}. \tag{24}$$

Proof We have for all $v \in \mathbb{R}^p$

$$\mathbb{E}_{\boldsymbol{\phi}}[\min_{\hat{\gamma}\in\mathbb{R}^d} \|\mathbf{X}\beta - \mathbf{X}\boldsymbol{\phi}\hat{\gamma}\|_2^2] \le \mathbb{E}_{\boldsymbol{\phi}}[\|\mathbf{X}\beta - \mathbf{X}\boldsymbol{\phi}\boldsymbol{\phi}'v\|_2^2].$$

Which we can minimize over the whole set $\mathbb{R}^p$:

$$\mathbb{E}_{\boldsymbol{\phi}}[\min_{\hat{\gamma}\in\mathbb{R}^d} \|\mathbf{X}\beta - \mathbf{X}\boldsymbol{\phi}\hat{\gamma}\|_2^2] \le \min_{v\in\mathbb{R}^p}\mathbb{E}_{\boldsymbol{\phi}}[\|\mathbf{X}\beta - \mathbf{X}\boldsymbol{\phi}\boldsymbol{\phi}'v\|_2^2].$$

This last expression we can calculate following the same path as in Theorem 1:

$$\begin{aligned}
\mathbb{E}_{\boldsymbol{\phi}}[\|\mathbf{X}\beta - \mathbf{X}\boldsymbol{\phi}\boldsymbol{\phi}'v\|_2^2] =& \beta'\mathbf{X}'\mathbf{X}\beta - 2\beta'\mathbf{X}'\mathbf{X}\mathbb{E}_{\boldsymbol{\phi}}[\boldsymbol{\phi}\boldsymbol{\phi}']v \\
&+ v'\mathbb{E}_{\boldsymbol{\phi}}[\boldsymbol{\phi}\boldsymbol{\phi}'\mathbf{X}'\mathbf{X}\boldsymbol{\phi}\boldsymbol{\phi}']v \\
=& \beta'\mathbf{X}'\mathbf{X}\beta - 2\beta'\mathbf{X}'\mathbf{X}v \\
&+ (1+1/d)v'\mathbf{X}'\mathbf{X}v + \frac{\operatorname{trace}(\Sigma)}{d}\|v\|_2^2,
\end{aligned}$$

where $\Sigma = X'X$. Next we minimize the above expression w.r.t v. For this we take the derivative w.r.t. v and then we zero the whole expression. This yields

$$2\Big(1+\frac{1}{d}\Big)\Sigma v + 2\frac{\operatorname{trace}(\Sigma)}{d} I_{p\times p} v - 2\Sigma\beta = 0.$$

Hence we have

$$v = \bigg(\Big(1+\frac{1}{d}\Big)\Sigma + \frac{\operatorname{trace}(\Sigma)}{d} I_{p\times p}\bigg)^{-1}\Sigma\beta,$$

which is element wise equal to

$$v_i = \frac{\beta_i\lambda_i}{(1+1/d)\lambda_i + \operatorname{trace}(\Sigma)/d}.$$

Define the notation $s = \operatorname{trace}(\Sigma)$. We now plug this back into the original expression and get

$$\begin{aligned}
\min_{v\in\mathbb{R}^p}\mathbb{E}_{\boldsymbol{\phi}}[\|\mathbf{X}\beta - \mathbf{X}\boldsymbol{\phi}\boldsymbol{\phi}'v\|_2^2] =& \beta'\Sigma\beta - 2\beta'\Sigma v \\
&+ (1+1/d)v'\Sigma v + \frac{s}{d}\|v\|_2^2
\end{aligned}$$

$$
\begin{aligned}
&= \sum_{i=1}^{p} \beta_i^2\lambda_i - 2\beta_i v_i\lambda_i + (1+1/d)v_i^2\lambda_i + s/dv_i^2 \\
&= \sum_{i=1}^{p} \Big(\beta_i^2\lambda_i - 2\beta_i^2\lambda_i \frac{\lambda_i}{(1+1/d)\lambda_i + s/d} \\
&\quad + \beta_i^2\lambda_i(1+1/d)\frac{\lambda_i^2}{((1+1/d)\lambda_i + s/d)^2} \\
&\quad + \beta_i^2\lambda_i \frac{s}{d}\frac{\lambda_i}{((1+1/d)\lambda_i + s/d)^2} \Big) \\
&= \sum_{i=1}^{p} \beta_i^2\lambda_i w_i,
\end{aligned}
$$

by combining the summands we get for w_i the expression mentioned in the theorem. □

Theorem 3 *Assume* Rank($\mathbf{X}$) $\geq d$*, then the MSE (4) equals*

$$
\mathbb{E}_{\boldsymbol{\phi}}[\mathbb{E}_{\varepsilon}[\|\mathbf{X}\beta - \mathbf{X}\hat{\beta}_d^{\boldsymbol{\phi}}\|_2^2]] = \sigma^2 d + \sum_{i=1}^{p} \beta_i^2\lambda_i \Big(1 - \frac{\lambda_i}{\eta_i}\Big). \tag{25}
$$

Furthermore we have

$$
\sum_{i=1}^{p} \frac{\lambda_i}{\eta_i} = d. \tag{26}
$$

Proof Calculating the expectation yields

$$
\mathbb{E}_{\boldsymbol{\phi}}[\mathbb{E}_{\varepsilon}[\|\mathbf{X}\beta - \mathbf{X}\hat{\beta}_d\|_2^2]] = \beta'\Sigma\beta - 2\beta'\Sigma T_d^{\phi}\Sigma\beta + \mathbb{E}_{\boldsymbol{\phi}}[\mathbb{E}_{\varepsilon}[Y'\mathbf{X}\phi_d^{\mathbf{X}}\mathbf{X}'Y]].
$$

Going through these terms we get:

$$
\begin{aligned}
\beta'\Sigma\beta &= \sum_{i=1}^{p} \beta_i^2\lambda_i \\
\beta'\Sigma T_d^{\phi}\Sigma\beta &= \sum_{i=1}^{p} \beta_i^2 \frac{\lambda_i^2}{\eta_i} \\
\mathbb{E}_{\boldsymbol{\phi}}[\mathbb{E}_{\varepsilon}[Y'\mathbf{X}\phi_d^{\mathbf{X}}\mathbf{X}'Y]] &= \beta'\Sigma\mathbb{E}_{\boldsymbol{\phi}}[\phi_d^{\mathbf{X}}]\Sigma\beta + \mathbb{E}_{\boldsymbol{\phi}}[\mathbb{E}_{\varepsilon}[\varepsilon'\mathbf{X}\phi_d^{\mathbf{X}}\mathbf{X}'\varepsilon]].
\end{aligned}
$$

The first term in the last line equals $\sum_{i=1}^{p} \beta_i^2 \lambda_i^2/\eta_i$. The second can be calculated in two ways, both relying on the shuffling property of the trace operator:

$$\begin{aligned}
\mathbb{E}_{\phi}[\mathbb{E}_{\varepsilon}[\varepsilon' \mathbf{X} \phi_d^{\mathbf{X}} \mathbf{X}' \varepsilon]] &= \mathbb{E}_{\varepsilon}[\varepsilon' \mathbf{X} T_d^{\mathbf{X}} \mathbf{X}' \varepsilon]] = \sigma^2 \operatorname{trace}(\mathbf{X} T_d^{\mathbf{X}} \mathbf{X}') \\
&= \sigma^2 \operatorname{trace}(\Sigma T_d^{\mathbf{X}}) = \sum_{i=1}^{p} \frac{\lambda_i}{\eta_i}. \\
\mathbb{E}_{\phi}[\mathbb{E}_{\varepsilon}[\varepsilon' \mathbf{X} \phi_d^{\mathbf{X}} \mathbf{X}' \varepsilon]] &= \sigma^2 \mathbb{E}_{\phi}[\operatorname{trace}(\mathbf{X} \phi_d^{\mathbf{X}} \mathbf{X}')] = \sigma^2 \mathbb{E}_{\phi}[\operatorname{trace}(\Sigma \phi_d^{\mathbf{X}})] \\
&= \sigma^2 \mathbb{E}_{\phi}[\operatorname{trace}(I_{d \times d})] = \sigma^2 d.
\end{aligned}$$

Adding the first version to the expectation from above we get the exact expected mean-squared error. Setting both versions equal we get the equation

$$d = \sum_{i=1}^{p} \frac{\lambda_i}{\eta_i} \quad .$$

□

Theorem 4 *Assume* Rank(**X**) $\geq d$*, then there exists a real number* $\tau \in [d^2/p, d]$ *such that the AMSE of* $\hat{\beta}_d$ *can be bounded from above by*

$$\mathbb{E}_{\phi}[\mathbb{E}_{\varepsilon}[\|\mathbf{X}\beta - \mathbf{X}\hat{\beta}_d\|_2^2]] \leq \sigma^2 \tau + \sum_{i=1}^{p} \beta_i^2 \lambda_i w_i^2,$$

where the w_i*'s are given as*

$$w_i = \frac{(1 + 1/d)\lambda_i^2 + (1 + 2/d)\lambda_i \operatorname{trace}(\Sigma) + \operatorname{trace}(\Sigma)^2/d}{(d + 2 + 1/d)\lambda_i^2 + 2(1 + 1/d)\lambda_i \operatorname{trace}(\Sigma) + \operatorname{trace}(\Sigma)^2/d}$$

and

$$\tau \in [d^2/p, d].$$

Proof First a simple calculation [10] using the closed form solution gives the following equation:

$$\mathbb{E}_{\phi}[\mathbb{E}_{\varepsilon}[\|\mathbf{X}\beta - \mathbf{X}\hat{\beta}_d\|_2^2]] = \sigma^2 \sum_{i=1}^{p} \Big(\frac{\lambda_i}{\eta_i}\Big)^2 + \sum_{i=1}^{p} \beta_i^2 \lambda_i \Big(1 - \frac{\lambda_i}{\eta_i}\Big)^2. \tag{27}$$

Now using the corollary from the last section we can bound the second term by the following way:

$$\left(1 - \frac{\lambda_i}{\eta_i}\right)^2 \leq w_i^2. \tag{28}$$

For the first term we write

$$\tau = \sum_{i=1}^{p} \left(\frac{\lambda_i}{\eta_i}\right)^2. \tag{29}$$

Now note that since $\lambda_i/\eta_i \leq 1$ we have

$$\left(\frac{\lambda_i}{\eta_i}\right)^2 \leq \frac{\lambda_i}{\eta_i} \tag{30}$$

and thus we get the upper bound by

$$\sum_{i=1}^{p} \left(\frac{\lambda_i}{\eta_i}\right)^2 \leq \sum_{i=1}^{p} \frac{\lambda_i}{\eta_i} = d. \tag{31}$$

For the lower bound of τ we consider an optimization problem. Denote $t_i = \frac{\lambda_i}{\eta_i}$, then we want to find $t \in \mathbb{R}^p$ such that

$$\sum_{i=1}^{p} t_i^2 \text{ is minimal}$$

under the restrictions that

$$\sum_{i=1}^{p} t_i = d \text{ and } 0 \leq t_i \leq 1.$$

The problem is symmetric in each coordinate and thus $t_i = c$. Plugging this into the linear sum gives $c = d/p$ and we calculate the quadratic term to give the result claimed in the theorem. □

References

1. Achlioptas, D.: Database-friendly random projections: Johnson-Lindenstrauss with binary coins. J. Comput. Syst. Sci. **66**(4), 671–687 (2003)
2. Ailon, N., Chazelle, B.: Approximate nearest neighbors and the fast Johnson-Lindenstrauss transform. In: Proceedings of the 38th Annual ACM Symposium on Theory of Computing (2006)

3. Blocki, J., Blum, A., Datta, A., and Sheffet, O.: The Johnson-Lindenstrauss transform itself preserves differential privacy. In: 2012 IEEE 53rd Annual Symposium on Foundations of Computer Science (FOCS), pp. 410–419. IEEE, Washington, DC (2012)
4. Cook, R.D.: Detection of influential observation in linear regression. Technometrics **19**, 15–18 (1977)
5. Dasgupta, S., Gupta, A.: An elementary proof of a theorem of Johnson and Lindenstrauss. Random Struct. Algoritm. **22**, 60–65 (2003)
6. Dhillon, P.S., Foster, D.P., Kakade, S.: A risk comparison of ordinary least squares vs ridge regression. J. Mach. Learn. Res. **14**, 1505–1511 (2013)
7. Dhillon, P., Lu, Y., Foster, D.P., Ungar, L.: New subsampling algorithms for fast least squares regression. In: Burges, C.J.C., Bottou, L., Welling, M., Ghahramani, Z., Weinberger, K.Q. (eds.) Advances in Neural Information Processing Systems, vol. 26, pp. 360–368. Curran Associates, Inc. (2013). http://papers.nips.cc/paper/5105-new-subsampling-algorithms-for-fast-least-squares-regression.pdf
8. Indyk, P. and Motwani, R.: Approximate nearest neighbors: towards removing the curse of dimensionality. In: Proceedings of the 30th Annual ACM Symposium on Theory of Computing (1998)
9. Johnson, W., Lindenstrauss, J.: Extensions of Lipschitz mappings into a Hilbert space. In: Contemporary Mathematics: Conference on Modern Analysis and Probability (1984)
10. Kabán, A.: A new look at compressed ordinary least squares. In: 2013 IEEE 13th International Conference on Data Mining Workshops, pp. 482–488 (2013). doi:10.1109/ICDMW.2013.152, ISSN:2375-9232
11. Lu, Y., Dhillon, P.S., Foster, D., Ungar, L.: Faster ridge regression via the subsampled randomized hadamard transform. In: Proceedings of the 26th International Conference on Neural Information Processing Systems, pp. 369-377. Curran Associates Inc., Lake Tahoe (2013). http://dl.acm.org/citation.cfm?id=2999611.2999653
12. Mahoney, M.W., Drineas, P.: CUR matrix decompositions for improved data analysis. Proc. Natl. Acad. Sci. **106**(3), 697–702 (2009)
13. Maillard, O.-A., Munos, R.: Compressed least-squares regression. In: Bengio, Y., Schuurmans, D., Lafferty, J.D., Williams, C.K.I., Culotta, A. (eds.) Advances in Neural Information Processing Systems, vol. 22, pp. 1213–1221. Curran Associates, Inc. (2009). http://papers.nips.cc/paper/3698-compressed-least-squares-regression.pdf
14. Marzetta, T., Tucci, G., Simon, S.: A random matrix-theoretic approach to handling singular covariance estimates. IEEE Trans. Inf. Theory **57**(9), 6256–6271 (2011)
15. McWilliams, B., Krummenacher, G., Lučić, M., and Buhmann, J.M.: Fast and robust least squares estimation in corrupted linear models. In: NIPS (2014)
16. McWilliams, B., Heinze, C., Meinshausen, N., Krummenacher, G., Vanchinathan, H.P.: Loco: distributing ridge regression with random projections. arXiv preprint arXiv:1406.3469 (2014)
17. Tropp, J.A.: Improved analysis of the subsampled randomized Hadamard transform. arXiv:1011.1595v4 [math.NA] (2010)
18. Zhang, L., Mahdavi, M., Jin, R., Yang, T., Zhu, S.: Recovering optimal solution by dual random projection. arXiv preprint arXiv:1211.3046 (2012)
19. Zhou, S., Lafferty, J., Wasserman, L.: Compressed and privacy-sensitive sparse regression. IEEE Trans. Inf. Theory. **55**(2), 846-866 (2009). doi:10.1109/TIT.2008.2009605. ISSN:0018-9448

Testing in the Presence of Nuisance Parameters: Some Comments on Tests Post-Model-Selection and Random Critical Values

Hannes Leeb and Benedikt M. Pötscher

Abstract We point out that the ideas underlying some test procedures recently proposed for testing post-model-selection (and for some other test problems) in the econometrics literature have been around for quite some time in the statistics literature. We also sharpen some of these results in the statistics literature. Furthermore, we show that some intuitively appealing testing procedures, that have found their way into the econometrics literature, lead to tests that do not have desirable size properties, not even asymptotically.

1 Introduction

Suppose we have a sequence of statistical experiments given by a family of probability measures $\{P_{n,\alpha,\beta} : \alpha \in A, \beta \in B\}$ where α is a "parameter of interest", and β is a "nuisance-parameter". Often, but not always, A and B will be subsets of the Euclidean space. Suppose the researcher wants to test the null hypothesis $H_0 : \alpha = \alpha_0$ using the real-valued test-statistic $T_n(\alpha_0)$, with large values of $T_n(\alpha_0)$ being taken as indicative for violation of H_0.[1] Suppose further that the distribution of $T_n(\alpha_0)$ under H_0 depends on the nuisance parameter β. This leads to the key question: How should the critical value then be chosen? [Of course, if another, pivotal, test-statistic is available, this one could be used. However, we consider here the case where a (non-trivial) pivotal test-statistic either does not exist or where the researcher—for better or worse—insists on using $T_n(\alpha_0)$.] In this situation a standard way (see, e.g., [3, p.170]) to deal with this problem is to choose as critical

[1]This framework obviously allows for "one-sided" as well as for "two-sided" alternatives (when these concepts make sense) by a proper definition of the test-statistic.

H. Leeb (✉) • B.M. Pötscher
Department of Statistics, University of Vienna, Vienna, Austria
e-mail: hannes.leeb@univie.ac.at

© Springer International Publishing AG 2017

S.E. Ahmed (ed.), *Big and Complex Data Analysis*, Contributions to Statistics,
DOI 10.1007/978-3-319-41573-4_4

value

$$c_{n,\sup}(\delta) = \sup_{\beta \in B} c_{n,\beta}(\delta), \tag{1}$$

where $0 < \delta < 1$ and where $c_{n,\beta}(\delta)$ satisfies $P_{n,\alpha_0,\beta}\left(T_n(\alpha_0) > c_{n,\beta}(\delta)\right) = \delta$ for each $\beta \in B$, i.e., $c_{n,\beta}(\delta)$ is *a* $(1-\delta)$-quantile of the distribution of $T_n(\alpha_0)$ under $P_{n,\alpha_0,\beta}$. [We assume here the existence of such a $c_{n,\beta}(\delta)$, but we do not insist that it is chosen as the smallest possible number satisfying the above condition, although this will usually be the case.] In other words, $c_{n,\sup}(\delta)$ is the "worst-case" critical value. While the resulting test, which rejects H_0 for

$$T_n(\alpha_0) > c_{n,\sup}(\delta), \tag{2}$$

certainly is a level δ test (i.e., has size $\leq \delta$), the conservatism caused by taking the supremum in (1) will often result in poor power properties, especially for values of β for which $c_{n,\beta}(\delta)$ is much smaller than $c_{n,\sup}(\delta)$. The test obtained from (1) and (2) above (more precisely, an asymptotic variant thereof) is what Andrews and Guggenberger [1] call a "size-corrected fixed critical value" test.[2]

An alternative idea, which has some intuitive appeal and which is much less conservative, is to use $c_{n,\hat{\beta}_n}(\delta)$ as a random critical value, where $\hat{\beta}_n$ is an estimator for β (taking its values in B), and to reject H_0 if

$$T_n(\alpha_0) > c_{n,\hat{\beta}_n}(\delta) \tag{3}$$

obtains (measurability of $c_{n,\hat{\beta}_n}(\delta)$ being assumed). This choice of critical value can be viewed as a parametric bootstrap procedure. Versions of $c_{n,\hat{\beta}_n}(\delta)$ have been considered by Williams [14] or, more recently, by Liu [9]. However,

$$P_{n,\alpha_0,\beta}\left(T_n(\alpha_0) > c_{n,\hat{\beta}_n}(\delta)\right) \geq P_{n,\alpha_0,\beta}\left(T_n(\alpha_0) > c_{n,\sup}(\delta)\right)$$

clearly holds for every β, indicating that the test using the random critical value $c_{n,\hat{\beta}_n}(\delta)$ may *not* be a level δ test, but may have size larger than δ. This was already noted by Loh [8]. A precise result in this direction, which is a variation of Theorem 2.1 in [8], is as follows:

Proposition 1 *Suppose that there exists a* $\beta_n^{\max} = \beta_n^{\max}(\delta)$ *such that* $c_{n,\beta_n^{\max}}(\delta) = c_{n,\sup}(\delta)$. *Then*

$$P_{n,\alpha_0,\beta_n^{\max}}\left(c_{n,\hat{\beta}_n}(\delta) < T_n(\alpha_0) \leq c_{n,\sup}(\delta)\right) > 0 \tag{4}$$

[2] While Andrews and Guggenberger [1] do not consider a finite-sample framework but rather a "moving-parameter" asymptotic framework, the underlying idea is nevertheless exactly the same.

implies

$$\sup_{\beta\in B} P_{n,\alpha_0,\beta}\left(T_n(\alpha_0) > c_{n,\hat{\beta}_n}(\delta)\right) > \delta, \tag{5}$$

i.e., the test using the random critical value $c_{n,\hat{\beta}_n}(\delta)$ *does not have level* δ. *More generally, if* $\hat{c}_n$ *is any random critical value satisfying* $\hat{c}_n \leq c_{n,\beta_n^{\max}}(\delta)(= c_{n,\sup}(\delta))$ *with* $P_{n,\alpha_0,\beta_n^{\max}}$*-probability* 1, *then (4) still implies (5) if in both expressions* $c_{n,\hat{\beta}_n}(\delta)$ *is replaced by* $\hat{c}_n$. *[The result continues to hold if the random critical value* $\hat{c}_n$ *also depends on some additional randomization mechanism.]*

Proof Observe that $c_{n,\hat{\beta}_n}(\delta) \leq c_{n,\sup}(\delta)$ always holds. But then the l.h.s. of (5) is bounded from below by

$$\begin{aligned}
&P_{n,\alpha_0,\beta_n^{\max}}\left(T_n(\alpha_0) > c_{n,\hat{\beta}_n}(\delta)\right) \\
&= P_{n,\alpha_0,\beta_n^{\max}}\left(T_n(\alpha_0) > c_{n,\sup}(\delta)\right) + P_{n,\alpha_0,\beta_n^{\max}}\left(c_{n,\hat{\beta}_n}(\delta) < T_n(\alpha_0) \leq c_{n,\sup}(\delta)\right) \\
&= P_{n,\alpha_0,\beta_n^{\max}}\left(T_n(\alpha_0) > c_{n,\beta_n^{\max}}(\delta)\right) + P_{n,\alpha_0,\beta_n^{\max}}\left(c_{n,\hat{\beta}_n}(\delta) < T_n(\alpha_0) \leq c_{n,\sup}(\delta)\right) \\
&= \delta + P_{n,\alpha_0,\beta_n^{\max}}\left(c_{n,\hat{\beta}_n}(\delta) < T_n(\alpha_0) \leq c_{n,\sup}(\delta)\right) > \delta,
\end{aligned}$$

the last inequality holding in view of (4). The proof for the second claim is completely analogous. ∎

To better appreciate condition (4) consider the case where $c_{n,\beta}(\delta)$ is uniquely maximized at $\beta_n^{\max}$ and $P_{n,\alpha_0,\beta_n^{\max}}(\hat{\beta}_n \neq \beta_n^{\max})$ is positive. Then

$$P_{n,\alpha_0,\beta_n^{\max}}(c_{n,\hat{\beta}_n}(\delta) < c_{n,\sup}(\delta)) > 0$$

holds and therefore we can expect condition (4) to be satisfied, unless there exists a quite strange dependence structure between $\hat{\beta}_n$ and $T_n(\alpha_0)$. The same argument applies in the more general situation where there are multiple maximizers $\beta_n^{\max}$ of $c_{n,\beta}(\delta)$ as soon as $P_{n,\alpha_0,\beta_n^{\max}}(\hat{\beta}_n \notin \arg\max c_{n,\beta}(\delta)) > 0$ holds for one of the maximizers $\beta_n^{\max}$.

In the same vein, it is also useful to note that Condition (4) can equivalently be stated as follows: The conditional cumulative distribution function $P_{n,\alpha_0,\beta_n^{\max}}(T_n(\alpha_0) \leq \cdot \mid \hat{\beta}_n)$ of $T_n(\alpha_0)$ given $\hat{\beta}_n$ puts positive mass on the interval $(c_{n,\hat{\beta}_n}(\delta), c_{n,\sup}(\delta)]$ for a set of $\hat{\beta}_n$'s that has positive probability under $P_{n,\alpha_0,\beta_n^{\max}}$. [Also note that Condition (4) implies that $c_{n,\hat{\beta}_n}(\delta) < c_{n,\sup}(\delta)$ must hold with positive $P_{n,\alpha_0,\beta_n^{\max}}$-probability.] A sufficient condition for this then clearly is that for a set of $\hat{\beta}_n$'s of positive $P_{n,\alpha_0,\beta_n^{\max}}$-probability we have that (i) $c_{n,\hat{\beta}_n}(\delta) < c_{n,\sup}(\delta)$, and (ii) the conditional cumulative distribution function $P_{n,\alpha_0,\beta_n^{\max}}(T_n(\alpha_0) \leq \cdot \mid \hat{\beta}_n)$ puts positive mass on *every* non-empty interval. The analogous result holds for the case where $\hat{c}_n$ replaces $c_{n,\hat{\beta}_n}(\delta)$ (and conditioning is w.r.t. $\hat{c}_n$), see Lemma 5 in the Appendix for a formal statement.

The observation that the test (3) based on the random critical value $c_{n,\hat{\beta}_n}(\delta)$ typically will not be a level δ test has led Loh [8] and subsequently Berger and Boos [2] and Silvapulle [13] to consider the following procedure (or variants thereof) which leads to a level δ test that is somewhat less "conservative" than the test given by (2)[3]: Let I_n be a random set in B satisfying

$$\inf_{\beta \in B} P_{n,\alpha_0,\beta}\left(\beta \in I_n\right) \geq 1 - \eta_n,$$

where $0 \leq \eta_n < \delta$. That is, I_n is a confidence set for the nuisance parameter β with infimal coverage probability not less than $1 - \eta_n$ (provided $\alpha = \alpha_0$). Define a random critical value via

$$c_{n,\eta_n,\mathrm{Loh}}(\delta) = \sup_{\beta \in I_n} c_{n,\beta}(\delta - \eta_n). \tag{6}$$

Then we have

$$\sup_{\beta \in B} P_{n,\alpha_0,\beta}\left(T_n(\alpha_0) > c_{n,\eta_n,\mathrm{Loh}}(\delta)\right) \leq \delta.$$

This can be seen as follows: For every $\beta \in B$

$$\begin{aligned} P_{n,\alpha_0,\beta}\left(T_n(\alpha_0) > c_{n,\eta_n,\mathrm{Loh}}(\delta)\right) &= P_{n,\alpha_0,\beta}\left(T_n(\alpha_0) > c_{n,\eta_n,\mathrm{Loh}}(\delta), \beta \in I_n\right) \\ &\quad + P_{n,\alpha_0,\beta}\left(T_n(\alpha_0) > c_{n,\eta_n,\mathrm{Loh}}(\delta), \beta \notin I_n\right) \\ &\leq P_{n,\alpha_0,\beta}\left(T_n(\alpha_0) > c_{n,\beta}(\delta - \eta_n), \beta \in I_n\right) + \eta_n \\ &\leq P_{n,\alpha_0,\beta}\left(T_n(\alpha_0) > c_{n,\beta}(\delta - \eta_n)\right) + \eta_n \\ &= \delta - \eta_n + \eta_n = \delta. \end{aligned}$$

Hence, the random critical value $c_{n,\eta_n,\mathrm{Loh}}(\delta)$ results in a test that is guaranteed to be level δ. In fact, its size can also be lower bounded by $\delta - \eta_n$ provided there exists a $\beta_n^{\max}(\delta - \eta_n)$ satisfying $c_{n,\beta_n^{\max}(\delta-\eta_n)}(\delta - \eta_n) = \sup_{\beta \in B} c_{n,\beta}(\delta - \eta_n)$: This follows since

$$\begin{aligned} &\sup_{\beta \in B} P_{n,\alpha_0,\beta}\left(T_n(\alpha_0) > c_{n,\eta_n,\mathrm{Loh}}(\delta)\right) \\ &\quad \geq \sup_{\beta \in B} P_{n,\alpha_0,\beta}\left(T_n(\alpha_0) > \sup_{\beta \in B} c_{n,\beta}(\delta - \eta_n)\right) \end{aligned}$$

[3] Loh [8] actually considers the random critical value $c_{n,\eta_n,\mathrm{Loh}^*}(\delta)$ given by $\sup_{\beta \in I_n} c_{n,\beta}(\delta)$, which typically does not lead to a level δ test in finite samples in view of Proposition 1 (since $c_{n,\eta_n,\mathrm{Loh}^*}(\delta) \leq c_{n,\sup}(\delta)$). However, Loh [8] focuses on the case where $\eta_n \to 0$ and shows that then the size of the test converges to δ; that is, the test is asymptotically level δ if $\eta_n \to 0$. See also Remark 4.

$$= \sup_{\beta \in B} P_{n,\alpha_0,\beta} \left(T_n(\alpha_0) > c_{n,\beta_n^{\max}(\delta-\eta_n)}(\delta - \eta_n) \right)$$

$$\geq P_{n,\alpha_0,\beta_n^{\max}(\delta-\eta_n)} \left(T_n(\alpha_0) > c_{n,\beta_n^{\max}(\delta-\eta_n)}(\delta - \eta_n) \right)$$

$$= \delta - \eta_n. \tag{7}$$

The critical value (6) (or asymptotic variants thereof) has also been used in econometrics, e.g., by DiTraglia [4], McCloskey [10, 11], and Romano et al. [12].

The test based on the random critical value $c_{n,\eta_n,\mathrm{Loh}}(\delta)$ may have size strictly smaller than δ. This suggests that this test will not improve over the conservative test based on $c_{n,\sup}(\delta)$ for *all* values of β: We can expect that the test based on (6) will sacrifice some power when compared with the conservative test (2) when the true β is close to $\beta_n^{\max}(\delta)$ or $\beta_n^{\max}(\delta - \eta_n)$; however, we can often expect a power gain for values of β that are "far away" from $\beta_n^{\max}(\delta)$ and $\beta_n^{\max}(\delta - \eta_n)$, as we then typically will have that $c_{n,\eta_n,\mathrm{Loh}}(\delta)$ is smaller than $c_{n,\sup}(\delta)$. Hence, each of the two tests will typically have a power advantage over the other in certain parts of the parameter space B.

It is thus tempting to try to construct a test that has the power advantages of both these tests by choosing as a critical value the smaller one of the two critical values, i.e., by choosing

$$\hat{c}_{n,\eta_n,\min}(\delta) = \min \left(c_{n,\sup}(\delta), c_{n,\eta_n,\mathrm{Loh}}(\delta) \right) \tag{8}$$

as the critical value. While both critical values $c_{n,\sup}(\delta)$ and $c_{n,\eta_n,\mathrm{Loh}}(\delta)$ lead to level δ tests, this is, however, unfortunately not the case in general for the test based on the random critical value (8). To see why, note that by construction the critical value (8) satisfies

$$\hat{c}_{n,\eta_n,\min}(\delta) \leq c_{n,\sup}(\delta),$$

and hence can be expected to fall under the wrath of Proposition 1 given above. Thus it can be expected to not deliver a test that has level δ, but has a size that exceeds δ. So while the test based on the random critical value proposed in (8) will typically reject more often than the tests based on (2) or on (6), it does so by violating the size constraint. Hence it suffers from the same problems as the parametric bootstrap test (3). [We make the trivial observation that the lower bound (7) also holds if $\hat{c}_{n,\eta_n,\min}(\delta)$ instead of $c_{n,\eta_n,\mathrm{Loh}}(\delta)$ is used, since $\hat{c}_{n,\eta_n,\min}(\delta) \leq c_{n,\eta_n,\mathrm{Loh}}(\delta)$ holds.] As a point of interest we note that the construction (8) has actually been suggested in the literature, see McCloskey [10].[4] In fact, McCloskey [10] suggested a random critical value $\hat{c}_{n,\mathrm{McC}}(\delta)$ which is the minimum of critical values of the form (8) with η_n running through a finite set of values; it is thus less than or equal to the individual $\hat{c}_{n,\eta_n,\min}$'s, which exacerbates the size distortion problem even further.

[4]This construction is no longer suggested in [11].

While Proposition 1 shows that tests based on random critical values like $c_{n,\hat{\beta}_n}(\delta)$ or $\hat{c}_{n,\eta_n,\min}(\delta)$ will typically not have level δ, it leaves open the possibility that the overshoot of the size over δ may converge to zero as sample size goes to infinity, implying that the test would then be at least *asymptotically* of level δ. In sufficiently "regular" testing problems this will indeed be the case. However, for many testing problems where nuisance parameters are present such as testing post-model- selection, it turns out that this is typically *not* the case: In the next section we illustrate this by providing a prototypical example where the overshoot does *not* converge to zero for the tests based on $c_{n,\hat{\beta}_n}(\delta)$ or $\hat{c}_{n,\eta_n,\min}(\delta)$, and hence these tests are not level δ *even asymptotically*.

2 An Illustrative Example

In the following we shall—for the sake of exposition—use a very simple example to illustrate the issues involved. Consider the linear regression model

$$y_t = \alpha x_{t1} + \beta x_{t2} + \epsilon_t \qquad (1 \le t \le n) \tag{9}$$

under the "textbook" assumptions that the errors ϵ_t are i.i.d. $N(0, \sigma^2)$, $\sigma^2 > 0$, and the nonstochastic $n\times 2$ regressor matrix X has full rank (implying $n > 1$) and satisfies $X'X/n \to Q > 0$ as $n \to \infty$. The variables y_t, x_{ti}, as well as the errors ϵ_t can be allowed to depend on sample size n (in fact may be defined on a sample space that itself depends on n), but we do not show this in the notation. For simplicity, we shall also assume that the error variance σ^2 is known and equals 1. It will be convenient to write the matrix $(X'X/n)^{-1}$ as

$$(X'X/n)^{-1} = \begin{pmatrix} \sigma^2_{\alpha,n} & \sigma_{\alpha,\beta,n} \\ \sigma_{\alpha,\beta,n} & \sigma^2_{\beta,n} \end{pmatrix}.$$

The elements of the limit of this matrix will be denoted by $\sigma^2_{\alpha,\infty}$, etc. It will prove useful to define $\rho_n = \sigma_{\alpha,\beta,n}/(\sigma_{\alpha,n}\sigma_{\beta,n})$, i.e., ρ_n is the correlation coefficient between the least-squares estimators for α and β in model (9). Its limit will be denoted by ρ_∞. Note that $|\rho_\infty| < 1$ holds, since $Q > 0$ has been assumed.

As in [7] we shall consider two candidate models from which we select on the basis of the data: The unrestricted model denoted by U which uses both regressors x_{t1} and x_{t2}, and the restricted model denoted by R which uses only the regressor x_{t1} (and thus corresponds to imposing the restriction $\beta = 0$). The least-squares estimators for α and β in the unrestricted model will be denoted by $\hat{\alpha}_n(U)$ and $\hat{\beta}_n(U)$, respectively. The least-squares estimator for α in the restricted model will be denoted by $\hat{\alpha}_n(R)$, and we shall set $\hat{\beta}_n(R) = 0$. We shall decide between the competing models U and R depending on whether $|\sqrt{n}\hat{\beta}(U_n)/\sigma_{\beta,n}| > c$ or not, where $c > 0$ is a user-specified cut-off point independent of sample size (in line with the fact that we consider conservative model selection). That is, we select the model $\hat{M}_n$ according to

$$\hat{M}_n = \begin{cases} U \text{ if } |\sqrt{n}\hat{\beta}_n(U)/\sigma_{\beta,n}| > c, \\ R \qquad \text{otherwise.} \end{cases}$$

We now want to test the hypothesis $H_0 : \alpha = \alpha_0$ versus $H_1 : \alpha > \alpha_0$ and we insist, for better or worse, on using the test-statistic

$$T_n(\alpha_0) = \left[n^{1/2}\left(\hat{\alpha}(R) - \alpha_0\right) / \left(\sigma_{\alpha,n}\left(1 - \rho_n^2\right)^{1/2}\right)\right] \mathbf{1}(\hat{M}_n = R)$$
$$+ \left[n^{1/2}\left(\hat{\alpha}(U) - \alpha_0\right) / \sigma_{\alpha,n}\right] \mathbf{1}(\hat{M}_n = U).$$

That is, depending on which of the two models has been selected, we insist on using the corresponding textbook test-statistic (for the known-variance case). While this could perhaps be criticized as somewhat simple-minded, it describes how such a test may be conducted in practice when model selection precedes the inference step. It is well known that if one uses this test-statistic and naively compares it to the usual normal-based quantiles acting as if the selected model were given a priori, this results in a test with severe size distortions, see, e.g., [5] and the references therein. Hence, while sticking with $T_n(\alpha_0)$ as the test-statistic, we now look for appropriate critical values in the spirit of the preceding section and discuss some of the proposals from the literature. Note that the situation just described fits into the framework of the preceding section with β as the nuisance parameter and $B = \mathbb{R}$.

Calculations similar to the ones in [7] show that the finite-sample distribution of $T_n(\alpha_0)$ under H_0 has a density that is given by

$$h_{n,\beta}(u) = \Delta\left(n^{1/2}\beta/\sigma_{\beta,n}, c\right) \phi\left(u + \rho_n\left(1 - \rho_n^2\right)^{-1/2} n^{1/2}\beta/\sigma_{\beta,n}\right)$$
$$+ \left(1 - \Delta\left(\left(1 - \rho_n^2\right)^{-1/2}\left(n^{1/2}\beta/\sigma_{\beta,n} + \rho_n u\right), \left(1 - \rho_n^2\right)^{-1/2} c\right)\right) \phi\left(u\right),$$

where $\Delta(a, b) = \Phi(a + b) - \Phi(a - b)$ and where ϕ and Φ denote the density and cdf, respectively, of a standard normal variate. Let $H_{n,\beta}$ denote the cumulative distribution function (cdf) corresponding to $h_{n,\beta}$.

Now, for given significance level δ, $0 < \delta < 1$, let $c_{n,\beta}(\delta) = H_{n,\beta}^{-1}(1-\delta)$ as in the preceding section. Note that the inverse function exists, since $H_{n,\beta}$ is continuous and is strictly increasing as its density $h_{n,\beta}$ is positive everywhere. As in the preceding section let

$$c_{n,\sup}(\delta) = \sup_{\beta \in \mathbb{R}} c_{n,\beta}(\delta) \tag{10}$$

denote the conservative critical value (the supremum is actually a maximum in the interesting case $\delta \leq 1/2$ in view of Lemmata 6 and 7 in the Appendix).

Let $c_{n,\hat{\beta}_n(U)}(\delta)$ be the parametric bootstrap-based random critical value. With η satisfying $0 < \eta < \delta$, we also consider the random critical value

$$c_{n,\eta,\mathrm{Loh}}(\delta) = \sup_{\beta \in I_n} c_{n,\beta}(\delta - \eta) \tag{11}$$

where

$$I_n = \left[\hat{\beta}_n(U) \pm n^{-1/2}\sigma_{\beta,n}\Phi^{-1}(1 - (\eta/2))\right]$$

is an $1 - \eta$ confidence interval for β. [Again the supremum is actually a maximum.] We choose here η *independent* of n as in [4, 10, 11] and comment on sample size dependent η below. Furthermore define

$$\hat{c}_{n,\eta,\min}(\delta) = \min\left(c_{n,\sup}(\delta), c_{n,\eta,\mathrm{Loh}}(\delta)\right). \tag{12}$$

Recall from the discussion in Sect. 1 that these critical values have been used in the literature in the contexts of testing post-model-selection, post-moment-selection, or post-model-averaging. Among the critical values $c_{n,\sup}(\delta)$, $c_{n,\hat{\beta}_n(U)}(\delta)$, $c_{n,\eta,\mathrm{Loh}}(\delta)$, and $\hat{c}_{n,\eta,\min}(\delta)$, we already know that $c_{n,\sup}(\delta)$ and $c_{n,\eta,\mathrm{Loh}}(\delta)$ lead to tests that are valid level δ tests. We next confirm—as suggested by the discussion in the preceding section—that the random critical values $c_{n,\hat{\beta}_n(U)}(\delta)$ and $\hat{c}_{n,\eta,\min}(\delta)$ (at least for some choices of η) do *not* lead to tests that have level δ (i.e., their size is strictly larger than δ). Moreover, we also show that the sizes of the tests based on $c_{n,\hat{\beta}_n(U)}(\delta)$ or $\hat{c}_{n,\eta,\min}(\delta)$ do *not* converge to δ as $n \to \infty$, implying that the asymptotic sizes of these tests exceed δ. These results a fortiori also apply to any random critical value that does not exceed $c_{n,\hat{\beta}_n(U)}(\delta)$ or $\hat{c}_{n,\eta,\min}(\delta)$ (such as $\hat{c}_{n,\mathrm{McC}}(\delta)$ in [10] or $c_{n,\eta,\mathrm{Loh}^*}(\delta)$). In the subsequent theorem we consider for simplicity only the case $\rho_n \equiv \rho$, but the result extends to the more general case where ρ_n may depend on n.

Theorem 2 *Suppose $\rho_n \equiv \rho \neq 0$ and let $0 < \delta \leq 1/2$ be arbitrary. Then*

$$\inf_{n>1} \sup_{\beta \in \mathbb{R}} P_{n,\alpha_0,\beta}\left(T_n(\alpha_0) > c_{n,\hat{\beta}_n(U)}(\delta)\right) > \delta. \tag{13}$$

Furthermore, for each fixed η, $0 < \eta < \delta$, that is sufficiently small we have

$$\inf_{n>1} \sup_{\beta \in \mathbb{R}} P_{n,\alpha_0,\beta}\left(T_n(\alpha_0) > \hat{c}_{n,\eta,\min}(\delta)\right) > \delta. \tag{14}$$

Proof We first prove (14). Introduce the abbreviation $\gamma = n^{1/2}\beta/\sigma_{\beta,n}$ and define $\hat{\gamma}(U) = n^{1/2}\hat{\beta}(U)/\sigma_{\beta,n}$. Observe that the density $h_{n,\beta}$ (and hence the cdf $H_{n,\beta}$) depends on the nuisance parameter β only via γ, and otherwise is independent of sample size n (since $\rho_n = \rho$ is assumed). Let $\bar{h}_\gamma$ be the density of $T_n(\alpha_0)$ when expressed in the reparameterization γ. As a consequence, the quantiles satisfy

$c_{n,\beta}(v) = \bar{c}_{\gamma}(v)$ for every $0 < v < 1$, where $\bar{c}_{\gamma}(v) = \bar{H}_{\gamma}^{-1}(1-v)$ and $\bar{H}_{\gamma}$ denotes the cdf corresponding to $\bar{h}_{\gamma}$. Furthermore, for $0 < \eta < \delta$, observe that $c_{n,\eta,\mathrm{Loh}}(\delta) = \sup_{\beta \in I_n} c_{n,\beta}(\delta - \eta)$ can be rewritten as

$$c_{n,\eta,\mathrm{Loh}}(\delta) = \sup_{\gamma \in \left[\hat{\gamma}(U) \pm \Phi^{-1}(1-(\eta/2))\right]} \bar{c}_{\gamma}(\delta - \eta).$$

Now define $\gamma^{\max} = \gamma^{\max}(\delta)$ as a value of γ such that $\bar{c}_{\gamma^{\max}}(\delta) = \bar{c}_{\sup}(\delta) := \sup_{\gamma \in \mathbb{R}} \bar{c}_{\gamma}(\delta)$. That such a maximizer exists follows from Lemmata 6 and 7 in the Appendix. Note that $\gamma^{\max}$ does not depend on n. Of course, $\gamma^{\max}$ is related to $\beta_n^{\max} = \beta_n^{\max}(\delta)$ via $\gamma^{\max} = n^{1/2}\beta_n^{\max}/\sigma_{\beta,n}$. Since $\bar{c}_{\sup}(\delta) = \bar{c}_{\gamma^{\max}}(\delta)$ is strictly larger than

$$\lim_{|\gamma| \to \infty} \bar{c}_{\gamma}(\delta) = \Phi^{-1}(1-\delta)$$

in view of Lemmata 6 and 7 in the Appendix, we have for all sufficiently small η, $0 < \eta < \delta$, that

$$\lim_{|\gamma| \to \infty} \bar{c}_{\gamma}(\delta - \eta) = \Phi^{-1}(1-(\delta-\eta)) < \bar{c}_{\sup}(\delta) = \bar{c}_{\gamma^{\max}}(\delta). \tag{15}$$

Fix such an η. Let now $\varepsilon > 0$ satisfy $\varepsilon < \bar{c}_{\sup}(\delta) - \Phi^{-1}(1-(\delta-\eta))$. Because of the limit relation in the preceding display, we see that there exists $M = M(\varepsilon) > 0$ such that for $|\gamma| > M$ we have $\bar{c}_{\gamma}(\delta - \eta) < \bar{c}_{\sup}(\delta) - \varepsilon$. Define the set

$$A = \left\{x \in \mathbb{R} : |x| > \Phi^{-1}(1-(\eta/2)) + M\right\}.$$

Then on the event $\{\hat{\gamma}(U) \in A\}$ we have that $\hat{c}_{n,\eta,\min}(\delta) \le \bar{c}_{\sup}(\delta) - \varepsilon$. Furthermore, noting that $P_{n,\alpha_0,\beta_n^{\max}}\left(T_n(\alpha_0) > c_{n,\sup}(\delta)\right) = P_{n,\alpha_0,\beta_n^{\max}}\left(T_n(\alpha_0) > \bar{c}_{\sup}(\delta)\right) = \delta$, we have

$$\begin{aligned}
&\sup_{\beta \in \mathbb{R}} P_{n,\alpha_0,\beta}\left(T_n(\alpha_0) > \hat{c}_{n,\eta,\min}(\delta)\right) \ge P_{n,\alpha_0,\beta_n^{\max}}\left(T_n(\alpha_0) > \hat{c}_{n,\eta,\min}(\delta)\right) \\
&\quad = P_{n,\alpha_0,\beta_n^{\max}}\left(T_n(\alpha_0) > \bar{c}_{\sup}(\delta)\right) + P_{n,\alpha_0,\beta_n^{\max}}\left(\hat{c}_{n,\eta,\min}(\delta) < T_n(\alpha_0) \le \bar{c}_{\sup}(\delta)\right) \\
&\quad \ge \delta + P_{n,\alpha_0,\beta_n^{\max}}\left(\hat{c}_{n,\eta,\min}(\delta) < T_n(\alpha_0) \le \bar{c}_{\sup}(\delta), \hat{\gamma}(U) \in A\right) \\
&\quad \ge \delta + P_{n,\alpha_0,\beta_n^{\max}}\left(\bar{c}_{\sup}(\delta) - \varepsilon < T_n(\alpha_0) \le \bar{c}_{\sup}(\delta), \hat{\gamma}(U) \in A\right).
\end{aligned}$$

We are hence done if we can show that the probability in the last line is positive and independent of n. But this probability can be written as follows:[5]

$$
\begin{aligned}
&P_{n,\alpha_0,\beta_n^{\max}}\left(\bar{c}_{\sup}(\delta)-\varepsilon<T_n(\alpha_0)\leq\bar{c}_{\sup}(\delta),\hat{\gamma}(U)\in A\right)\\
&\quad=P_{n,\alpha_0,\beta_n^{\max}}\left(\bar{c}_{\sup}(\delta)-\varepsilon<T_n(\alpha_0)\leq\bar{c}_{\sup}(\delta),\hat{\gamma}(U)\in A,|\hat{\gamma}(U)|\leq c\right)\\
&\qquad+P_{n,\alpha_0,\beta_n^{\max}}\left(\bar{c}_{\sup}(\delta)-\varepsilon<T_n(\alpha_0)\leq\bar{c}_{\sup}(\delta),\hat{\gamma}(U)\in A,|\hat{\gamma}(U)|>c\right)\\
&\quad=P_{n,\alpha_0,\beta_n^{\max}}\left(\bar{c}_{\sup}(\delta)\geq n^{1/2}\left(\hat{\alpha}(R)-\alpha_0\right)/\left(\sigma_{\alpha,n}\left(1-\rho^2\right)^{1/2}\right)\right.\\
&\quad\left.>\bar{c}_{\sup}(\delta)-\varepsilon,\hat{\gamma}(U)\in A,|\hat{\gamma}(U)|\leq c\right)\\
&\qquad+P_{n,\alpha_0,\beta_n^{\max}}\left(\bar{c}_{\sup}(\delta)\geq n^{1/2}\left(\hat{\alpha}(U)-\alpha_0\right)/\sigma_{\alpha,n}\right.\\
&\quad\left.>\bar{c}_{\sup}(\delta)-\varepsilon,\hat{\gamma}(U)\in A,|\hat{\gamma}(U)|>c\right)\\
&\quad=\left[\Phi(\bar{c}_{\sup}(\delta)+\rho\left(1-\rho^2\right)^{-1/2}\gamma^{\max})-\Phi(\bar{c}_{\sup}(\delta)+\rho\left(1-\rho^2\right)^{-1/2}\gamma^{\max}-\varepsilon)\right]\\
&\qquad\times\Pr\left(Z_2\in A,|Z_2|\leq c\right)+\Pr\left(\bar{c}_{\sup}(\delta)\geq Z_1>\bar{c}_{\sup}(\delta)-\varepsilon,Z_2\in A,|Z_2|>c\right),
\end{aligned}
$$

where we have made use of independence of $\hat{\alpha}(R)$ and $\hat{\gamma}(U)$, cf. Lemma A.1 in [6], and of the fact that $n^{1/2}\left(\hat{\alpha}(R)-\alpha_0\right)$ is distributed as $N(-\sigma_{\alpha,n}\rho\gamma^{\max},\sigma_{\alpha,n}^2\left(1-\rho^2\right))$ under $P_{n,\alpha_0,\beta_n^{\max}}$. Furthermore, we have used the fact that $\left(n^{1/2}\left(\hat{\alpha}(U)-\alpha_0\right)/\sigma_{\alpha,n},\hat{\gamma}(U)\right)'$ is under $P_{n,\alpha_0,\beta_n^{\max}}$ distributed as $(Z_1,Z_2)'$ where

$$
(Z_1,Z_2)'\sim N\left((0,\gamma^{\max})',\begin{pmatrix}1&\rho\\\rho&1\end{pmatrix}\right),
$$

which is a non-singular normal distribution, since $|\rho|<1$. It is now obvious from the final expression in the last but one display that the probability in question is strictly positive and is independent of n. This proves (14).

We turn to the proof of (13). Observe that $c_{n,\hat{\beta}_n(U)}(\delta)=\bar{c}_{\hat{\gamma}(U)}(\delta)$ and that

$$
\bar{c}_{\sup}(\delta)=\bar{c}_{\gamma^{\max}}(\delta)>\lim_{|\gamma|\to\infty}\bar{c}_{\gamma}(\delta)=\Phi^{-1}(1-\delta)
$$

in view of Lemmata 6 and 7 in the Appendix. Choose $\varepsilon>0$ to satisfy $\varepsilon<\bar{c}_{\sup}(\delta)-\Phi^{-1}(1-\delta)$. Because of the limit relation in the preceding display, we see that there exists $M=M(\varepsilon)>0$ such that for $|\gamma|>M$ we have $\bar{c}_{\gamma}(\delta)<\bar{c}_{\sup}(\delta)-\varepsilon$. Define the set

$$
B=\{x\in\mathbb{R}:|x|>M\}.
$$

[5]The corresponding calculation in previous versions of this paper had erroneously omitted the term $\rho\left(1-\rho^2\right)^{-1/2}\gamma^{\max}$ from the expression on the far right-hand side of the subsequent display. This is corrected here by accounting for this term. Alternatively, one could drop the probability involving $|\hat{\gamma}(U)|\leq c$ altogether from the proof and work with the resulting lower bound.

Then on the event $\{\hat{\gamma}(U) \in B\}$ we have that $c_{n,\hat{\beta}_n(U)}(\delta) = \bar{c}_{\hat{\gamma}(U)}(\delta) \leq \bar{c}_{\sup}(\delta) - \varepsilon$. The rest of the proof is then completely analogous to the proof of (14) with the set A replaced by B. ■

Remark 3

(i) Inspection of the proof shows that (14) holds for every η, $0 < \eta < \delta$, that satisfies (15).
(ii) It is not difficult to show that the suprema in (13) and (14) actually do *not* depend on n.

Remark 4 If we allow η to depend on n, we may choose $\eta = \eta_n \to 0$ as $n \to \infty$. Then the test based on $\hat{c}_{n,\eta_n,\min}(\delta)$ still has a size that strictly overshoots δ for every n, but the overshoot will go to zero as $n \to \infty$. While this test then "approaches" the conservative test that uses $c_{n,\sup}(\delta)$, it does not respect the level for any finite-sample size. [The same can be said for Loh's [8] original proposal $c_{n,\eta_n,\mathrm{Loh}^*}(\delta)$, cf. footnote 3.] Contrast this with the test based on $c_{n,\eta_n,\mathrm{Loh}}(\delta)$ which holds the level for each n, and also "approaches" the conservative test if $\eta_n \to 0$. Hence, there seems to be little reason for preferring $\hat{c}_{n,\eta_n,\min}(\delta)$ (or $c_{n,\eta_n,\mathrm{Loh}^*}(\delta)$) to $c_{n,\eta_n,\mathrm{Loh}}(\delta)$ in this scenario where $\eta_n \to 0$.

Appendix

Lemma 5 *Suppose a random variable $\hat{c}_n$ satisfies* $\Pr(\hat{c}_n \leq c^*) = 1$ *for some real number c^* as well as* $\Pr(\hat{c}_n < c^*) > 0$. *Let S be real-valued random variable. If for every non-empty interval J in the real line*

$$\Pr(S \in J \mid \hat{c}_n) > 0 \tag{16}$$

holds almost surely, then

$$\Pr\left(\hat{c}_n < S \leq c^*\right) > 0.$$

The same conclusion holds if in (16) the conditioning variable $\hat{c}_n$ is replaced by some variable w_n, say, provided that $\hat{c}_n$ is a measurable function of w_n.

Proof Clearly

$$\Pr\left(\hat{c}_n < S \leq c^*\right) = E\left[\Pr\left(S \in (\hat{c}_n, c^*] \mid \hat{c}_n\right)\right] = E\left[\Pr\left(S \in (\hat{c}_n, c^*] \mid \hat{c}_n\right) \mathbf{1}\left(\hat{c}_n < c^*\right)\right],$$

the last equality being true, since the first term in the product is zero on the event $\hat{c}_n = c^*$. Now note that the first factor in the expectation on the far right-hand side of the above equality is positive almost surely by (16) on the event $\{\hat{c}_n < c^*\}$, and that the event $\{\hat{c}_n < c^*\}$ has positive probability by assumption. ■

Recall that $\bar{c}_\gamma(v)$ has been defined in the proof of Theorem 2.

Lemma 6 *Assume $\rho_n \equiv \rho \neq 0$. Suppose $0 < v < 1$. Then the map $\gamma \to \bar{c}_\gamma(v)$ is continuous on $\mathbb{R}$. Furthermore, $\lim_{\gamma\to\infty} \bar{c}_\gamma(v) = \lim_{\gamma\to-\infty} \bar{c}_\gamma(v) = \Phi^{-1}(1-v)$.*

Proof If $\gamma_l \to \gamma$, then $\bar{h}_{\gamma_l}$ converges to $\bar{h}_\gamma$ pointwise on $\mathbb{R}$. By Scheffé's Lemma, $\bar{H}_{\gamma_l}$ then converges to $\bar{H}_\gamma$ in total variation distance. Since $\bar{H}_\gamma$ is strictly increasing on $\mathbb{R}$, convergence of the quantiles $\bar{c}_{\gamma_l}(v)$ to $\bar{c}_\gamma(v)$ follows. The second claim follows by the same argument observing that $\bar{h}_\gamma$ converges pointwise to a standard normal density for $\gamma \to \pm\infty$. ■

Lemma 7 *Assume $\rho_n \equiv \rho \neq 0$.*

(i) Suppose $0 < v \leq 1/2$. Then for some $\gamma \in \mathbb{R}$ we have that $\bar{c}_\gamma(v)$ is larger than $\Phi^{-1}(1-v)$.
(ii) Suppose $1/2 \leq v < 1$. Then for some $\gamma \in \mathbb{R}$ we have that $\bar{c}_\gamma(v)$ is smaller than $\Phi^{-1}(1-v)$.

Proof Standard regression theory gives

$$\hat{\alpha}_n(U) = \hat{\alpha}_n(R) + \rho\sigma_{\alpha,n}\hat{\beta}_n(U)/\sigma_{\beta,n},$$

with $\hat{\alpha}_n(R)$ and $\hat{\beta}_n(U)$ being independent; for the latter cf., e.g., [6], Lemma A.1. Consequently, it is easy to see that the distribution of $T_n(\alpha_0)$ under $P_{n,\alpha_0,\beta}$ is the same as the distribution of

$$T' = T'(\rho,\gamma) = \left(\sqrt{1-\rho^2}W + \rho Z\right)\mathbf{1}\{|Z+\gamma| > c\} + \left(W - \rho\frac{\gamma}{\sqrt{1-\rho^2}}\right)\mathbf{1}\{|Z+\gamma| \leq c\},$$

where, as before, $\gamma = n^{1/2}\beta/\sigma_{\beta,n}$, and where W and Z are independent standard normal random variables.

We now prove (i): Let q be shorthand for $\Phi^{-1}(1-v)$ and note that $q \geq 0$ holds by the assumption on v. It suffices to show that $\Pr(T' \leq q) < \Phi(q)$ for some γ. We can now write

$$\begin{aligned}\Pr\left(T' \leq q\right) &= \Pr\left(\sqrt{1-\rho^2}W + \rho Z \leq q\right) - \Pr\left(|Z+\gamma| \leq c, W \leq \frac{q-\rho Z}{\sqrt{1-\rho^2}}\right) \\ &\quad + \Pr\left(|Z+\gamma| \leq c, W \leq q + \frac{\rho\gamma}{\sqrt{1-\rho^2}}\right) \\ &= \Phi(q) - \Pr(A) + \Pr(B).\end{aligned}$$

Here, A and B are the events given in terms of W and Z. Picturing these two events as subsets of the plane (with the horizontal axis corresponding to Z and the vertical axis corresponding to W), we see that A corresponds to the vertical band where

$|Z + \gamma| \leq c$, truncated above the line where $W = (q - \rho Z)/\sqrt{1 - \rho^2}$; similarly, B corresponds to the same vertical band $|Z + \gamma| \leq c$, truncated now above the horizontal line where $W = q + \rho\gamma/\sqrt{1 - \rho^2}$.

We first consider the case where $\rho > 0$ and distinguish two cases:

Case 1: $\rho c \leq \left(1 - \sqrt{1 - \rho^2}\right) q.$

In this case the set B is contained in A for every value of γ, with $A \backslash B$ being a set of positive Lebesgue measure. Consequently, $\Pr(A) > \Pr(B)$ holds for every γ, proving the claim.

Case 2: $\rho c > \left(1 - \sqrt{1 - \rho^2}\right) q.$

In this case choose γ so that $-\gamma - c \geq 0$, and, in addition, such that also $(q - \rho(-\gamma - c))/\sqrt{1 - \rho^2} < 0$, which is clearly possible. Recalling that $\rho > 0$, note that the point where the line $W = (q - \rho Z)/\sqrt{1 - \rho^2}$ intersects the horizontal line $W = q + \rho\gamma/\sqrt{1 - \rho^2}$ has as its first coordinate $Z = -\gamma + (q/\rho)(1 - \sqrt{1 - \rho^2})$, implying that the intersection occurs in the right half of the band where $|Z + \gamma| \leq c$. As a consequence, $\Pr(B) - \Pr(A)$ can be written as follows:

$$\Pr(B) - \Pr(A) = \Pr(B \backslash A) - \Pr(A \backslash B)$$

where

$$B \backslash A = \Big\{ -\gamma + (q/\rho)(1 - \sqrt{1 - \rho^2}) \leq Z \leq -\gamma + c,$$
$$(q - \rho Z)/\sqrt{1 - \rho^2} < W \leq q + \rho\gamma/\sqrt{1 - \rho^2} \Big\}$$

and

$$A \backslash B = \Big\{ -\gamma - c \leq Z \leq -\gamma + (q/\rho)(1 - \sqrt{1 - \rho^2}),$$
$$q + \rho\gamma/\sqrt{1 - \rho^2} < W \leq (q - \rho Z)/\sqrt{1 - \rho^2} \Big\}.$$

Picturing $A \backslash B$ and $B \backslash A$ as subsets of the plane as in the preceding paragraph, we see that these events correspond to two triangles, where the triangle corresponding to $A \backslash B$ is larger than or equal (in Lebesgue measure) to that corresponding to $B \backslash A$. Since γ was chosen to satisfy $-\gamma - c \geq 0$ and $(q - \rho(-\gamma - c))/\sqrt{1 - \rho^2} < 0$, we see that each point in the triangle corresponding to $A \backslash B$ is closer to the origin than any point in the triangle corresponding to $B \backslash A$. Because the joint Lebesgue density of (Z, W), i.e., the bivariate standard Gaussian density, is spherically symmetric and radially monotone, it follows that $\Pr(B \backslash A) - \Pr(A \backslash B) < 0$, as required.

The case $\rho < 0$ follows because $T'(\rho, \gamma)$ has the same distribution as $T'(-\rho, -\gamma)$.

Part (ii) follows, since $T'(\rho, \gamma)$ has the same distribution as $-T'(-\rho, \gamma)$. ■

Remark 8 If $\rho_n \equiv \rho \neq 0$ and $v = 1/2$, then $\bar{c}_0(1/2) = \Phi^{-1}(1/2) = 0$, since $\bar{h}_0$ is symmetric about zero.

Remark 9 If $\rho_n \equiv \rho = 0$, then $T_n(\alpha_0)$ is standard normally distributed for every value of β, and hence $\bar{c}_\gamma(v) = \Phi^{-1}(1-v)$ holds for every γ and v.

References

1. Andrews, D.W.K., Guggenberger, P.: Hybrid and size-corrected subsampling methods. Econometrica **77**, 721–762 (2009)
2. Berger, R.L., Boos, D.D.: P values maximized over a confidence set for the nuisance parameter. J. Am. Stat. Assoc. **89** 1012–1016 (1994)
3. Bickel, P.J., Doksum, K.A.: Mathematical Statistics: Basic Ideas and Selected Topics. Holden-Day, Oakland (1977)
4. DiTraglia, F.J.: Using invalid instruments on purpose: focused moment selection and averaging for GMM. Working Paper, Version November 9, 2011 (2011)
5. Kabaila, P., Leeb, H.: On the large-sample minimal coverage probability of confidence intervals after model selection. J. Am. Stat. Assoc. **101**, 619–629 (2006)
6. Leeb, H., Pötscher, B.M.: The finite-sample distribution of post-model-selection estimators and uniform versus non-uniform approximations. Economet. Theor. **19**, 100–142 (2003)
7. Leeb, H., Pötscher, B.M.: Model selection and inference: facts and fiction. Economet. Theor. **21**, 29–59 (2005)
8. Loh, W.-Y.: A new method for testing separate families of hypotheses. J. Am. Stat. Assoc. **80**, 362–368 (1985)
9. Liu, C.-A.: A plug-in averaging estimator for regressions with heteroskedastic errors. Working Paper, Version October 29, 2011 (2011)
10. McCloskey, A.: Powerful procedures with correct size for test statistics with limit distributions that are discontinuous in some parameters. Working Paper, Version October 2011 (2011)
11. McCloskey, A.: Bonferroni-based size correction for nonstandard testing problems. Working Paper, Brown University (2012)
12. Romano, J.P., Shaikh, A., Wolf, M.: A practical Two-step method for testing moment inequalities. Econometrica **82**, 1979–2002 (2014)
13. Silvapulle, M.J.: A test in the presence of nuisance parameters. J. Am. Stat. Assoc. **91**, 1690–1693 (1996) (Correction, ibidem 92 (1997) 801)
14. Williams, D.A.: Discrimination between regression models to determine the pattern of enzyme synthesis in synchronous cell cultures. Biometrics **26**, 23–32 (1970)

Analysis of Correlated Data with Error-Prone Response Under Generalized Linear Mixed Models

Grace Y. Yi, Zhijian Chen, and Changbao Wu

Abstract Measurements of variables are often subject to error due to various reasons. Measurement error in covariates has been discussed extensively in the literature, while error in response has received much less attention. In this paper, we consider generalized linear mixed models for clustered data where measurement error is present in response variables. We investigate asymptotic bias induced by nonlinear error in response variables if such error is ignored, and evaluate the performance of an intuitively appealing approach for correction of response error effects. We develop likelihood methods to correct for effects induced from response error. Simulation studies are conducted to evaluate the performance of the proposed methods, and a real data set is analyzed with the proposed methods.

1 Introduction

Generalized linear mixed models (GLMMs) have been broadly used to analyze correlated data, such as clustered/familial data, longitudinal data, and multivariate data. GLMMs provide flexible tools to accommodate normally or non-normally distributed data through various link functions between the response mean and a set of predictors. For longitudinal studies, in which repeated measurements of a response variable are collected on the same subject over time, GLMMs can be used as a convenient analytic tool to account for subject-specific variations [e.g., 5].

Standard statistical analysis with GLMMs is typically developed under the assumption that all variables are precisely observed. However, this assumption is commonly violated in applications. There has been much interest in statistical inference pertaining to error-in-covariates, and a large body of methods have been developed [e.g., 3, 17, 18]. Measurement error in response, however, has received

G.Y. Yi (✉) • C. Wu
Department of Statistics and Actuarial Science, University of Waterloo, Waterloo, ON, Canada N2L 3G1
e-mail: yyi@uwaterloo.ca; cbwu@uwaterloo.ca

Z. Chen
Bank of Nova Scotia, 4 King Street West, Toronto, ON, Canada M5H 1A1
e-mail: zhijian.chen@scotiabank.com

© Springer International Publishing AG 2017
S.E. Ahmed (ed.), *Big and Complex Data Analysis*, Contributions to Statistics,
DOI 10.1007/978-3-319-41573-4_5

much less attention, and this is partially attributed to a misbelief that ignoring response error would still lead to valid inferences. Unfortunately, this is only true in some special cases, e.g., the response variable follows a linear regression model and is subject to additive measurement error. With nonlinear response models or nonlinear error models, inference results can be seriously biased if response error is ignored. Buonaccorsi [1] conducted numerical studies to illustrate induced biases under linear models with nonlinear response measurement error. With binary responses subject to error, several authors, such as Neuhaus [10] and Chen et al. [4], demonstrated that naive analysis ignoring measurement error may lead to incorrect inference results.

Although there is some research on this topic, systematic studies on general clustered/longitudinal data with response error do not seem available. It is the goal of this paper to investigate the asymptotic bias induced by the error in response and to develop valid inference procedures to account for such biases. We formulate the problem under flexible frameworks where GLMMs are used to feature various response processes and nonlinear models are adopted to characterize response measurement error.

Our research is partly motivated by the Framingham Heart Study, a large scale longitudinal study concerning the development of cardiovascular disease. It is well known that certain variables, such as blood pressure, are difficult to measure accurately due to the biological variability and that their values are greatly affected by the change of environment. There has been a large body of work on the analysis of data from the Framingham Heart Study, accounting for measurement error in covariates. For example, Carroll et al. [2] considered binary regression models to relate the probability of developing heart disease to risk factors including error-contaminated systolic blood pressure. Within the framework of longitudinal analysis, the impact of covariate measurement error and missing data on model parameters has been examined. Yi [16] and Yi et al. [19] proposed estimation and inference methods that account for measurement error and missing response observations. Other work can be found in [7, 20], among others. Relative to the extensive analysis of data with covariate error, there is not much work on accounting for measurement error in continuous responses using the data from the Framingham Heart Study.

The remainder of the paper is organized as follows. In Sect. 2, we formulate the response and the measurement error processes. In Sect. 3, we investigate the estimation bias in two analyses: the naive analysis that completely ignores response measurement error, and a partial-adjustment method that fits model to transformed surrogate responses. In Sect. 4, we develop likelihood-based methods to cover two useful situations: measurement error parameters are known, or measurement error parameters are unknown. In Sect. 5, we evaluate the performances of various approaches through simulation studies. In Sect. 6, we illustrate the proposed method using a real data set from the Framingham Heart Study. Discussion and concluding remarks are given in Sect. 7.

2 Model Formulation

2.1 Response Model

Suppose data from a total of n independent clusters are collected. Let Y_{ij} denote the response for the jth subject in cluster i, $i = 1, \ldots, n$, $j = 1, \ldots, m_i$. Let $\mathbf{X}_{ij}$ and $\mathbf{Z}_{ij}$ be vectors of covariates for subject j and cluster i, respectively, and write $\mathbf{X}_i = (\mathbf{X}_{i1}^{\mathrm{T}}, \ldots, \mathbf{X}_{im_i}^{\mathrm{T}})^{\mathrm{T}}$ and $\mathbf{Z}_i = (\mathbf{Z}_{i1}^{\mathrm{T}}, \ldots, \mathbf{Z}_{im_i}^{\mathrm{T}})^{\mathrm{T}}$. Here we use upper case letters and the corresponding lower case letters to denote random variables and their realizations, respectively.

Conditional on random effects $\mathbf{b}_i$ and covariates $\{\mathbf{X}_i, \mathbf{Z}_i\}$, the $Y_{ij}(j = 1, \ldots, m_i)$ are assumed to be conditionally independent and follow a distribution from the exponential family with the probability density or mass function

$$f_{y|x,z,b}(y_{ij}|\mathbf{x}_{ij}, \mathbf{z}_{ij}, \mathbf{b}_i) = \exp[\{y_{ij}\alpha_{ij} - a_1(\alpha_{ij})\}/a_2(\phi) + a_3(y_{ij}, \phi)], \quad (1)$$

where functions $a_1(\cdot)$, $a_2(\cdot)$, and $a_3(\cdot)$ are user-specified, ϕ is a dispersion parameter, and α_{ij} is the canonical parameter which links the conditional mean, $\mu_{ij}^b = E(Y_{ij}|\mathbf{X}_i, \mathbf{Z}_i, \mathbf{b}_i)$, via the identity $\mu_{ij}^b = \partial a_1(\alpha_{ij})/\partial \alpha_{ij}$.

A generalized linear mixed model (GLMM) relates μ_{ij}^b to the covariates and random effects via a regression model

$$g(\mu_{ij}^b) = \mathbf{X}_{ij}^{\mathrm{T}}\boldsymbol{\beta} + \mathbf{Z}_{ij}^{\mathrm{T}}\mathbf{b}_i, \quad (2)$$

where $\boldsymbol{\beta}$ is a vector of regression coefficients for the fixed effects, and $g(\cdot)$ is a link function. Random effects $\mathbf{b}_i$ are assumed to have a distribution, say, $f_b(\mathbf{b}_i; \boldsymbol{\sigma}_{\mathbf{b}})$, with an unknown parameter vector $\boldsymbol{\sigma}_{\mathbf{b}}$. The link function $g(\cdot)$ is monotone and differentiable, and its form can be differently specified for individual applications. For instance, for binary Y_{ij}, $g(\cdot)$ can be chosen as a logit, probit, or complementary log-log link, while for Poisson or Gamma variables Y_{ij}, $g(\cdot)$ is often set as a log link.

A useful class of models belonging to GLMMs is linear mixed models (LMM) where $g(\cdot)$ in (2) is set to be the identity function, leading to

$$Y_{ij} = \mathbf{X}_{ij}^{\mathrm{T}}\boldsymbol{\beta} + \mathbf{Z}_{ij}^{\mathrm{T}}\mathbf{b}_i + \epsilon_{ij} \quad (3)$$

where the error term ϵ_{ij} is often assumed to be normally distributed with mean 0 and unknown variance ϕ.

Let $\boldsymbol{\theta} = (\boldsymbol{\beta}^{\mathrm{T}}, \boldsymbol{\sigma}_b^{\mathrm{T}}, \phi)^{\mathrm{T}}$ be the vector of model parameters. In the absence of response error, estimation of $\boldsymbol{\theta}$ is based on the likelihood for the observed data:

$$\mathscr{L}(\boldsymbol{\theta}) = \prod_{i=1}^{n} \mathscr{L}_i(\boldsymbol{\theta}),$$

where

$$\mathscr{L}_i(\boldsymbol{\theta}) = \int \prod_{j=1}^{m_i} f_{y|x,z,b}(y_{ij}|\mathbf{x}_{ij}, \mathbf{z}_{ij}, \mathbf{b}_i; \boldsymbol{\theta}) f_b(\mathbf{b}_i; \boldsymbol{\sigma}_{\mathbf{b}}) d\mathbf{b}_i \tag{4}$$

is the marginal likelihood for cluster i, and $f_{y|x,z,b}(y_{ij}|\mathbf{x}_{ij}, \mathbf{z}_{ij}, \mathbf{b}_i; \boldsymbol{\theta})$ is determined by (1) in combination with (2). Maximizing $\mathscr{L}(\boldsymbol{\theta})$ with respect to $\boldsymbol{\theta}$ gives the maximum likelihood estimator of $\boldsymbol{\theta}$.

2.2 *Measurement Error Models*

When Y_{ij} is subject to measurement error, we observe a value that may differ from the true value; let S_{ij} denote such an observed measurement for Y_{ij}, and we call it a surrogate variable. In this paper we consider the case where Y_{ij} is a continuous variable only. Let $f_{s|y,x,z}(S_{ij}|\mathbf{y}_i, \mathbf{x}_i, \mathbf{z}_i)$ or $f_{s|y,x,z}(S_{ij}|y_{ij}, \mathbf{x}_{ij}, \mathbf{z}_{ij})$ denote the conditional probability density (or mass) function for S_{ij} given $\{\mathbf{Y}_i, \mathbf{X}_i, \mathbf{Z}_i\}$ or $\{Y_{ij}, \mathbf{X}_{ij}, \mathbf{Z}_{ij}\}$, respectively. It is often assumed that

$$f_{s|y,x,z}(s_{ij}|\mathbf{y}_i, \mathbf{x}_i, \mathbf{z}_i) = f_{s|y,x,z}(s_{ij}|y_{ij}, \mathbf{x}_{ij}, \mathbf{z}_{ij}).$$

This assumption says that given the true variables $\{Y_{ij}, \mathbf{X}_{ij}, \mathbf{Z}_{ij}\}$ for each subject j in a cluster i, the observed measurement S_{ij} is independent of variables $\{Y_{ik}, \mathbf{X}_{ik}, \mathbf{Z}_{ik}\}$ of other subjects in the same cluster for $k \neq j$.

Parametric modeling can be invoked to feature the relationship between the true response variable Y_{ij} and its surrogate measurement S_{ij}. One class of useful models are specified as

$$S_{ij} = h(Y_{ij}, \mathbf{X}_{ij}, \mathbf{Z}_{ij}; \boldsymbol{\gamma}_i) + e_{ij}, \tag{5}$$

where the stochastic noise term e_{ij} has mean zero. Another class of models are given by

$$S_{ij} = h(Y_{ij}, \mathbf{X}_{ij}, \mathbf{Z}_{ij}; \boldsymbol{\gamma}_i) \cdot e_{ij}, \tag{6}$$

where the stochastic term e_{ij} has mean 1. These models basically modulate the mean structure of the surrogate variable S_{ij}:

$$E(S_{ij}|\mathbf{Y}_i, \mathbf{X}_i, \mathbf{Z}_i) = h(Y_{ij}, \mathbf{X}_{ij}, \mathbf{Z}_{ij}; \boldsymbol{\gamma}_i), \tag{7}$$

where the function form $h(\cdot)$ can be chosen differently to facilitate various applications, and $\boldsymbol{\gamma}_i$ is a vector of error parameters for cluster i. For cases where the measurement error process is homogeneous, e.g., same measuring system is used across clusters, we replace $\boldsymbol{\gamma}_i$ with a common parameter vector $\boldsymbol{\gamma}$.

Specification of $h(\cdot)$ reflects the feature of the measurement error model. For example, if $h(\cdot)$ is set as a linear function, model (5) gives a linear relationship between the response and surrogate measurements:

$$S_{ij} = \gamma_0 + \gamma_1 Y_{ij} + \gamma_2^{\mathrm{T}} \mathbf{X}_{ij} + \gamma_3^{\mathrm{T}} \mathbf{Z}_{ij} + e_{ij},$$

where parameters γ_0, γ_1, γ_2, and γ_3 control the dependence of surrogate measurement S_{ij} on the response and covariate variables; in the instance where both γ_2 and γ_3 are zero vectors, surrogate measurement S_{ij} is not affected by the measurements of the covariates and depends on the true response variable Y_{ij} only. More complex relationships can be delineated by employing nonlinear function forms for $h(\cdot)$. In our following simulation studies and data analysis, linear, exponential, and logarithmic functions are considered for $h(\cdot)$.

We call (5) *additive error models*, and (6) *multiplicative error models* to indicate how noise terms e_{ij} act relative to the mean structure of S_{ij}. Commonly, noise terms e_{ij} are assumed to be independent of each other, of the true responses as well as of the covariates. Let $f(e_{ij}; \boldsymbol{\sigma}_e)$ denote the probability density function of e_{ij}, where $\boldsymbol{\sigma}_e$ is an associated parameter vector. With model (5), the e_{ij} are often assumed to be normally distributed, while for model (6), a log normal or a Gamma distribution may be considered.

3 Asymptotic Bias Analysis

In this section we investigate asymptotic biases caused by response error under the two situations: (1) response error is totally ignored in estimation procedures, and (2) an intuitively compelling correction method is applied to adjust for measurement error in response.

3.1 *Naive Analysis of Ignoring Measurement Error*

We consider a naive analysis which fits the GLMM (1) to the observed raw data (hereafter referred to as NAI1), i.e., we assume that the S_{ij} are linked with covariates via the same random effects model. Let $\boldsymbol{\theta}^* = (\boldsymbol{\beta}^{*\mathrm{T}}, \boldsymbol{\sigma}_b^{*\mathrm{T}}, \phi^*)^{\mathrm{T}}$ denote the corresponding parameter vector, and the corresponding working likelihood contributed from cluster i is given by

$$\mathcal{L}_i^w(\boldsymbol{\theta}^*) = \int \prod_{j=1}^{m} f_{y|x,z,b}(s_{ij}|\mathbf{x}_{ij}, \mathbf{z}_{ij}, \mathbf{b}_i^*; \boldsymbol{\theta}^*) f_b(\mathbf{b}_i^*; \boldsymbol{\sigma}_b^*) d\mathbf{b}_i^*.$$

Maximizing $\sum_{i=1}^{n} \log \mathcal{L}_i^w(\boldsymbol{\theta}^*)$ with respect to $\boldsymbol{\theta}^*$ gives an estimator, say $\hat{\boldsymbol{\theta}}^*$, of $\boldsymbol{\theta}^*$.

Adapting the arguments of White [14] it can be shown that under certain regularity conditions, as $n \to \infty$, $\hat{\boldsymbol{\theta}}^*$ converges in probability to a limit that is the solution to a set of estimating equations

$$\mathrm{E}_{\text{true}}\left\{\sum_{i=1}^{n} \partial \log \mathscr{L}_i^w(\boldsymbol{\theta}^*)/\partial \boldsymbol{\theta}^*\right\} = \mathbf{0}, \tag{8}$$

where the expectation is taken with respect to the true joint distribution of the associated random variables. The evaluation of (8) involves integration over the nonlinear error functions which are often intractable.

To gain insights into the impact of ignoring error in response, we consider a LMM

$$Y_{ij} = \beta_0 + (\beta_1 + b_i)X_{ij} + \epsilon_{ij}, \tag{9}$$

where β_0 and β_1 are regression parameters, the ϵ_{ij} are independent of each other and of other variables, $\epsilon_{ij} \sim N(0, \phi)$ with variance ϕ, and $b_i \sim \text{Normal}(0, \sigma_b^2)$ with variance σ_b^2. We consider the additive error model (5), where the e_{ij} are independent of each other and of other variables, $e_{ij} \sim N(0, \sigma_e^2)$, and the mean error structures are, respectively, specified as one of the following two cases.

Case 1 *Linear measurement error.*

Commonly seen in epidemiologic studies, this structure specifies a linear form for the measurement error

$$h(Y_{ij}, \mathbf{X}_{ij}, \mathbf{Z}_{ij}; \boldsymbol{\gamma}) = \gamma_0 + \gamma_1 Y_{ij},$$

where $\boldsymbol{\gamma} = (\gamma_0, \gamma_1)$, γ_0 represents a systematic error of the measuring device at $Y_{ij} = 0$, and γ_1 is a scale factor. It can be easily shown that simple relationship between the true and working parameters is

$$\beta_0^* = \gamma_0 + \gamma_1\beta_0, \ \beta_1^* = \gamma_1\beta_1, \ \sigma_b^{*2} = \gamma_1^2\sigma_b^2,$$

and

$$\phi^* = \gamma_1^2\phi + \sigma_e^2.$$

These results suggest that estimation of fix effect β_1 and variance component σ_b^2 is generally attenuated or inflated by factor γ_1, a factor which governs the difference between the true response Y_{ij} and surrogate measurement S_{ij}. When γ_1 equals 1, even if there is systematic measurement error involved with measuring Y_{ij} (i.e., $\gamma_0 \neq 0$), disregarding error in Y_{ij} does not bias point estimates of fix effect β_1 and variance component σ_b^2, but may reduce estimation precision.

Case 2 *Exponential measurement error.*

The second error structure specifies an exponential form for the measurement error

$$h(Y_{ij}, \mathbf{X}_{ij}, \mathbf{Z}_{ij}; \gamma) = \exp(\gamma Y_{ij}),$$

which may be useful to feature transformed response variables that are not measured precisely.

The bias in the naive estimator for fixed effect β_1 does not have an analytic form when the response is subject to nonlinear measurement error. To illustrate the induced bias in estimation of β_1 with response error ignored, we undertake a numerical study. The covariates X_{ij} are independently generated from a normal distribution $N(0, 1)$. We fix the values of β_0 and ϕ at -1 and 0.01, respectively, and consider values of σ_b^2 to be 0.01, 0.25, and 1, respectively. The error parameters are, respectively, specified as $\gamma = 0.5$ and 1, and $\sigma_e^2 = 0.01, 0.25,$ and 0.75.

As shown in Fig. 1, the relationship between the naive limit β_1^* and the value of β_1 is nonlinear. For instance, when $\gamma = 0.5$, the naive estimate is attenuated for small values of β_1 but is inflated for large values of β_1. In general, the direction and magnitude of the bias induced by nonlinear response error depend on the function form of $h(\cdot)$ as well as the magnitude of the parameters in the measurement error process.

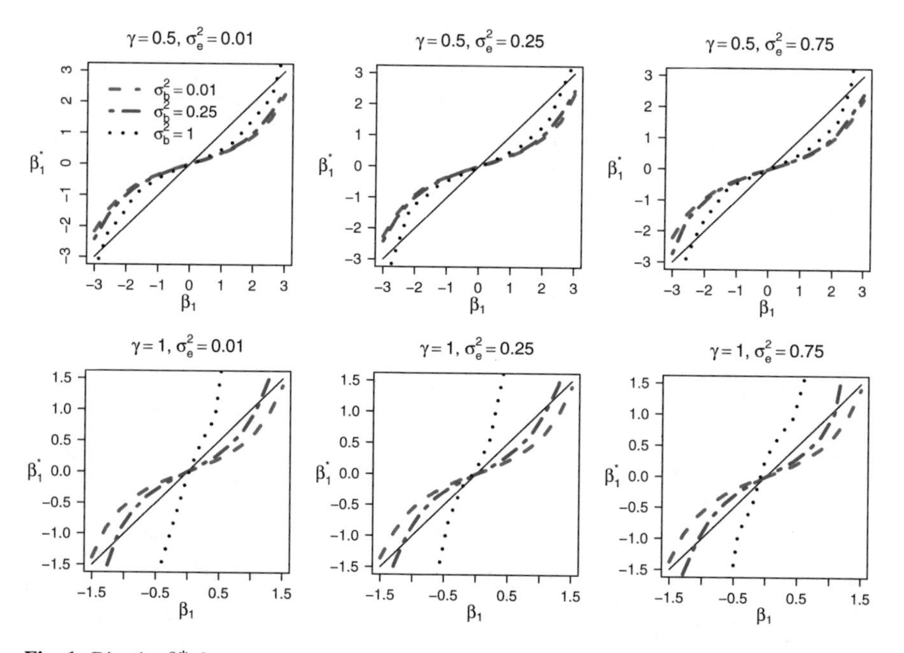

Fig. 1 Bias in β_1^* from the completely naive approach induced by an exponential error model. The *dashed, two-dash*, and *dotted lines* correspond to $\sigma_b^2 = 0.01, 0.25,$ and 1, respectively

3.2 Analysis of Transformed Data

With the response process modeled by an LMM, Buonaccorsi [1] considered an intuitively tempting method to correct for response error in estimation. The idea is to employ a two-step approach to correct for response error effects. In the first step, keeping the covariates fixed, we use the mean function $h(\cdot)$ of the measurement error model and find its inverse function $h^{-1}(\cdot)$, and then calculate a pseudo-response

$$\tilde{Y}_{ij} = h^{-1}(S_{ij}; \boldsymbol{\gamma}).$$

In the second step, we perform standard statistical analysis with $\tilde{Y}_{ij}$ taken as a response variable. This approach (hereafter referred to as NAI2) is generally preferred over NAI1, as it reduces a certain amount of bias induced by response measurement error. However, this method does not completely remove the biases induced from response error.

To evaluate the performance of using pseudo-response in estimation procedures, we may follow the same spirit of Sect. 3.1 to conduct bias analysis. As it is difficult to obtain analytic results for general models, here we perform empirical studies by employing the same response model (9) and the measurement error model for Case 2 as in Sect. 3.1.

It is seen that as expected, the asymptotic bias, displayed in Fig. 2, is smaller than that from the NAI1 analysis. This confirms that the NAI2 method outperforms

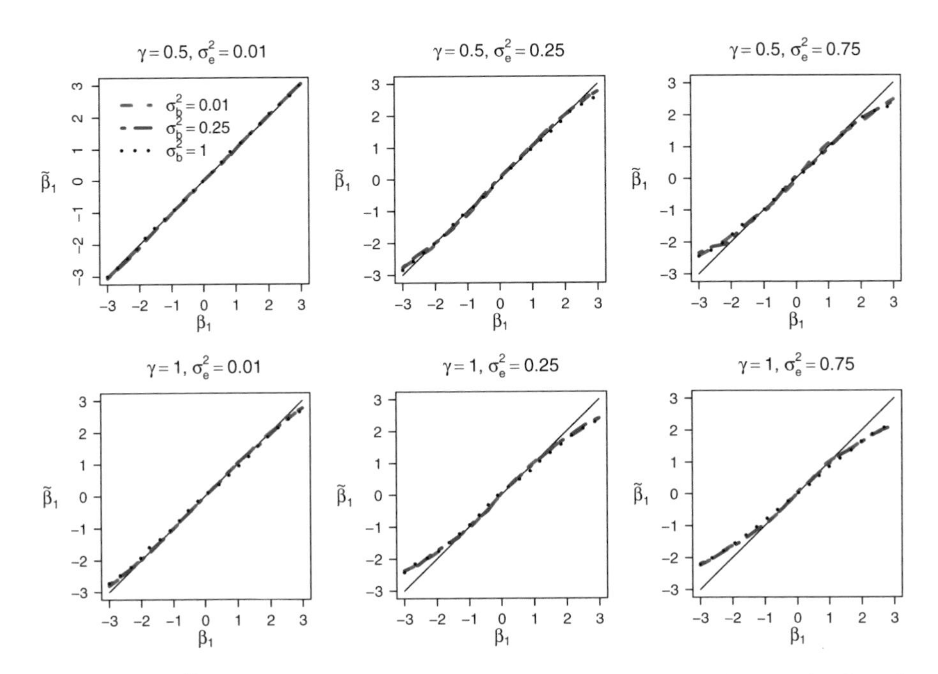

Fig. 2 Bias in $\tilde{\beta}_1$ from NAI2 analyses with response subject to exponential error. The *dashed*, *two-dash*, and *dotted lines* are for $\sigma_b^2 = 0.01, 0.25$, and 1, respectively

the NAI1 method. However, the NAI2 method does not completely remove the bias induced in the response error. The asymptotic bias involved in the NAI2 method is affected by the size of the covariate effect as well as the degree of response error. The asymptotic bias increases as the size of β_1 increases. Furthermore, the values of the error parameters γ and σ_e^2 have significant impact on the bias; the size of the bias tends to increase as σ_e^2 increases.

4 Inference Methods

The analytic and numerical results in Sect. 3 demonstrate that disregarding response error may yield biased estimation results. To account for the response error effects, in this section we develop valid inference methods for the response model parameter vector $\boldsymbol{\theta}$. Our development accommodates different scenarios pertaining to the knowledge of response measurement error. Let $\boldsymbol{\eta}$ denote the parameter vector associated with a parametric model of the response measurement error process. Estimation of $\boldsymbol{\theta}$ may suffer from nonidentifiability issues in the presence of measurement error in the variables. To circumvent this potential problem, we consider three useful situations: (i) $\boldsymbol{\eta}$ is known, (ii) $\boldsymbol{\eta}$ is unknown but a validation subsample is available, and (iii) $\boldsymbol{\eta}$ is unknown but replicates for the surrogates are available.

The first situation highlights the idea of addressing the difference between the surrogate measurements and the response variables without worrying about model nonidentifiability issues. The second and third scenarios reflect useful practical settings where error model parameter $\boldsymbol{\eta}$ is often unknown, but estimable from additional data sources such as a validation subsample or replicated surrogate measurements. For each of these three situations, we propose strategies for estimating the response model parameters and derive the asymptotic properties of the resulting estimators.

4.1 η Is Known

In some applications, the value of $\boldsymbol{\eta}$ is known to be $\boldsymbol{\eta}_0$, say, from a priori study, or specified by the analyst for sensitivity analyses. Inference about $\boldsymbol{\theta}$ is then carried out based on the marginal likelihood of the observed data:

$$\mathcal{L}(\boldsymbol{\theta}, \boldsymbol{\eta}_0) = \prod_{i=1}^{n} \mathcal{L}_i(\boldsymbol{\theta}, \boldsymbol{\eta}_0)$$

where

$$\mathscr{L}_i(\boldsymbol{\theta}, \boldsymbol{\eta}) = \int \left\{ \prod_{j=1}^{m_i} \int f_{s|y,x,z}(s_{ij}|y_{ij}, \mathbf{x}_{ij}, \mathbf{z}_{ij}; \boldsymbol{\eta}) \times f_{y|x,z,b}(y_{ij}|\mathbf{x}_{ij}, \mathbf{z}_{ij}, \mathbf{b}_i; \boldsymbol{\theta}) dy_{ij} \right\} f_b(\mathbf{b}_i; \boldsymbol{\sigma}_b) d\mathbf{b}_i,$$

which requires the conditional independence assumption

$$f_{s|y,x,z,b}(s_{ij}|y_{ij}, \mathbf{x}_{ij}, \mathbf{z}_{ij}, \mathbf{b}_i; \boldsymbol{\eta}) = f_{s|y,x,z}(s_{ij}|y_{ij}, \mathbf{x}_{ij}, \mathbf{z}_{ij}; \boldsymbol{\eta}); \tag{10}$$

$f_{s|y,x,z,b}(s_{ij}|y_{ij}, \mathbf{x}_{ij}, \mathbf{z}_{ij}, \mathbf{b}_i; \boldsymbol{\eta})$ and $f_{s|y,x,z}(s_{ij}|y_{ij}, \mathbf{x}_{ij}, \mathbf{z}_{ij}; \boldsymbol{\eta})$ represent the conditional probability density function of S_{ij} given $\{Y_{ij}, \mathbf{X}_{ij}, \mathbf{Z}_{ij}, \mathbf{b}_i\}$ and $\{Y_{ij}, \mathbf{X}_{ij}, \mathbf{Z}_{ij}\}$, respectively.

Maximizing $\sum_{i=1}^{n} \log \mathscr{L}_i(\boldsymbol{\theta}, \boldsymbol{\eta}_0)$ with respect to the parameter $\boldsymbol{\theta}$ gives the maximum likelihood estimator $\hat{\boldsymbol{\theta}}$ of $\boldsymbol{\theta}$. Let $\mathbf{U}_i(\boldsymbol{\theta}, \boldsymbol{\eta}_0) = \partial \log \mathscr{L}_i(\boldsymbol{\theta}, \boldsymbol{\eta}_0)/\partial \boldsymbol{\theta}$. From standard likelihood theory, under regularity conditions, $\hat{\boldsymbol{\theta}}$ is a consistent estimator for $\boldsymbol{\theta}$. As $n \to \infty$, $n^{1/2}(\hat{\boldsymbol{\theta}} - \boldsymbol{\theta})$ is asymptotically normally distributed with mean $\mathbf{0}$ and variance $\mathscr{I}^{-1}$, where $\mathscr{I} = E\{-\partial \mathbf{U}_i(\boldsymbol{\theta}, \boldsymbol{\eta}_0)/\partial \boldsymbol{\theta}^{\mathrm{T}}\}$. By the Bartlett identity and the Law of Large Numbers, $\mathscr{I}$ can be consistently estimated by $n^{-1} \sum_{i=1}^{n} \mathbf{U}_i(\hat{\boldsymbol{\theta}}, \boldsymbol{\eta}_0) \mathbf{U}_i^{\mathrm{T}}(\hat{\boldsymbol{\theta}}, \boldsymbol{\eta}_0)$.

4.2 η Is Estimated from Validation Data

In many applications, $\boldsymbol{\eta}$ is often unknown and must be estimated from additional data sources, such as a validation subsample or replicates of measurements of Y_{ij}. Here we consider the case that a validation subsample is available, and in the next section we discuss the situation with replicated measurements.

Assume that the validation subsample is randomly selected, and let $\delta_{ij} = 1$ if Y_{ij} is available and $\delta_{ij} = 0$ otherwise. Specifically, if $\delta_{ij} = 1$, then measurements $\{y_{ij}, s_{ij}, \mathbf{x}_{ij}, \mathbf{z}_{ij}\}$ are available; when $\delta_{ij} = 0$, measurements $\{s_{ij}, \mathbf{x}_{ij}, \mathbf{z}_{ij}\}$ are available. Let $N_v = \sum_{i=1}^{n} \sum_{j=1}^{m_i} \delta_{ij}$ be the number of the measurements in the validation subsample. The full marginal likelihood of the main data and the validation data contributed from cluster i is given by

$$\mathscr{L}_{Fi}(\boldsymbol{\theta}, \boldsymbol{\eta}) = \int \left[\prod_{j=1}^{m_i} \{f_{s|x,z,b}(s_{ij}|\mathbf{x}_{ij}, \mathbf{z}_{ij}, \mathbf{b}_i; \boldsymbol{\theta}, \boldsymbol{\eta})\}^{1-\delta_{ij}} \times \{f_{s,y|x,z,b}(s_{ij}, y_{ij}|\mathbf{x}_{ij}, \mathbf{z}_{ij}, \mathbf{b}_i; \boldsymbol{\theta}, \boldsymbol{\eta})\}^{\delta_{ij}} \right] f_b(\mathbf{b}_i; \boldsymbol{\sigma}_b) d\mathbf{b}_i, \tag{11}$$

where $f_{s,y|x,z,b}(s_{ij}, y_{ij}|\mathbf{x}_{ij}, \mathbf{z}_{ij}, \mathbf{b}_i; \boldsymbol{\theta}, \boldsymbol{\eta})$ represents the conditional probability density functions of $\{S_{ij}, Y_{ij}\}$, given the covariates $\{\mathbf{x}_{ij}, \mathbf{z}_{ij}\}$ and random effects $\mathbf{b}_i$.

Under the conditional independence assumption (10), we obtain

$$f_{s|x,z,b}(s_{ij}|\mathbf{x}_{ij},\mathbf{z}_{ij},\mathbf{b}_i;\boldsymbol{\theta},\boldsymbol{\eta}) = \int f_{s|y,x,z}(s_{ij}|y_{ij},\mathbf{x}_{ij},\mathbf{z}_{ij};\boldsymbol{\eta})f_{y|x,z,b}(y_{ij}|\mathbf{x}_{ij},\mathbf{z}_{ij},\mathbf{b}_i;\boldsymbol{\theta})dy_{ij},$$

and

$$f_{s,y|x,z,b}(s_{ij},y_{ij}|\mathbf{x}_{ij},\mathbf{z}_{ij},\mathbf{b}_i;\boldsymbol{\theta},\boldsymbol{\eta}) = f_{s|y,x,z}(s_{ij}|y_{ij},\mathbf{x}_{ij},\mathbf{z}_{ij};\boldsymbol{\eta})f_{y|x,z,b}(y_{ij}|\mathbf{x}_{ij},\mathbf{z}_{ij},\mathbf{b}_i;\boldsymbol{\theta}),$$

where $f_{s|y,x,z}(s_{ij}|y_{ij},\mathbf{x}_{ij},\mathbf{z}_{ij};\boldsymbol{\eta})$ is the conditional probability density function determined by the measurement error model such as (5) or (6), and $f_{y|x,z,b}(y_{ij}|\mathbf{x}_{ij},\mathbf{z}_{ij},\mathbf{b}_i;\boldsymbol{\theta})$ is the conditional probability density function specified by the GLMM (1) in combination with (2).

Let

$$\mathscr{L}_{\theta i}(\boldsymbol{\theta},\boldsymbol{\eta}) = \int \left[\prod_{j=1}^{m_i} \left\{f_{s|x,z,b}(s_{ij}|\mathbf{x}_{ij},\mathbf{z}_{ij},\mathbf{b}_i;\boldsymbol{\theta},\boldsymbol{\eta})\right\}^{1-\delta_{ij}} \times \left\{f_{y|x,z,b}(y_{ij}|\mathbf{x}_{ij},\mathbf{z}_{ij},\mathbf{b}_i;\boldsymbol{\theta})\right\}^{\delta_{ij}} \right] f_b(\mathbf{b}_i;\boldsymbol{\sigma}_b)d\mathbf{b}_i,$$

and

$$\mathscr{L}_{\eta i}(\boldsymbol{\eta}) = \prod_{j=1}^{m_i} \left\{f_{s|y,x,z}(s_{ij}|y_{ij},\mathbf{x}_{ij},\mathbf{z}_{ij};\boldsymbol{\eta})\right\}^{\delta_{ij}},$$

then $\mathscr{L}_{Fi}(\boldsymbol{\theta},\boldsymbol{\eta}) = \mathscr{L}_{\theta i}(\boldsymbol{\theta},\boldsymbol{\eta})\,\mathscr{L}_{\eta i}(\boldsymbol{\eta})$.

Inference about $\{\boldsymbol{\theta},\boldsymbol{\eta}\}$ can, in principle, be conducted by maximizing $\prod_{i=1}^n \mathscr{L}_{Fi}(\boldsymbol{\theta},\boldsymbol{\eta})$, or $\sum_{i=1}^n \log \mathscr{L}_{Fi}(\boldsymbol{\theta},\boldsymbol{\eta})$, with respect to $\{\boldsymbol{\theta},\boldsymbol{\eta}\}$. When the dimension of $\{\boldsymbol{\theta},\boldsymbol{\eta}\}$ is large, direct maximization of $\sum_{i=1}^n \log \mathscr{L}_{Fi}(\boldsymbol{\theta},\boldsymbol{\eta})$ with respect to $\boldsymbol{\theta}$ and $\boldsymbol{\eta}$ can be computationally demanding. We propose to use a two-stage estimation procedure as an alternative to the joint maximization procedure.

Let $\mathbf{U}_i^*(\boldsymbol{\theta},\boldsymbol{\eta}) = \partial \log \mathscr{L}_{\theta i}(\boldsymbol{\theta},\boldsymbol{\eta})/\partial\boldsymbol{\theta}$ and $\mathbf{Q}_i(\boldsymbol{\eta}) = \partial \log \mathscr{L}_{\eta i}(\boldsymbol{\eta})/\partial\boldsymbol{\eta}$. In the first stage, estimator for $\boldsymbol{\eta}$, denoted by $\hat{\boldsymbol{\eta}}$, is obtained by solving

$$\sum_{i=1}^n \mathbf{Q}_i(\boldsymbol{\eta}) = \mathbf{0}.$$

In the second stage, replace $\boldsymbol{\eta}$ with $\hat{\boldsymbol{\eta}}$ and solve

$$\sum_{i=1}^n \mathbf{U}_i^*(\boldsymbol{\theta},\hat{\boldsymbol{\eta}}) = \mathbf{0} \tag{12}$$

for $\boldsymbol{\theta}$. Let $\hat{\boldsymbol{\theta}}_p$ denote the solution to (12).

Assume that the size of the validation sample is increasing with the sample size n on the same scale, i.e., as $n \to \infty$ and $N_v/n \to \rho$ for a positive constant ρ. Then under regularity conditions, $\sqrt{n}(\hat{\boldsymbol{\theta}}_p - \boldsymbol{\theta})$ is asymptotically normally distributed with mean 0 and variance given by

$$\Sigma^* = \left[-E\{\partial \mathbf{U}_i^*(\boldsymbol{\theta},\boldsymbol{\eta})/\partial \boldsymbol{\theta}^{\mathrm{T}}\}\right]^{-1} + \left[E\{\partial \mathbf{U}_i^*(\boldsymbol{\theta},\boldsymbol{\eta})/\partial \boldsymbol{\theta}^{\mathrm{T}}\}\right]^{-1} E\{\partial \mathbf{U}_i^*(\boldsymbol{\theta},\boldsymbol{\eta})/\partial \boldsymbol{\eta}^{\mathrm{T}}\}$$
$$\times \left[E\{\partial \mathbf{Q}_i(\boldsymbol{\eta})/\partial \boldsymbol{\eta}^{\mathrm{T}}\}\right]^{-1} \left[E\{\partial \mathbf{U}_i^*(\boldsymbol{\theta},\boldsymbol{\eta})/\partial \boldsymbol{\eta}^{\mathrm{T}}\}\right]^{\mathrm{T}} \left[E\{\partial \mathbf{U}_i^*(\boldsymbol{\theta},\boldsymbol{\eta})/\partial \boldsymbol{\theta}^{\mathrm{T}}\}\right]^{-1}.$$

The proof is outlined in the Appendix. An estimate of $\boldsymbol{\Sigma}^*$ can be obtained by replacing $E\{\partial \mathbf{U}_i^*(\boldsymbol{\theta},\boldsymbol{\eta})/\partial \boldsymbol{\theta}^{\mathrm{T}}\}$, $E\{\partial \mathbf{U}_i^*(\boldsymbol{\theta},\boldsymbol{\eta})/\partial \boldsymbol{\eta}^{\mathrm{T}}\}$, and $E\{\partial \mathbf{Q}_i(\boldsymbol{\eta})/\partial \boldsymbol{\eta}^{\mathrm{T}}\}$ with their empirical counterparts $n^{-1}\sum_{i=1}^{n} \partial \mathbf{U}_i^*(\hat{\boldsymbol{\theta}}_p, \hat{\boldsymbol{\eta}})/\partial \boldsymbol{\theta}^{\mathrm{T}}$, $n^{-1}\sum_{i=1}^{n} \partial \mathbf{U}_i^*(\hat{\boldsymbol{\theta}}_p, \hat{\boldsymbol{\eta}})/\partial \boldsymbol{\eta}^{\mathrm{T}}$, and $n^{-1}\sum_{i=1}^{n} \partial \mathbf{Q}_i(\hat{\boldsymbol{\eta}})/\partial \boldsymbol{\eta}^{\mathrm{T}}$, respectively.

4.3 Inference with Replicates

In this section we discuss inferential procedures for the setting with replicates of the surrogate measurements for Y_{ij}. Suppose the response variable for each subject in a cluster is measured repeatedly, and let S_{ijr} denote the rth observed measurement for subject j in cluster i, $r = 1, \ldots, d_{ij}$, where the replicate number d_{ij} can vary from subject to subject. For $r \neq r'$, S_{ijr} and $S_{ijr'}$ are assumed to be conditionally independent, given $\{\mathbf{Y}_i, \mathbf{X}_i, \mathbf{Z}_i, \mathbf{b}_i\}$. The marginal likelihood contributed from cluster i is given by

$$\mathscr{L}_{Ri}(\boldsymbol{\theta},\boldsymbol{\eta}) = \int f_b(\mathbf{b}_i;\boldsymbol{\sigma}_b) \prod_{j=1}^{m_i} \left\{ \int f_{y|x,z,b}(y_{ij}|\mathbf{x}_{ij}, \mathbf{z}_{ij}, \mathbf{b}_i;\boldsymbol{\theta}) \right.$$
$$\left. \times \prod_{r=1}^{d_{ij}} f_{s|y,x,z,b}(s_{ijr}|y_{ij}, \mathbf{x}_{ij}, \mathbf{z}_{ij}, \mathbf{b}_i;\boldsymbol{\eta}) dy_{ij} \right\} d\mathbf{b}_i.$$

Unlike the two-stage estimation procedure for the case with validation data, estimation for $\boldsymbol{\theta}$ and $\boldsymbol{\eta}$ generally cannot be separated from each other, because information on the underlying true responses and the measurement process is mixed together. A joint estimation procedure for $\{\boldsymbol{\theta},\boldsymbol{\eta}\}$ by maximizing $\prod_{i=1}^{n} \mathscr{L}_{Ri}(\boldsymbol{\theta},\boldsymbol{\eta})$ is particularly required.

Specifically, let

$$\mathscr{U}_i(\boldsymbol{\theta},\boldsymbol{\eta}) = \partial \log \mathscr{L}_{Ri}(\boldsymbol{\theta},\boldsymbol{\eta})/\partial \boldsymbol{\theta}, \quad \text{and} \quad \mathscr{Q}_i(\boldsymbol{\theta},\boldsymbol{\eta}) = \partial \log \mathscr{L}_{Ri}(\boldsymbol{\theta},\boldsymbol{\eta})/\partial \boldsymbol{\eta}$$

be the score functions. Define

$$\Psi_{Ri}(\boldsymbol{\theta},\boldsymbol{\eta}) = \begin{pmatrix} \mathscr{Q}_i(\boldsymbol{\theta},\boldsymbol{\eta}) \\ \mathscr{U}_i(\boldsymbol{\theta},\boldsymbol{\eta}) \end{pmatrix}.$$

The maximum likelihood estimators for $\boldsymbol{\theta}$ and η is obtained by solving

$$\sum_{i=1}^{n} \Psi_{Ri}(\boldsymbol{\theta}, \boldsymbol{\eta}) = \mathbf{0};$$

we let $(\hat{\boldsymbol{\theta}}_R, \hat{\boldsymbol{\eta}}_R)$ denote the solution.

Under suitable regularity conditions, $n^{1/2}\begin{pmatrix} \hat{\boldsymbol{\theta}}_R - \boldsymbol{\theta} \\ \hat{\boldsymbol{\eta}}_R - \boldsymbol{\eta} \end{pmatrix}$ is asymptotically normally distributed with mean $\mathbf{0}$ and covariance matrix $[E\{\Psi_{Ri}(\boldsymbol{\theta}, \boldsymbol{\eta})\Psi_{Ri}^{\mathrm{T}}(\boldsymbol{\theta}, \boldsymbol{\eta})\}]^{-1}$.

4.4 Numerical Approximation

To implement the proposed methods, numerical approximations are often needed because integrals involved in the likelihood formulations do not have analytic forms in general. With low dimensional integrals, Gaussian–Hermite quadratures may be invoked to handle integrals without a closed form. For example, the integral with an integrand of form $\exp(-u^2)f(u)$ is approximated by a sum

$$\int_{-\infty}^{\infty} \exp(-u^2)f(u)du \approx \sum_{k=1}^{K} w_k f(t_k),$$

where $f(\cdot)$ is a given function, K is the number of selected points, and t_k and w_k are the value and the weight of the kth designated point, respectively. The approximation accuracy relies on the order of the quadrature approximations. We found in our simulation that a quadrature approximation with order 5 performs adequately well for a single integral; as the number of random components increases, more quadrature points are required in order to obtain a good approximation. When $f(\cdot)$ is a symmetric or nearly symmetric function, the approximation is generally good, even when the number of quadrature points is chosen to be small.

Computation quickly becomes infeasible as the number of nested random components grows [9]. The convergence of an optimization procedure can be very slow if the dimension of the random components is high. One approach to deal with such integrals is to linearize the model with respect to the random effects, e.g., using a first-order population-averaged approximation to the marginal distribution by expanding the conditional distribution about the average random effect [12]. Alternatively, Laplace's approximation can be useful to obtain an approximate likelihood function with a closed form [12, 15]. The basic form of linearization using Laplace's approximation is a second-order Taylor series expansion of the integrand $f(\mathbf{u})$ and is given by $\int_{\mathbb{R}^d} f(\mathbf{u})d\mathbf{u} \approx (2\pi)^{d/2} f(\mathbf{u}_0)\left|-\partial^2 \log f(\mathbf{u}_0)/\partial\mathbf{u}\partial\mathbf{u}^{\mathrm{T}}\right|^{-1/2}$, where d is the dimension of $\mathbf{u}$, and $\mathbf{u}_0$ is the mode of $f(\mathbf{u})$, i.e., the solution to $\partial \log f(\mathbf{u})/\partial\mathbf{u} = \mathbf{0}$. To construct Laplace's approximation, the first two derivatives of $\log f(\mathbf{u})$ are basically required.

5 Simulation Studies

We conduct simulation studies to assess the performance of the proposed likelihood-based methods. We consider the setting with $n = 100$ and $m_i = 5$ for $i = 1, \ldots, n$. The covariates X_{ij} are simulated from the standard normal distribution, and random effects b_i are generated from a normal distribution with mean 0 and variance $\sigma_b^2 = 0.04$. The response measurements are generated from the model

$$Y_{ij} = \beta_0 + \beta_1 X_{ij} + b_i X_{ij} + \epsilon_{ij},$$

where $\epsilon_{ij} \sim N(0, \phi)$, and the parameter values are set as $\beta_0 = -1$, $\beta_1 = \log(0.5)$, and $\phi = 0.04$.

We consider two models for the measurement error process. That is, surrogate measurements S_{ij} are simulated from one of the two measurement error models:

(M1). $S_{ij} = \exp(\gamma Y_{ij}) + e_{ij}$,
(M2). $S_{ij} = \gamma_0 + \gamma_1 Y_{ij} + e_{ij}$,

where e_{ij} is independent of $\mathbf{Y}_i$ and $\mathbf{X}_i$, and follows a normal distribution with mean 0 and variance $\sigma_e^2 = 0.04$. For error model (M1), the error parameters are specified as $\gamma = 0.5$. For error model (M2), the parameters are specified as $\gamma_0 = 0.5$ and $\gamma_1 = 0.5$.

Let $\boldsymbol{\eta}$ denote the vector of associated parameters for the measurement error model. Specifically, in error model (M1), $\boldsymbol{\eta} = (\gamma, \sigma_e^2)^{\mathrm{T}}$; while in error model (M2), $\boldsymbol{\eta} = (\gamma_0, \gamma_1, \sigma_e^2)^{\mathrm{T}}$. We evaluate the proposed methods under two scenarios regarding the knowledge of $\boldsymbol{\eta}$: (i) $\boldsymbol{\eta}$ is treated as known, and (ii) $\boldsymbol{\eta}$ is estimated from internal validation data. For scenario (ii), we obtain a validation subsample by randomly selecting one subject from each cluster. We use Gaussian quadrature of order 15 in the numerical approximation for the likelihood-based approaches. Two thousand simulations are run for each parameter configuration.

We conduct three analyses for each simulated data set: the two naive approaches described in Sects. 3.1 and 3.2 and the proposed methods described in Sect. 4. We report the simulation results based on four measures: relative bias in percent (Bias%), sample standard deviation of the estimates (SD), average of model-based standard errors (ASE), and coverage probability of the 95 % confidence interval (CP%).

Table 1 reports the results for the exponential measurement error model (M1). As expected, the NAI1 approach produces very biased (attenuated) estimates of the fixed-effect parameter β_1, and the coverage rates of the 95 % confidence interval are close to 0. The NAI2 approach, which analyzes transformed surrogate responses, produces slightly better estimates of β_1. The magnitude of the relative bias, although smaller than that from NAI1, is still substantial. In contrast, the proposed likelihood approaches give consistent estimates for β_1 in both scenarios, and the coverage rates of its 95 % confidence intervals are close to the nominal value.

Table 2 reports the results for the linear measurement error model (M2). Again the estimates for β_1 from the NAI1 approach are biased, and the values are scaled

Table 1 Simulation results for cases with measurement error model (M1) (2000 simulations)

	NAI1[a]				NAI2[b]				Proposed[c]			
	Bias%	SD	ASE	CP%	Bias%	SD	ASE	CP%	Bias%	SD	ASE	CP%
	Scenario (i): η is known											
β_0	−164.5	0.011	0.010	< 0.1	16.7	0.051	0.046	5.0	−0.56	0.037	0.035	94.2
β_1	−67.7	0.013	0.014	< 0.1	16.0	0.064	0.060	52.9	−0.83	0.040	0.039	94.9
σ_b^2	−80.3	0.003	0.184	100.0	235.8	0.090	0.253	94.3	−2.13	0.016	0.018	93.8
ϕ	17.6	0.003	0.035	100.0	2439.1	0.234	0.035	< 0.1	3.65	0.022	0.025	96.0
	Scenario (ii): η is estimated from internal validation data											
β_0	–	–	–	–	13.7	0.072	0.042	19.8	−0.04	0.040	0.042	94.8
β_1	–	–	–	–	13.1	0.067	0.054	61.0	0.32	0.053	0.049	94.6
σ_b^2	–	–	–	–	183.4	0.079	0.242	96.4	4.57	0.024	0.028	95.7
ϕ	–	–	–	–	1975.9	0.220	0.035	< 0.1	−3.14	0.017	0.014	93.3

[a]NAI1: naive LMM analysis of observed data ignoring measurement error.
[b]NAI2: naive LMM analysis of the constructed pseudo-response data.
[c]Proposed: the proposed likelihood method that accounts for measurement error.

Table 2 Simulation results for cases with linear measurement error model (M2) (2000 simulations)

	NAI1[a]				NAI2[b]				Proposed[c]			
	Bias%	SD	ASE	CP%	Bias%	SD	ASE	CP%	Bias%	SD	ASE	CP%
	Scenario (i): η is known											
β_0	−100.0	0.010	0.010	< 0.1	−0.04	0.021	0.021	95.2	−0.04	0.021	0.022	95.8
β_1	−50.0	0.015	0.015	< 0.1	0.08	0.030	0.030	94.3	0.10	0.030	0.030	94.8
σ_b^2	−75.0	0.003	0.162	100.0	−0.01	0.012	0.162	100.0	−3.28	0.012	0.013	94.9
ϕ	25.0	0.003	0.035	100.0	400.12	0.014	0.035	< 0.1	−0.96	0.014	0.014	95.1
	Scenario (ii): η is estimated from internal validation data											
β_0	–	–	–	–	−0.13	0.037	0.021	75.3	−0.11	0.031	0.030	94.3
β_1	–	–	–	–	0.44	0.043	0.030	84.0	0.22	0.039	0.041	95.6
σ_b^2	–	–	–	–	0.96	0.013	0.161	100.0	−2.72	0.017	0.017	94.8
ϕ	–	–	–	–	406.53	0.025	0.035	< 0.1	−2.02	0.018	0.022	95.7

[a]NAI1: naive LMM analysis of observed data ignoring measurement error.
[b]NAI2: naive LMM analysis of the constructed pseudo-response data.
[c]Proposed: the proposed likelihood method that accounts for measurement error.

approximately by a factor of γ_1, which is in agreement with the analytical result shown in Sect. 3. The NAI2 approach yields good estimates for β_0, β_1, and σ_b^2 with small finite sample biases. The NAI2 estimates for ϕ, however, are very biased, resulting in coverage rates of corresponding confidence intervals far from the nominal value of 95 %. In contrast, the proposed likelihood-based approach gives consistent estimators for the fixed-effect and variance component, and the associated standard errors are similar to the empirical standard deviations. As a result, the coverage rates of the 95 % confidence intervals are close to the nominal value.

6 Application

We illustrate our proposed methods by analyzing the data from the Framingham Heart Study. The data set includes exams #2 and #3 for $n = 1615$ male subjects aged 31–65 [3]. Two systolic blood pressure (SBP) readings were taken during each exam. One of the clinical interests is to understand the relationship between SBP and potential risk factors such as baseline smoking status and age [6, 8, 11]. The risk factors, however, may not have linear effects on SBP directly.

Preliminary exploration shows that SBP measurements are skewed, and using a square-root transformation to $(T_{ij} - 50)$ is reasonably satisfactory for obtaining a symmetric data distribution, where T_{ij} represents the true SBP measurement for subject i at time j, where $j = 1$ corresponds to exam #2, and $j = 2$ for exam #3, and $i = 1, \ldots, n$. We now let Y_{ij} denote such a transformed variable, i.e., $Y_{ij} = \sqrt{T_{ij} - 50}$. We assume that the Y_{ij} follow the model

$$Y_{ij} = \beta_0 + \beta_{\text{age}} X_{ij1} + \beta_{\text{smoke}} X_{ij2} + \beta_{\text{exam}} X_{ij3} + b_i + \epsilon_{ij}, \quad j = 1, 2, \; i = 1, \ldots, n,$$

where X_{ij1} is the baseline age of subject i at exam #2, X_{ij2} is the indicator variable for baseline smoking status of subject i at exam #1, X_{ij3} is 1 if $j = 2$ and 0 otherwise, and b_i and ϵ_{ij} are assumed to be independently and normally distributed with means 0 and variances given by σ_b^2 and ϕ, respectively.

Because a subject's SBP changes over time, the two individual SBP readings at each exam are regarded as replicated surrogates. Several measurement error models for SBP reading have been proposed by different researchers [2, 7, 13]. Let T_{ijr}^* be the rth observed SBP reading for subject i at time j, $i = 1, \ldots, n, j = 1, 2, r = 1, 2$. We consider an error model $\log(T_{ijr}^* - 50) = \log(T_{ij} - 50) + e_{ijr}$, suggested by Wang et al. [13], where the e_{ijr} are assumed to be independent of each other and of other variables, and are normally distributed with mean 0 and variance σ_e^2. Let S_{ijr} denote $\log(T_{ijr}^* - 50)$, then the measurement error model is equivalently given by

$$S_{ijr} = 2\log(Y_{ij}) + e_{ijr}.$$

Table 3 Analysis of data from the Framingham Heart Study

	NAI1[a]			NAI2[b]			Proposed[c]		
	Est.	SE	p-value	Est.	SE	p-value	Est.	SE	p-value
β_0	4.117	0.030	< 0.001	7.727	0.140	< 0.001	7.729	0.156	< 0.001
β_{age}	0.006	0.001	< 0.001	0.029	0.003	< 0.001	0.027	0.003	< 0.001
β_{smoke}	−0.027	0.012	0.031	−0.122	0.057	0.032	−0.120	0.061	0.048
β_{exam}	−0.020	0.004	< 0.001	−0.086	0.018	< 0.001	−0.087	0.017	< 0.001
σ_b^2	0.036	0.021	0.083	0.782	0.020	< 0.001	0.754	0.040	< 0.001
ϕ	0.013	0.018	0.474	0.248	0.018	< 0.001	0.120	0.007	< 0.001

[a]NAI1: naive LMM analysis of observed data ignoring measurement error.
[b]NAI2: naive LMM analysis of the constructed pseudo-response data.
[c]Proposed: the proposed likelihood method that accounts for measurement error.

Table 3 reports results from analyses using the proposed method and the two naive approaches. The estimated regression coefficients β_{age}, β_{smoke}, and β_{exam} from the proposed method are 0.027, −0.120, and −0.087, respectively. At the 5 % significance level, age is significantly associated with increasing blood pressure. The negative coefficient for smoking status may suggest an effect of smoking on decreasing blood pressure. As expected, the results from the NAI2 approach are similar to those from the proposed method due to the small value of the measurement error variance. The NAI1 estimates, however, are not comparable to those from the NAI2 and the proposed method, possibly in part due to a different scale of the response variable.

7 Discussion

In this paper, we exploit analysis of response-error-contaminated clustered data within the framework of generalized linear mixed models. Although in some situations ignoring error in response does not alter point estimates of regression parameters, ignoring error in response does affect inference results for general circumstances. Error in response can produce seriously biased results.

In this paper we perform asymptotic bias analysis to assess the impact of ignoring error in response. We investigate the performance of a partial-error-correction method that was intuitively used in the literature [1]. To fully account for error effects, we develop valid inferential procedures for various practical settings which pertain to the information on response error. Simulation studies demonstrate satisfactory performance of the proposed methods under various settings.

Appendix

Let $\Psi_i(\boldsymbol{\theta}, \boldsymbol{\eta}) = \begin{pmatrix} \mathbf{Q}_i(\boldsymbol{\eta}) \\ \mathbf{U}_i^*(\boldsymbol{\theta}, \boldsymbol{\eta}) \end{pmatrix}$. Because $(\hat{\boldsymbol{\theta}}_p, \hat{\boldsymbol{\eta}})$ is a solution to $\Psi_i(\boldsymbol{\theta}, \boldsymbol{\eta}) = 0$, by first-order Taylor series approximation, we have

$$n^{1/2} \begin{pmatrix} \hat{\boldsymbol{\eta}} - \boldsymbol{\eta} \\ \hat{\boldsymbol{\theta}}_p - \boldsymbol{\theta} \end{pmatrix} = - \begin{pmatrix} E\{\partial \mathbf{Q}_i(\boldsymbol{\eta})/\partial \boldsymbol{\eta}^{\mathrm{T}}\} & 0 \\ E\{\partial \mathbf{U}_i^*(\boldsymbol{\theta}, \boldsymbol{\eta})/\partial \boldsymbol{\eta}^{\mathrm{T}}\} & E\{\partial \mathbf{U}_i^*(\boldsymbol{\theta}, \boldsymbol{\eta})/\partial \boldsymbol{\theta}^{\mathrm{T}}\} \end{pmatrix}^{-1}$$

$$\times\, n^{-1/2} \sum_{i=1}^{n} \Psi_i(\boldsymbol{\theta}, \boldsymbol{\eta}) + o_p(1).$$

It follows that $n^{1/2}(\hat{\boldsymbol{\theta}}_p - \boldsymbol{\theta})$ equals

$$-n^{-1/2} \left[E\{\partial \mathbf{U}_i^*(\boldsymbol{\theta}, \boldsymbol{\eta})/\partial \boldsymbol{\theta}^{\mathrm{T}}\}\right]^{-1} \left\{ \sum_{i=1}^{n} \mathbf{U}_i^*(\boldsymbol{\theta}, \boldsymbol{\eta}) - E\{\partial \mathbf{U}_i^*(\boldsymbol{\theta}, \boldsymbol{\eta})/\partial \boldsymbol{\eta}^{\mathrm{T}}\} \right.$$

$$\left. \times \left[E\{\partial \mathbf{Q}_i(\boldsymbol{\eta})/\partial \boldsymbol{\eta}^{\mathrm{T}}\}\right]^{-1} \sum_{i=1}^{n} \mathbf{Q}_i(\boldsymbol{\eta}) \right\} + o_p(1) = -n^{-1/2} \Gamma^{-1}(\boldsymbol{\theta}, \boldsymbol{\eta})$$

$$\sum_{i=1}^{n} \Omega_i(\boldsymbol{\theta}, \boldsymbol{\eta}) + o_p(1),$$

where $\Omega_i(\boldsymbol{\theta}, \boldsymbol{\eta}) = \mathbf{U}_i^*(\boldsymbol{\theta}, \boldsymbol{\eta}) - E\{\partial \mathbf{U}_i^*(\boldsymbol{\theta}, \boldsymbol{\eta})/\partial \boldsymbol{\eta}^{\mathrm{T}}\}[E\{\partial \mathbf{Q}_i(\boldsymbol{\eta})/\partial \boldsymbol{\eta}^{\mathrm{T}}\}]^{-1}\mathbf{Q}_i(\boldsymbol{\eta})$, and $\Gamma(\boldsymbol{\theta}, \boldsymbol{\eta}) = E\{\partial \mathbf{U}_i^*(\boldsymbol{\theta}, \boldsymbol{\eta})/\partial \boldsymbol{\theta}^{\mathrm{T}}\}$.

Applying the Central Limit Theorem, we can show that $n^{1/2}(\hat{\boldsymbol{\theta}}_p - \boldsymbol{\theta})$ is asymptotically normally distributed with mean 0 and asymptotic covariance matrix given by $\Gamma^{-1}\Sigma(\Gamma^{-1})^{\mathrm{T}}$, where $\Sigma = E\{\Omega_i(\boldsymbol{\theta}, \boldsymbol{\eta})\Omega_i^{\mathrm{T}}(\boldsymbol{\theta}, \boldsymbol{\eta})\}$. But under suitable regularity conditions and correct model specification, $E\{\mathbf{U}_i^*(\boldsymbol{\theta}, \boldsymbol{\eta})\mathbf{U}_i^{*\mathrm{T}}(\boldsymbol{\theta}, \boldsymbol{\eta})\} = E\{-\partial \mathbf{U}_i^*(\boldsymbol{\theta}, \boldsymbol{\eta})/\partial \boldsymbol{\theta}^{\mathrm{T}}\}$, $E\{\mathbf{Q}_i(\boldsymbol{\eta})\mathbf{Q}_i^{\mathrm{T}}(\boldsymbol{\eta})\} = E\{-\partial \mathbf{Q}_i(\boldsymbol{\eta})/\partial \boldsymbol{\eta}^{\mathrm{T}}\}$, and $E\{\mathbf{U}_i^*(\boldsymbol{\theta}, \boldsymbol{\eta})\mathbf{Q}_i^{\mathrm{T}}(\boldsymbol{\eta})\} = E\{-\partial \mathbf{U}_i^*(\boldsymbol{\theta}, \boldsymbol{\eta})/\partial \boldsymbol{\eta}^{\mathrm{T}}\}$. Thus,

$$\Sigma = E\{-\partial \mathbf{U}_i^*(\boldsymbol{\theta}, \boldsymbol{\eta})/\partial \boldsymbol{\theta}^{\mathrm{T}}\} + E\{\partial \mathbf{U}_i^*(\boldsymbol{\theta}, \boldsymbol{\eta})/\partial \boldsymbol{\eta}^{\mathrm{T}}\} \left[E\{\partial \mathbf{Q}_i(\boldsymbol{\eta})/\partial \boldsymbol{\eta}^{\mathrm{T}}\}\right]^{-1}$$

$$\times \left[E\{\partial \mathbf{U}_i^*(\boldsymbol{\theta}, \boldsymbol{\eta})/\partial \boldsymbol{\eta}^{\mathrm{T}}\}\right]^{\mathrm{T}}.$$

Therefore, the asymptotic covariance matrix for $n^{1/2}(\hat{\boldsymbol{\theta}}_p - \boldsymbol{\theta})$ is

$$\Sigma^* = \left[E\{-\partial \mathbf{U}_i^*(\boldsymbol{\theta}, \boldsymbol{\eta})/\partial \boldsymbol{\theta}^{\mathrm{T}}\}\right]^{-1} + \left[E\{-\partial \mathbf{U}_i^*(\boldsymbol{\theta}, \boldsymbol{\eta})/\partial \boldsymbol{\theta}^{\mathrm{T}}\}\right]^{-1} E\{\partial \mathbf{U}_i^*(\boldsymbol{\theta}, \boldsymbol{\eta})/\partial \boldsymbol{\eta}^{\mathrm{T}}\}$$

$$\times \left[E\{\partial \mathbf{Q}_i(\boldsymbol{\eta})/\partial \boldsymbol{\eta}^{\mathrm{T}}\}\right]^{-1} \left[E\{\partial \mathbf{U}_i^*(\boldsymbol{\theta}, \boldsymbol{\eta})/\partial \boldsymbol{\eta}^{\mathrm{T}}\}\right]^{\mathrm{T}} \left[E\{-\partial \mathbf{U}_i^*(\boldsymbol{\theta}, \boldsymbol{\eta})/\partial \boldsymbol{\theta}^{\mathrm{T}}\}\right]^{-1}.$$

Acknowledgements This research was supported by grants from the Natural Sciences and Engineering Research Council of Canada (G. Y. Yi and C. Wu).

References

1. Buonaccorsi, J.P.: Measurement error in the response in the general linear model. J. Am. Stat. Assoc. **91**, 633–642 (1996)
2. Carroll, R.J., Spiegelman, C.H., Gordon, K.K., Bailey, K.K., Abbott, R.D.: On errors-in-variables for binary regression models. Biometrika **71**, 19–25 (1984)
3. Carroll, R.J., Ruppert, D., Stefanski, L.A., Crainiceanu, C.M.: Measurement error in nonlinear models: a modern perspective, 2nd edn. Chapman and Hall/CRC, London (2006)
4. Chen, Z., Yi, G.Y., Wu, C.: Marginal methods for correlated binary data with misclassified responses. Biometrika **98**, 647–662 (2011)
5. Diggle, P.J., Heagerty, P., Liang, K.Y., Zeger, S.L.: Analysis of Longitudinal Data, 2nd edn. Oxford University Press, New York (2002)
6. Ferrara, L.A., Guida, L., Iannuzzi, R., Celentano, A., Lionello, F.: Serum cholesterol affects blood pressure regulation. J. Hum. Hypertens. **16**, 337–343 (2002)
7. Hall, P., Ma, Y.Y.: Semiparametric estimators of functional measurement error models with unknown error. J. R. Stat. Soc. Ser. B **69**, 429–446 (2007)
8. Jaquet, F., Goldstein, I.B., Shapiro, D.: Effects of age and gender on ambulatory blood pressure and heart rate. J. Hum. Hypertens. **12**, 253–257 (1998)
9. McCulloch, C.E., Searle, S.R.: Generalized, Linear, and Mixed Models. Wiley, New York (2001)
10. Neuhaus, J.M.: Bias and efficiency loss due to misclassified responses in binary regression. Biometrika **86**, 843–855 (1996)
11. Primatesta, P., Falaschetti, E., Gupta, S., Marmot, M.G., Poulter, N.R.: Association between smoking and blood pressure - evidence from the health survey for England. Hypertension **37**, 187–193 (2001)
12. Vonesh, E.F.: A note on the use of Laplace's approximation for nonlinear mixed-effects models. Biometrika **83**, 447–452 (1996)
13. Wang, N., Lin, X., Gutierrez, R.G., Carroll, R.J.: Bias analysis and SIMEX approach in generalized linear mixed measurement error models. J. Am. Stat. Assoc. **93**, 249–261 (1998)
14. White, H.: Maximum likelihood estimation of misspecified models. Econometrica **50**, 1–25 (1982)
15. Wolfinger, R.: Laplace's approximation for nonlinear mixed models. Biometrika **80**, 791–795 (1993)
16. Yi, G.Y.: A simulation-based marginal method for longitudinal data with dropout and mismeasured covariates. Biostatistics **9**, 501–512 (2008)
17. Yi, G.Y.: Measurement error in life history data. Int. J. Stat. Sci. **9**, 177–197 (2009)
18. Yi, G.Y., Cook, R.J. Errors in the measurement of covariates. In: The Encyclopedia of Biostatistics, 2nd edn., vol. 3, pp. 1741–1748. Wiley, New York (2005)
19. Yi, G.Y., Liu, W., Wu, L.: Simultaneous inference and bias analysis for longitudinal data with covariate measurement error and missing responses. Biometrics 67, 67–75 (2011)
20. Zucker, D.M.: A pseudo-partial likelihood method for semiparametric survival regression with covariate errors. J. Am. Stat. Assoc. **100**, 1264–1277 (2005)

Bias-Reduced Moment Estimators of Population Spectral Distribution and Their Applications

Yingli Qin and Weiming Li

Abstract In this paper, we propose a series of bias-reduced moment estimators for the Population Spectral Distribution (PSD) of large covariance matrices, which are fundamentally important for modern high-dimensional statistics. In addition, we derive the limiting distributions of these moment estimators, which are then adopted to test the order of PSDs. The simulation study demonstrates the desirable performance of the order test in conjunction with the proposed moment estimators for the PSD of large covariance matrices.

Keywords Asymptotically normal • Consistency • Covariance matrix • High-dimension • Hypothesis testing • Moment estimator • Population spectral distribution

1 Introduction

Statistical inference concerning large covariance matrices is developing rapidly, due to the wide availability of high-dimensional data from a variety of scientific, economic, and social studies. Some specific structural assumptions about covariance matrices are often considered, e.g., sparsity in terms of population eigenvalues and eigenvectors or sparsity in terms of the entries of covariance matrices. Johnstone [11] proposes that there only exist a fixed number r of population eigenvalues separated from the bulk. In an even more extreme case, Berthet and Rigollet [4] assume $r = 1$ and the covariance matrix can be modeled as $I + \theta \nu \nu^T$, where ν is a unit length sparse vector and $\theta \in \mathbb{R}^+$. Birnbaum et al. [5] propose adaptive estimation of $r \geq 1$ individual leading eigenvectors when the ordered entries of each eigenvector decay rapidly.

Y. Qin
Department of Statistics and Actuarial Science, University of Waterloo, Waterloo, ON, Canada N2L 3G1
e-mail: yingli.qin@uwaterloo.ca

W. Li (✉)
Shanghai University of Finance and Economics, Shanghai, China
e-mail: liwm601@gmail.com

© Springer International Publishing AG 2017

S.E. Ahmed (ed.), *Big and Complex Data Analysis*, Contributions to Statistics,
DOI 10.1007/978-3-319-41573-4_6

In high-dimensional framework, where the dimension p and the sample size n are both large, estimating Population Spectral Distribution (PSD) H_p of covariance matrix Σ_p has attracted much attention recently, see [3, 9, 12, 14, 15, 19]. In [15], the estimation is designed for discrete PSDs with finite support. In [9], the proposed method is evaluated by three simple models considered in their simulation study: $\Sigma_p = I_p$, $H_p = 0.5\delta_1 + 0.5\delta_2$, and a Toeplitz covariance matrix. For the first model, all population eigenvalues are equal to 1, which is a special case of order 1 discrete PSDs, i.e., $H_p = \delta_1$, while the second model is of order 2 (with mass points 1 and 2) and the third is of order p (i.e., continuous PSD as $p \to \infty$).

In this paper, our main contribution is to propose bias-reduced moment estimators for the PSD of large covariance matrices. These moment estimators can be proved to enjoy some desirable theoretical properties. We then adopt the test in [18] in conjunction with the proposed moment estimators to test the order of PSDs.

Specifically, we assume that under the null hypothesis, there are k distinct population eigenvalues $a_1, \ldots, a_k$, and their multiplicities are $p_1, \ldots, p_k$, respectively. Then the PSD H_p can be expressed as

$$H_p = w_1\delta_{a_1} + \cdots + w_k\delta_{a_k}, \tag{1}$$

where $w_i = p_i/p$ and thus $\sum_{i=1}^{k} w_i = 1$. This model has been considered in [3, 12, 14, 15, 19], where the estimation of H_p is developed by assuming the order $k = k_0$ is known. This assumption does not cause any serious problem if the true order k is smaller than k_0, since the model with higher order contains the (smaller) true model. But if $k > k_0$, then any estimation based on $k = k_0$ can surely lead to erroneous result. Another closely related work is [7], in which the authors develop a cross-validation type procedure to estimate the order k. However, their estimators cannot be used to test the order of PSDs because of the lack of asymptotic distributions. Qin and Li [18] consider the following hypotheses to find statistical evidence to support that there are no more than k_0 distinct mass points in H_p.

$$H_0 : k \leq k_0 \quad \text{v.s.} \quad H_1 : k > k_0, \quad k_0 \in \mathbb{N}. \tag{2}$$

The rest of the paper is organized as follows. In the next section, we discuss the bias-reduced estimation of moments of PSDs. In Sect. 3, we reformulate the test in [18] with our proposed moment estimators. Section 4 reports simulation results. Concluding remarks are presented in Sect. 5 and proofs of the main theorems are postponed to the last section.

2 Moments of a PSD and Their Bias-Reduced Estimators

Let $\mathbf{x}_1, \ldots, \mathbf{x}_n$, $\mathbf{x}_i \in \mathbb{R}^p$, be a sequence of independent and identically distributed zero mean random vectors with a common population covariance matrix Σ_p. The sample covariance matrix is

$$S_n = \frac{1}{n}\sum_{i=1}^{n} \mathbf{x}_i\mathbf{x}_i'.$$

Note that the population mean is assumed to be zero for simplicity, if not, one may replace S_n with its centralized version.

Let H_p be the PSD of Σ_p and F_n be the empirical spectral distribution (ESD) of S_n. Integer moments of H_p and F_n are, respectively, defined as

$$\gamma_k := \int t^k dH_p(t) \quad \text{and} \quad \hat{\beta}_k := \int x^k dF_n(x),$$

$k = 0, 1, 2, \ldots$. Unbiased estimators of γ_k's based on $\hat{\beta}_k$'s under normality are provided in [10, 21]. However, their results are limited to $k \leq 4$. In [3, 12, 13], more general moment estimators are introduced. However, their estimators are biased. Moreover, their asymptotic means and variances have no explicit forms, and are expressed through contour integrals only. In this paper, we present an explicit bias-reduced version of the estimators in [3].

Our main assumptions are listed as follows. These three assumptions are conventional conditions for the central limit theorem of linear spectral statistics, see [1, 2].

Assumption (a) The sample size n and the dimension p both tend to infinity such that $c_n := p/n \to c \in (0, \infty)$.

Assumption (b) There is a doubly infinite array of i.i.d. random variables (w_{ij}), $i, j \geq 1$, satisfying

$$E(w_{11}) = 0, \;\; E(w_{11}^2) = 1, \;\; E(w_{11}^4) < \infty,$$

such that for every given p, n pair, $W_n = (w_{ij})_{1\leq i\leq p, 1\leq j\leq n}$. Hence, the observed data vectors can be represented as $\mathbf{x}_j = \Sigma_p^{1/2} w_{\cdot j}$ where $w_{\cdot j} = (w_{ij})_{1\leq i\leq p}$ denotes the jth column of W_n.

Assumption (c) The PSD H_p of Σ_p weakly converges to a probability distribution H, as $p \to \infty$, and the sequence of spectral norms $(||\Sigma_p||)$ is bounded.

Under the assumptions (a)–(c), the ESD F_n converges in distribution to a determinate distribution $F^{c,H}$ [20], called the limiting spectral distribution (LSD), and the moments γ_k and $\hat{\beta}_k$ also converge,

$$\gamma_k \to \tilde{\gamma}_k := \int t^k dH(t) \quad \text{and} \quad \hat{\beta}_k \to \tilde{\beta}_k := \int x^k dF^{c,H}(x).$$

Moreover, these limiting moments $\tilde{\gamma}_k$'s and $\tilde{\beta}_k$'s are linked through a series of recursive formulas [16],

$$\begin{aligned}
\tilde{\gamma}_1 &= \tilde{\beta}_1, \\
\tilde{\gamma}_2 &= \tilde{\beta}_2 - c\tilde{\gamma}_1^2, \\
\tilde{\gamma}_k &= \tilde{\beta}_k - \frac{1}{c}\sum (c\tilde{\gamma}_1)^{i_1}(c\tilde{\gamma}_2)^{i_2}\cdots(c\tilde{\gamma}_{k-1})^{i_{k-1}}\phi(i_1,\ldots,i_{k-1}), \quad k \geq 2,
\end{aligned}$$

where the sum runs over the following partitions of k:

$$(i_1,\ldots,i_{k-1}) : k = i_1 + 2i_2 + \cdots + (k-1)i_{k-1}, \quad i_l \in \mathbb{N},$$

and the coefficient $\phi(i_1,\ldots,i_{k-1}) = k!/[i_1!\cdots i_{k-1}!(k+1-i_1-\cdots i_{k-1})!]$.

Bai et al. [3] just plug $\hat{\beta}_k$'s into these recursive formulas to get the estimators of γ_k's (also estimators of $\tilde{\gamma}_k$'s).

It's obvious that the mapping from $\tilde{\beta}_k$'s to $\tilde{\gamma}_k$'s,

$$g : (\tilde{\beta}_1,\ldots,\tilde{\beta}_k)' \to (\tilde{\gamma}_1,\ldots,\tilde{\gamma}_k)', \tag{3}$$

is one-to-one and its Jacobian matrix $\partial g(\beta)/\partial\beta$ is a lower-triangular matrix with unit determinant. Therefore, the properties of the plug-in estimators are fully determined by those of $\hat{\beta}_k$'s which actually, as estimators of $\tilde{\beta}_k$'s when $H_p = H$ and $c_n = c$, are biased by the order of $O(1/p)$ [1]. In this paper, our main contribution is to correct the bias and propose bias-reduced moment estimators.

Let $q_{s,t}$ be the coefficient of z^t in the Taylor expansion of $(1+z)^{-s}$ at $z = 0$ and define three power series $P(z)$, $Q(z)$, and $R(z)$ as

$$P(z) = -1 - c\sum_{l=1}^{\infty} \tilde{\gamma}_l(-z)^l, \tag{4}$$

$$Q(z) = c\sum_{l=0}^{\infty} q_{3,l}\tilde{\gamma}_{l+2}z^l, \quad R(z) = 1 - c\sum_{l=0}^{\infty} q_{2,l}\tilde{\gamma}_{l+2}z^{l+2}. \tag{5}$$

Let μ_k ($k \geq 1$) be the coefficient of z^{k-2} in the Taylor expansion of function $P^k(z)Q(z)/R(z)$ at $z = 0$. Apparently $\mu_1 = 0$. When calculating μ_k for $k \geq 2$, it's enough to keep the terms of z^l for $l \leq k-2$ in the series P, Q, and R since higher order terms, after taking derivatives of order $k-2$, are all zero at $z = 0$. Therefore, μ_k is a function of $c, \tilde{\gamma}_1,\ldots,\tilde{\gamma}_k$, and thus a function of $c, \tilde{\beta}_1,\ldots,\tilde{\beta}_k$.

It will be shown that μ_k/p is approximately the leading term of the bias contained in $\hat{\beta}_k$, and hence we modify this estimator to

$$\hat{\beta}_k^* = \hat{\beta}_k - \frac{1}{p}\hat{\mu}_k,$$

where $\hat{\mu}_k = \mu_k(c_n, \hat{\beta}_1, \ldots, \hat{\beta}_k)$, $k = 1, 2, \ldots$. The correction can be conducted iteratively by updating $\hat{\mu}_k$ from $\hat{\beta}_k^*$'s to reduce the bias to the order of $o(1/p)$. As a consequence, we obtain bias-reduced estimators of the moments γ_k's, referred to as $\hat{\gamma}_k$'s,

$$(\hat{\gamma}_1, \ldots, \hat{\gamma}_k)' = g(\hat{\beta}_1^*, \ldots, \hat{\beta}_k^*), \tag{6}$$

$k = 1, 2, \ldots$.

Theorem 1 *Suppose that the assumptions* (a)–(c) *hold, then*

(i) *the estimator $\hat{\gamma}_k$ $(k \geq 1)$ is strongly consistent, i.e.,*

$$\hat{\gamma}_k - \gamma_k \xrightarrow{a.s.} 0.$$

(ii) *If in addition $E(w_{11}^4) = 3$, then*

$$p\,(\hat{\gamma}_1 - \gamma_1, \ldots, \hat{\gamma}_k - \gamma_k)' \xrightarrow{D} N_k(0, \Psi(k)), \tag{7}$$

where $\Psi(k) = ABA'$, A is the Jacobian matrix $\partial g(\beta)/\partial \beta$ at $\beta = (\tilde{\beta}_k)$, and $B = (b_{ij})_{1 \leq i,j \leq k}$ with its entries

$$b_{ij} = 2\sum_{l=0}^{i-1}(i-l)\alpha_{i,l}\alpha_{j,i+j-l},$$

where $\alpha_{s,t}$ is the coefficient of z^t in the Taylor expansion of $P^s(z)$, the sth power of $P(z)$ defined in (4) .

Theorem 1 establishes the consistency and asymptotic normality of the proposed bias-reduced moment estimators $\hat{\gamma}_k$'s. Compared with the estimators in [3], our proposed moment estimators have two main advantages: One is that the limiting mean vector in (7) is zero, which implies that our estimators reduce biases to the order of $o(1/p)$; The other is that the limiting covariance matrix in (7) is explicitly formulated.

3 Test Procedure

Define a $(k+1) \times (k+1)$ Hankel matrix $\Gamma(G,k)$ related to a distribution G,

$$\Gamma(G,k) = \begin{pmatrix} g_0 & g_1 & \cdots & g_k \\ g_1 & g_2 & \cdots & g_{k+1} \\ \vdots & \vdots & & \vdots \\ g_k & g_{k+1} & \cdots & g_{2k} \end{pmatrix},$$

where g_j is the jth moment of G, $j = 0, \ldots, 2k$. Write $D(k) = \det(\Gamma(H_p,k))$ then, from Proposition 1 in [12], $D(k_0) = 0$ if the null hypothesis in (2) holds, otherwise $D(k_0) > 0$. On the other hand, from Theorem 1, a plug-in estimator of this determinant, denoted by $\widehat{D}(k_0)$, can be obtained by replacing γ_k in $D(k_0)$ with $\hat{\gamma}_k$, defined in (6), for $k = 1, \ldots, 2k_0$, i.e.,

$$\widehat{D}(k_0) = \begin{vmatrix} \hat{\gamma}_0 & \hat{\gamma}_1 & \cdots & \hat{\gamma}_{k_0} \\ \hat{\gamma}_1 & \hat{\gamma}_2 & \cdots & \hat{\gamma}_{k_0+1} \\ \vdots & \vdots & & \vdots \\ \hat{\gamma}_{k_0} & \hat{\gamma}_{k_0+1} & \cdots & \hat{\gamma}_{2k_0} \end{vmatrix}.$$

We may thus reject the null hypothesis if $\widehat{D}(k_0)$ is significantly greater than zero. Applying Theorem 1 and the main theorem in [18], we may immediately derive the asymptotic distribution of $\widehat{D}(k_0)$.

Theorem 2 *Suppose that the assumptions* (a)–(c) *hold, then the statistic* $\widehat{D}(k_0)$ *is asymptotically normal, i.e.,*

$$p\left(\widehat{D}(k_0) - D(k_0)\right) \xrightarrow{D} N(0, \sigma_{k_0}^2),$$

where $\sigma_{k_0}^2 = \alpha' V \Omega V' \alpha$ *with* $\alpha = vec(adj(\Gamma(H,k_0)))$, *the vectorization of the adjugate matrix of* $\Gamma(H,k_0)$. *The* $(2k_0+1) \times (2k_0+1)$ *matrix* Ω *consists of the first row and column zero and the remaining submatrix* $\Psi(2k_0)$ *defined in* (7), *and the* $(k_0+1)^2 \times (2k_0+1)$ *matrix* $V = (v_{ij})$ *is a 0-1 matrix with only* $v_{i,a_i} = 1$, $a_i = i - \lfloor (i-1)/(k_0+1) \rfloor k_0$, $i = 1, \ldots, (k_0+1)^2$, *where* $\lfloor x \rfloor$ *denotes the greatest integer not exceeding* x.

To present the limiting null distribution and guarantee the consistency of the order test, we need the following assumption:

Assumption (d) The order of H_p is consistent with the order of H, that is, they simultaneously satisfy the null hypothesis or the alternative in (2).

This assumption is a generalized version of the condition that the order of H_p is equal to that of its limit H, which requires the weight parameters $w_i = p_i/p$ of H_p in (1) all converge to some positive constants, which, for example, excludes the spike model $H_p = (1 - 1/p)\delta_1 + (1/p)\delta_a$, for some $a \neq 1$, see [11]. Notice that the order of H_p for their spike model is always 2 but that of H is 1.

From Theorem 1, the unknown parameters involved in the limiting variance $\sigma^2_{k_0}$ are $c, \tilde{\gamma}_1, \ldots, \tilde{\gamma}_{4k_0}$. Under the null hypothesis and Assumption (d), $\tilde{\gamma}_k$ for $k \geq 2k_0$ is a function of $\tilde{\gamma}_1, \tilde{\gamma}_2, \ldots, \tilde{\gamma}_{2k_0-1}$. A numerical algorithm for obtaining $\tilde{\gamma}_k$ from the lower moments is introduced in [12]. Therefore, under the null hypothesis, a strongly consistent estimator of $\sigma^2_{k_0}$ is $\sigma^2_{k_0}(c_n, \hat{\gamma}_1, \ldots, \hat{\gamma}_{2k_0-1})$, denoted by $\hat{\sigma}^2_{H_0}$.

Theorem 3 *Suppose that the assumptions* (a)–(d) *hold then, under the null hypothesis,*

$$\frac{p\widehat{D}(k_0)}{\hat{\sigma}_{H_0}} \xrightarrow{D} N(0, 1),$$

where $\hat{\sigma}_{H_0}$ *is the square root of* $\hat{\sigma}^2_{H_0}$.

Theorem 4 *Suppose that the assumptions* (a)–(d) *hold, then the asymptotic power of the order test tends to 1, as* $(n, p) \to \infty$.

4 Simulation

4.1 Case of Testing for Order Two PSDs

We report on simulations carried out to evaluate the performance of the order test. Samples are drawn from zero mean multivariate normal population $N_p(0, \Sigma)$. The sample size is $n = 100, 200, 300, 400, 500$ and the dimension to sample size ratio is $c = 1, 3, 5, 7$. The number of independent replications is 10,000.

We first examine empirical sizes of the test. The model under the null hypothesis is

$$H_p = w_1\delta_{a_1} + w_2\delta_{a_2},$$

where the distinct mass points are fixed at $(a_1, a_2) = (1, 4)$ and their weights are $(w_1, w_2) = (0.95, 0.05)$, $(0.9, 0.1)$, $(0.8, 0.2)$, and $(0.5, 0.5)$. Results collected in Table 1 show that, when $n = 100$, the empirical sizes are a bit smaller than the targeted nominal level 0.05; as the sample size increases, all empirical sizes approach 0.05.

Table 1 Empirical sizes in percentages of the test for PSDs of order two

	$H_p = 0.95\delta_1 + 0.05\delta_4$				$H_p = 0.9\delta_1 + 0.1\delta_4$			
n	$c = 1$	$c = 3$	$c = 5$	$c = 7$	$c = 1$	$c = 3$	$c = 5$	$c = 7$
100	2.47	3.68	3.82	4.19	3.30	3.81	4.31	4.32
200	4.00	4.70	4.94	4.11	4.85	4.74	5.10	4.14
300	4.35	4.87	4.92	4.55	4.86	4.72	4.89	4.89
400	4.89	4.76	4.73	4.99	5.03	4.99	4.90	5.05
	$H_p = 0.8\delta_1 + 0.2\delta_4$				$H_p = 0.5\delta_1 + 0.5\delta_4$			
n	$c = 1$	$c = 3$	$c = 5$	$c = 7$	$c = 1$	$c = 3$	$c = 5$	$c = 7$
100	3.52	4.30	4.44	4.56	4.57	4.36	4.34	4.25
200	4.92	4.59	4.55	5.02	5.25	4.90	4.68	4.86
300	5.27	5.07	4.51	5.15	4.95	5.33	4.97	5.06
400	5.12	5.50	4.91	4.46	5.12	4.92	4.71	5.18

The dimension to sample size ratio $c = 1, 3, 5, 7$. The nominal significant level is $\alpha = 0.05$ and the number of independent replications is 10,000

We also observe that, for small p and n, the performance of the order test in conjunction with the bias-reduced moment estimators varies slightly when the mixture proportions of H_p change. This is due to the fact that our test statistic is dependent upon the moment estimators of H_p, which are affected by the changing mixture proportions.

Next, we examine the power of the order test. Four models under the alternative hypothesis are employed:

Model 1: $H_p = 0.8\delta_1 + 0.1\delta_4 + 0.1\delta_7$,
Model 2: $H_p = 0.8\delta_1 + 0.1\delta_3 + 0.05\delta_7 + 0.05\delta_{10}$,
Model 3: $H_p = 0.8\delta_1 + 0.2 \cdot U(4, 10)$,
Model 4: $H_p = U(1, 25)$,

where $U(a, b)$ stands for a uniform distribution on the interval $(a, b) \subset \mathbb{R}^+$. The fist two models are discrete PSDs and their orders are, respectively, 3 and 4. Model 3 can be seen as a mixture of a discrete distribution and a continuous one, where 80 % of the population eigenvalues are 1 and the remaining 20 % are drawn from $U(4, 10)$. The last model is completely continuous.

Notice that the test statistic is invariant to orthonormal transformation. Hence, without loss of generality, we set Σ_p to be diagonal. For discrete PSDs, we set the diagonal entries of Σ_p according to the mixture proportions and corresponding distinct mass points, then use this (same) Σ_p for all 10,000 replications; while for continuous PSDs or PSDs with a continuous mixture component, for each of 10,000 replications, we generate a (different) set of diagonal entries for Σ_p accordingly.

Figure 1 exhibits the empirical power for Models 1–4. The results exhibit a trend that the power tends to 1 as the sample size increases, while the power deteriorates as the ratio c increases. This demonstrates that the increased dimension makes the order detection harder to achieve. The power for Model 2 is better than that for Model 1, which can be attributed to the fact that, compared with Model 1, Model

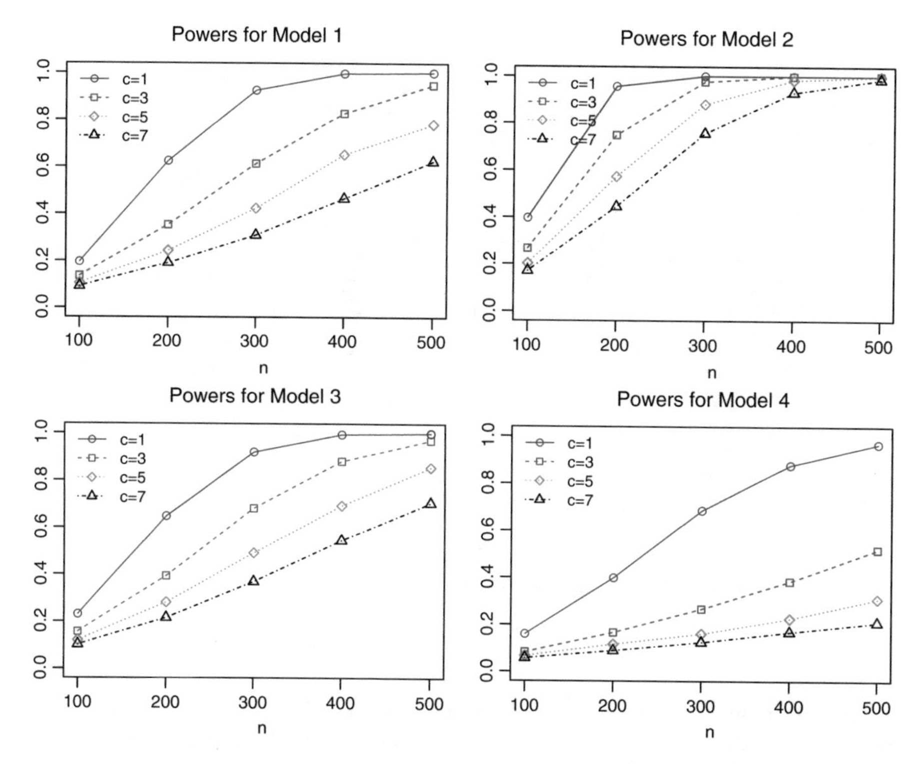

Fig. 1 Empirical powers of the test for Models 1–4 with the dimensional ratio $c = 1, 3, 5, 7$. The nominal significant level is $\alpha = 0.05$ and the number of independent replications is 10,000

2 is further away from the null hypothesis due to the existence of the largest mass point 10. Another phenomena is that the power for the pure continuous model grows slowly compared with the others, although its true order is infinity in the limit, which seems far away from the null hypothesis. A possible reason is that the moment estimators of this continuous PSD have large fluctuations comparing to those of the other discrete PSDs.

4.2 *Case of Testing for Order Three PSDs*

Qin and Li [18] do not provide simulation results on order three PSDs due to the unavailability of higher order moment estimators. Given the proposed bias-reduced moment estimators in this paper, we will be able to test for any order of PSDs. In this section, we examine the performance of the test for order three hypothesis. Samples are still drawn from zero mean multivariate normal population. The sample size is taken as $n = 300, 400, 500, 600$ and the dimension to sample size ratio is set to be $c = 0.3, 0.6, 0.9, 1.2$. The number of independent replications is 10,000.

Table 2 Empirical sizes in percentages of the test for PSDs of order three

	$H_p = 0.4\delta_1 + 0.4\delta_4 + 0.2\delta_7$				$H_p = 0.4\delta_1 + 0.4\delta_5 + 0.2\delta_{10}$			
n	$c = 0.3$	$c = 0.6$	$c = 0.9$	$c = 1.2$	$c = 0.3$	$c = 0.6$	$c = 0.9$	$c = 1.2$
300	2.78	4.00	4.77	4.09	3.18	4.36	4.94	4.65
400	4.13	4.82	5.00	5.32	4.24	4.91	5.18	5.92
500	4.96	5.52	5.53	5.38	4.59	5.11	5.77	5.79
600	4.92	5.39	5.51	5.82	4.83	5.65	5.51	6.00
	$H_p = 0.5\delta_1 + 0.3\delta_4 + 0.2\delta_7$				$H_p = 0.5\delta_1 + 0.3\delta_5 + 0.2\delta_{10}$			
n	$c = 0.3$	$c = 0.6$	$c = 0.9$	$c = 1.2$	$c = 0.3$	$c = 0.6$	$c = 0.9$	$c = 1.2$
300	3.05	4.56	4.44	4.70	3.37	4.71	5.13	5.45
400	4.39	5.45	5.68	5.73	4.62	5.37	6.07	5.97
500	4.54	5.84	5.90	6.03	4.86	5.72	5.66	6.19
600	5.04	5.68	5.95	5.89	5.46	5.89	6.00	6.15

The dimension to sample size ratio $c = 0.3, 0.6, 0.9, 1.2$. The nominal significant level is $\alpha = 0.05$ and the number of independent replications is 10,000

The model under the null hypothesis is

$$H_p = w_1\delta_{a_1} + w_2\delta_{a_2} + w_3\delta_{a_3},$$

where the distinct mass points are $(a_1, a_2, a_3) = (1, 4, 7), (1, 5, 10)$ and their weights are $(w_1, w_2, w_3) = (0.4, 0.4, 0.2), (0.5, 0.3, 0.2)$. Results in Table 2 show that the empirical sizes are all close to the nominal level, though their fluctuation is a bit larger than that in the test of order two.

Next, we examine the power of the order test using four models under the alternative.

Model 5: $H_p = 0.4\delta_1 + 0.3\delta_5 + 0.2\delta_{15} + 0.1\delta_{25}$,
Model 6: $H_p = 0.4\delta_1 + 0.3\delta_5 + 0.2\delta_{15} + (1/15)\delta_{25} + (1/30)\delta_{30}$,
Model 7: $H_p = 0.4\delta_1 + 0.4\delta_5 + 0.2U(10, 20)$,
Model 8:$H_p = 0.4\delta_1 + 0.3\delta_5 + 0.2\delta_{15} + 0.1U(20, 30)$.

The fist two models are discrete PSDs of orders 4 and 5, respectively, and the last two models are mixture distributions of discrete and continuous. Figure 2 illustrates the power curves for Models 5–8. It shows that this test is more difficult to gain power than the order two test since we need to estimate higher order moments of PSDs. However, we still can see that the power increases along with the increasing (n, p), which again demonstrates the consistency of the test.

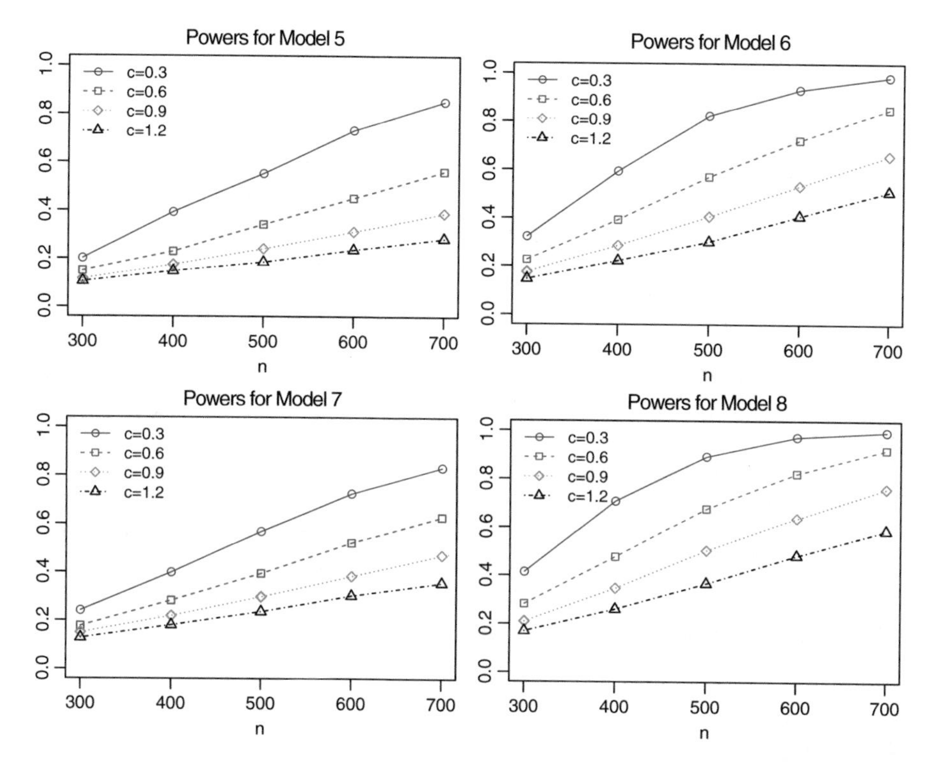

Fig. 2 Empirical powers of the test for Models 5–8 with the dimensional ratio $c = 0.3, 0.6, 0.9, 1.2$. The nominal significant level is $\alpha = 0.05$ and the number of independent replications is 10,000

5 Conclusions and Remarks

In this paper we propose bias-reduced moment estimators of PSDs, which are originally introduced in [3]. The proposed estimators successfully remove all $O(1/p)$ terms in the biases such that the asymptotic normal distributions regain zero mean. We adopt these bias-reduced estimators to a test procedure for the order of PSDs, proposed by Qin and Li [18]. Asymptotic distributions of the test statistic are presented under both the null and the alternative hypotheses as $(n, p) \to \infty$ with their ratio $p/n \to c \in (0, \infty)$. We have observed in the simulation study that the order test maintains desired nominal level and its power tends to 1 as (n, p) tend to infinity.

Recall that unbiased estimators of the first fourth moments of the PSD are given in [10, 21], referred to as $\hat{\gamma}_k^{(u)}, k = 1, 2, 3, 4$. Corresponding estimators in [3] are referred as to $\hat{\gamma}_k^{(b)}$. Some elementary calculations reveal that

$$\hat{\gamma}_1 = \hat{\gamma}_1^{(b)} = \hat{\gamma}_1^{(u)}, \quad \hat{\gamma}_2 = \hat{\gamma}_2^{(b)}\left(1 - \frac{1}{n}\right) = \hat{\gamma}_2^{(u)}\left(1 - \frac{3}{n^2} + \frac{2}{n^3}\right),$$

$$\hat{\gamma}_3 = \hat{\gamma}_3^{(b)}\left(1 - \frac{3}{n}\right) = \hat{\gamma}_3^{(u)}\left(1 - \frac{17}{n^2} + \frac{12}{n^3} + \frac{52}{n^4} - \frac{48}{n^5}\right),$$

$$\hat{\gamma}_4 = \hat{\gamma}_4^{(b)} + O_p\left(\frac{1}{n}\right) = \hat{\gamma}_4^{(u)} + O_p\left(\frac{1}{n^2}\right),$$

from which we can clearly see that these estimators are all asymptotically equivalent, while $\hat{\gamma}_k^{(b)}$ has a bias of order $O(1/p)$ and $\hat{\gamma}_k$ keeps a bias of order $O(1/p^2)$, $k = 2, 3, 4$.

It is worth noticing that the central limiting theorems of all these estimators heavily rely on the moment conditions, say $E(w_{11}^4) = 3$, of the underlying distribution. If the fourth moment is not equal to 3, then there are two additional terms appearing in the limiting mean and covariance matrix, see [17]. Moreover, these two terms are functions of both eigenvalues and eigenvectors of Σ_p (unless Σ_p is diagonal), which are currently hard to be estimated.

6 Proofs

6.1 *Proof of Theorem 1*

Suppose that the assumptions (a)–(c) hold, from [20], the ESD F_n converges weakly to the LSD $F^{c,H}$, and moreover the Stieltjes transform $s_n(z)$ of the ESD F_n converges almost surely to $s(z)$, the Stieltjes transform of $F^{c,H}$. Let $(\beta_1, \ldots, \beta_k)' = g^{-1}(\gamma_1, \ldots, \gamma_k)$ then,

$$\beta_j = \int t^j dF^{c_n,H_p}(t) \to \tilde{\beta}_j := \int t^j dF^{c,H}(t), \quad j \geq 1,$$

where F^{c_n,H_p} is an LSD derived from $F^{c,H}$ by replacing c and H with c_n and H_p, respectively.

When the support of H is bounded, the support of $F^{c,H}$ is also bounded. Thus, for any $z \in \mathbb{C}$ with $|z|$ large, the Stieltjes transform $s_n(z)$ and $s(z)$ can be expanded as Laurent series, and we have

$$s_n(z) = \int \frac{1}{x - z} dF_n(x) = \sum_{l=0}^{\infty} \frac{-1}{z^{l+1}} \hat{\beta}_l \xrightarrow{a.s.} s(z) = \sum_{l=0}^{\infty} \frac{-1}{z^{l+1}} \tilde{\beta}_l.$$

From this we get $\hat{\beta}_j^* - \beta_j = \hat{\beta}_j - \hat{\mu}_j/p - \beta_j \xrightarrow{a.s.} 0$, and hence

$$\hat{\gamma}_j - \gamma_j \xrightarrow{a.s.} 0, \quad j = 1, 2, \ldots,$$

as $(n, p) \to \infty$, which is the first conclusion.

For the second conclusion, applying Theorem 1.1 in [1] with $f_j(z) = z^j$, $j = 1, \ldots, k$, for real case, we obtain

$$p\left(\hat{\beta}_1 - \beta_1, \ldots, \hat{\beta}_k - \beta_k\right) \xrightarrow{D} N_k(\mu, B),$$

where the mean vector $\mu = (\mu_j)$ with

$$\mu_j = -\frac{1}{2\pi \mathrm{i}} \oint_{C_1} \frac{cz^j \underline{s}^3(z) \int t^2(1 + t\underline{s}(z))^{-3} dH(t)}{(1 - c\int \underline{s}^2(z)t^2(1 + t\underline{s}(z))^{-2} dH(t))^2} dz, \tag{8}$$

and the covariance $B = (b_{ij})$ with its entries

$$b_{ij} = -\frac{1}{2\pi^2} \oint_{C_2} \oint_{C_1} \frac{z_1^i z_2^j}{(\underline{s}(z_1) - \underline{s}(z_2))^2} \underline{s}'(z_1)\underline{s}'(z_2) dz_1 dz_2, \tag{9}$$

where

$$\underline{s}(z) = -\frac{1-c}{z} + cs(z)$$

is companion Stieltjes transform of $F^{c,H}$ satisfying

$$z = -\frac{1}{\underline{s}(z)} + c \int \frac{t}{1 + t\underline{s}(z)} dH(t). \tag{10}$$

The contours C_1 and C_2 in (8) and (9) are simple, closed, non-overlapping, taken in the positive direction in the complex plane, and each enclosing the support of $F^{c,H}$. Then the second conclusion of this theorem follows from a standard application of the Delta method, and the remaining works are to calculate the contour integrals in (8) and (9).

Without loss of generality, let the contour C_2 enclose C_1 and both of them be away from the support S_F of $F^{c,H}$ such that

$$\max_{t \in S_H, z \in C_i} |t\underline{s}(z)| < 1,$$

where S_H is the support of H. In such a situation, for any $z \in C_1 \cup C_2$,

$$P(\underline{s}(z)) = -1 - c\sum_{l=1}^{\infty}(-\underline{s}(z))^l\tilde{\gamma}_l = -1 + c\int \frac{t\underline{s}(z)}{1 + t\underline{s}(z)}dH(t),$$

$$Q(\underline{s}(z)) = c\sum_{l=0}^{\infty} q_{3,l}\tilde{\gamma}_{l+2}\underline{s}^l(z) = c\int \frac{t^2}{(1 + t\underline{s}(z))^3}dH(t),$$

$$R(\underline{s}(z)) = 1 - c\sum_{l=0}^{\infty} q_{2,l}\tilde{\gamma}_{l+2}\underline{s}^{l+2}(z) = 1 - c\int \frac{(zt)^2}{(1 + tz)^2}dH(t),$$

and from (10) we also get $P(\underline{s}(z)) = z\underline{s}(z)$, where the functions P, Q, and R are defined in (4)–(5). On the other hand, denote the image of C_i under $\underline{s}(z)$ be

$$\underline{s}(C_i) = \{\underline{s}(z) : z \in C_i\}, i = 1, 2.$$

Notice that $\underline{s}(z)$ is a univalent analytic function on $\mathbb{C} \setminus (S_F \cup \{0\})$, and thus C_i and $\underline{s}(C_i)$ are homeomorphic, which implies $\underline{s}(C_1)$ and $\underline{s}(C_2)$ are also simple, closed, and non-overlapping. In addition, from the open mapping theorem and the fact $\underline{s}(z) \to 0$ as $|z| \to \infty$, we may conclude that $\underline{s}(C_2)$ encloses $\underline{s}(C_1)$, and both of them have negative direction and enclose zero.

Based on these knowledge and by the equality

$$\frac{\underline{s}^2(z)}{\underline{s}'(z)} = 1 - c\int \frac{t^2\underline{s}^2(z)}{(1 + t\underline{s}(z))^2}dH(t), \tag{11}$$

the integral in (8) becomes

$$\begin{aligned}
\mu_j &= -\frac{1}{2\pi i}\oint_{C_1} \frac{cz^j\underline{s}(z)\underline{s}'(z)\int t^2(1 + t\underline{s}(z))^{-3}dH(t)}{1 - c\int \underline{s}^2(z)t^2(1 + t\underline{s}(z))^{-2}dH(t)}dz \\
&= \frac{1}{2\pi i}\oint_{\underline{s}(C_1)} \frac{P^j(\underline{s})Q(\underline{s})}{\underline{s}^{j-1}R(\underline{s})}d\underline{s} \\
&= \begin{cases} 0, & j = 1, \\ \frac{1}{(j-2)!}\left[P^j(z)Q(z)/R(z)\right]^{(j-2)}\Big|_{z=0}, & 2 \le j \le k, \end{cases}
\end{aligned} \tag{12}$$

where the equality in (11) is obtained by taking the derivative of z on both sides of the Eq. (10), and the results in (12) are from the Cauchy integral theorem.

Finally, the integral in (9) can be simplified as

$$b_{ij} = -\frac{1}{2\pi^2}\oint_{C_2}\oint_{C_1} \frac{z_1^i z_2^j}{(\underline{s}(z_1) - \underline{s}(z_2))^2}d\underline{s}(z_1)d\underline{s}(z_2)$$

$$= -\frac{1}{2\pi^2} \oint_{\underline{s}(C_2)} \oint_{\underline{s}(C_1)} \frac{P_i(\underline{s}_1)P_j(\underline{s}_2)}{\underline{s}_1^i \underline{s}_2^j (\underline{s}_1 - \underline{s}_2)^2} d\underline{s}_1 d\underline{s}_2$$

$$= -\frac{1}{2\pi^2} \oint_{\underline{s}(C_2)} \frac{P_j(\underline{s}_2)}{\underline{s}_2^j} \left(\oint_{\underline{s}(C_1)} \frac{P_i(\underline{s}_1)}{\underline{s}_1^i (\underline{s}_1 - \underline{s}_2)^2} d\underline{s}_1 \right) d\underline{s}_2.$$

By the Cauchy integral theorem,

$$\oint_{\underline{s}(C_1)} \frac{P_i(\underline{s}_1)}{\underline{s}_1^i (\underline{s}_1 - \underline{s}_2)^2} d\underline{s}_1 = \sum_{l=0}^{i-1} \oint_{\underline{s}(C_1)} \frac{\alpha_{i,l}}{\underline{s}_1^{i-l} (\underline{s}_1 - \underline{s}_2)^2} d\underline{s}_1$$

$$= -2\pi \mathrm{i} \sum_{l=0}^{i-1} \frac{\alpha_{i,l}(i-l)}{\underline{s}_2^{i-l+1}}.$$

From similar arguments, we get

$$b_{ij} = -\frac{1}{\pi \mathrm{i}} \sum_{l=0}^{i-1} (i-l)\alpha_{i,l} \oint_{\underline{s}(C_2)} \frac{P_j(\underline{s}_2)}{\underline{s}_2^{i+j-l+1}} d\underline{s}_2$$

$$= 2\sum_{l=0}^{i-1} (i-l)\alpha_{i,l}\alpha_{j,i+j-l},$$

$i, j = 1, \ldots, k$.

6.2 *Proof of Theorem 4*

Under the alternative hypothesis and the assumption of this theorem, we have $D(k_0) = \det(\Gamma(H_p, k_0)) \to \det(\Gamma(H, k_0)) > 0$ and

$$\hat{\sigma}_{H_0}^2 \xrightarrow{a.s.} \sigma_{H_0}^2 := \sigma_{k_0}^2(c, \tilde{\gamma}_1, \ldots, \tilde{\gamma}_{2k_0-1}, \gamma_{2k_0}^*, \ldots, \gamma_{4k_0}^*) > 0,$$

as $(n, p) \to \infty$, where γ_k^*, $2k_0 \le k \le 4k_0$, is the kth moment of a discrete random variable with only k_0 different masses, determined by its first $2k_0 - 1$ moments $\tilde{\gamma}_1, \ldots, \tilde{\gamma}_{2k_0-1}$. Therefore, for large p and n, $\hat{\sigma}_{H_0}$ exists and is positive, and

$$P\left(\frac{\widehat{D}(k_0)}{\hat{\sigma}_{H_0}/p} > z_\alpha\right) = P\left(\frac{\widehat{D}(k_0) - D(k_0)}{\sigma_{k_0}/p} > z_\alpha \frac{\hat{\sigma}_{H_0}}{\sigma_{k_0}} - \frac{D(k_0)}{\sigma_{k_0}/p}\right)$$

$$= 1 - \Phi\left(z_\alpha \frac{\sigma_{H_0}}{\sigma_{k_0}} - \frac{\det(\Gamma(H, k_0))}{\sigma_{k_0}/p}\right) + o_p(1)$$

$$\to 1,$$

as $(n, p) \to \infty$, where σ_{k_0} is the square root of $\sigma_{k_0}^2$ defined in Theorem 2 and z_α is the $1 - \alpha$ quantile of standard normal population.

Acknowledgements We would like to thank Dr. S. Ejaz Ahmed for organizing this Springer refereed volume. We appreciate his tremendous efforts. Comments by the anonymous referees led to substantial improvement of the manuscript. Yingli Qin's research is partly supported by Research Incentive Fund grant No. 115953 and Natural Sciences and Engineering Research Council of Canada (NSERC) grant No. RGPIN-2016-03890. Weiming Li's research is supported by National Natural Science Foundation of China, No. 11401037 and Program for IRTSHUFE.

References

1. Bai, Z.D., Silverstein, J.W.: CLT for linear spectral statistics of large-dimensional sample covariance matrices. Ann. Probab. **32**, 553–605 (2004)
2. Bai, Z. D., Silverstein, J. W. (2010). *Spectral Analysis of Large Dimensional Random Matrices* (2nd ed.). New York: Springer.
3. Bai, Z.D., Chen, J.Q., Yao, J.F.: On estimation of the population spectral distribution from a high-dimensional sample covariance matrix. Aust. N. Z. J. Stat. **52**, 423–437 (2010)
4. Berthet, Q., Rigollet, P.: Optimal detection of sparse principal components in high dimension. Ann. Statist. **41**, 1780–1815 (2013)
5. Birnbaum, A., Johnstone, I.M., Nadler, B., Paul, D.: Minimax bounds for sparse PCA with noisy high-dimensional data. Ann. Statist. **41**, 1055–1084 (2013)
6. Cai, T.T., Ma, Z.M., Wu, Y.H.: Sparse PCA: Optimal rates and adaptive estimation. Ann. Statist. **41**, 3074–3110 (2013)
7. Chen, J.Q., Delyon, B., Yao, J.F.: On a model selection problem from high-dimensional sample covariance matrices. J. Multivar. Anal. **102**, 1388–1398 (2011)
8. Dudoit, S., Fridlyand, J., Speed, T.P.: Comparison of discrimination methods for the classification of tumors using gene expression data. J. Am. Stat. Assoc. **97**, 77–87 (2002)
9. El Karoui, N.: Spectrum estimation for large dimensional covariance matrices using random matrix theory. Ann. Statist. **36**, 2757–2790 (2008)
10. Fisher, T.J., Sun, X., Gallagher, C.M.: A new test for sphericity of the covariance matrix for high dimensional data. J. Multivar. Anal. **101**, 2554–2570 (2010)
11. Johnstone, I.M.: On the distribution of the largest eigenvalue in principal components analysis. Ann. Statist. **29**, 295–327 (2001)
12. Li, W.M., Yao, J.F.: A local moment estimator of the spectrum of a large dimensional covariance matrix. Stat. Sin. **24**, 919–936 (2014)
13. Li, W.M., Yao, J.F.: On generalized expectation-based estimation of a population spectral distribution from high-dimensional data. Ann. Inst. Stat. Math. **67**, 359–373 (2015)
14. Li, W.M., Chen, J.Q., Qin, Y.L., Yao, J.F., Bai, Z.D.: Estimation of the population spectral distribution from a large dimensional sample covariance matrix. J. Stat. Plan. Inference **143**, 1887–1897 (2013)
15. Mestre, X.: Improved estimation of eigenvalues and eigenvectors of covariance matrices using their sample estimates. IEEE Trans. Inf. Theory **54**, 5113–5129 (2008)
16. Nica, A., Speicher, R.: Lectures on the Combinatorics of Free Probability. Cambridge University Press, New York (2006)
17. Pan, G.M., Zhou, W.: Central limit theorem for signal-to-interference ratio of reduced rank linear receiver. Ann. Appl. Probab. **18**, 1232–1270 (2008)
18. Qin, Y.L., Li, W.M.: Testing the order of a population spectral distribution for high-dimensional data. Comput. Stat. Data Anal. **95**, 75–82 (2016)

19. Rao, N.R., Mingo, J.A., Speicher, R., Edelman, A.: Statistical eigen-inference from large Wishart matrices. Ann. Statist. **36**, 2850–2885 (2008)
20. Silverstein, J.W.: Strong convergence of the empirical distribution of eigenvalues of large-dimensional random matrices. J. Multivar. Anal. **55**, 331–339 (1995)
21. Srivastava, M.S.: Some tests concerning the covariance matrix in high dimensional data. J. Japan Stat. Soc. **35**, 251–272 (2005)

Part II
Network Analysis and Big Data

Statistical Process Control Charts as a Tool for Analyzing Big Data

Peihua Qiu

Abstract Big data often take the form of data streams with observations of certain processes collected sequentially over time. Among many different purposes, one common task to collect and analyze big data is to monitor the longitudinal performance/status of the related processes. To this end, statistical process control (SPC) charts could be a useful tool, although conventional SPC charts need to be modified properly in some cases. In this paper, we introduce some basic SPC charts and some of their modifications, and describe how these charts can be used for monitoring different types of processes. Among many potential applications, dynamic disease screening and profile/image monitoring will be discussed in some detail.

Keywords Curve data • Data stream • Images • Longitudinal data • Monitoring • Profiles • Sequential process • Surveillance

1 Introduction

Recent advances in data acquisition technologies have led to massive amounts of data being collected routinely in different scientific disciplines (e.g., [30, 45]). In addition to volume, big data often have complicated structures. In applications, they often take the form of data streams. Examples of big sets of data streams include those obtained from complex engineering systems (e.g., production lines), sequences of satellite images, climate data, website transaction logs, credit card records, and so forth. In many such applications, one major goal to collect and analyze big data is to monitor the longitudinal performance/status of the related processes. For such big data applications, statistical process control (SPC) charts could be a useful tool. This paper tries to build a connection between SPC and big data analysis, by introducing some representative SPC charts and by describing their (potential) use in various big data applications.

P. Qiu (✉)
Department of Biostatistics, University of Florida, Gainesville, FL, USA
e-mail: pqiu@phhp.ufl.edu

© Springer International Publishing AG 2017

S.E. Ahmed (ed.), *Big and Complex Data Analysis*, Contributions to Statistics,
DOI 10.1007/978-3-319-41573-4_7

SPC charts are widely used in manufacturing and other industries for monitoring sequential processes (e.g., production lines, internet traffics, operation of medical systems) to make sure that they work stably and satisfactorily (cf., [18, 36]). Since the first control chart was proposed in 1931 by Walter A. Shewhart, many control charts have been proposed in the past more than 80 years, including different versions of the Shewhart chart, CUSUM chart, EWMA chart, and the chart based on change-point detection (CPD). See, for instance, [8, 12, 13, 16, 19, 28, 31, 46, 48] and [51]. Control charts discussed in these and many other relatively early papers are based on the assumptions that the process distribution is normal and process observations at different time points are independent. Some recent SPC charts are more flexible in the sense that they can accommodate data autocorrelation and non-normality (e.g., [3, 35, 37, 38]).

The conventional control charts mentioned above are designed mainly for monitoring processes whose observations at individual time points are scalars/vectors and whose observation distributions are unchanged when the processes run stably. In applications, especially in those with big data involved, process observations could be images or other types of profiles (see Sect. 4 for a detailed description). When processes are stable, their observation distributions could change over time due to seasonality and other reasons. To handle such applications properly, much research effort has been made in the literature to extend/generalize the conventional control charts. After some basic SPC concepts and control charts are discussed in Sect. 2, these extended/generalized control charts will be discussed in Sects. 3 and 4. Some remarks conclude the article in Sect. 5.

2 Conventional SPC Charts

In the past several decades, SPC charts were mainly used for monitoring production lines in the manufacturing industry, although they also found many applications in infectious disease surveillance, environment monitoring, and other areas. When a production line is first installed, SPC charts can be used to check whether the quality of a relatively small amount of products produced by the production line meets the quality requirements. If some products are detected to be defective, then the root causes need to be figured out and the production line is adjusted accordingly. After the proper adjustment, a small amount of products is produced again for quality inspection. This trial-and-adjustment process continues until all assignable causes are believed to be removed and the production line works stably. This stage of process control is often called *phase-I SPC* in the literature. At the end of phase-I SPC, a clean dataset is collected under stable operating conditions of the production line for estimating the distribution of the quality variables when the process is *in-control (IC)*. This dataset is called an IC dataset hereafter. The estimated IC distribution can then be used for designing a control chart for online monitoring of the production line operation. The online monitoring phase is called *phase-II SPC*. Its major goal is to guarantee that the production line is IC, and give a signal as quickly as possible after the observed data provide a sufficient evident that the production line has become *out-of-control (OC)*. Most big data applications with data streams involved concern phase-II SPC only because new observations are collected in daily basis. However, the IC distribution of the quality variables still needs to be properly estimated beforehand in a case-by-case basis. See related discussions in Sects. 3 and 4 for some examples.

Next, we introduce some basic control charts for phase-II SPC. We start with cases with only one quality variable X involved. Its distribution is assumed to be normal, and its observations at different time points are assumed independent. When the process is IC, the process mean and standard deviation are assumed to be μ_0 and σ_0, respectively. These parameters are assumed known in phase-II SPC. But, they need to be estimated from an IC dataset in practice, as mentioned above. At time n, for $n \geq 1$, assume that there is a batch of m observations of X, denoted as $X_{n1}, X_{n2}, \ldots, X_{nm}$. Then, by the $\overline{X}$ Shewhart chart, the process has a mean shift if

$$|\overline{X}_n - \mu_0| > Z_{1-\alpha/2}\frac{\sigma_0}{\sqrt{m}}, \tag{1}$$

where α is a significance level and $Z_{1-\alpha/2}$ is the $(1-\alpha/2)$-th quantile of the standard normal distribution. In the SPC literature, the performance of a control chart is often measured by the IC average run length (ARL), denoted as ARL_0, and the OC ARL, denoted as ARL_1. ARL_0 is the average number of observations from the beginning of process monitoring to the signal time when the process is IC, and ARL_1 is the average number of observations from the occurrence of a shift to the signal time after the process becomes OC. Usually, the value of ARL_0 is pre-specified, and the chart performs better for detecting a given shift if the value of ARL_1 is smaller. For the $\overline{X}$ chart (1), it is obvious that $\text{ARL}_0 = 1/\alpha$. For instance, when α is chosen 0.0027 (i.e., $Z_{1-\alpha/2} = 3$), $\text{ARL}_0 = 370$.

The $\overline{X}$ chart (1) detects a mean shift at the current time n using the observed data at that time point alone. This chart is good for detecting relatively large shifts. Intuitively, when a shift is small, it should be better to use all available data by the time point n, including those at time n and all previous time points. One such chart is the cumulative sum (CUSUM) chart proposed by Page [31], which gives a signal of mean shift when

$$C_n^+ > h \text{ or } C_n^- < -h, \qquad \text{for } n \geq 1, \tag{2}$$

where $h > 0$ is a control limit,

$$C_n^+ = \max\left(0, C_{n-1}^+ + (\overline{X}_n - \mu_0)\frac{\sqrt{m}}{\sigma_0} - k\right), \quad C_n^- = \min\left(0, C_{n-1}^- + (\overline{X}_n - \mu_0)\frac{\sqrt{m}}{\sigma_0} + k\right), \tag{3}$$

and $k > 0$ is an allowance constant. From the definition of C_n^+ and C_n^- in (3), it can be seen that (1) both of them use all available observations by the time n, and (2) a re-starting mechanism is introduced in their definitions so that C_n^+ (C_n^-) is reset to 0 each time when there is little evidence of an upward (downward) mean shift. For the CUSUM chart (2), the allowance constant k is often pre-specified, and its control limit h is chosen such that a pre-specified ARL_0 level is reached.

An alternative control chart using all available observations is the exponentially weighted moving average (EWMA) chart originally proposed by Roberts [46]. This chart gives a signal of mean shift if

$$|E_n| > \rho_E \sqrt{\frac{\lambda}{2-\lambda}}, \qquad \text{for } n \geq 1, \tag{4}$$

where $\rho_E > 0$ is a parameter,

$$E_n = \lambda(\overline{X}_n - \mu_0)\frac{\sqrt{m}}{\sigma_0} + (1-\lambda)E_{n-1}, \tag{5}$$

$E_0 = 0$, and $\lambda \in (0, 1]$ is a weighting parameter. Obviously, $E_n = \lambda \sum_{i=1}^{n}(1-\lambda)^{n-i}(\overline{X}_n - \mu_0)\sqrt{m}/\sigma_0$ is a weighted average of $\{(\overline{X}_i - \mu_0)\sqrt{m}/\sigma_0, i \leq n\}$ with the weights decay exponentially fast when i moves away from n. In the chart (4), λ is usually pre-specified, and ρ_E is chosen such that a given ARL_0 level is reached.

All the charts (1), (2), and (4) assume that the IC parameters μ_0 and σ_0 have been properly estimated beforehand. The CPD chart proposed by Hawkins et al. [19] does not require this assumption. However, its computation is more demanding, compared to that involved in the charts (1), (2), and (4), which makes it less feasible for big data applications. For this reason, it is not introduced here.

Example 1 The data shown in Fig. 1a denote the Ethernet data lengths (in log scale) of the one million Ethernet packets received by a computing facility. The x-axis denotes the time (in seconds) since the start of the trace. The Ethernet data lengths smaller than 64 or larger than 1518 were not included in the dataset. The data with $x \leq 250$ look unstable and they are excluded from this analysis. Then, the data with $250 < x \leq 1000$ are used as an IC dataset, from which μ_0 and σ_0 are estimated. Their estimators are used for monitoring the data with $x > 1000$ (i.e., the phase-II data). The blue vertical dashed line in Fig. 1a separates the IC dataset from the phase-II data. In phase-II monitoring, we treat every five consecutive observations as a batch of $m = 5$ observations, the means of their Ethernet data lengths and arrival times are both computed, and the mean of the Ethernet data lengths is monitored. We group the data in batches in this example to shrink the data size so that the related plots can be better presented for the demonstration purpose. In practice, the control charts can be applied to the original data with a single observation at each time point. Figure 1b shows the $\overline{X}$ chart (1) with $Z_{1-\alpha/2} = 3.09$ (or, $\alpha = 0.002$), where the dots are batch means of the Ethernet data lengths, and the horizontal blue dotted lines are the control limits $\mu_0 \pm Z_{1-\alpha/2}\frac{\sigma_0}{\sqrt{m}}$. The ARL_0 value of this chart is $1/0.002 = 500$. From Fig. 1b, it can be seen that no signal is given by the $\overline{X}$ chart. The CUSUM chart (2) with $k = 1$ and with h chosen such that $\text{ARL}_0 = 500$ is

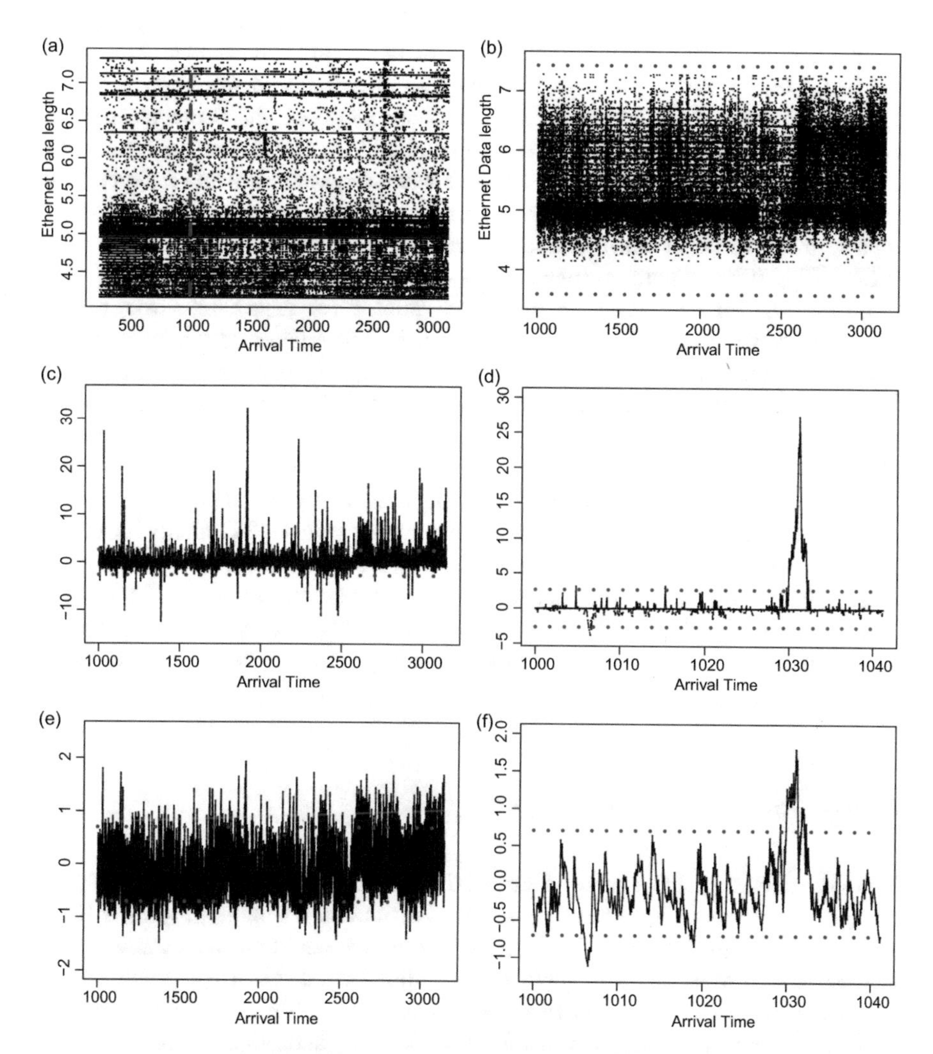

Fig. 1 (**a**) Original observations of the Ethernet data lengths, with the *vertical blue dashed line* separating the IC dataset from the phase II observations. (**b**) $\overline{X}$ chart with $\text{ATS}_0 = 500$ for monitoring the mean of every five consecutive observations. (**c**) CUSUM chart with $k = 1$ and $\text{ARL}_0 = 500$. (**d**) First $1/50$-th of the plot (**c**). (**e**) EWMA chart with $\lambda = 0.1$ and $\text{ARL}_0 = 500$. (**f**) First $1/50$-th of the plot (**e**). The *horizontal blue dotted lines* in plots (**b**)–(**f**) are control limits

shown in Fig. 1c, where the horizontal blue dotted lines are the control limits h and $-h$. Because this chart is quite crowded, the first $1/50$-th is shown in Fig. 1d. From both plots, we can see that many signals are given by the CUSUM chart, and the signals come and go, implying that the mean shifts are isolated instead of persistent. The corresponding results of the EWMA chart (4) with $\lambda = 0.1$ are shown in Fig. 1e and f. If we compare the results from the CUSUM chart with those from the EWMA chart, we can see some consistency in their patterns.

In Example 1, parameter determination of the control charts (1), (2), and (4) are based on the assumptions that the process observation distribution is normal and the observations at different time points are independent. These assumptions could be invalid. For instance, from Fig. 1a and b, it is obvious that the observation distribution is skewed to the right. In cases when the normality and independence assumptions are invalid, it has been demonstrated in the literature that the performance of the related control charts is generally unreliable in the sense that their actual ATS_0 values could be substantially different from the assumed ATS_0 value (e.g., [3, 39]). In such cases, many nonparametric (or distribution-free) control charts and control charts that can accommodate autocorrelation have been proposed. See, for instance, [1, 2, 4, 6, 9, 17, 29, 47, 49, 55, 59]. More recent research on nonparametric SPC can be found in Chaps. 8 and 9 of [36] and the special issue of *Quality and Reliability Engineering International* that was edited by Chakraborti et al. [7].

In applications, especially in those with big data involved, the number of quality variables could be large. In such cases, many multivariate SPC charts have been proposed (cf., [36, Chap. 7]). Most early ones are based on the normality assumption (e.g., [16, 20, 28, 53]. Some recent ones are nonparametric or distribution-free (e.g., [27, 35, 37, 38, 60]). There are also some multivariate SPC charts proposed specifically for cases with a large number of quality variables, based on LASSO and some other variable selection techniques (e.g., [5, 52, 58, 65]).

3 Dynamic Statistical Screening

The conventional SPC charts described in the previous section are mainly for monitoring processes with a stable process distribution when the process is IC. In many applications, however, the process distribution would change even when the process is IC. For instance, in applications with infectious disease surveillance, the incidence rate of an infectious disease would change over time even in time periods without disease outbreaks, due mainly to seasonality and other reasons. For such applications, the conventional SPC charts cannot be applied directly. Recently, [40] proposed a new method called *dynamic screening system (DySS)* for handling these applications, which is discussed in this section. A completely nonparametric version is discussed recently in [26]. A multivariate DySS procedure is proposed in [41]. Its applications for monitoring the incidence rates of the hand, foot, and mouth disease in China and the AIDS epidemic in the USA are discussed in [56, 57].

The DySS method is a generalization of the conventional SPC charts for cases when the IC mean and variance change over time. It can be used in the following two different scenarios. First, it can be used for early detection of diseases based on the longitudinal pattern of certain disease predictors. In this scenario, if each person is regarded as a process, then many processes are involved. The IC (or regular) longitudinal pattern of the disease predictors can be estimated from an observed dataset of a group of people who do not have the disease in question. Then, we can sequentially monitor the disease predictors of a given person, and use the cumulative difference between her/his longitudinal pattern of the disease predictors and the estimated regular longitudinal pattern for disease early detection. The related sequential monitoring problem in this scenario is called *dynamic screening (DS)* in [36]. Of course, the DS problem exists in many other applications, including performance monitoring of durable goods (e.g., airplanes, cars). For instance, we are required to check many mechanical indices of an airplane each time when it arrives a city, and some interventions should be made if the observed values of the indices are significantly worse than those of a well-functioning airplane of the same type and age. Second, the DySS method can also be used for monitoring a single process whose IC distribution changes over time. For instance, suppose we are interested in monitoring the incidence rate of an infectious disease in a region over time. As mentioned in the previous paragraph, the incidence rate will change over time even in years when no disease outbreaks occur. For such applications, by the DySS method, we can first estimate the regular longitudinal pattern of the disease incidence rate from observed data in time periods without disease outbreaks, and the estimated regular longitudinal pattern can then be used for future disease monitoring.

From the above brief description, the DySS method consists of three main steps described below.

(1) Estimation of the regular longitudinal pattern of the quality variables from a properly chosen IC dataset.
(2) Standardization of the longitudinal observations of a process in question for sequential monitoring of its quality variables, using the estimated regular longitudinal pattern obtained in step (1).
(3) Dynamic monitoring of the standardized observations of the process, and giving a signal as soon as all available data suggest a significant shift in its longitudinal pattern from the estimated regular pattern.

In the DySS method, step (1) tries to establish a standard for comparison purposes in step (2). By standardizing the process observations, step (2) actually compares the process in question cross-sectionally and longitudinally with other well-functioning processes (in scenario 1) or with the same process during the time periods when it is IC (in scenario 2). Step (3) tries to detect the significant difference between the longitudinal pattern of the process in question and the regular longitudinal pattern based on their cumulative difference. Therefore, the DySS method has made use of the current data and all history data in its decision-making process. It should provide an effective tool for solving the DS and other related problems.

Example 2 We demonstrate the DySS method using a dataset obtained from the SHARe Framingham Heart Study of the National Heart Lung and Blood Institute (cf., [14, 36]). Assume that we are interested in early detecting stroke based on the longitudinal pattern of people's total cholesterol level (in mg/100 ml). In the data, there are 1028 non-stroke patients. Each of them was followed seven times, and the total cholesterol level, denoted as y, was recorded at each time. The observation times of different patients are all different. So, by the DySS method, we first need to estimate the regular longitudinal pattern of y based on this IC data. We assume that the IC data follow the model

$$y(t_{ij}) = \mu(t_{ij}) + \varepsilon(t_{ij}), \qquad \text{for } j = 1, 2, \ldots, J_i, \; i = 1, 2, \ldots, m, \tag{6}$$

where t_{ij} is the jth observation time of the ith patient, $y(t_{ij})$ is the observed value of y at t_{ij}, $\mu(t_{ij})$ is the mean of $y(t_{ij})$, and $\varepsilon(t_{ij})$ is the error term. In the IC data, $m = 1028$, $J_i = 7$, for all i, and t_{ij} take theirs values in the interval $[9, 85]$ years old. We further assume that the error term $\varepsilon(t)$, for any $t \in [9, 85]$, consists of two independent components, i.e., $\varepsilon(t) = \varepsilon_0(t) + \varepsilon_1(t)$, where $\varepsilon_0(\cdot)$ is a random process with mean 0 and covariance function $V_0(s, t)$, for any $s, t \in [9, 85]$, and $\varepsilon_1(\cdot)$ is a noise process satisfying the condition that $\varepsilon_1(s)$ and $\varepsilon_1(t)$ are independent for any $s, t \in [9, 85]$. In this decomposition, $\varepsilon_1(t)$ denotes the pure measurement error, and $\varepsilon_0(t)$ denotes all possible covariates that may affect y but are not included in model (6). In such cases, the covariance function of $\varepsilon(\cdot)$ is

$$V(s, t) = \text{Cov}\,(\varepsilon(s), \varepsilon(t)) = V_0(s, t) + \sigma_1^2(s) I(s = t), \qquad \text{for any } s, t \in [9, 85],$$

where $\sigma_1^2(s) = \text{Var}(\varepsilon_1(s))$, and $I(s = t) = 1$ when $s = t$ and 0 otherwise. In model (6), observations of different individuals are assumed to be independent. By the four-step procedure discussed in [36], we can obtain estimates of the IC mean function $\mu(t)$ and the IC variance function $\sigma_y^2(t) = V_0(t, t) + \sigma_1^2(t)$, denoted as $\widehat{\mu}(t)$ and $\widehat{\sigma}_y^2(t)$, respectively.

The estimated regular longitudinal pattern of y can then be described by $\widehat{\mu}(t)$ and $\widehat{\sigma}_y^2(t)$. For a new patient, assume that his/her y observations are $\{y(t_j^*), j = 1, 2, \ldots\}$, and their standardized values are

$$\widehat{\epsilon}(t_j^*) = \frac{y(t_j^*) - \widehat{\mu}(t_j^*)}{\widehat{\sigma}_y(t_j^*)}, \qquad \text{for } j = 1, 2, \ldots. \tag{7}$$

Then, we can apply the upward version of the CUSUM chart (2) and (3) (i.e., it gives a signal when $C_n^+ > h$) to the standardized data for detecting upward mean shifts. The upward version of the CUSUM chart (2) and (3) is considered here because we are mainly concerned about upward mean shift in the total cholesterol level in this example. For the ten patients in the data who had atleast one stroke during the study, their CUSUM charts are shown in Fig. 2. In each CUSUM chart, (k, h) are chosen to be $(0.1, 0.927)$. In such cases, the average time to signal is about 25 years for a non-stroke patient. From the figure, it can be seen that the first patient does not receive a signal, the second patient receives a signal at the second observation time, and so forth. In this example, we only monitor ten patients for a demonstration. In practice, the same method can be used for monitoring millions of patients in exactly the same way.

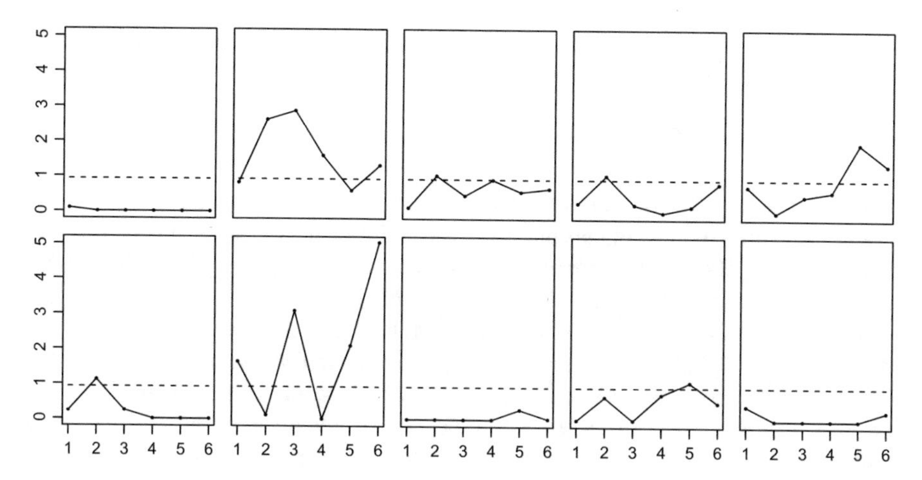

Fig. 2 The upward CUSUM chart with the charting statistic C_n^+ defined in (3) for the ten stroke patients in a dataset from the SHARe Framingham Heart Study. In the chart, (k, h) are chosen to be $(0.1, 0.927)$

4 Profiles/Images Monitoring

In the previous two sections, process observations are assumed to be scalars (i.e., univariate SPC) or vectors (i.e., multivariate SPC). In some applications, product quality is reflected in the relationship among two or more variables. In such cases, one observes a set of data points (or called a *profile*) of these variables for each sampled product. The major goal of SPC is to check the stability of the relationship over time based on the observed profile data. This is the so-called *profile monitoring* problem in the literature [36, Chap. 10].

The early research in profile monitoring is under the assumption that the relationship among variables is linear, which is called linear profile monitoring in the literature (e.g., [22, 24, 25, 61]). For a given product, assume that we are concerned about the relationship between a response variable y and a predictor x. For the i-th sampled product, the observed profile data are assumed to follow the linear regression model

$$y_{ij} = a_i + b_i x_{ij} + \varepsilon_{ij}, \qquad \text{for } j = 1, 2, \ldots, n_i, \quad i = 1, 2, \ldots, \tag{8}$$

where a_i and b_i are coefficients, and $\{\varepsilon_{ij}, j = 1, 2, \ldots, n_i\}$ are random errors. In such cases, monitoring the stability of the relationship between x and y is equivalent to monitoring the stability of $\{(a_i, b_i), i = 1, 2, \ldots\}$. Then, the IC values of a_i and b_i can be estimated from an IC dataset, and the linear profile monitoring can be accomplished by using a bivariate SPC chart.

In some applications, the linear regression model (8) is too restrictive to properly describe the relationship between x and y. Instead, we can use a nonlinear model based on certain physical/chemical theory. In such cases, the linear model (8) can be generalized to the nonlinear model

$$y_{ij} = f(x_{ij}, \boldsymbol{\theta}_i) + \varepsilon_{ij}, \qquad \text{for } j = 1, 2, \ldots, n_i, \quad i = 1, 2, \ldots, \tag{9}$$

where $f(x, \boldsymbol{\theta})$ is a known parametric function with parameter vector $\boldsymbol{\theta}$. For such a nonlinear profile monitoring problem, we can estimate the IC value of $\boldsymbol{\theta}$ from an IC dataset, and apply a conventional SPC chart to the sequence $\{\boldsymbol{\theta}_i, i = 1, 2, \ldots\}$ for monitoring their stability (e.g., [10, 15, 21, 23, 62]).

In many applications, the linear profile model (8) is inappropriate and it is difficult to specify the nonlinear profile model (9) either. For instance, Fig. 3 is about a manufacturing process of aluminum electrolytic capacitors (AECs) considered in [43]. This process transforms raw materials, such as anode aluminum foil, cathode aluminum foil, and plastic tube, into AECs that are appropriate to use in low leakage circuits and are well adapted to a wide range of environmental temperatures. The quality of AECs is reflected in the relationship between the dissipation factor (DF) and the environmental temperature. The figure shows three AEC profiles along with an estimator of the IC profile function (see the related discussion below). In this example, the profiles look nonlinear and a parametric function for describing their pattern is unavailable. For such applications, a number of nonparametric profile monitoring approaches have been proposed (e.g., [43, 44, 63, 64]). In [44], the following nonparametric mixed-effects model is used for describing the relationship between x and y:

$$y_{ij} = g(x_{ij}) + f_i(x_{ij}) + \varepsilon_{ij}, \qquad \text{for } j = 1, 2, \ldots, n_i, \quad i = 1, 2, \ldots, \tag{10}$$

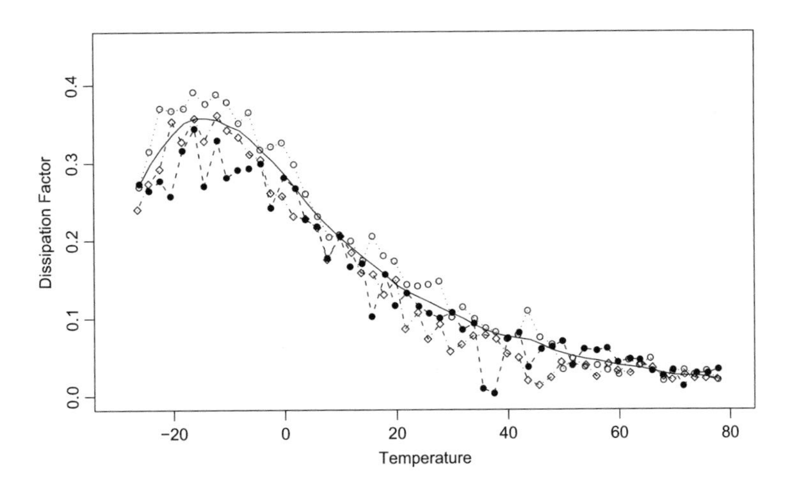

Fig. 3 Three AEC profiles (*lines* connecting points with *three different symbols*) and a nonparametric estimator (*solid curve*) of the IC profile function

where g is the population profile function (i.e., the fixed-effects term), f_i is the random-effects term describing the deviation of the i-th individual profile from g, $\{(x_{ij}, y_{ij}), i = 1, 2, \ldots, n_j\}$ is the sample collected for the i-th profile, and $\{\varepsilon_{ij}, j = 1, 2, \ldots, n_i\}$ are i.i.d. random errors with mean 0 and variance σ^2. In model (10), it is routinely assumed that the random-effects term f_i and the random errors ε_{ij} are independent of each other, and f_i is a realization of a mean 0 process with a common covariance function

$$\gamma(x_1, x_2) = E[f_i(x_1)f_i(x_2)], \qquad \text{for any } x_1, x_2.$$

Then, the IC functions of $g(x)$ and $\gamma(x_1, x_2)$, denoted as $g_0(x)$ and $\gamma_0(x_1, x_2)$, and the IC value of σ^2, denoted as σ_0^2, can be estimated from an IC dataset. At the current time point t, we can estimate g by minimizing the following local weighted negative-log likelihood:

$$WL(a, b; s, \lambda, t) = \sum_{i=1}^{t} \sum_{j=1}^{n_i} [y_{ij} - a - b(x_{ij} - s)]^2 K_h\left(x_{ij} - s\right) (1 - \lambda)^{t-i} / \nu^2(x_{ij}),$$

where $\lambda \in (0, 1]$ is a weighting parameter, and $\nu^2(x) = \gamma(x, x) + \sigma^2$ is the variance function of the response. Note that $WL(a, b; s, \lambda, t)$ combines the local linear kernel smoothing procedure (cf., Subsection 2.8.5, [36]) with the exponential weighting scheme used in EWMA through the term $(1 - \lambda)^{t-i}$. At the same time, it takes into account the heteroscedasticity of observations by using $\nu^2(x_{ij})$. Then, the local linear kernel estimator of $g(s)$, defined as the solution to a of the minimization problem $\min_{a,b} WL(a, b; s, \lambda, t)$ and denoted as $\widehat{g}_{t,h,\lambda}$, can be obtained. Process monitoring can then be performed based on the charting statistic

$$T_{t,h,\lambda} = \int \frac{[\widehat{g}_{s,h,\lambda} - g_0(s)]^2}{\nu^2(s)} \Gamma_1(s) ds,$$

where Γ_1 is some pre-specified density function.

In some applications, there are multiple response variables. For instance, Fig. 4 shows a forging machine with four strain gages. The strain gages can record the tonnage force at the four dies located at the four corners of the machine during a forging process, resulting in data with four profiles. For such examples, models (8)–(10) can still be used for describing observed profile data, except that the response variable and the related coefficients and mean function are vectors in the current setup. Research on this *multivariate profile monitoring* problem just gets started. See, for instance, [32, 33] for related discussions.

In modern industries and scientific research, image data become more and more popular [34]. For instance, NASA's satellites send us images about the earth surface constantly for monitoring the earth surface resources. Magnetic resonance imaging (MRI) has become a major tool for studying the brain functioning. Manufacturing companies monitor the quality of certain products (e.g., metal) by

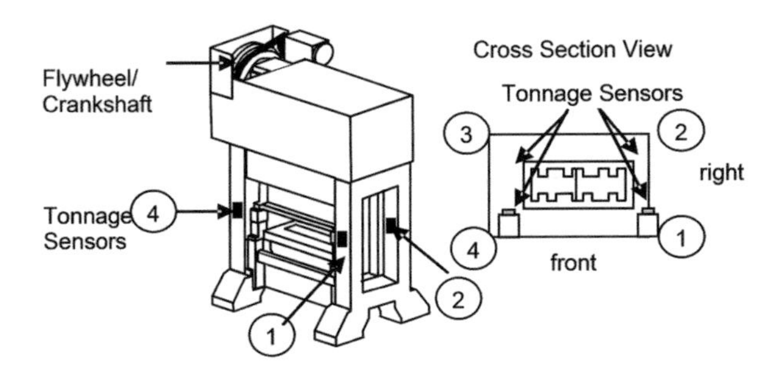

Fig. 4 A forging machine with four strain gages

taking images of the products. A central task in all these applications involves image processing and monitoring. In the literature, there has been some existing research on effective *image monitoring* (cf., [11, 50]). Most existing methods construct their control charts based on some summary statistics of the observed images or some detected image features. Some important (spatial) structures of the image sequences, however, have not been well accommodated yet in these methods, and no general SPC methods and practical guidelines have been proposed/provided for image monitoring. Therefore, in my opinion, the image monitoring area is still mostly open. Next, I will use one example to address one important issue that has not been taken into account in the existing research.

Example 3 The US Geological Survey and NASA have launched eight satellites since 1972 to gather earth resource data and for monitoring changes in the earth's land surface and in the associated environment (http://landsat.gsfc.nasa.gov). The most recent satellite Landsat-8 can give us images of different places in the entire earth every 16 days. In about a year, we can get 23 images of a given place of interest. These images have been widely used in studying agriculture, forestry and range resources, land use and mapping, geology, hydrology, coastal resources, and environmental monitoring. Figure 8 in [54] shows two satellite images of the San Francisco bay area, taken in 1990 and 1999, respectively. Assume that we are interested in detecting earth surface change over time in this area. To detect the earth surface change in the bay area between 1990 and 1999, a simple and commonly used method is to compute the difference of the two images, which is shown in the left panel of Fig. 5. From this "difference" image, it seems that the bay area changed quite dramatically from 1990 to 1999. But, if we check the two original images and their "difference" image carefully, then we can find that much of the pattern in the "difference" image is due to the geometric mis-alignment between the two images caused by the fact that the relative position between the satellite camera and earth at the two time points changed slightly. In the image processing literature, the research area called *image registration* is specially for handling this problem (e.g., [42]). After the two original images are aligned using the image registration method in [42], the "difference" image is shown in the right panel of Fig. 5. It can be seen that the pattern in this image is much weaker than that in the image shown in the

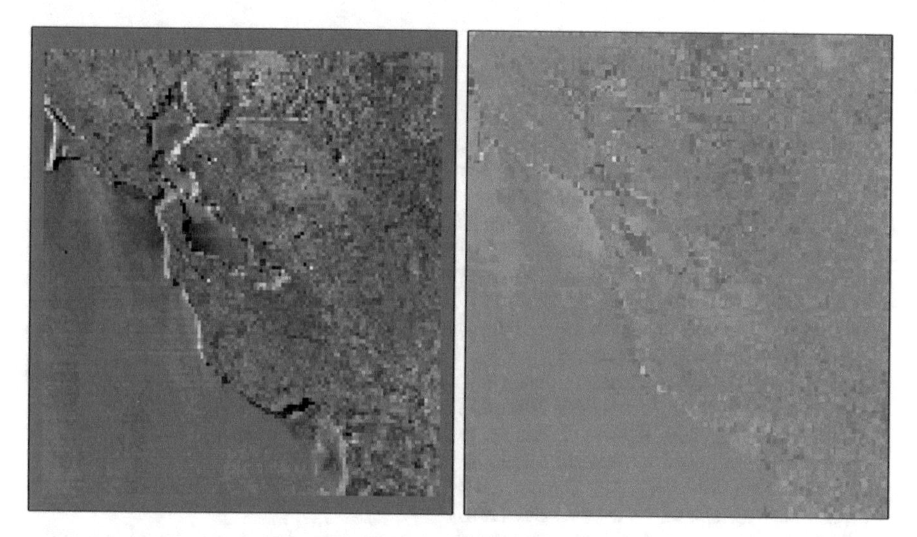

Fig. 5 The *left panel* is the difference of two satellite images of the San Francisco bay area taken in 1990 and 1999 (cf., [54, Fig. 8]). The *right panel* is their difference after a proper image registration

left panel. Therefore, when we sequentially monitor the satellite image sequence, image registration should be taken into account. In the image monitoring literature, however, this issue has not received much attention yet.

5 Concluding Remarks

Data stream is a common format of big data. In applications with data streams involved, one common research goal is to monitor the data stream and detect any longitudinal shifts and changes. For such applications, SPC charts would be an efficient statistical tool, although not many people in the big data area are familiar with this tool yet. In this paper, we have briefly introduced certain SPC charts that are potentially useful for analyzing big data. However, much future research is needed to make the existing SPC charts be more appropriate for big data applications. In this regard, fast and efficient computation, dimension reduction, and other topics about big data management and analysis are all relevant.

Acknowledgements This research is supported in part by a US National Science Foundation grant. The author thanks the invitation of the book editor Professor Ejaz Ahmed, and the review of an anonymous referee.

References

1. Albers, W., Kallenberg, W.C.M.: Empirical nonparametric control charts: estimation effects and corrections. J. Appl. Stat. **31**, 345–360 (2004)
2. Amin, R.W., Widmaier, O.: Sign control charts with variable sampling intervals. Commun. Stat. Theory Meth. **28**, 1961–1985 (1999)
3. Apley, D.W., Lee, H.C.: Design of exponentially weighted moving average control charts for autocorrelated processes with model uncertainty. Technometrics **45**, 187–198 (2003)
4. Bakir, S.T.: Distribution-free quality control charts based on signed-rank-like statistics. Commun. Stat. Theory Meth. **35**, 743–757 (2006)
5. Capizzi, G., Masarotto, G.: A least angle regression control chart for multidimensional data. Technometrics **53**, 285–296 (2011)
6. Chakraborti, S., van der Laan, P., Bakir, S.T.: Nonparametric control charts: an overview and some results. J. Qual. Technol. **33**, 304–315 (2001)
7. Chakraborti, S., Qiu, P., Mukherjee, A. (eds.): Special issue on nonparametric statistical process control charts. Qual. Reliab. Eng. Int. **31**, 1–151 (2015)
8. Champ, C.W., Woodall, W.H.: Exact results for Shewhart control charts with supplementary runs rules. Technometrics **29**, 393–399 (1987)
9. Chatterjee, S., Qiu, P.: Distribution-free cumulative sum control charts using bootstrap- based control limits. Ann. Appl. Stat. **3**, 349–369 (2009)
10. Chicken, E., Pignatiello, J.J. Jr., Simpson, J.R.: Statistical process monitoring of nonlinear profiles using wavelets. J. Qual. Technol. **41**, 198–212 (1998)
11. Chiu, D., Guillaud, M., Cox, D., Follen, M., MacAulay, C.: Quality assurance system using statistical process control: an implementation for image cytometry. Cell. Oncol. **26**, 101–117 (2004)
12. Crosier, R.B.: Multivariate generalizations of cumulative sum quality-control schemes. Technometrics **30**, 291–303 (1988)
13. Crowder, S.V.: Design of exponentially weighted moving average schemes. J. Qual. Technol. **21**, 155–162 (1989)
14. Cupples, L.A., et al.: The Framingham heart study 100K SNP genome-wide association study resource: overview of 17 phenotype working group reports. BMC Med. Genet. **8**, S1 (2007)
15. Ding, Y., Zeng, L., Zhou, S.: Phase I analysis for monitoring nonlinear profiles in manufacturing processes. J. Qual. Technol. **38**, 199–216 (2006)
16. Hawkins, D.M.: Multivariate quality control based on regression-adjusted variables. Technometrics **33**, 61–75 (1991)
17. Hawkins, D.M., Deng, Q.: A nonparametric change-point control chart. J. Qual. Technol. **42**, 165–173 (2010)
18. Hawkins, D.M., Olwell, D.H.: Cumulative Sum Charts and Charting for Quality Improvement. Springer, New York (1998)
19. Hawkins, D.M., Qiu, P., Kang, C.W.: The changepoint model for statistical process control. J. Qual. Technol. **35**, 355–366 (2003)
20. Healy, J.D.: A note on multivariate CUSUM procedures. Technometrics **29**, 409–412 (1987)
21. Jensen, W.A., Birch, J.B.: Profile monitoring via nonlinear mixed models. J. Qual. Technol. **41**, 18–34 (2009)
22. Jensen, W.A., Birch, J.B., Woodall, W.H.: Monitoring correlation within linear profiles using mixed models. J. Qual. Technol. **40**, 167–183 (2008)
23. Jin, J., Shi, J.: Feature-preserving data compression of stamping tonnage information using wavelets. Technometrics **41**, 327–339 (1999)
24. Kang, L., Albin, S.L.: On-line monitoring when the process yields a linear profile. J. Qual. Technol. **32**, 418–426 (2000)
25. Kim, K., Mahmoud, M.A., Woodall, W.H.: On the monitoring of linear profiles. J. Qual. Technol. **35**, 317–328 (2003)

26. Li, J., Qiu, P.: Nonparametric dynamic screening system for monitoring correlated longitudinal data. IIE Trans. **48**, 772–786 (2016)
27. Liu, R.Y.: Control charts for multivariate processes. J. Am. Stat. Assoc. **90**, 1380–1387 (1995)
28. Lowry, C.A., Woodall, W.H., Champ, C.W., Rigdon, S.E.: A multivariate exponentially weighted moving average control chart. Technometrics **34**, 46–53 (1992)
29. Lu, C.W., Reynolds, M.R. Jr.: Control charts for monitoring the mean variance of autocorrelated processes. J. Qual. Technol. **31**, 259–274 (1999)
30. Martin, H., Priscila, L.: The world's technological capacity to store, communicate, and compute information. Science **332**, 60–65 (2011)
31. Page, E.S.: Continuous inspection scheme. Biometrika **41**, 100–115 (1954)
32. Paynabar, K., Jin, J., Pacella, M.: Analysis of multichannel nonlinear profiles using uncorrelated multilinear principal component analysis with applications in fault detection and diagnosis. IIE Trans. **45**, 1235–1247 (2013)
33. Paynabar, K., Qiu, P., Zou, C.: A change point approach for phase-I analysis in multivariate profile monitoring and diagnosis. Technometrics **58**, 191–204 (2016)
34. Qiu, P.: Image Processing and Jump Regression Analysis. Wiley, New York (2005)
35. Qiu, P.: Distribution-free multivariate process control based on log-linear modeling. IIE Trans. **40**, 664–677 (2008)
36. Qiu, P.: Introduction to Statistical Process Control. Chapman Hall/CRC, Boca Raton, FL (2014)
37. Qiu, P., Hawkins, D.M.: A rank based multivariate CUSUM procedure. Technometrics **43**, 120–132 (2001)
38. Qiu, P., Hawkins, D.M.: A nonparametric multivariate CUSUM procedure for detecting shifts in all directions. J. R. Stat. Soc. -D (The Statistician) **52**, 151–164 (2003)
39. Qiu, P., Li, Z.: On nonparametric statistical process control of univariate processes. Technometrics **53**, 390–405 (2011)
40. Qiu, P., Xiang, D.: Univariate dynamic screening system: an approach for identifying individuals with irregular longitudinal behavior. Technometrics **56**, 248–260 (2014)
41. Qiu, P., Xiang, D.: Surveillance of cardiovascular diseases using a multivariate dynamic screening system. Stat. Med. **34**, 2204–2221 (2015)
42. Qiu, P., Xing, C.: On nonparametric image registration. Technometrics **55**, 174–188 (2013)
43. Qiu, P., Zou, C.: Control chart for monitoring nonparametric profiles with arbitrary design. Stat. Sin. **20**, 1655–1682 (2010)
44. Qiu, P., Zou, C., Wang, Z.: Nonparametric profile monitoring by mixed effects modeling (with discussions). Technometrics **52**, 265–293 (2010)
45. Reichman, O.J., Jones, M.B., Schildhauer, M.P.: Challenges and opportunities of open data in ecology. Science **331**, 703–705 (2011)
46. Roberts, S.V.: Control chart tests based on geometric moving averages. Technometrics **1**, 239–250 (1959)
47. Ross, G.J., Tasoulis, D.K., Adams, N.M.: Nonparametric monitoring of data streams for changes in location and scale. Technometrics **53**, 379–389 (2011)
48. Shewhart, W.A.: Economic Control of Quality of Manufactured Product. D. Van Nostrand Company, New York (1931)
49. Timmer, D.H., Pignatiello, J., Longnecker, M.: The development and evaluation of CUSUM-based control charts for an AR(1) process. IIE Trans. **30**, 525–534 (1998)
50. Tong, L.-I., Wang, C.-H., Huang, C.-L.: Monitoring defects in IC fabrication using a Hotelling T2 control chart. IEEE Trans. Semicond. Manuf. **18**, 140–147 (2005)
51. Tracy, N.D., Young, J.C., Mason, R.L.: Multivariate control charts for individual observations. J. Qual. Technol. **24**, 88–95 (1992)
52. Wang, K., Jiang, W.: High-dimensional process monitoring and fault isolation via variable selection. J. Qual. Technol. **41**, 247–258 (2009)
53. Woodall, W.H., Ncube, M.M.: Multivariate CUSUM quality-control procedures. Technometrics **27**, 285–292 (1985)

54. Xing, C., Qiu, P.: Intensity-based image registration by nonparametric local smoothing. IEEE Trans. Pattern Anal. Mach. Intell. **33**, 2081–2092 (2011)
55. Yashchin, E.: Statistical control schemes: methods, applications and generalizations. Int. Stat. Rev. **61**, 41–66 (1993)
56. Zhang, J., Kang, Y., Yang, Y., Qiu, P.: Statistical monitoring of the hand, foot and mouth disease in China. Biometrics **71**, 841–850 (2015)
57. Zhang, J., Qiu, P., Chen, X.: Statistical monitoring-based alarming systems in modeling the AIDS epidemic in the US, 1985–2011. Curr. HIV Res. **14**, 130–137 (2016)
58. Zou, C., Qiu, P.: Multivariate statistical process control using LASSO. J. Am. Stat. Assoc. **104**, 1586–1596 (2009)
59. Zou, C., Tsung, F.: Likelihood ratio-based distribution-free EWMA control charts. J. Qual. Technol. **42**, 1–23 (2010)
60. Zou, C., Tsung, F.: A multivariate sign EWMA control chart. Technometrics **53**, 84–97 (2011)
61. Zou, C., Zhang, Y., Wang, Z.: Control chart based on change-point model for monitoring linear profiles. IIE Trans. **38**, 1093–1103 (2006)
62. Zou, C., Tsung, F., Wang, Z.: Monitoring general linear profiles using multivariate EWMA schemes. Technometrics **49**, 395–408 (2007)
63. Zou, C., Tsung, F., Wang, Z.: Monitoring profiles based on nonparametric regression methods. Technometrics **50**, 512–526 (2008)
64. Zou, C., Qiu, P., Hawkins, D.: Nonparametric control chart for monitoring profiles using change point formulation and adaptive smoothing. Stat. Sin. **19**, 1337–1357 (2009)
65. Zou, C., Jiang, W., Wang, Z., Zi, X.: An efficient on-line monitoring method for high-dimensional data streams. Technometrics **57**, 374–387 (2015)

Fast Community Detection in Complex Networks with a K-Depths Classifier

Yahui Tian and Yulia R. Gel

Abstract We introduce a notion of data depth for recovery of community structures in large complex networks. We propose a new data-driven algorithm, K-depths, for community detection using the L_1-depth in an unsupervised setting. We evaluate finite sample properties of the K-depths method using synthetic networks and illustrate its performance for tracking communities in online social media platform Flickr. The new method significantly outperforms the classical K-means and yields comparable results to the regularized K-means. Being robust to low-degree vertices, the new K-depths method is computationally efficient, requiring up to 400 times less CPU time than the currently adopted regularization procedures based on optimizing the Davis–Kahan bound.

1 Introduction

The explosive growth of online social networking and recent advances on modeling of massive and complex data has led to a skyrocketing interest in analysis of graph-structured data and, particularly, in discovering network communities. Indeed, many real-world networks—from brain connectivity to ecosystems to gang formation and money laundering—exhibit a phenomena where certain features tend to cluster into local cohesive groups. Community detection has been extensively studied in statistics, computer science, social sciences and domain knowledge disciplines and nowadays still remains one of the most hottest research areas in network analysis (for overview of algorithms, see, e.g., [5, 11, 13, 21, 22, 37, 42, 46, 50, 68], and the references therein).

The current paper is motivated by three overarching questions. First, there exists no unique and agreed upon definition of *network community*, typically a community is thought of a cohesive set of vertices that have stronger or better internal connections within the set than with external vertices [37, 44]. Second, community discovery is further aggravated in a presence of (usually multiple) outliers, and until recently the two tightly woven problems of outlier detection

Y. Tian • Y.R. Gel (✉)
University of Texas at Dallas, 800 W Campbell Rd, Richardson TX 75080, USA
e-mail: yxt120830@utdallas.edu; ygl@utdallas.edu

© Springer International Publishing AG 2017

S.E. Ahmed (ed.), *Big and Complex Data Analysis*, Contributions to Statistics,
DOI 10.1007/978-3-319-41573-4_8

and network clustering have been studied as independent problems [5, 15, 48]. Third, vertices with a low degree (or the so-called parasitic outliers of the spectrum [35]) tend to produce multiple zero eigenvalues of the graph Laplacian, which results in a higher variability of spectral clustering and thus a reduced finite sample performance in community detection. Fourth, most of the currently available methods for community discovery within a spectral clustering framework are based on the Euclidean distance as a measure of "cohesion" or "closeness" among vertices, and thus do not explicably account for the underlying probabilistic geometry of the graph.

We propose to address the above challenges by introducing a concept of *data depth* into the network community detection that allows to integrate ideas on cohesion, centrality, outliers, and community discovery under a one systematized "roof." Data depth is a nonparametric and inherently geometric tool to analyze, classify, and visualize multivariate data without making prior assumptions about underlying probability distributions. A new impetus has been recently given to data depths due to their broad utility in high dimensional and functional data analysis (for overview, see, e.g., [9, 26, 27, 34, 40, 47, 58, 73], and the references therein.). Given a notion of data depth, we can measure the "depth" (or "outlyingness") of a given object or a set of objects with respect to an observed data cloud. A higher value of a data depth implies a deeper location or higher centrality in the data cloud. By plotting such a natural center-outward ordering of depth values that serves as a topological map of the data, the presence of clusters, outliers, and anomalies can be evaluated simultaneously in a quick and visual manner. A notion of data depth is novel to network studies. The only relevant paper on the topic is due to [14] who consider a random sample of graphs following the same probability model on the space of all graphs of a given size. This probabilistic framework, however, is not applicable to analysis of most real-world graph-structured data where the available data consists only of a *single network*. In this paper we primarily focus on utility of L_1-depth as the main tool for unsupervised community detection in a spectral setting. Although there exist numerous other depth alternatives, our choice of a depth function is motivated by simplicity and tractability of L_1-depth and the fact that it can be computed using a fast and monotonically converging algorithm [29, 30, 65]. This makes L_1-depth particularly attractive for community discovery in large complex networks.

The paper is organized as follows. Section 2 provides background on graphs, spectral clustering, and K-means algorithm. We introduce the new K-depths method based on the L_1-depth and discuss its properties in Sect. 3. simulation studies are presented in Sect. 4. Section 5 illustrates application of the K-depths method to tracking communities in online social media platform Flickr.

2 Preliminaries and Background

Graph Notations Consider an undirected and loopless graph $\mathcal{G} = (\mathcal{V}, \mathcal{E})$, with a vertex set $\mathcal{V}$ of cardinality n and an edge set $\mathcal{E}$. We assume that $\mathcal{G}$ consists of K non-overlapping communities and K is given. Let A be an $n \times n$-symmetric empirical adjacency matrix, i.e.,

$$A = \begin{cases} 1, & \text{if } (i,j) \in \mathcal{E} \\ 0, & \text{otherwise.} \end{cases}$$

The population counterpart of A is denoted by P. Let D be a diagonal matrix of degrees, i.e., $D_{ii} = \sum_{j=1}^{n} A_{ij}$. Then, the graph Laplacian is defined as

$$L = D^{-1/2} A D^{-1/2}. \tag{1}$$

Spectral Clustering For smaller networks, communities can be identified via optimizing various goodness of partition measures, for instance, Ratio Cut [19], Normalized Cut [60], and Modularity [45], which involve a search for optimal split over all possible partitions of vertices. However, such discrete optimization problems are typically NP-hard and thus are not feasible for larger networks. The computational challenges can be circumvented using spectral clustering (SC) that yields a continuous approximation to discrete optimization [67]. Hence, SC is now one of the most widely popular procedures for tracking communities in large complex networks [66].

The key idea of SC is to embed a graph $\mathcal{G}$ into a collection of multivariate sample points. Given K communities, we identify orthogonal eigenvectors $\mathbf{v}_{\cdot j}, j = 1, \ldots, K$ of the Laplacian L (or adjacency matrix A) that correspond to the largest K eigenvalues, and construct the $n \times K$-matrix $V = [\mathbf{v}_{\cdot 1}, \ldots, \mathbf{v}_{\cdot K}]$. Each row of V, $\mathbf{v}_i \equiv \mathbf{v}_{i\cdot}$, provides a representation in $\mathbb{R}^K$ of a vertex in $\mathcal{V}$. Given this embedding, we can now employ any appropriate classifier to cluster this multivariate data set into K communities, and the most conventional choice is a method of K-means [1, 31, 36, 51].

Given a set of data points $x_i \in \mathbb{R}^d$, for $i = 1, \ldots, n$, the method of K-means [41] aims to group observations into K sets $\mathbf{C} = \{C_1, \ldots, C_K\}$ in such a way that the within-cluster sum of squares is minimized, that is, we minimize

$$\underset{\mathbf{C}}{\operatorname{argmin}} \sum_{k=1}^{K} \sum_{x \in C_k} ||x - \mu_k||^2, \tag{2}$$

where μ_k is the mean of points in C_k, $||x - \mu_k||^2$ is the squared Euclidean distance between x and k-th group mean μ_k. The optimization (2) is highly computationally intensive. As an alternative, we can employ the Lloyd's algorithm (also known as Voronoi iteration or relaxation) for (2) that is based on iterative refinement and that allows to quickly identify an optimum (see the outline of the K-means 1). In this paper, the initial centers are chosen randomly from the data set.

Algorithm 1: The K-means algorithm

Input : a set of data points $\mathbf{X} = \{x_1, \ldots, x_n\}$, an initial set of K means $m_1, \ldots, m_K$.
Output: a partition of $\mathbf{X}$.

1 do

2 • Assign points to its nearest cluster in terms of squared Euclidean distance, for $k = 1, \ldots, K$:

$$C_k = \{x_i : ||x_i - m_k||^2 \leq ||x_i - m_j||^2, \forall j, 1 \leq j \leq K\}$$

• Update cluster centers as the mean of points in new clusters, for $k = 1, \ldots, K$:

$$m_k = \frac{1}{|C_k|} \sum_{x_i \in C_k} x_i.$$

3 until *the assignment no longer change*;

Regularization Low-degree vertices tend to produce multiple zero eigenvalues of a Laplacian L, which in turns increases clustering variability and adversely impacts a performance of the K-means algorithm. The problem is closely connected to the concentration of L, that is, the study on how close a sample Laplacian L to its expected value. Sparser networks tend to produce more low-degree vertices and do not concentrate. The idea of regularization in this context is to somehow diminish the impact of such vertices with low degrees, by viewing them as outliers and shrinking them toward the center of spectrum. As a result, regularization leads to a higher concentration. There are a number of regularization procedures ranging from brute-force trimming of outliers to sophisticated methods that are closely connected to regularization of covariance matrices (for more discussion and the most recent literature review see [35]). One of the most popular approaches, by analogy with a ridge regularization of covariance matrices, is to select some positive parameter τ and add τ/n to all entries of the adjacency matrix A [1], that is

$$A_\tau = A + \tau J,$$

where $J = 1/n\mathbf{1}$, $\mathbf{1}$ is $n \times n$-matrix with all elements 1. The resulting regularized Laplacian then takes a form

$$L_\tau = D_\tau^{-1/2} A_\tau D_\tau^{-1/2},$$

where $D_{ii,\tau} = \sum_{j=1}^{n} A_{ij} + \tau$. The optimal regularizer τ can then be selected by minimizing the Davis–Kahan bound, i.e., the bound on the distance between the sample and population Laplacians (for study on properties of regularized spectral clustering see, [31, 35], and the references therein). However, selecting an optimal regularizer τ is highly computationally expensive. In addition, the impact of small and weak communities on performance of regularized spectral clustering is not clear.

In this light, an interesting question arises on whether we can develop an alternative data-driven and computationally inexpensive method for taming "outliers" with low degrees and bypass the optimization stage of the Davis–Kahan bound? It seems natural to unitize here a statistical methodology that has been developed with a particular focus on analysis of outliers, that is, a notion of data depth.

3 Community Detection Using L_1 Data Depth

In this section, we propose a new unsupervised K-depths algorithm for network community detection based on iterative refinement with L_1 depth.

The L_1 Data Depth In this paper we consider an L_1-data depth of Vardi and Zhang [65]. Consider N distinct observations $x_1, \ldots, x_N$ in $\mathbb{R}^p$ which we need to partition into K clusters, and let $I(k)$ be a set of labels for observations in the k-th cluster. Let each observation x_i be associated with a scalar η_i, $i = 1, \ldots, N$, where η_i are viewed as weights or as "multiplicities" of x_i, and $\eta_i = 1$ if the data set has no ties. The multivariate L_1-median of a k-th cluster, $y_0(k)$, is then defined as

$$y_0(k) = \operatorname{argmin} C(y|k), \tag{3}$$

where $C(y|k)$ is the weighted sum of distances between y and points x_i in the k-th cluster

$$C(y|k) = \sum_{i \in I(k)} \eta_i ||x_i - y|| \qquad \forall k. \tag{4}$$

Here $||u - v||$, $u, v \in \mathbb{R}^p$, is the Euclidean distance in $\mathbb{R}^p$. If $x_1, \ldots, x_N$ are not multicollinear (which is the case of the considered spectral clustering framework), $C(y)$ is positive and strictly convex in $\mathbb{R}^p$. If the set $x_1, \ldots, x_N$ has ties, "multiplicities" η_i can be chosen in such a way that it preserves convexity of $C(y)$ (see [65], for further discussion).

The L_1 depth was proposed by Vardi and Zhang [65], based on the notion of a multivariate L_1-median (3), and the idea has been further extended to clustering and classification in multivariate and functional settings by López-Pintado and Jörnsten [39], Jörnsten [29]. Given a cluster assignment, the L_1 depth of point $x, x \in \mathbb{R}^K$ with respect to a k-th cluster is defined as

$$LD(x|k) = 1 - \max[0, ||\bar{e}(x|k)|| - f(x|k)]. \tag{5}$$

Here $f(x|k) = \eta(x)/\sum_{i\in I(k)} \eta_i$ with $\eta(x) = \sum_{i=1}^{N} \eta_i I(x = x_i)$ and $\bar{e}(x|k)$ is the average of the unit vectors from a point x to all observations in the k-th cluster and is defined as

$$\bar{e}(x|k) = \sum_{i\in I(k), x_i\neq x} \eta_i e_i(x) / \sum_{j\in I(k)} \eta_j,$$

where $e_i(x) = (x_i - x)/||x_i - x||$.

The idea of $1 - LD(x|k)$ is to quantify a minimal additional weight required to assign x so that x becomes the multivariate L_1-median of the k-th cluster $x \cup \{x_i, i \in I(k)\}$ [65]. Hence, L_1 depths as a robust representation of a topological structure of each cluster. Since L_1 is non-zero outside the convex hull of the data cloud, it is a feasible depth choice for comparing multiple clusters [29].

The K-Depths Method It is well known that K-means clustering algorithm is non-robust to outliers [16, 59, 69]. This partially is due to the fact that the K-means algorithm is based on a squared Euclidean norm as the measure of "distance" and only captures the information between a pair of points, i.e., a *candidate* center and another point (see Fig. 1a). Also to identify a cluster, the K-means algorithm uses a presumptive cluster center defined by a cluster mean, which makes it sensitive to anomalies and outliers. Although we update centers and clusters until the assignments no longer change, there is no guarantee that the global optimum for (2) can be found [49, 54].

Our idea is motivated by the two overarching questions. Is there an alternative "cohesion" measure to a squared Euclidean norm? Does such a measure allow to

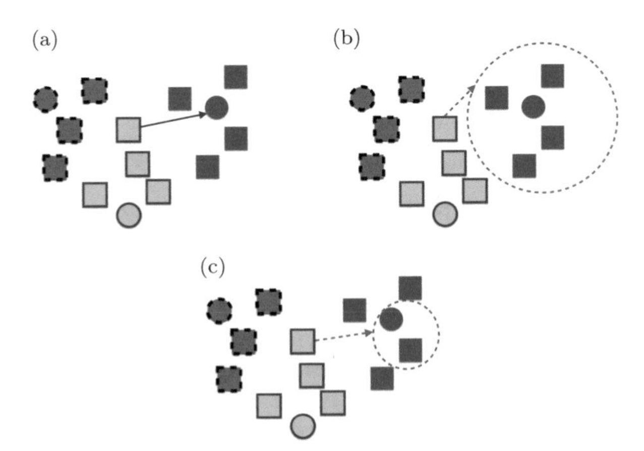

Fig. 1 Comparing K-means and K-depths algorithms. *Circles* denote cluster centers. Each cluster is identified by *colors* and *border* around points. (**a**) K-means. (**b**) K-depths. (**c**) Generalized K-depths

achieve a higher accuracy and stability by taking advantage of more information between clusters and points?

Indeed, such a "cohesion" measure exists, and it can be based on a data depth notion. As discussed earlier, a depth function evaluates how "deep" (or "central") a point is with respect to a group of data (i.e., a cluster). Hence, depth functions allow for more informative and robust "cohesion" (or "distance") measures than a squared Euclidean norm (Fig. 1b).

Our proposed approach is then to use a data depth (particularly, the L_1 depth) to find "nearest" clusters as a part of iterative refinement, and we call the new method "K-depths" clustering algorithm. That is, following the spectral clustering setting, we embed a graph into a collection of multivariate sample points. Then, given K communities, we identify orthogonal eigenvectors of the Laplacian L that correspond to the K largest eigenvalues of L, and construct an $n \times K$-matrix V that is formed by eigenvectors of L. We view each row of V as a representation of a network vertex in $\mathbb{R}^K$, and thus, we get n sample points in K-dimensional space. Clustering of these multivariate points using the K-depths yields a partition of networks into K communities. (The K-depths method is outlined in Algorithm 2. Note that we still use a squared Euclidean norm to initialize the K-depths iterative refinement.) Note that instead of Laplacian spectral embedding, we can also consider adjacency spectral embedding (see [36] and references therein).

Algorithm 2: Spectral clustering K-depths algorithm

Input : network $\mathcal{G}$; number of communities K, depth function LD.
Output: a partition of $\mathcal{G}$.

1 compute L using (1) ; `// Spectral Clustering`
2 construct V by combining the leading K eigenvectors of L;
3 view each row of V as a multivariate representation of each vertex in $\mathcal{V}$;
4 randomly select K points as initial centers $m_1^0, m_2^0, \ldots, m_K^0$; `// K-depths`
5 define initial clusters: $C_k^0 = \{x_i : ||x_i - m_k||^2 \leq ||x_i - m_j||^2, \forall j, 1 \leq j \leq K\}$;
6 **do**
7 extract inner p percent vertices: $I_k = \{x_i : LD(i|k) \geq LD(.|k)_{(p*n_k)}\}$ for $k = 1, \ldots, K$ update clusters: $C_k = \{x_i : LD(x_i|k) \geq LD(x_i|j), \forall j, 1 \leq j \leq K\}$;
8 **until** *the assignment no longer change*;

The K-depths algorithm presented above is closely related to the modified Weiszfeld algorithm of [65]. The idea of the K-depths is to evaluate "centrality" of any given point in respect to all points within a cluster (see Fig.1b), that is, in respect to points located inside the cluster and points located close to a cluster borderline. However, points that fall in-between clusters may provide redundant or noisy information, which leads a higher variability of the clustering algorithm. We therefore introduce the generalized K-depths measure which only accounts for the inner parts of a cluster to calculate depth values (Fig. 1c). Given a contour plot of a cluster, we compute L_1 depth values using points which are within an arbitrary percentage contour $p \in [0, 1]$. For instance, Fig. 1b is a special case of Fig. 1c where the *locality* parameter p is 1, i.e., all 100 % of available data are used in the K-depths algorithm. We can also view the locality parameter p as a trade-off of bias (i.e., detection accuracy) and variance (i.e., detection variability).

Remark The optimal choice of p, similarly to selection of optimal trimming, largely depends on a definition of outlier, types of anomalous behavior, proportion of contamination, and structure of the data. Conventionally, trimming and other robustifying parameters are chosen using various types of resampling, including V-fold crossvalidation, jackknife, and bootstrap (see [2, 24, 25]). Under the network setting, the problem is further aggravated by the lack of an agreed-upon definition of outliers and network anomalies and their dependence on the underlying network model structure (for overviews, see [3–5, 17, 18]). For instance, [5] discuss at least four kinds of outliers: mixed membership, hubs, small clusters, independent neutral nodes. Although selecting p using crossvalidation is likely to be affected by the presence of outliers in an observed network, we believe that one of the resampling ideas such as crossvalidation or bootstrap [12, 63] is still arguably the most feasible approach that allows to minimize parametric assumptions about the network model.

3.1 Properties of Spectral Clustering K-Depths Algorithm

Asymptotic properties of spectral clustering and, particularly, the K-means/ medians algorithms have been widely studied both in probability and statistics (for the most recent overviews, see, e.g., [28, 36, 52, 53], and the references therein). While most of the results focus on denser networks, most recently [36] derive an upper error bound for spectral clustering under moderately sparse stochastic block model with a maximum expected degree of order $\log n$ or higher.

The key result behind deriving all asymptotic properties of the K-means/ medians algorithms is to show that there exists a sequence $\epsilon_n, \epsilon_n \geq 0$ such that $\lim_{n\to\infty} \epsilon_n = 0$ and

$$z^{A_k} \leq (1 + \epsilon_n) z^*(\mathcal{G}), \; n \in Z^+ \tag{6}$$

where $z^{A_k}(\mathcal{G})$ is the approximate polynomial time solution from the K-means/medians algorithms and $z^*(\mathcal{G})$ is the optimal solution. If such a sequence ϵ_n exists, then [10] define asymptotic optimality of the K-medians algorithm.

Defining $z(\mathcal{G})$ in (6) in terms of a Frobenius norm of a distance between the K largest eigenvectors $U_1, \ldots, U_K$ of a population adjacency matrix P and their respective counterparts $\hat{U}_1, \ldots, \hat{U}_K$ from an empirical adjacency matrix A, [33] show that there exists an approximate polynomial time solution to the K-means algorithm with an error bound

$$||\hat{\Theta}\hat{X} - \hat{U}||_F^2 \leq (1+\epsilon) \min_{\substack{\Theta \in \mathbb{M}_{n,K} \\ X \in \mathbb{R}_{K\times K}}} ||U - \hat{U}||_F^2, \quad \hat{U},\ U \in \mathbb{R}^{n\times K},$$

where $U = [U_1, \ldots, U_K]$ and $\hat{U} = [\hat{U}_1, \ldots, \hat{U}_K]$. Here Θ is a true membership matrix such that Θ_{ig_i} is 1 where $g_i \in \{1, \ldots, K\}$ is the community membership of vertex i, and $\mathbb{M}_{n,K}$ is a collection of all $n \times K$-matrices where each row has exactly one 1 and the remaining $K-1$ entries are 0. For discussion on analogous results on existence of $(1+\epsilon)$-approximate solution for a k-medians algorithm in network applications see, for instance, [36].

Since statistical properties of median and L_1-depth are closed related (see [65]), we state the following conjecture about the error bound of the K-depths algorithm under the L_1 depth and adjacency spectral embedding.

Conjecture 1 There exists an Ω-approximate polynomial time solution to the K-depths method under adjacency spectral embedding which attains

$$||\hat{\Theta}\hat{X} - \hat{U}||_F^2 \leq \Omega \min_{\substack{\Theta \in \mathbb{M}_{n,K} \\ X \in \mathbb{R}_{K\times K}}} ||U - \hat{U}||_F^2, \tag{7}$$

where Ω is a positive constant and $(\hat{\Theta}, \hat{X}) \in \mathbb{M}_{n,K} \times \mathbb{R}_{K\times K}$ is the output of Ω-approximate K-depths algorithm.

Armed with (7), an upper bound on network community detection error of the K-depths algorithm 2 under adjacency spectral embedding can be derived for a stochastic block model (SBM), following derivations of [36, 52, 65]. This error bound for the K-depths increases with an increasing network sparsity and with the growing number of communities. In addition, assuming existence of a Σ-approximate solution to the K-depths algorithm, analogous error bounds can be derived under Laplacian spectral embedding [52, 53].

4 Simulations

In this section we evaluate a finite sample performance of the unsupervised K-depths classifier for detecting network communities and primarily focus on a case of two communities. To measure a goodness of clustering, we employ such standard criteria as misclassification rate and normalized mutual information (NMI). We define misclassification rate as the total percentage of mislabeled vertices, i.e.,

$$\gamma = \frac{1}{n}\sum_{i=1}^{K} |S_i|,$$

where $|S_i|$ is the number of misclassified vertices in the i-th community.

Given the two sets of clusters with a total of n vertices: $\mathbb{R} = \{r_1, \ldots, r_K\}$ and $\mathbb{C} = \{c_1, \ldots, c_J\}$, the NMI is given by Manning et al. [43]:

$$\text{NMI}(\mathbb{R}, \mathbb{C}) = \frac{I(\mathbb{R}; \mathbb{C})}{[H(\mathbb{R}) + H(\mathbb{C})]/2}.$$

Here I is mutual information

$$\begin{aligned} I(\mathbb{R}; \mathbb{C}) &= \sum_k \sum_j P(r_k \bigcap c_j) \log \frac{P(r_k \bigcap c_j)}{P(r_k)P(c_j))} \\ &= \sum_k \sum_j \frac{|r_k \bigcap c_j|}{n} \log \frac{n|r_k \bigcap c_j|}{|r_k||c_j|} \end{aligned}$$

where $P(r_k)$, $P(c_j)$, and $P(r_k \bigcap c_j)$ are the probabilities of a vertex being in cluster r_k, c_j and in the intersection of r_k and c_j, respectively, and H is entropy defined by

$$H(\mathbb{R}) = -\sum_k P(r_k) \log P(r_k) = -\sum \frac{|r_k|}{n} \log \frac{|r_k|}{n}.$$

NMI takes values between 0 and 1, and we prefer a clustering partition with a higher NMI.

4.1 Network Clustering with Two Groups

Here we use a benchmark simulation framework based on a 2-block stochastic block model (SBM)[61, 71]. SBM is a particular case of an inhomogeneous Erdös–Renyi model in which edges are formed independently and probability of an edge between two vertices is determined by group membership of vertices [23].

Following a simulation setting of Joseph and Yu [31], we generate 100 networks of order 3000 from an SBM with a block probability matrix

$$B = \begin{bmatrix} 0.01 & 0.0025 \\ 0.0025 & 0.003 \end{bmatrix}, \tag{8}$$

and assume that the connections within the k-th community follow an independent Bernoulli distribution with probability B_{kk}, $k = 1, 2$.

Table 1(a) summarizes clustering performance of the K-means and K-depths algorithms in terms of misclassification rate and NMI. We find that the K-depths method noticeably outperforms the K-means algorithm, delivering 36 % lower misclassification rate and more than four times higher NMI, although with a

Table 1 Performance of the K-means and K-depths algorithms in respect to misclassification rate γ and NMI, with standard deviation in (), under (a) SBM (8) and (b) Generalized SBM (GSBM). The locality parameter p for the K-depths algorithm is 0.1

Method	γ	NMI
(a)		
K-means	0.44	0.05
	(0.08)	(0.09)
K-depths	0.28	0.23
	(0.13)	(0.19)
(b)		
K-means	0.62	0.24
	(0.21)	(0.08)
K-depths	0.55	0.43
	(0.25)	(0.07)

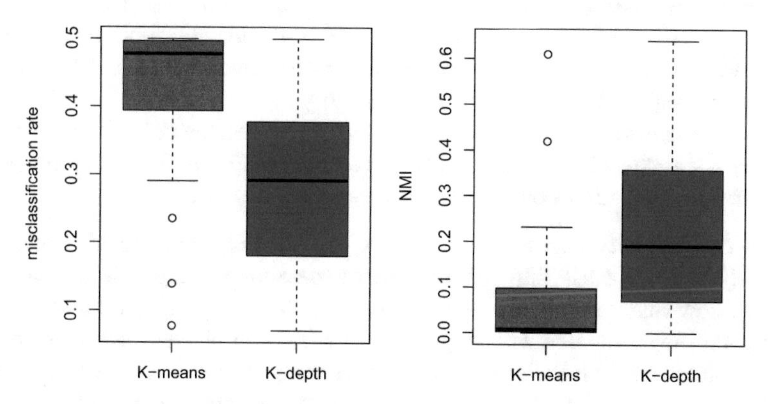

Fig. 2 Boxplots of clustering performance of the K-means and K-depths in terms of misclassification rate and NMI for the SBM (8)

somewhat higher variability. Remarkably, the boxplot for misclassification rate and NMI (see the left panel of Fig. 2) indicates that despite a higher variability, the lower quartile of the misclassification rates delivered by the K-depths algorithm is smaller than the upper quartile of the misclassification rates yielded by the K-means algorithm. A similar dynamics is also observed for NMI (see the right panel of Fig. 2).

We find that regularization of both K-means and K-depths where an optimal regularizer τ is selected using optimizing the Davis–Kahan bound as per [31] improves community discovery. That is, the regularized K-means outperforms the regularized K-depths in terms of misclassification rates, i.e., 0.16 vs. 0.22; and the regularized K-depths outperforms the regularized K-means in terms of NMI, i.e., 0.44 vs. 0.40. However, regularization turns out to be highly computationally

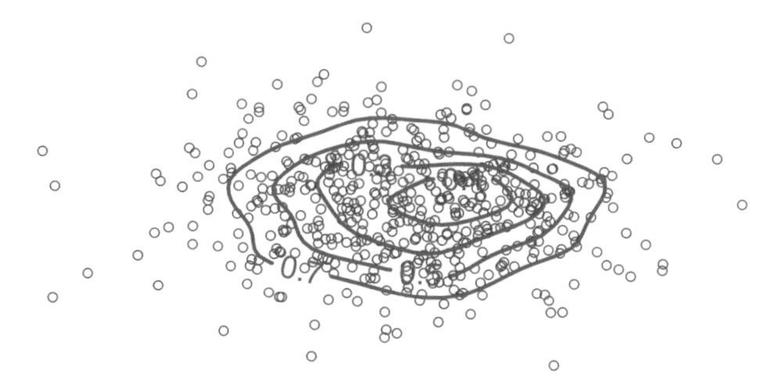

Fig. 3 Contour plots based on the L_1-data depth and varying data proportions p, i.e., p is 0.1, 0.3, 0.5, and 0.7

expensive, that is, finding an optimal regularization for a single network of 3000 vertices under SBM (8) requires 1800 s (with 1 additional sec for the K-means algorithm itself). In contrast, the unregularized K-depths algorithm takes only 4 s. (The elapsed time is assessed in R on an OS X 64 bit laptop with 1.4 GHz Intel Core i5 processor and 4 GB 1600 MHz DDR3 memory.)

Thus, being intrinsically robust to low-degree vertices, the new K-depths method provides a simple and computationally efficient alternative to the currently adopted regularization procedures based on optimizing the Davis–Kahan bound.

Choice of a Locality Parameter Let us explore the impact of a locality parameter p, $p \in [0, 1]$, on a clustering performance of the K-depths algorithm. Note that p controls how many points are selected to form the "deepest" sub-clusters which other points are compared with. Figure 3 visualizes sub-clusters and the respective contour plots based on the L_1-depth, corresponding to $p = (0.1,\ 0.3,\ 0.5,\ 0.7)$. If p is 1, the whole data cloud is used, while lower values of p lead to a higher concentration of points around the cluster center and aim to minimize the impact of outlying points or noise. Hence, a locality parameter p can be viewed as a trade-off between bias and variance. Figure 4 shows the performance of the K-depths algorithm in respect to varying p and the SBM (8). We find that in general both mean and variance of misclassification rates and NMI are stable and comparable for p of less than 0.5. As expected, higher values of p lead to a better performance in terms of average misclassification rates and NMI but also result in a substantially higher variability. In general, an optimal p can be selected via crossvalidation, and choice of p is likely to be linked with a sparsity of an observed network. However, given the stability of the K-depths performance, as a rule of thumb we suggest to use a p of 0.5 or less.

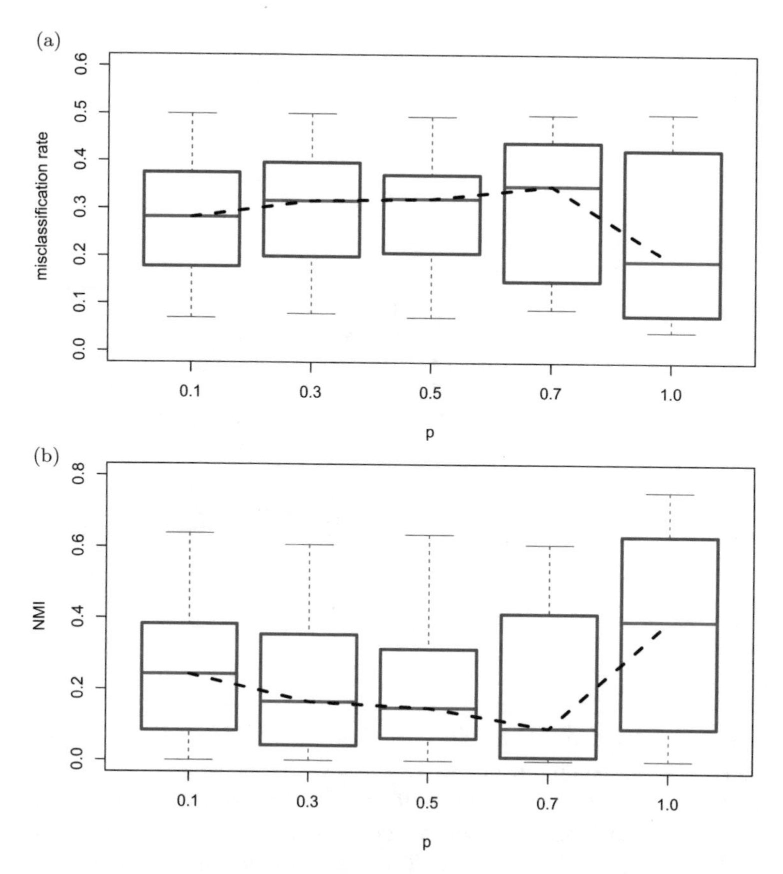

Fig. 4 Boxplots of misclassification rates (**a**) NMI (**b**) with various choices of locality parameter p. The dashed line connects medians for resulting misclassification rates and NMI for various locality parameters p, in plots (**a**) and (**b**) respectively

4.2 Network Clustering with Outliers

Now we evaluate the performance of the K-depths algorithm in respect to a network with outliers. In particular, we consider the so-called *Generalized Stochastic Block Model (GSBM)* of Cai and Li [5] which is based on incorporating small and weak communities (outliers) into a conventional SBM structure. More specifically, consider an undirected and loopless graph $\mathcal{G} = (\mathcal{V}, \mathcal{E})$ with $N = n + m$ vertices, where n is the number of "inliers" which follow the standard SBM framework and m is the number of "outliers" which connect with other vertices in random. Each inlier vertex is assigned to one of the two communities, while all outliers are placed into the 3rd community. An example of GSBM is shown in Fig. 5, two strong communities are colored by red and green within solid circles, the outliers (one weak and small community) are colored by blue within a dashed circle.

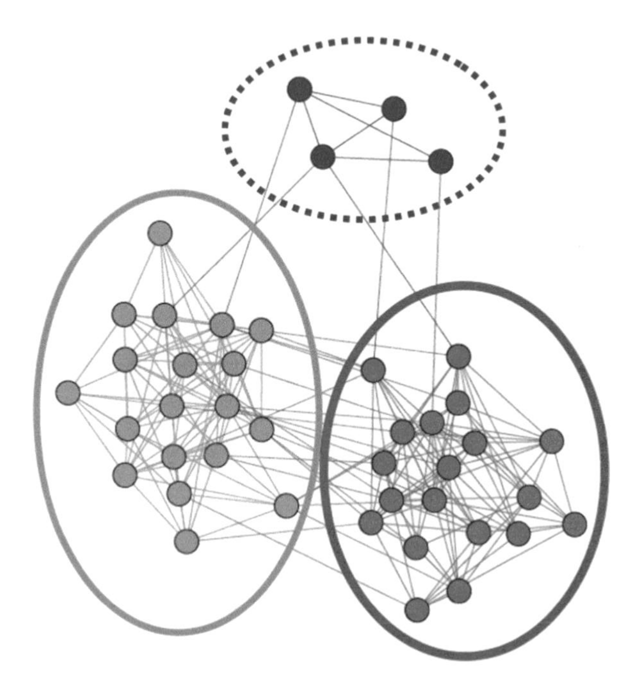

Fig. 5 Network with outliers, or small and weak community, under GSBM

In this section we consider a GSBM of Cai and Li [5] by adding 30 outliers (i.e., one small and weak community) into a standard 2-block SBM (8).

In particular, we set a probability of an edge between outliers to be of 0.01. Connection between inliers and outliers is defined by an arbitrary $(0, 1)$-matrix Z, $Z \in \mathbb{R}^{n \times m}$, such that $\mathbb{E}Z = \boldsymbol{\beta}\mathbf{1}^T = [\boldsymbol{\beta}, \ldots, \boldsymbol{\beta}]$ and the component of $\boldsymbol{\beta}$ are 3000 i.i.d. copies of U^2, where U is a uniform random variable on $[0, 0.0025]$.

Following [5], we define a misclassification rate based only on inliers in the dominant 1st and 2nd communities, i.e.,

$$\gamma = \frac{1}{n} \sum_{k=1}^{2} |S_k|,$$

where $|S_k|$ is a number of misclassified vertices in the k-th community and $k = 1, 2$. Similarly, NMI is defined calculated only on inliers and a number of clusters K are set to 3 for both K-means and K-depths algorithms.

Table 1(b) summarizes the results for misclassification rates and NMI delivered by the K-means and K-depths algorithms. In general, misclassification rates for both methods under the GSBM model are noticeably higher than the analogous rates under a standard SBM. However, the K-depths algorithm still outperforms the K-means method, yielding a 10 % lower misclassification rate. In turn, NMI delivered by the K-depths algorithm is almost twice higher than the corresponding NMI of the K-means method, i.e., 0.43 vs. 0.24, respectively. Remarkably, under

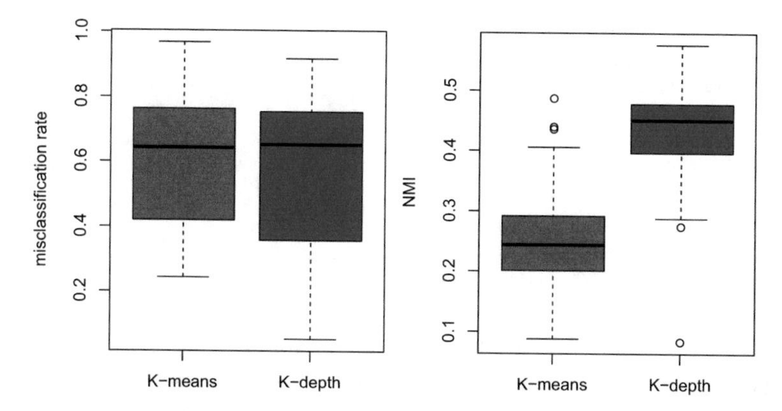

Fig. 6 Boxplots of clustering performance of the *K*-means and *K*-depths in terms of misclassification rate and NMI under the GSBM

the GSBM variability of both methods is very similar, while the upper quartile of NMI for the *K*-means algorithm is lower than almost all values of NMI delivered by the *K*-depths algorithm (see Fig. 6).

5 Application to Flickr Communities

In this section, we illustrate the *K*-depths algorithm to tracking communities in Flickr. Flickr is a popular website for users to share personal photographs and also an online platform. This data set contains the information of 80,513 Flickr bloggers, each blogger is viewed as a vertex, and the friendship between bloggers is represented by undirected edges. The data is available from [70]. Bloggers are divided into 195 groups depending on their interests. As discussed by Tang and Liu [62], the network is very sparse and scale-free (i.e., its degree distribution follows a power law).

In our study, we consider a subnetwork of Flickr by extracting vertices that belong to the second and third communities and edges within and in-between of these communities. Isolated vertices (vertices with no edges) are removed. The resulting data represents an undirected graph with 216 vertices and 996 edges; the second community contains 155 vertices and 753 edges, while the third community contains 61 vertices and 19 edges.

We now apply the *K*-means and *K*-depths algorithms to identify clusters in the Flickr subnetwork (see Table 2). We find that the *K*-depths algorithm delivers a misclassification rate of 0.35, which is more than 26 % lower than the misclassification rate of 0.47 yielded by the *K*-means algorithm. In turn, NMI yielded by the *K*-depths algorithm is comparable with NMI of the *K*-means algorithm.

Table 2 Misclassification rate (γ) and Normalized Mutual Information (NMI) criteria for the K-means and K-depths methods for the Flickr subnetwork

Method	γ	NMI
K-means	0.47	0.07
K-depths	0.35	0.07

The locality parameter p for the K-depths algorithm is 0.5

6 Conclusion and Future Work

In this paper, we introduce a new unsupervised approach to network community detection based on a nonparametric concept of data depth within a spectral clustering framework. In particular, we propose a data-driven K-depths algorithm based on iterative refinement of the L_1 depth. The new method is shown to substantially outperform the classical K-means and to deliver comparable results to the regularized K-means. The K-depths algorithm is simple and computationally efficient, requiring up to 400 times less CPU time than the currently adopted regularization procedures based on optimizing the Davis–Kahan bound. Moreover, the K-depths algorithm is intrinsically robust to low-degree vertices and accounts for the underlying geometrical structure of a graph, thus paving the way for using the L_1 depth and other depth functions as an alternative to computationally expensive selection of optimal regularizers.

In addition to asymptotic analysis of the K-depths clustering, in the future we plan to advance the K-depths approach to other types of depth functions, for example, the classical ones: half-space depth, Mahalanobis depth, random projection depth etc [38, 55–57, 72], and to the most recent such as Monge-Kantorovich depth [6, 20] and to explore utility of the K-depths method as initialization algorithm (for discussion, see [64] and the references therein). Another interesting direction is to investigate the relationship between properties of the K-depths approach and the trimmed K-means algorithms [7, 8, 32], both in networks and general multivariate clustering contexts.

Acknowledgements Authors are grateful to Robert Serfling, Ricardo Fraiman, and Rebecka Jörnsten for motivating discussions at various stages of this paper. Yulia R. Gel is supported in part by the National Science Foundation grant IIS 1633331. This work was made possible by the facilities of the Shared Hierarchical Academic Research Computing Network (SHARCNET) of Canada.

References

1. Amini, A.A., Chen, A., Bickel, P.J., Levina, E.: Pseudo-likelihood methods for community detection in large sparse networks. Ann. Stat. **41**, 2097–2122 (2013)
2. Arlot, S., Celisse, A., et al.: A survey of cross-validation procedures for model selection. Stat. Surv. **4**, 40–79 (2010)

3. Baddar, S.A.-H., Merlo, A., Migliardi, M.: Anomaly detection in computer networks: a state-of-the-art review. J. Wirel. Mob. Netw. Ubiquit. Comput. Dependable Appl. **5**(4), 29–64 (2014)
4. Bhuyan, M.H., Bhattacharyya, D.K., Kalita, J.K.: Network anomaly detection: methods, systems and tools. IEEE Commun. Surv. Tutorials **16**(1), 303–336 (2014)
5. Cai, T.T., Li, X.: Robust and computationally feasible community detection in the presence of arbitrary outlier nodes. Ann. Stat. **43**(3), 1027–1059 (2015)
6. Chernozhukov, V., Galichon, A., Hallin, M., Henry, M.: Monge-Kantorovich depth, quantiles, ranks, and signs. arXiv preprint arXiv:1412.8434 (2014)
7. Cuesta-Albertos, J., Gordaliza, A., Matrán, C., et al.: Trimmed k-means: An attempt to robustify quantizers. Ann. Stat. **25**(2), 553–576 (1997)
8. Cuesta-Albertos, J.A., Matrán, C., Mayo-Iscar, A.: Trimming and likelihood: robust location and dispersion estimation in the elliptical model. Ann. Stat. **36**(5), 2284–2318 (2008)
9. Cuevas, A., Febrero, M., Fraiman, R.: Robust estimation and classification for functional data via projection-based depth functions. Comput. Stat. **22**, 481–496 (2007)
10. Emelichev, V., Efimchik, N.: Asymptotic approach to the problem of k-median of a graph. Cybern. Syst. Anal. **30**(5), 726–732 (1994)
11. Estrada, E., Knight, P.A.: A First Course in Network Theory. Oxford University Press, Oxford (2015)
12. Fallani, F.D.V., Nicosia, V., Latora, V., Chavez, M.: Nonparametric resampling of random walks for spectral network clustering. Phys. Rev. E **89**(1), 012802 (2014)
13. Fortunato, S.: Community detection in graphs. Phys. Rep. **486**(3), 75–174 (2010)
14. Fraiman, D., Fraiman, F., Fraiman, R.: Statistics of dynamic random networks: a depth function approach. arXiv:1408.3584v3 (2015)
15. Gao, J., Liang, F., Fan, W., Wang, C., Sun, Y., Han, J.: On community outliers and their efficient detection in information networks. In: Proceedings of the 16th ACM SIGKDD International Conference on Knowledge Discovery and Data Mining (2010)
16. García-Escudero, L.Á., Gordaliza, A.: Robustness properties of k means and trimmed k means. J. Am. Stat. Assoc. **94**(447), 956–969 (1999)
17. Gogoi, P., Bhattacharyya, D., Borah, B., Kalita, J.K.: A survey of outlier detection methods in network anomaly identification. Comput. J. **54**(4) (2011)
18. Gupta, M., Gao, J., Han, J.: Community distribution outlier detection in heterogeneous information networks. In: Machine Learning and Knowledge Discovery in Databases, pp. 557–573. Springer, Berlin (2013)
19. Hagen, L., Kahng, A.B.: New spectral methods for ratio cut partitioning and clustering. IEEE Trans. Comput. Aided Des. Integr. Circuits Syst. **11**(9), 1074–1085 (1992)
20. Hallin, M.: Monge-Kantorovich ranks and signs. GOF DAYS 2015, p. 33 (2015)
21. Harenberg, S., Bello, G., Gjeltema, L., Ranshous, S., Harlalka, J., Seay, R., Padmanabhan, K., Samatova, N.: Community detection in large-scale networks: a survey and empirical evaluation. WIRE Comput. Stat. **6**, 426–439 (2014)
22. Harenberg, S., Bello, G., Gjeltema, L., Ranshous, S., Harlalka, J., Seay, R., Padmanabhan, K., Samatova, N.: Community detection in large-scale networks: a survey and empirical evaluation. Wiley Interdiscip. Rev. Comput. Stat. **6**(6), 426–439 (2014)
23. Holland, P., Laskey, K.B., Leinhardt, S.: Stochastic blockmodels: first steps. Soc. Networks **5**(2), 109–137 (1983)
24. Huber, P.J., Ronchetti, E.: Robust Statistics. Wiley, Hoboken vol. 10(1002). doi:9780470434697 (2009)
25. Hubert, M., Rousseeuw, P.J., Van Aelst, S.: High-breakdown robust multivariate methods. Stat. Sci. **23**(1), 92–119 (2008)
26. Hugg, J., Rafalin, E., Seyboth, K., Souvaine, D.: An experimental study of old and new depth measures. In: Proceedings of the Meeting on Algorithm Engineering & Experiments, pp. 51–64. Society for Industrial and Applied Mathematics (2006)
27. Hyndman, R.J., Shang, H.L.: Rainbow plots, bagplots, and boxplots for functional data. J. Comput. Graph. Stat. **19**, 29–45 (2010)
28. Jin, J.: Fast community detection by score. Ann. Stat. **43**(1), 57–89 (2015)

29. Jörnsten, R.: Clustering and classification based on the L 1 data depth. J. Multivar. Anal. **90**(1), 67–89 (2004)
30. Jörnsten, R., Vardi, Y., Zhange, C.-H.: A robust clustering method and visualization tool based on data depth. In: Dodge, Y. (ed.) Statistics in Industry and Technology: Statistical Data Analysis, pp. 353–366. Birkhäuser, Basel (2002)
31. Joseph, A., Yu, B.: Impact of regularization on spectral clustering. Ann. Stat. **44**(4), 1765–1791 (2016)
32. Kondo, Y., Salibian-Barrera, M., Zamar, R.: A robust and sparse k-means clustering algorithm. arXiv preprint arXiv:1201.6082 (2012)
33. Kumar, A., Sabharwal, Y., Sen, S.: A simple linear time $(1 + \epsilon)$-approximation algorithm for k-means clustering in any dimensions. In: Annual Symposium on Foundations of Computer Science, vol. 45, pp. 454–462. IEEE Computer Society Press, New York (2004)
34. Lange, T., Mosler, K.: Fast nonparametric classification based on data depth. Stat. Pap. **55**, 49–69 (2014)
35. Le, C.M., Vershynin, R.: Concentration and regularization of random graphs. arXiv preprint arXiv:1506.00669 (2015)
36. Lei, J., Rinaldo, A.: Consistency of spectral clustering in stochastic block models. Ann. Stat. **43**(1), 215–237 (2015)
37. Leskovec, J., Lang, K.J., Mahoney, M.: Empirical comparison of algorithms for network community detection. In: Proceedings of the 19th International Conference on World Wide Web, pp. 631–640. ACM, New York (2010)
38. Liu, R.Y., Parelius, J.M., Singh, K.: Special invited paper: multivariate analysis by data depth: descriptive statistica, graphics and inference. Ann. Stat. **27**(3), 783–858 (1999)
39. López-Pintado, S., Jörnsten, R.: Functional analysis via extensions of the band depth. In: Complex Datasets and Inverse Problems: Tomography, Networks and Beyond. Lecture Notes-Monograph Series, pp. 103–120. Beachwood, Ohio, USA (2007)
40. López-Pintado, S., Romo, J.: On the concept of depth for functional data. J. Am. Stat. Assoc. **104**, 718–734 (2009)
41. MacQueen, J., et al.: Some methods for classification and analysis of multivariate observations. In: Proceedings of the fifth Berkeley Symposium on Mathematical Statistics and Probability, vol. 1(14), pp. 281–297 (1967)
42. Malliaros, F.D., Vazirgiannis, M.: Clustering and community detection in directed networks: a survey. Phys. Rep. **533**, 95–142 (2013)
43. Manning, C.D., Raghavan, P., Schütze, H.: Introduction to Information Retrieval, vol. 1. Cambridge University Press, Cambridge (2008)
44. Newman, M., Clauset, A.: Structure and inference in annotated networks. arXiv preprint arXiv:1507.04001 (2015)
45. Newman, M.E.: Modularity and community structure in networks. Proc. Natl. Acad. Sci. **103**(23), 8577–8582 (2006)
46. Newman, M.E.J.: Networks: An Introduction. Oxford University Press, Oxford (2010)
47. Nieto-Reyes, A., Battey, H.: A topologically valid definition of depth for functional data. preprint. Stat. Sci. **31**(1), 61–79 (2016)
48. Ott, L., Pang, L., Ramos, F., Chawla, S.: On integrated clustering and outlier detection. In: Proceedings of NIPS (2014)
49. Pena, J.M., Lozano, J.A., Larranaga, P.: An empirical comparison of four initialization methods for the k-means algorithm. Pattern Recogn. Lett. **20**(10), 1027–1040 (1999)
50. Plantiè, M., Crampes, M.: Survey on social community detection. Social Media Retrieval Computer Communications and Networks (2012)
51. Qin, T., Rohe, K.: Regularized spectral clustering under the degree-corrected stochastic blockmodel. In: NIPS, pp. 3120–3128 (2013)
52. Rohe, K., Chatterjee, S., Yu, B.: Spectral clustering and the high-dimensional stochastic blockmodel. Ann. Stat. **39**, 1878–1915 (2011)
53. Sarkar, P., Bickel, P.: Role of normalization in spectral clustering for stochastic blockmodels. Ann. Stat. **43**, 962–990 (2013)

54. Selim, S.Z., Ismail, M.A.: *k*-means-type algorithms: a generalized convergence theorem and characterization of local optimality. IEEE Trans. Pattern Anal. Mach. Intell. **6**(1), 81–87 (1984)
55. Serfling, R.: Generalized quantile processes based on multivariate depth functions, with applications in nonparametric multivariate analysis. J. Multivar. Anal. **83**, 232–247 (2002)
56. Serfling, R.: Quantile functions for multivariate analysis: approaches and applications. Statistica Neerlandica **56**, 214–232 (2002)
57. Serfling, R.: Depth functions in nonparametric multivariate inference. In: Data Depth: Robust Multivariate Analysis, Computational Geometry and Applications. DIMACS Series in Discrete Mathematics and Theoretical Computer Science, vol. 72(1). American Mathematical Society, Providence, RI (2006)
58. Serfling, R., Wijesuriya, U.: Nonparametric description of functional data using the spatial depth approach (2015). Accessible at www.utdallas.edu/~serfling
59. Sharma, S., Yadav, R.L.: Comparative study of *k*-means and robust clustering. Int. J. Adv. Comput. Res. **3**(3), 207 (2013)
60. Shi, J., Malik, J.: Normalized cuts and image segmentation. IEEE Trans. Pattern Anal. Mach. Intell. **22**(8), 888–905 (2000)
61. Sussman, D.L., Tang, M., Fishkind, D.E., Priebe, C.E.: A consistent adjacency spectral embedding for stochastic blockmodel graphs. J. Am. Stat. Assoc. **107**(499), 1119–1128 (2012)
62. Tang, L., Liu, H.: Relational learning via latent social dimensions. In: Proceedings of the 15th ACM SIGKDD International Conference on Knowledge Discovery and Data Mining, pp. 817–826 (2009)
63. Thompson, M.E., Ramirez Ramirez, L.L., Lyubchich, V., Gel, Y.R.: Using the bootstrap for statistical inference on random graphs. Can. J. Stat. **44**, 3–24 (2016)
64. Torrente, A., Romo, J.: Refining *k*-means by bootstrap and data depth (2013). https://www.researchgate.net/profile/Juan_Romo/publication/242090768_Reflning_k-means_by_Bootstrap_and_Data_Depth/links/02e7e528daa72dc0a1000000.pdf
65. Vardi, Y., Zhang, C.-H.: The multivariate l1-median and associated data depth. Proc. Natl. Acad. Sci. **97**(4), 1423–1426 (2000)
66. von Luxburg, U.: A tutorial on spectral clustering. Stat. Comput. **17**(4), 395–416 (2007)
67. White, S., Smyth, P.: A spectral clustering approach to finding communities in graph. In: SDM, vol. 5, pp. 76–84 (2005)
68. Wilson, J.D., Wang, S., Mucha, P.J., Bhamidi, S., Nobel, A.B.: A testing based extraction algorithm for identifying significant communities in networks. Ann. Appl. Stat. **8**(3), 1853–1891 (2014)
69. Witten, D.M., Tibshirani, R.: A framework for feature selection in clustering. J. Am. Stat. Assoc. **105**(490), 713–726 (2012)
70. Zafarani, R., Liu, H.: Social computing data repository at ASU (2009)
71. Zhang, Y., Levina, E., Zhu, J.: Community detection in networks with node features. arXiv preprint arXiv:1509.01173 (2015)
72. Zhou, W., Serfling, R.: General notions of statistical depth function. Ann. Stat. **28**, 461–482 (2000)
73. Zuo, Y., Serfling, R.: General notions of statistical depth function. Ann. Stat. **28**, 461–482 (2000)

How Different Are Estimated Genetic Networks of Cancer Subtypes?

Ali Shojaie and Nafiseh Sedaghat

Abstract Genetic networks provide compact representations of interactions between genes, and offer a systems perspective into biological processes and cellular functions. Many algorithms have been developed to estimate such networks based on steady-state gene expression profiles. However, the estimated networks using different methods are often very different from each other. On the other hand, it is not clear whether differences observed between estimated networks in two different biological conditions are truly meaningful, or due to variability in estimation procedures. In this paper, we aim to answer these questions by conducting a comprehensive empirical study to compare networks obtained from different estimation methods and for different subtypes of cancer. We evaluate various network descriptors to assess complex properties of estimated networks, beyond their local structures, and propose a simple permutation test for comparing estimated networks. The results provide new insight into properties of estimated networks using different reconstruction methods, as well as differences in estimated networks in different biological conditions.

1 Introduction

Aberrations in biological networks have been associated with the onset and progression of complex diseases [1, 2]. Examples include changes in transcription regulation and cell signaling networks in cancer and cardiovascular diseases [3–5], as well as alterations in functional brain connectivity in neurological disorders [6, 7]. Over the past few years, biomedical researchers have thus started to develop new experimental procedures [8] to study changes in biological networks associated with complex diseases, and to move towards *differential network biology* [9–11].

A. Shojaie (✉)
Department of Biostatistics, University of Washington, Seattle, WA, USA
e-mail: ashojaie@u.washington.edu

N. Sedaghat
Computer Engineering Department, Iran University of Science and Technology, Tehran, Iran

© Springer International Publishing AG 2017

S.E. Ahmed (ed.), *Big and Complex Data Analysis*, Contributions to Statistics,
DOI 10.1007/978-3-319-41573-4_9

The increasing evidence on the association of changes in biological networks with different diseases has sparked an interest in computational biology and bioinformatics to obtain estimates of biological network for different disease conditions using high throughput biological data [12–18]. Such *condition-specific* network estimates are then used to generate new hypotheses about changes in biological networks associated with complex diseases [1–7]. In fact, given the cost of experimental procedures for obtaining condition-specific network information—e.g., knockout experiments—and the heterogeneity of complex diseases, computational methods are viable and efficient alternatives for studying how networks change in disease conditions.

Graphical models [19, 20] are commonly used to model and analyze biological networks [21, 22]. A graphical model defines a probability distribution $\mathcal{P}$ over a graph $\mathcal{G} = (V, E)$, with the node set $V = \{1, \ldots, p\}$ and edge set $E \subseteq V \times V$. In the setting of genetic networks, the nodes of the graph represent random variables $X_1, \ldots, X_p$ corresponding to, e.g., gene expression levels of p genes. The edge set E then encodes some type of dependency between the nodes. Obtaining condition-specific estimates of biological networks thus requires the estimation of E from n observations of $X_1, \ldots, X_p$ in a given disease state or biological condition.

Over the past decade, significant advances have been made in development of new methods for estimation of large biological networks from high throughput measurements. In particular, a number of penalized estimation methods [13–18] have been proposed for estimation of graphical models in high dimensions—when $p \gg n$—imposing different assumptions on the probability distribution $\mathcal{P}$. Consider, for simplicity, the setting of two biological conditions, say, *cases* and *controls*. A first step in differential analysis of biological networks is to obtain condition-specific estimates of the edge sets E^{cases} and E^{controls}. Penalized estimation methods have been recently used for this task [15, 23]. However, the vast majority of existing approaches do not quantify the uncertainty of estimated networks. In particular, it is unclear whether differences observed among estimated networks are statistically meaningful, or can be attributed to estimation variation. On the other hand, networks encode a vast amount of information, beyond the presence/absence of edges. To delineate the consequences of local differences in E^{cases} and E^{controls} from a systems perspective, it is therefore necessary to understand how network properties change as edges are removed/added in the network.

Motivated by the previous studies comparing different network estimation methods [24, 25], this paper aims to address the above questions through an empirical comparison of estimated networks of estrogen-receptor-positive (ER$^+$) and estrogen-receptor-negative (ER$^-$) subtypes of breast cancer, using data from The Cancer Genome Atlas (TCGA) (https://tcga-data.nci.nih.gov/tcga). We start by comparing the edge structures of ER$^+$ and ER$^-$ networks. We then compare a wide range of network descriptors to better understand the differences between estimated ER$^+$ and ER$^-$ networks. To determine whether the choice of network estimation method affects the observed patterns of differences, we include various estimation methods, ranging from simple to complex procedures.

The rest of the paper is organized as follows. In Sect. 2, we briefly describe different estimation methods used in this analysis. Section 3 describes the summary measures used for evaluating similarities among networks. Results of comparing networks from different estimation methods are presented in Sect. 4, while Sect. 5 contains the results of comparing estimated networks of ER^+ and ER^-. We summarize our findings in Sect. 6, and comment on future research directions.

2 Network Reconstruction Methods

As pointed out in the Introduction, graphical models have been widely used to reconstruct biological networks. This includes both directed and undirected graphical models [21, 26–28]. Directed networks are often used to encode causal relationships among variables [29], and provide valuable information on how variables (e.g., genes) in a graphical model *influence* each other. Unfortunately, estimation of such causal networks is in general an NP-complete problem [30]. More importantly, it is often not possible to estimate directed networks from *observational data*, and data from perturbation screens [31, 32] and/or time-course experiments [31, 33, 34] are needed to determine the direction of edges in the network. Thus, even though directed networks are of main interest in many applications, in this paper, we focus on undirected graphical models.

Undirected graphical models for estimation of biological networks can be broadly categorized into two classes, based on whether they encode *marginal* or *conditional* associations [22]. A *marginal association graph* is estimated by calculating the marginal association between every two pairs of random variables X_j and X_k corresponding to genes j and k. An edge is then drawn between nodes j and k if the magnitude of marginal association exceeds some threshold. Different measures of dependence—ranging from simple Pearson correlation [35] to mutual information [36] to more complex measure of non-linear associations [37]—can be used to quantify the degree of marginal association between two variables. The widely used WGCNA [13] approach—described in Sect. 2.1—is based on the Pearson correlations among pairs of nodes.

Despite their simplicity and computational advantages, marginal association graphs suffer from a major shortcoming: if X_j and $X_{j'}$ are both highly associated with a third variable X_k, they will also have a large marginal associations. For instance, if two genes are co-regulated by the same *transcription factor*, they would be most likely connected in an undirected network based on marginal associations, even though their association is due to their joint connection to the transcription factor. Recognizing this limitation, a number of approaches have been proposed to remove the false positive edges corresponding to indirect associations; among these ARACNE [38] uses the so-called *data processing inequality* and has been used successfully in a number of applications [39]. The post-processing step of ARACNE limits the number of possible edges in estimated networks [24]. Therefore, despite its popularity, we do not consider ARACNE in our comparisons.

In *conditional association graphs* an edge is drawn between j and k if the magnitude of association between X_j and X_k, after adjusting for all other variables, exceeds some threshold. Thus, conditional association graphs are deemed more appropriate in biological settings, as they capture relevant dependencies. However, compared to marginal association graphs, conditional association graphs are more difficult to estimate, both computationally, and also in terms of the number of samples required to estimate the conditional dependencies.

The computational complexity of estimating conditional independence graphs becomes more amenable in the setting of multivariate normal distributions corresponding to Gaussian graphical models (GGM). This stems from the fact that if $(X_1, \ldots, X_p) \sim N_p(0, \Sigma)$, then X_j and X_k are conditionally independent, given all other variables, if and only if $\Sigma^{-1}_{jk} = 0$ [19]. Thus, in this case, conditional associations can be obtained from *partial correlations*, by estimating the inverse covariance, or concentration, matrix of $(X_1, \ldots, X_p)$. Utilizing this connection, a number of methods have been proposed over the past decade for penalized estimation of high-dimensional GGMs [23, 40]. The graphical lasso (GLASSO) [15] algorithm of Sect. 2.3 is one such method.

The neighborhood selection (NS) [14] and Sparse PArtial Correlation Estimation (SPACE) [16] methods of Sects. 2.2 and 2.4 are alternatives to GLASSO, that instead estimate the partial correlations using p penalized linear regressions. Interestingly, under mild regularity conditions, assuming linear dependency among variables is equivalent to multivariate normality [18], which is not expected to hold in many application settings. Violations of this assumption can significantly affect the accuracy of estimates for estimation of GGMs. A few of methods have been recently proposed to address this shortcoming; the nonparanormal framework (NPN) [41] and SPArse Conditional graph Estimation with Joint Additive Models (SPACE JAM) [18] in Sects. 2.5 and 2.6 relax the normality assumption by considering marginal (copula) transformations of the original variables and directly estimating non-linear associations among variables, respectively.

In this paper, we consider various methods for estimation of undirected graphical models, including both marginal and conditional associations, as well as methods based on linear and non-linear dependencies, to provide a comprehensive assessment of differences between genetic networks of ER^+ and ER^- samples. In the remainder of this section, we briefly describe each of the estimation methods considered.

2.1 Weighted Gene Correlation Network Analysis

Weighted Gene Correlation Network Analysis (WGCNA) [13] determines the presence of edges between pairs of edges based on the magnitude of their Pearson correlation s_{ij}, which is a marginal measure of linear associations. Pearson correlation values are first transformed by applying a power adjacency function $|s_{ij}|^\beta$, where the exponent β is selected to obtain a network with a scale-free topology [42, 43], which is expected to better represent real-world biological networks. The presence of an edge between a pair of genes i and j is then determined by thresholding the value of $|s_{ij}|^\beta$ at a prespecified cutoff τ. WGCNA also facilitates identification of gene modules by converting co-expression values into the topology overlap measure (TOM), which represents the relative interconnectedness of pair of genes in the network. While the identification of gene modules is certainly of interest, it is outside the scope of this paper.

WGCNA is implemented in an R-package with the same name, and an estimate of the network is obtained using the function *adjacency*(.). The output of this function is the weighted adjacency matrix of the network; the number of edges in the network can thus be controlled by applying different thresholds τ to this matrix.

2.2 Neighborhood Selection

Neighborhood selection (NS) [14] is a simple approach for estimation of sparse graphical models. In this approach, the neighborhood of node j is estimated using a lasso-penalized regression of X_j on all other nodes, X_{-j}. Specifically,

$$\hat{ne}_j^\lambda = \{k \in V : \hat{\theta}_k^{j,\lambda} \neq 0\}, \tag{1}$$

where λ is a penalty parameter, $V = \{1, \ldots, p\}$ is the set of nodes in $\mathcal{G}$, and

$$\hat{\theta}^{j,\lambda} = \min_{\theta \in \mathbb{R}^{p-1}} \left\{ n^{-1} \|X_j - X_{-j}\theta\|_2^2 + \lambda \sum_{k \neq j} |\theta_k| \right\}, \tag{2}$$

In (2), $\sum_{k \neq j} |\theta_k| \equiv \|\theta\|_1$ denotes the ℓ_1 norm of the coefficient matrix and forces some of the entries of the estimated $\hat{\theta}^{j,\lambda}$ to be exactly zero. Larger values of the tuning parameter λ result in sparser estimates $\hat{\theta}^{j,\lambda}$ and hence a smaller neighborhood $\hat{ne}_j^\lambda$.

The neighborhood selection estimation procedure in Eqs. (1) and (2) does not make specific assumptions about the distribution of random variables X_j. However, it turns out that assuming linear relationships among variables is (almost) equivalent to assuming multivariate normality; see [18] for more details.

Under multivariate normality, $X = (X_1, X_2, \ldots, X_p) \sim N_p(0, \Sigma)$, θ_k^j defines the partial correlation between X_j and X_k. It can thus be shown that the neighborhood $\hat{ne}_j^\lambda$ gives a consistent estimate of the set of variables that are conditionally dependent on X_j, given all other nodes. However, the above equation strategy may give asymmetric estimates of edge weights between two nodes. It may even happen that $k \in \hat{ne}_j^\lambda$ but $j \notin \hat{ne}_k^\lambda$. A symmetric estimate of the network can be obtained from considering either the union or intersection of the estimated neighborhoods. The NS approach is implemented in the R-package `glasso`; specifically, the gene network can be estimated using the function `glasso(.)` with the option `approx=TRUE`.

2.3 Graphical Lasso

Graphical lasso (GLASSO) [15] builds on a basic property of multivariate normal random variables, that two variables X_j and X_k are conditionally independent of each other, given all other variables, if and only if their corresponding entry of the inverse covariance, or concentration, matrix Σ^{-1} is zero. Thus, assuming multivariate normality, the graph of conditional independence relations among the genes can be estimated based on the nonzero elements of the estimated inverse covariance matrix. To achieve this, GLASSO estimates a sparse concentration matrix by maximizing the ℓ_1-penalized log-likelihood function for a p-dimensional multivariate normal distribution, $N_p(0, \Sigma)$ given by

$$\log \det(\Sigma^{-1}) - \mathrm{tr}(S\Sigma^{-1}) - \lambda \|\Sigma^{-1}\|_1, \tag{3}$$

Here, $\mathrm{tr}(A)$ denotes the trace of matrix A, S is the empirical covariance matrix, and the ℓ_1 penalty $\|\Sigma^{-1}\|_1$ is the sum of absolute values of elements of Σ^{-1}. This penalty enforces sparsity in the estimate of Σ^{-1} by setting some of its entries to zero. The tuning parameter λ is a positive number controlling the degree of sparsity.

The above optimization problem is concave, and can hence be solved using an iterative coordinate-descent algorithm. In each iteration of the algorithm, one row of Σ is updated, given most recent estimates of the remaining rows. This algorithm is implemented in the R-package `glasso`, and an estimate of the gene network can be obtained based on the estimated inverse covariance matrix using the function `glasso(.)` with the option `approx=FALSE`.

2.4 SPACE

Sparse PArtial Correlation Estimation (SPACE) [16] converts the estimation of concentration matrix into a regression problem, based on the loss function

$$L_n(\theta, \sigma, X) = \frac{1}{2}\left(\sum_{j=1}^{p} \omega_j \|X_j - \sum_{k \neq j} \rho^{jk} \sqrt{\frac{\sigma^{kk}}{\sigma^{jj}}} X_k\|^2\right), \tag{4}$$

where $X_j = (X_j^1, \ldots, X_j^n)^T, j = 1, \ldots, p$ are vectors of n independent observations for the jth variable (gene) and $(X_1, \ldots, X_p) \sim N_p(0, \Sigma)$. Here, $\theta = (\rho^{12}, \ldots, \rho^{(p-1)p})^T$ where ρ^{jk} is the partial correlation between X_j and X_k. Finally, $\sigma = \{\sigma^{jk}\}_{1 \le j,k \le p}$ are the diagonal entries of the concentration matrix, and $w = \{\omega_j\}_{j=1}^p$ are nonnegative weights.

To address the estimation of parameters in the high-dimensional, low-sample-size setting ($p \gg n$), the authors consider minimizing the penalized loss function

$$L_n(\theta, \sigma, Y) = L_n(\theta, \sigma, Y) + \lambda \|\theta\|_1 = \lambda \sum_{1 \le j < k \le p} |\rho^{ij}|, \tag{5}$$

where the ℓ_1 penalty $\|\theta\|_1 = \lambda \sum_{1 \le j < k \le p} |\rho^{jk}|$ encourages sparse estimates of θ and $\lambda > 0$ is a tuning parameter.

In summary, SPACE minimizes a penalized loss function with symmetric constraint by performing joint lasso regressions of variables on the others. Numerical experiments indicate that this approach may be preferred over competing methods, in settings where the network includes "hub" nodes, i.e., genes connected to many other genes. The algorithm for solving the above optimization problem is implemented in the R-package `space`, where the function `space.joint()` can be used to obtain an estimate of the concentration matrix. The tuning parameter λ controls the sparsity level, or the number of edges in the network.

2.5 *Nonparanormal*

The nonparanormal (NPN) [17, 41] is a penalized maximum likelihood estimation method, which generalizes the estimation of sparse concentration matrices to non-Gaussian distributions. In particular, nonparanormal distribution replaces the original random variables $X = (X_1, \ldots, X_p)$ by the transformed random variable $f(X) = (f_1(X_1), \ldots, f_p(X_p))$, and assume that $f(X)$ has a multivariate normal distribution. The proposed semiparametric approach applies a Gaussian copula transformation where variables are marginally transformed by smooth monotone functions. The estimate of the gene network is obtained by solving the graphical lasso optimization problem (3), for the transformed variables $f_1(X_1), \ldots, f_p(X_p)$.

More recently, it has been shown that the NPN estimate can be obtained by using rank-based measures of association, i.e., Spearman correlation or Kendal's τ, instead of the usual Pearson correlation in the graphical lasso problem [44, 45]. Using this observation, the NPN estimate is obtained by plugging in a (transformed version of) the Kendal's τ correlation matrix in place of the empirical covariance matrix S in (3). Both estimation procedures are implemented in the R-package `huge` (High-dimensional Undirected Graph Estimation) [17], where function `huge()` returns an adjacency matrix. As in graphical lasso, the sparsity level of the graph is controlled through the tuning parameter λ in (3).

2.6 *SPACE JAM*

SPArse Conditional graph Estimation with Joint Additive Models (SPACE JAM) [18] is a semiparametric approach that estimates conditional independence relationships using joint additive models. This is achieved by estimating the conditional means $E_{X_j}(X_j|\{X_k : (j,k) \in E\})$ using an additive model $X_j|\{X_k, k \neq j\} = \sum_{k \neq j} f_{jk}(X_k) + \varepsilon_j$ where ε_j is a mean-zero term.

To encourage sparsity in the conditional independence graph, the authors apply a group lasso penalty [46, 47], by linking p individual sparse additive models, and estimating $f_{jk}(.)$ by solving the following optimization problem:

$$\min_{f_{jk}, 1 \leq j,k \leq p} \left\{ \frac{1}{2n} \sum_{j=1}^{p} \|X_j - \sum_{k \neq j} f_{jk}(X_k)\|_2^2 + \lambda \sum_{k>j} \{\|f_{jk}(X_k)\|_2^2 + \|f_{kj}(X_j)\|_2^2\}^{\frac{1}{2}} \right\}. \quad (6)$$

The optimization problem in (6) is convex and is solved using a block coordinate-descent algorithm implemented in the R-package `spacejam`; the adjacency matrix of the network is obtained using the function `SJ(.)`, and the tuning parameter λ controls the sparsity level of the network.

3 Network Descriptors

An edge between two nodes in a network estimated using the procedures of Sect. 2 represents marginal or conditional independence relations among the corresponding pairs of variables. The collection of these edges describes the global relationships of variables in the network. Clearly, these complex relationships cannot be understood from investigating the presence/absence of edges alone. Therefore, to understand the global properties of estimated networks, and delineate similarities and differences between them, we consider a wide range of network descriptors. These descriptors explain different aspects of estimated networks, and provide insight into various network properties. The network descriptors considered in this paper can be categorized into the following five categories:

1. simple summary measures of the *degree distribution*;
2. descriptors of network *connectedness*, including the number of clusters, cluster coefficients, centrality degree, Zagreb index, and graph energy;
3. descriptors of *spread of information* and node influence on networks, including diameter, centrality betweenness and closeness, and graph vertex complexity;
4. descriptors of network *symmetry*, including Bertz index and the topological information content;
5. various *network motifs* involving 3, 4, and 5 nodes (see Fig. 1).

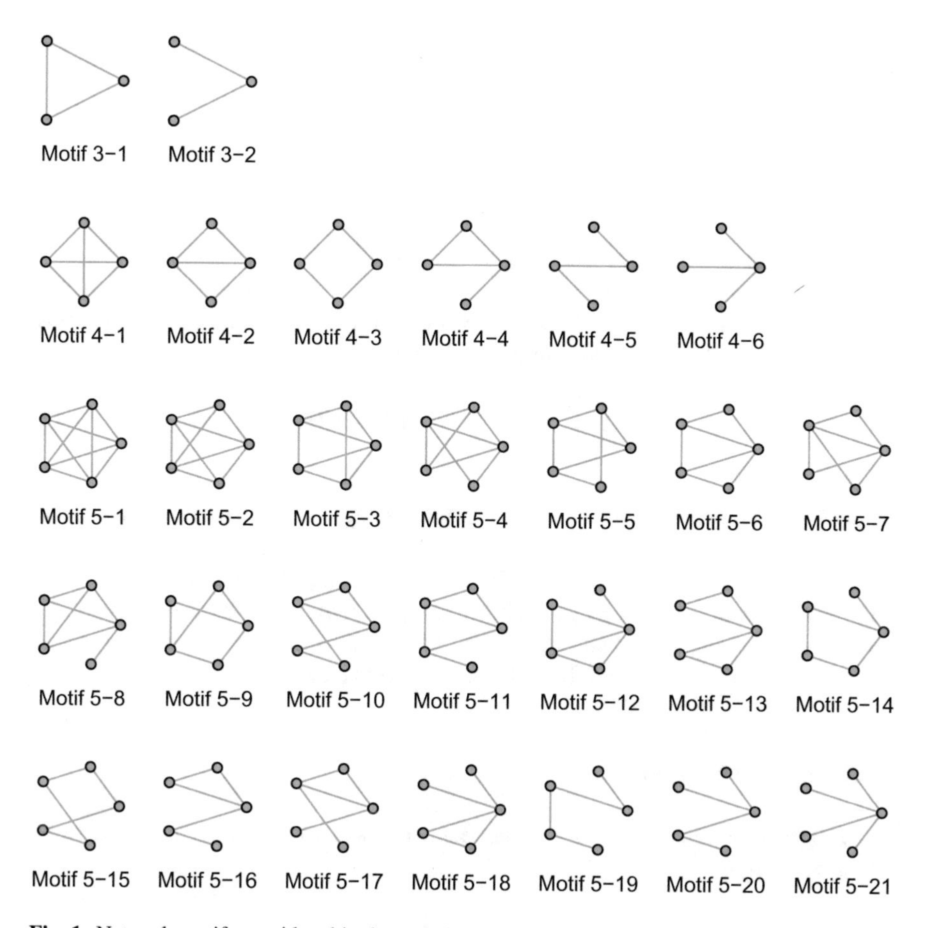

Fig. 1 Network motifs considered in the experiments

In addition to the above descriptors, we will also utilize the network *structural correlation* to quantify the degree of similarity of two networks with each other. Next, we briefly describe the network descriptors in each of the above categories.

3.1 Degree Distribution Summary Statistics

The degree distribution is often used as the first tool for obtaining insight into network properties. We consider select simple summary measures of degree distribution, including the first quartile, median, third quartile, and maximum degree, as well as the interquartile range (IQR). We also consider the number of nodes with degree zero and one. Given the network estimates are set to have a fixed number of edges, we do not include the mean degree. We also do not include the minimum degree, which is equal to zero for all estimated networks.

3.2 Descriptors of Network Connectedness

3.2.1 Graph Centralization Based on Degree

The centralization of a graph G measures the absolute deviation between the most central node and the other nodes in graph; formally,

$$C(G) = \sum_{i \in V(G)} | \max_{v \in V(G)} C(v) - C(i)|, \tag{7}$$

where $C(v)$ is any *centrality* measures, including degree, betweenness, or closeness [48].

A small centrality degree measure indicates that a majority of nodes have similar degrees. On the other hand, a large centrality degree indicates that the graph includes few nodes with degrees much larger than others. This often implies that there is at least one *hub* node (node with high degree) in the network.

3.2.2 Zagreb Group Index

The Zagreb group index [49, 50] is also defined based on node degrees in the graph and is given by

$$ZI(G) = \sum_{(v_i, v_j) \in E(G)} deg(v_i)deg(v_j). \tag{8}$$

In a graph with a large *ZI* value, high degree nodes are connected to each other. In other words, in graphs with large *ZI*, many dense subgraphs exist in the network. Such interaction patterns are not expected to be less common in biological networks, where many genes are expected to be connected to hub genes, and each hub gene is connected to very few other hub genes [51].

3.2.3 Graph Energy

The eigenvalues of a graph characterize the topological structure of the graph; for instance, the first nonzero eigenvalue λ_1 takes a larger value in networks with higher overall connectivity than sparse networks. On the other hand, graphs with a large number of shared eigenvalues have more similar structures. Graph energy [52] is a eigenvalue-based measures, defined as the sum of eigenvalues of the adjacency matrix

$$E(G) = \sum_{j=1}^{p} \lambda_j. \tag{9}$$

3.2.4 Clustering Coefficient and Number of Clusters

Biological networks have a modular nature, i.e., many cellular processes are governed by subsets of biomolecules that form an interaction module. The clustering coefficient [53] measures the tendency of the network to be divided into clusters, i.e., subset of highly connected vertices. As expected, biological networks have a significantly higher average clustering coefficient compared to simple random networks.

Suppose node $j \in V(G)$ has degree $deg(j) = k$ and that there are e edges between the k neighbors of j in G. The *local clustering coefficient* of j in G is then defined as $C_j = \frac{2e}{k(k-1)}$. Thus, C_j measures the ratio of the number of edges between the neighbors of j to the total possible number of such edges, $\frac{k(k-1)}{2}$; clearly, $0 \leq C_j \leq 1$.

The *average clustering coefficient* of the network C_{average} is given by

$$C_{\text{avg}} = \frac{1}{p} \sum_{j=1}^{p} C_j, \tag{10}$$

where $p = |V|$ is the number of nodes. The closer the local clustering coefficient is to 1, the more likely it is for the network to form clusters.

In contrast to the clustering coefficient, the *number of clusters* in the network is simply the number of connected components in the graph, which provides less information about the connectivity of each of the clusters.

3.2.5 Medium Articulation

Medium articulation (MA_g) is a graph complexity measure proposed initially by Wilhelm and Hollunder [54] for directed graphs. Kim and Wilhelm [55] extended this measure to undirected graphs. MA_g is a powerful discriminator between graphs with equal number of nodes and edges in terms of the graph topology, and is calculated as the product of *redundancy* MA_R and *mutual information* MA_I of the graph G. Mutual information is zero in a minimally articulated graph, i.e., when each node has inputs/outputs from/to other nodes, while redundancy is zero in a maximally articulated graph, i.e., when each node has exactly one input and one output, but network is still connected. The product of these two measures, MA_g, is thus zero in both extremes and gets the maximum value in between, i.e., graphs with a medium number of edges; see [56] for more information about MA_R and MA_I.

For instance, since the clique is a fully connected subgraph, it has high redundancy, while its mutual information is lowest. On the other hand, a path has the lowest redundancy and the highest mutual information. This is why cliques and paths are the basic elements of defining MA_g [55], which is given by

$$MA_g(G) = MA_R(G)MA_I(G), \tag{11}$$

where the redundancy MA_R is defined as

$$MA_R(G) = 4\left(\frac{R(G) - R_{\text{path}}(G)}{R_{\text{clique}}(G) - R_{\text{path}}(G)}\right)\left(1 - \frac{R(G) - R_{\text{path}}(G)}{R_{\text{clique}}(G) - R_{\text{path}}(G)}\right) \tag{12}$$

$$R(G) = \frac{1}{|E|}\sum_{j,k<i} \log(deg(j)deg(k)) \tag{13}$$

$$R_{\text{clique}}(G) = 2\log(p-1), \tag{14}$$

$$R_{\text{path}}(G) = 2\left(\frac{p-2}{p-1}\right)\log 2, \tag{15}$$

and the mutual information MA_I is defined as

$$MA_I(G) = 4\left(\frac{I(G) - I_{\text{path}}(G)}{I_{\text{path}}(G) - I_{\text{clique}}(G)}\right)\left(1 - \frac{I(G) - I_{\text{path}}(G)}{I_{\text{path}}(G) - I_{\text{clique}}(G)}\right), \tag{16}$$

$$I(G) = \frac{1}{|E|}\sum_{j,k<j} \log\left(\frac{2|E|}{d_i d_j}\right), \tag{17}$$

$$I_{\text{clique}}(G) = \log\left(\frac{p}{p-1}\right), \tag{18}$$

$$I_{\text{path}}(G) = \log(p-1) - \left(\frac{p-3}{p-1}\right)\log 2. \tag{19}$$

3.3 Descriptors Related to Spread of Information in Network

The spread of information in a network is one of its important properties. The descriptors presented in this section measure the spread of the network in terms of distances and lengths of shortest paths between nodes.

3.3.1 Diameter

Diameter is one of the most popular descriptors in this category. It measures the length of the longest shortest path between nodes in a connected graph or longest shortest path in the connected components of a disconnected graph.

3.3.2 Graph Centrality Based on Closeness and Betweenness

The base formula for centrality closeness and betweenness is the same as centrality based on degree in (7). In other words, centrality closeness and betweenness measure the absolute deviation between the most central node and the other nodes in graph. However, the "centrality" $C(j)$ is defined differently for each of these measures. Betweenness centrality of a node measures how many times a node is in the shortest paths between other nodes in the graph. In the other words, it indicates to the importance of the node in terms of being on the shortest connection between other nodes; a node with high centrality betweenness acts like a bridge in the network. Closeness centrality, on the other hand, measures how close a node is to the other nodes in the graph. Formally, it is calculated as the inverse of average distance of the shortest path from the node to the other nodes. In other words, closeness shows how efficient a node is in spreading the information to other nodes.

In networks with higher centrality closeness, there is a large difference between the largest closeness and other nodes' closeness. This large gap suggests that there the network contains few efficient nodes that are well positioned to spread information to the other nodes. In contrast, the other nodes are, in general, less efficient [48, 57] in spreading information through the network. Such connectivity patterns can be expected in real biological networks with many hubs.

3.3.3 Graph Vertex Complexity Index

Graph vertex complexity [58] is an information-theoretic measure that summarizes the amount of information passed through k-neighbors of each node in the network; k-neighbors of a node are those that are k steps away. The graph vertex complexity for a graph with p nodes is defined as

$$I_{VC}(G) = \frac{1}{p} \sum_{i=1}^{p} v_i^c, \tag{20}$$

where v_i^c is the vertex complexity for node i given by

$$v_i^c = - \sum_{j=0}^{\sigma(v_i)} \frac{k_j^i}{p} \log\left(\frac{k_j^i}{p}\right). \tag{21}$$

In this formula, $\sigma(v_i)$ is the eccentricity of vertex i—the maximum graph distance between i and any other node in G—and k_j^i is the number of nodes j steps way from node i. Note that I_{VC} does not take into account the magnitude of the distance and only considers the number of nodes with a particular distance.

3.4 Descriptors of Network Symmetry

Real-world networks, including biological networks, are known to demonstrate high levels of symmetry [59]. More symmetric graphs contain redundant structures that renders them more robust against environmental perturbations. Symmetry characterizes the extent to which the graph is invariant under various transformations. The most common such transformation is (vertex) automorphism [60]. An *automorphism* of a graph is a permutation of its vertex set that preserves incidences of vertices and edges. In this regard, the *orbit* of vertex j of a graph G is the set of all vertices $k \in V(G)$ such that for an automorphism ϕ it holds that $\phi(j) = k$ [61]. Two commonly used measures of network symmetry are Bertz index, BI, and the topological information content [62].

3.4.1 Bertz Index

The Bertz index [63], BI, uses the size of graph as well as orbits in the entropy formulation and is defined as

$$BI(G) = 2|Z|\log(|Z|) - \sum_{i=1}^{m} |Z_i|\log(|Z_i|).$$

where Z is an arbitrary graph invariant, such as vertices, edges, degrees, $|.|$ denotes the set cardinality and Z_i is the ith orbit, corresponding to the invariant Z.

When graph vertices are considered as invariant Z, BI reduces to

$$BI(G) = 2p\log(p) - \sum_{i=1}^{m} |N_i|\log(|N_i|), \tag{22}$$

where p is the number of nodes in G and $|N_i|$ is the number of nodes in the ith orbit. The first term in (22) stands for the size of the graph, whereas the second term accounts for graph symmetry [62, 64]. Smaller BI values correspond to more symmetric networks.

3.4.2 Topological Information Content

Topological information content [65], similar to *BI*, measures the symmetry of the network using the entropy formulation and is defined as:

$$I_{\text{orb}}(G) = -\sum_{i=1}^{m} \frac{|N_i|}{p} \log\left(\frac{|N_i|}{p}\right), \tag{23}$$

where $|N_i|$ is the number of nodes in the ith orbit. Less symmetric graphs G have relatively larger values of topological information content, as most of the orbits in G tend to be singleton partitions. On the other hand, topological information content of a highly symmetric graph with fewer partitions is relatively low.

3.5 *Network Motifs*

In complex networks, including biological networks, specific connectivity patterns often occur at significantly higher rates than simple random networks. Network motifs help uncover basic structural elements of the network. In particular, understanding biological units and their interactions is one of the important goals of systems biology, which helps researchers determine the function of biological units in a living cell [66, 67]. Abundance of various network motifs are important network descriptors that can be used to classify network models [68] and predict interactions among nodes [69]. However, counting general network motifs in large networks is computationally challenging. Thus, in this paper we focus only on (undirected) motifs consisting of 3, 4, or 5 nodes (see Fig. 1). Given the similarity in patterns of the number of motifs with the same number of nodes, in Sects. 4 and 5, we present the results for the first motif from each of the classes in Fig. 1, and include the results for other motifs in the Supplementary Material.

3.6 *Structural Correlation*

The structural correlation coefficient measures the similarity between the structures of two graphs G and H by maximizing the correspondence between their edge sets. Specifically,

$$\text{scor}(G, H|L_G, L_H) = \max_{L_G, L_H} \text{cor}(\psi(G), \psi(H)), \tag{24}$$

where $\psi(G)$ is a permutation/relabeling of G, $\psi(G) \in L_G$ and L_G is the support of ψ, called accessible permutations of G; a relabeling/permutation of G is a transformation of G which relabels its vertex set by ψ. Further, $\text{cor}(G, H)$ is the

Pearson correlation between the adjacency matrices of the graphs, obtained by vectorizing each of the adjacency matrices. The set of accessible permutations for a given graph is determined by the *theoretical exchangeability* of its vertices; two vertices are considered to be theoretically exchangeable if relabeling of the vertices does not modify the structure of the graphs [70].

Because the set of accessible permutations is of order $O(p!)$, (p is the number of vertices in graph), searching for maximum correlation in large networks is computationally expensive. So, many methods try to estimate the structural correlation using random search algorithms, such as hill climbing and simulated annealing [71].

4 Comparison of Network Estimates From Different Procedures

4.1 Data Preprocessing

We use gene expression profiles (level 3.0) from breast cancer tumor samples available through The Cancer Genome Atlas (TCGA) (https://tcga-data.nci.nih.gov/tcga). The data contain expression levels of 17,814 genes over 530 breast cancer samples. After removing three samples corresponding to metastatic tumors and genes mapped to sex chromosomes, we retained a data set containing 17,296 genes and 527 samples. Upon examination of the clinical data available for 520 samples, we grouped the data into two classes: 403 ER^+ samples and 117 ER^- samples. Finally, given that we aim to study genetic interactions in cancer, we restricted our analysis to genes in three main KEEG pathways associated with breast cancer, namely the "p53 signaling pathway," the "breast cancer pathway," and "cancer pathway." The final data set consists of expression values for $p = 358$ genes and $n = 520$ samples. We then imputed six missing expression values using a K-Nearest Neighbor (KNN) imputation method with $K = 10$. Prior to estimating genetic networks, we standardized the data so that the expression values for each gene have mean 0 and standard deviation 1.

4.2 Results

To assess similarities and differences among networks estimated using procedures of Sect. 2, here we focus on the ER^+ samples from TCGA. This choice is in part due to availability of larger sample sizes in the ER^+ data, but also aims to simplify the presentation of the results. Results for ER^- samples are presented in the Supplementary Material.

Figures 2, 3, 4, 5, 6 and 7 compare the values of various classes of descriptors for networks estimated using the methods of Sect. 2 with the number of edges ranging

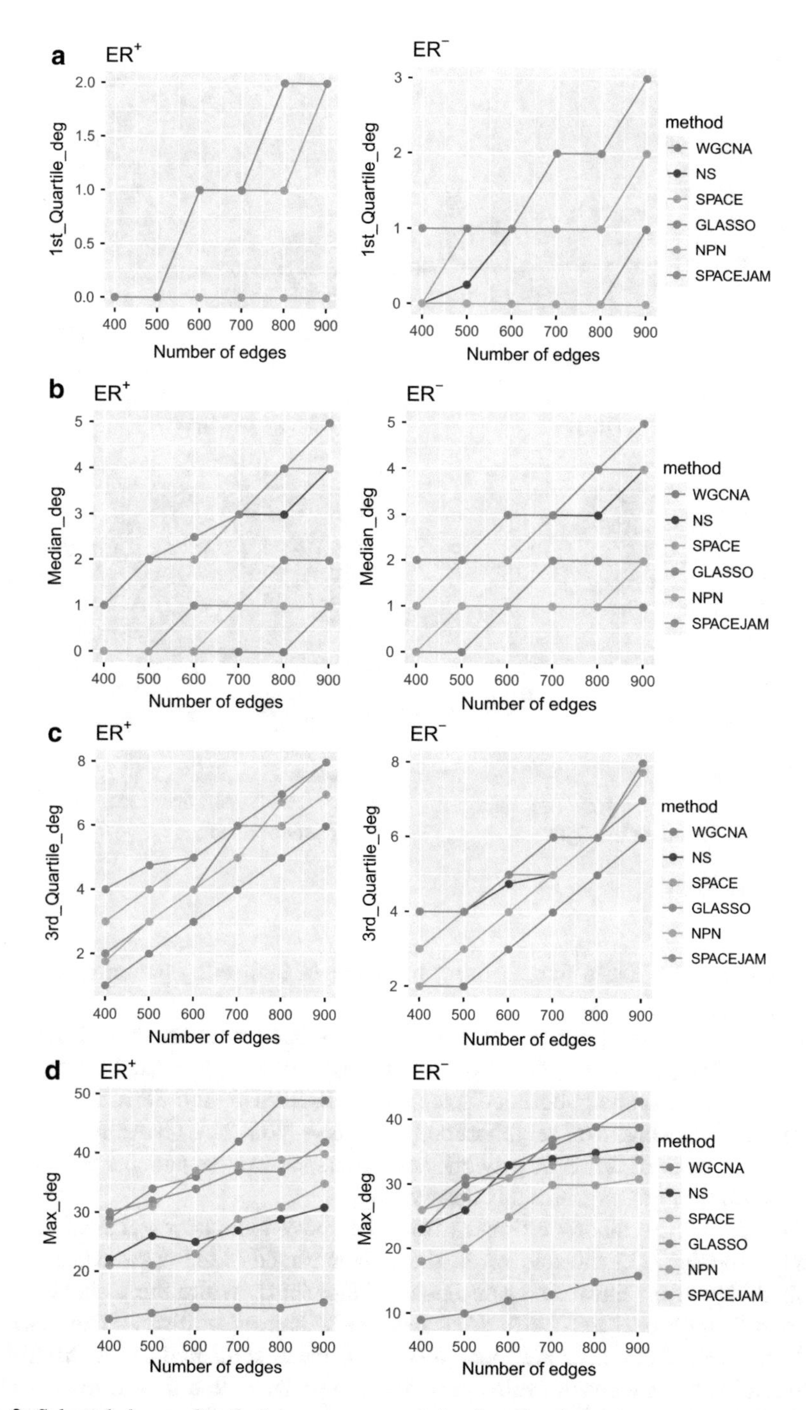

Fig. 2 Selected *degree distribution* summary statistics for all estimated networks for the ER^+ and ER^- data. Rows 1–6 show first quartile, median, third quartile, maximum, interquartile range (IQR) and the number of nodes with degree one in networks with different number of edges

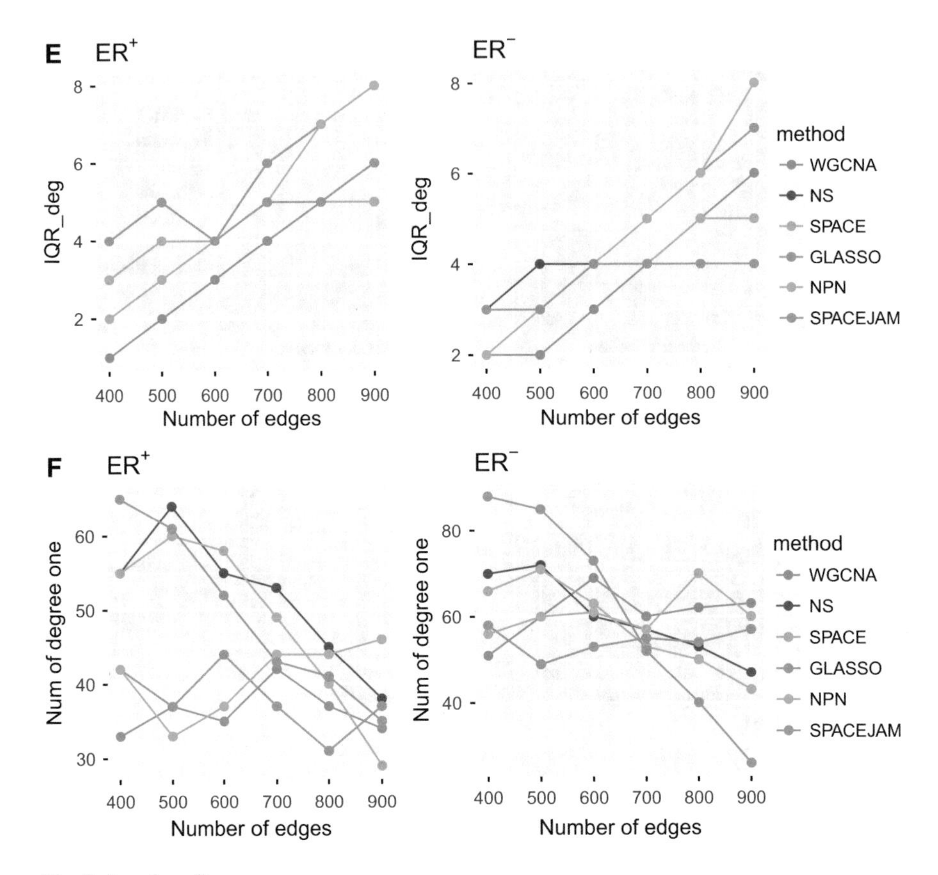

Fig. 2 (continued)

from 400 to 900. These figures show a number of interesting patterns, which we briefly comment on next.

Overall, the results indicate that despite significant differences in formulation and estimation procedures, the methods considered in this paper can be categorized into those based on neighborhood selection—NS, SPACE, and SPACE JAM—and those that are not based on neighborhood selection—WGCNA, GLASSO, and NPN. Examining plots of different network descriptors, as well as patterns of structural correlations in Fig. 7, verifies this observation.

The similarities among estimates from the above two classes of methods may seem surprising. On the one hand, the neighborhood-based approaches include methods based on linear and non-linear relationships. While the estimates from the non-linear model in SPACE JAM seem to be somewhat distinct from NS and SPACE, these differences are much less pronounced compared to the differences between the two classes of estimators. On the other hand, non-neighborhood-based methods differ both in terms of measure of association and the use of conditional versus marginal associations. Nonetheless, our numerical results indicate that the

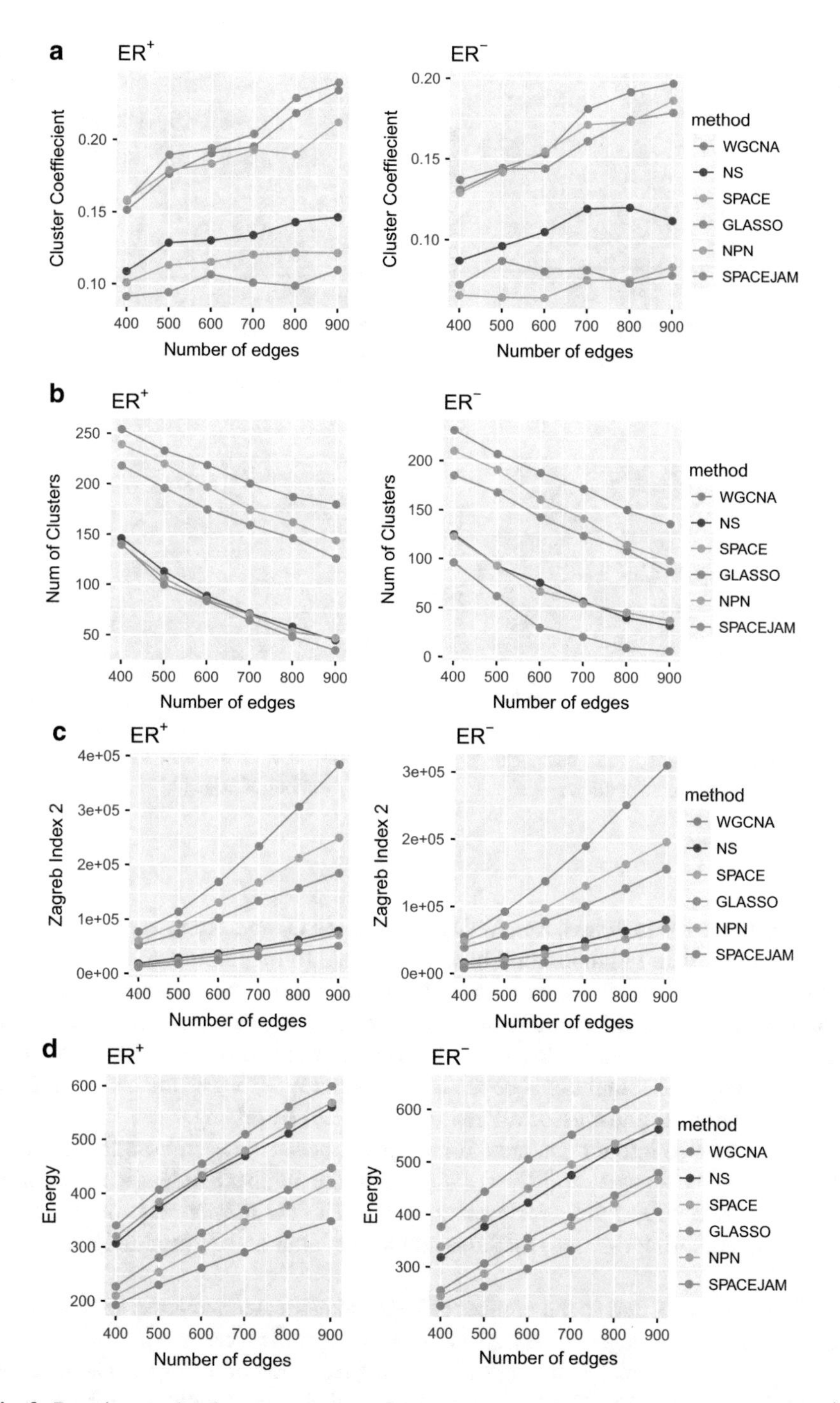

Fig. 3 Descriptors related to *connectedness* of the network for all estimated networks for the ER^+ and ER^- data. Rows 1–6 show cluster coefficient, number of clusters, Zagreb index, energy, degree centrality and medium articulation of networks with different number of edges

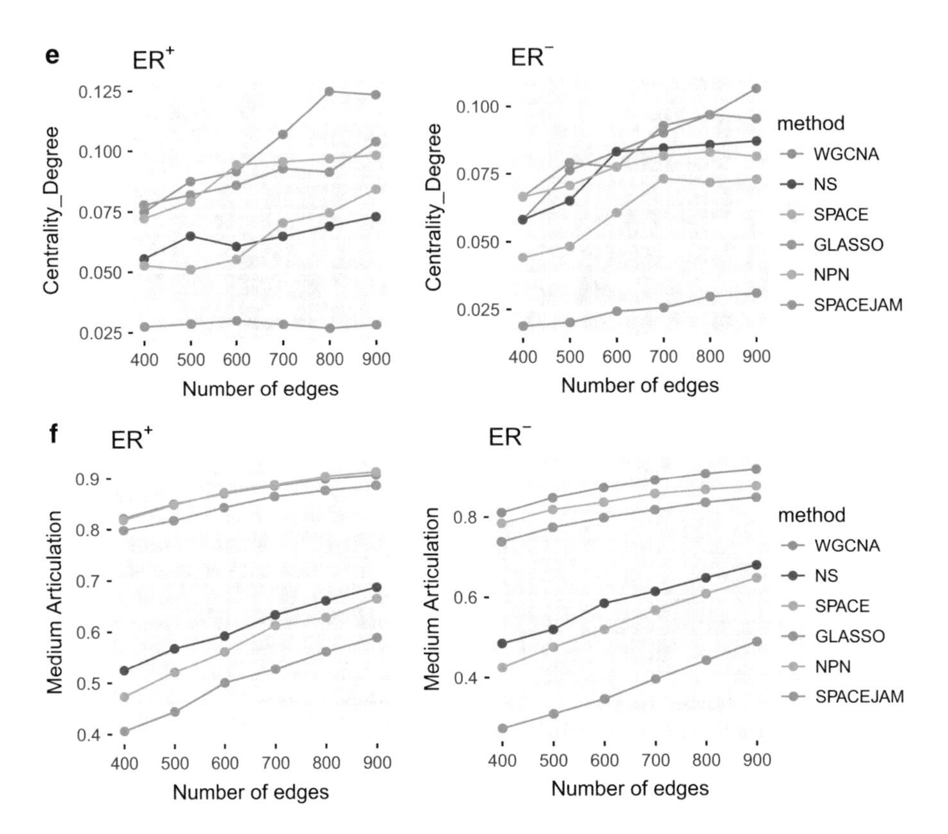

Fig. 3 (continued)

three methods in this class, i.e., WGCNA, GLASSO, and NPN, are more similar to each other than neighborhood-based methods. The similarity of WGCNA and GLASSO can be partially explained by recent results that establish a connection between GLASSO and simple thresholding of the sample covariance matrix [72–74]. However, the high level of similarity between NPN estimates—which are based on non-linear conditional dependencies—and WGCNA estimates—which are based on marginal linear associations—seems rather surprising.

We next delve into the patterns of changes in network descriptors for estimates from each of the above two classes of models, as the number of edges in the network increases from 400 to 900. For brevity, we refer to the former class of estimators as NB (neighborhood-based) methods and to the latter as NN (non-neighborhood) methods.

Figure 2 shows that as the number of edges in estimated networks increases, the first quantile of the degree distribution for NB methods increases, whereas it stays at zero for the NN estimates. In other words, the proportion of nodes with zero degree is not decreasing in the NN estimates. A somewhat similar pattern can be seen by looking at the median degree. Further, the number of nodes with degree one stays

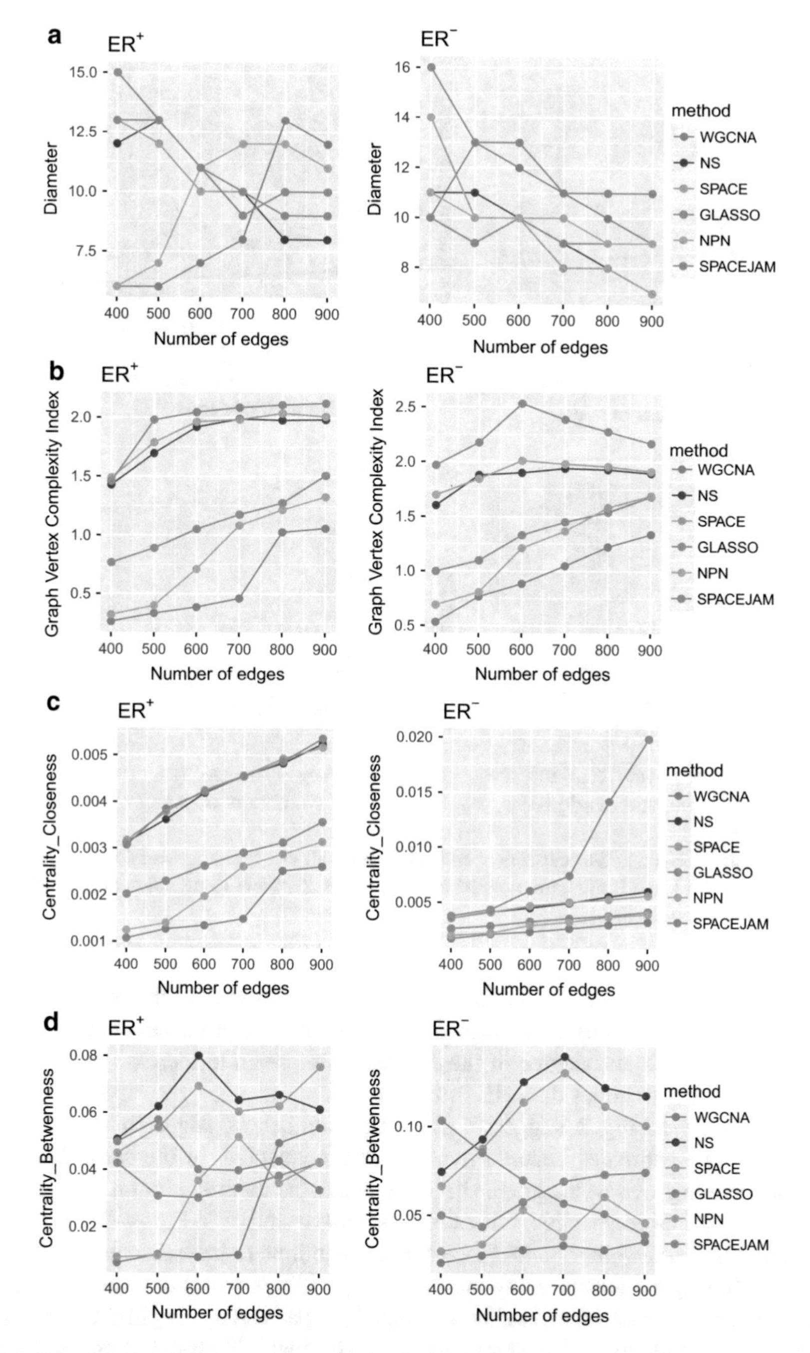

Fig. 4 Descriptors related to *spread* of information and node influence of the network for all estimated networks for the ER^+ and ER^- data. Rows 1–4 show diameter, graph vertex complexity index, closeness centrality and betweenness centrality of in networks with different number of edges

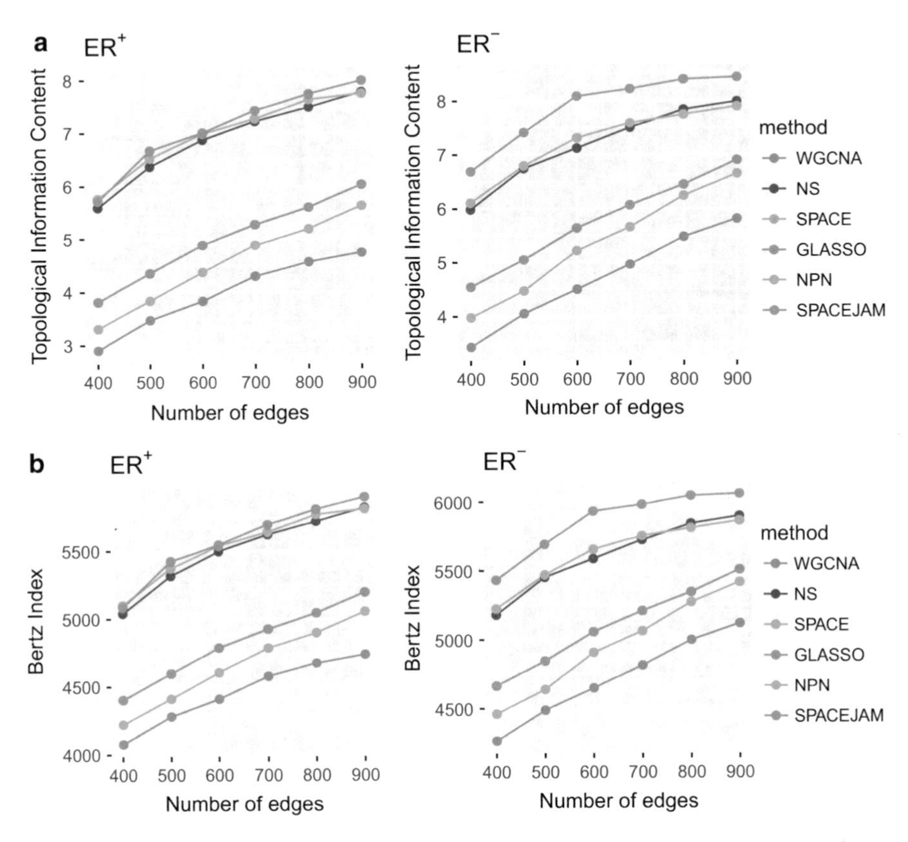

Fig. 5 Descriptors related to network *symmetry*, among all estimated networks for the ER^+ and ER^- data. Rows 1 and 2 show topological information content and Bertz index of networks with different number of edges

the same for NN estimates, but decreases for NB methods. On the other hand, the estimates seem to be similar in terms of the third quantile of the degree distribution, whereas the maximum degree of the NN estimates seem to increase more rapidly with the number of edges than NB estimates.

The results in Fig. 2 suggest that as the number of edges in the networks increases, NB estimates become overall more connected, in the sense that their median degree grows as the graphs become denser but their maximum degree grows slowly. From this perspective, NB estimates behave similar to Erdös–Rényi random graphs [75]. On the other hand, NN estimates continue to have disconnected nodes and few highly connected components. These findings corroborate with the plots for most measures of connectedness in Fig. 3. In particular, the plots of clustering coefficient and number of clusters together verify that NN estimates are comprised of many highly connected components, whereas NB methods tend to produce estimates in which more nodes are reachable from each other. The plots of the

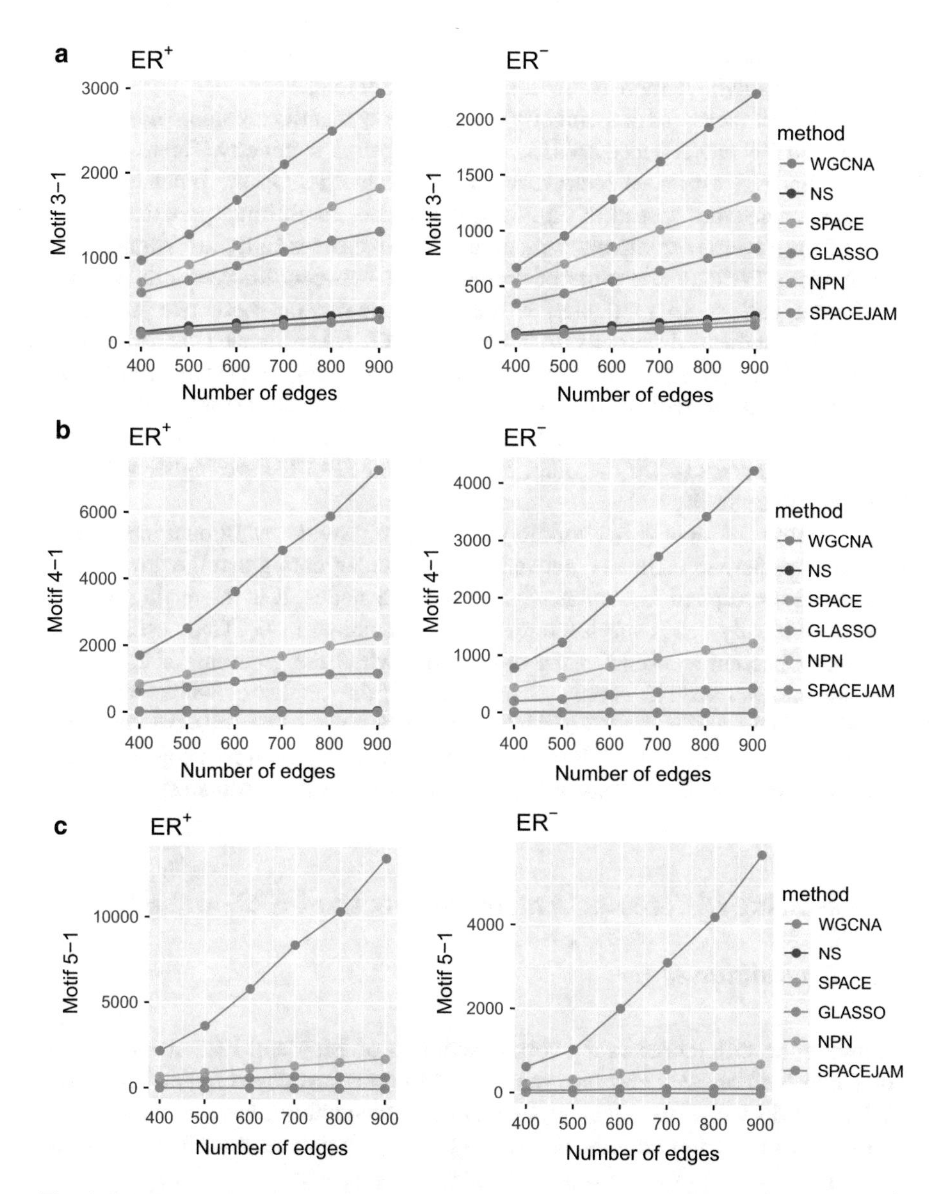

Fig. 6 Selected *network motifs* with 3, 4, and 5 nodes for all estimated networks for the ER^+ and ER^- data. Rows 1–3 show the number of motifs 3-1, 4-1 and 5-1 in networks with different number of edges

Zagreb index and energy also match the categorization of estimated networks to NB and NN. The only notable exceptions are the degree centrality plots, which suggest that node degrees in SPACE JAM estimates are significantly more concentrated than the other two NB methods. This may be due to the fact that SPACE JAM is the only method considered here which allows for truly non-linear relationships among nodes, and is solving a more difficult estimation problem.

The plots of measures of symmetry in Fig. 5 show that the grouping of estimated networks to NN and NB also holds in terms of network symmetry. The results also suggest that NN estimates seem to be more symmetric. On the other hand, the measures of network spread in Fig. 4 require a more careful interpretation. While plots of graph vertex complexity index and closeness centrality are aligned with our previous findings, the plots of diameter and betweenness centrality indicate a different pattern. In particular, it seems that based on these two measures, information spreads differently in NPN and WGCNA estimates than the other four estimates. Further, the plot of betweenness centrality indicates that NPN and WGCNA estimates with fewer edges have very low levels of betweenness, but become more similar to GLASSO and SPACE JAM as the number of edges in the network increases. On the other hand, NS and SPACE have higher values of betweenness centrality.

Examining the plots of network motifs in Fig. 6 provides additional insight into the local structure of estimated networks. In particular, noting that the three motifs considered correspond to cliques with 3, 4, and 5 nodes, it is interesting that the number of locally dense substructures seems to increase in WGCNA estimates as the graphs become denser. On the other hand, while the grouping of estimation methods into NN and NB is only clear in terms of the number of 3-node cliques—triangles—in the graph, the NN and NB classification can still be observed in 4- and 5-node cliques. Specifically, NB methods do not contain any cliques consisting of 4 or 5 nodes, whereas these dense substructures do exist in NN estimates.

5 Assessing Differences Among Networks of ER^+ and ER^-

5.1 Preliminaries

To assess the differences in network descriptors of ER^+ and ER^- networks, we compared the observed absolute values of differences in descriptors of ER^+ and ER^- networks with those obtained from $B = 500$ randomly generated pairs of data sets by permuting the samples in ER^+ and ER^-. To prevent any differences due to sample sizes, all $B = 500$ pairs of samples were generated with $n_{\mathrm{pos}} = 403$ and $n_{\mathrm{neg}} = 117$ samples in each of the two groups. Further, in each replication, the tuning parameters for different estimation methods were chosen so that the networks contained the same number of edges. The plots in Figs. 8, 9, 10, 11, 12 show the distribution of absolute differences of network descriptors for randomly generated ER^+ and ER^- samples $|desc_{ER^+} - desc_{ER^-}|$. The dot in each boxplot shows the absolute difference of *true values* of the same descriptor in the original ER^+ and ER^- networks.

Table 1 shows the p-values obtained by comparing the observed (absolute) differences in network descriptors with the null distribution obtained from pairs of networks with 500 edges based on randomly permuted samples. Formally,

$$p\text{-value} = \frac{1}{B}\sum_{k=1}^{B} |desc_{ER+} - desc_{ER-}| \leq |desc^{k}_{\text{pos}} - desc^{k}_{\text{neg}}|. \quad (25)$$

P-values for networks with other values of total number of edges are given in the Supplementary Material.

5.2 *Results*

The plots in Figs. 8, 9, 10, 11, 12 and the p-values in Table 1 point to a number of interesting findings. Most importantly, while the estimated ER^+ and ER^- networks seem to have significantly fewer common edges compared to pairs of networks from random samples, more global properties of estimated networks do not seem to be completely different from those based on random samples. This observation can have two explanations. First, differences in estimated structures are local and do not affect the global properties of the networks. This can be perhaps due to the fact that significant changes in global structure of biological networks may not be biologically viable. The second explanation is that unlike presence/absence of edges, global properties of estimated networks are more representative of the estimation procedure than the source of samples. In other words, while the local structures of estimated ER^+ and ER^- networks are different, both networks are estimated using the *same procedure*; therefore, their global properties are not very distinct.

The p-values in Table 1 also suggest that, compared to NB methods, ER^+ and ER^- estimates from WGCNA, NPN, and GLASSO have more different descriptors. This difference is particularly pronounced for WGNCA and NPN estimates. Examining the boxplots in Figs. 8, 9, 10, 11 and 12 suggests that this difference is not due to differences in variability of descriptors in estimated networks from NB and NN methods. The lower number of significant differences in structures of NB estimates may be due to the fact that the node degrees are more evenly spread in these estimates, and that the estimates contain fewer clusters of highly connected components.

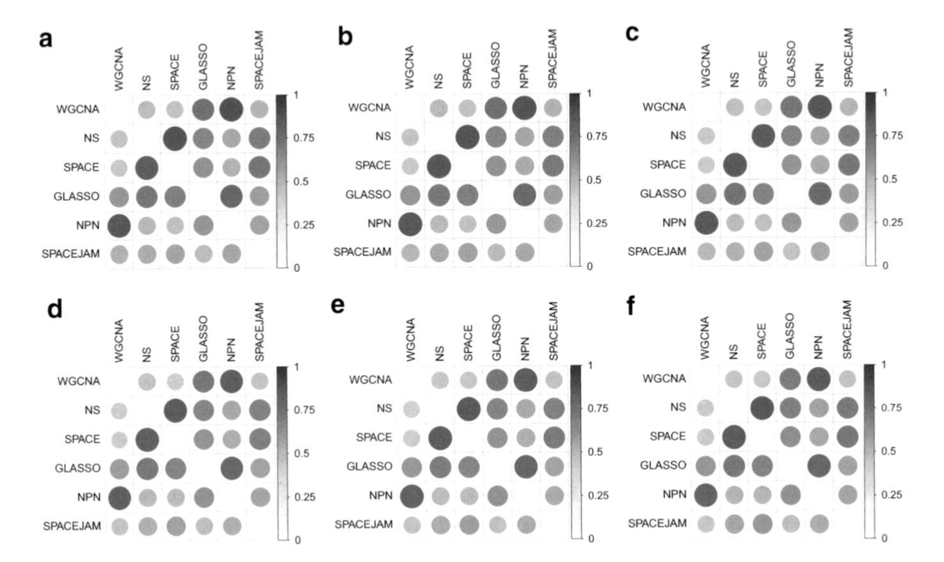

Fig. 7 *Structural correlation* matrix for ER^+ (upper triangular part) and ER^- (lower triangular part) networks: (**a**) 400 edges, (**b**) 500 edges, (**c**) 600 edges, (**d**) 700 edges, (**e**) 800 edges, (**f**) 900 edges

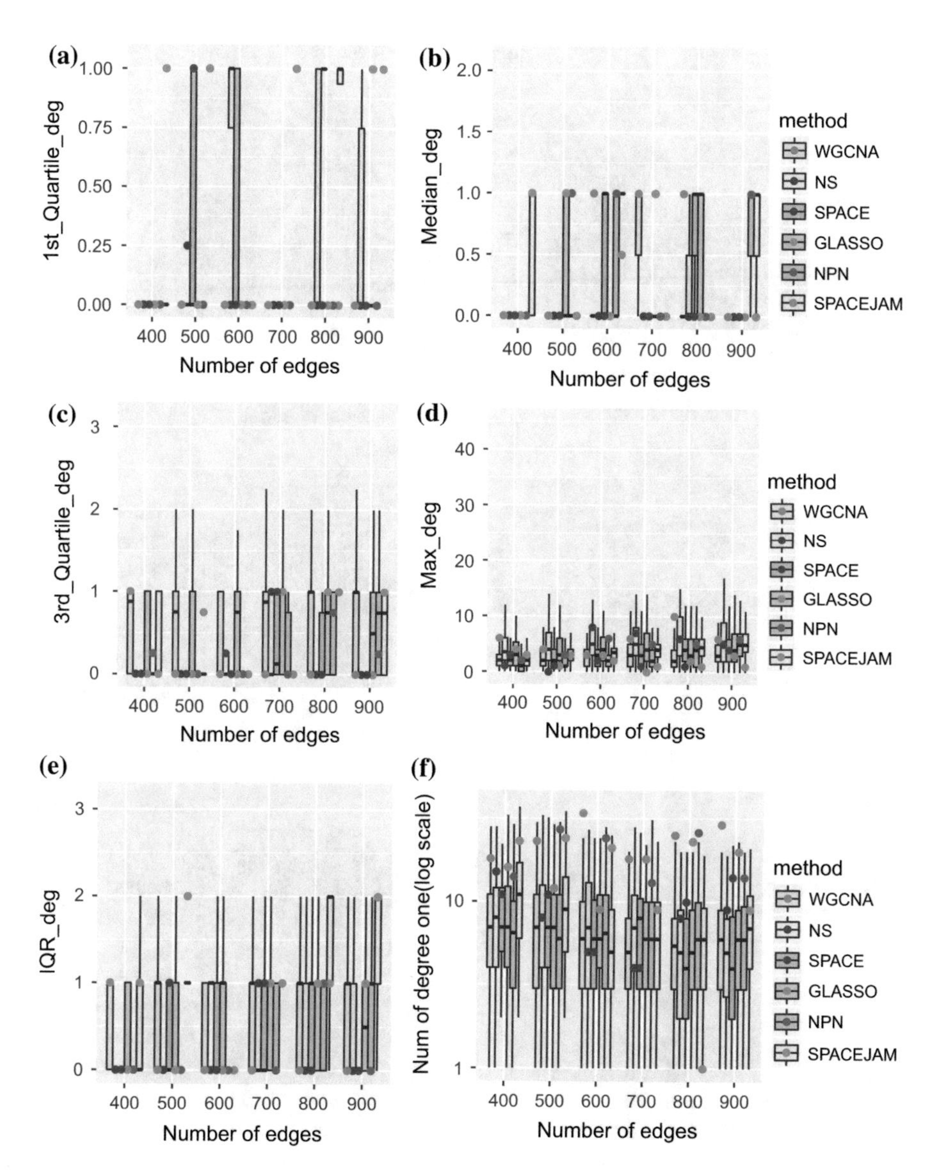

Fig. 8 Comparison of distribution of absolute differences of *degree distribution* summary statistics in estimated ER^+ and ER^- networks. Plots in (**a**)–(**f**) show the distribution of absolute differences of first quartile of degrees (**a**), median of degrees (**b**), third quartile of degrees (**c**), maximum of degrees (**d**), interquartile range of degrees (**e**) and number of nodes with degree one (**f**) in networks with different number of edges

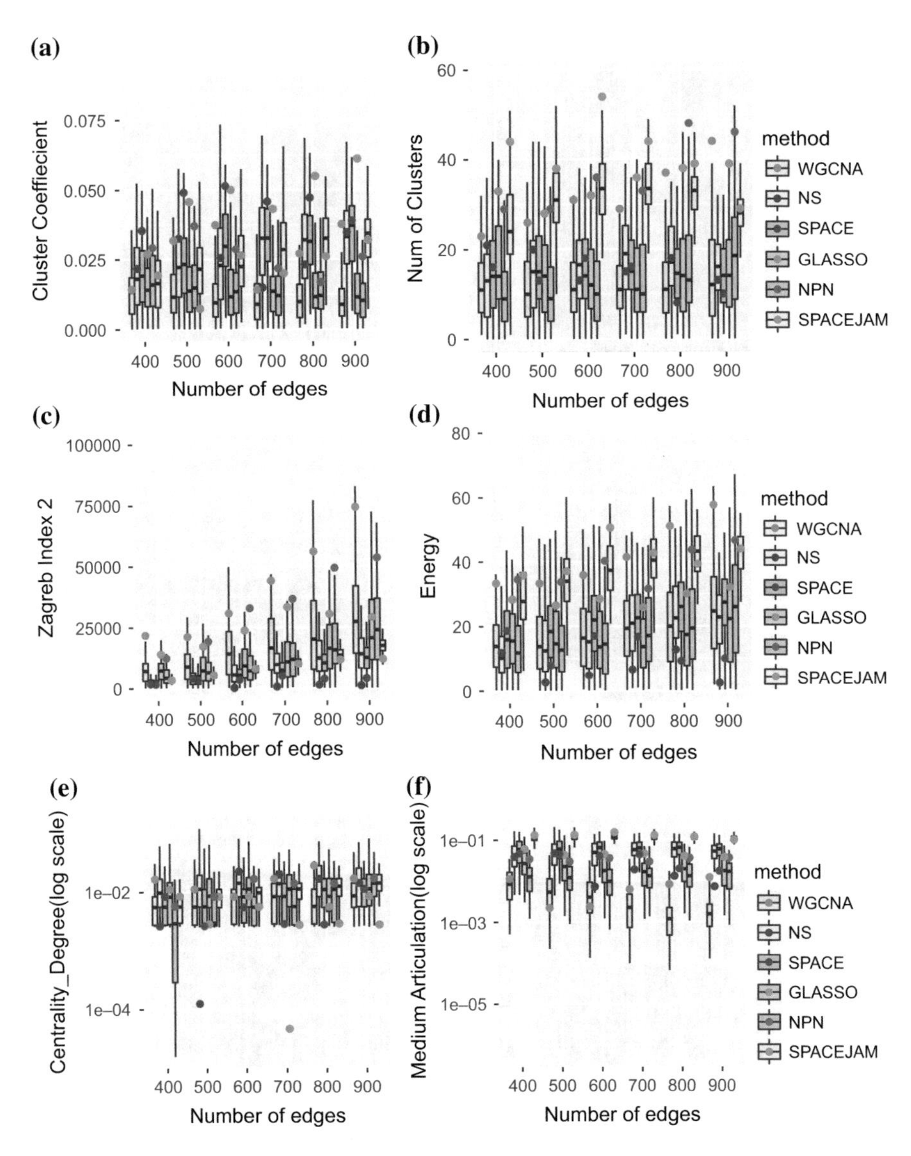

Fig. 9 Comparison of distribution of absolute differences of *connectedness* descriptors in estimated ER^+ and ER^- networks. Plots in (**a**)–(**f**) show the distribution of absolute differences of the cluster coefficient (**a**), number of clusters (**b**), Zagreb index (**c**), energy (**d**), degree centrality (**e**) medium articulation (**f**) in networks with different number of edges

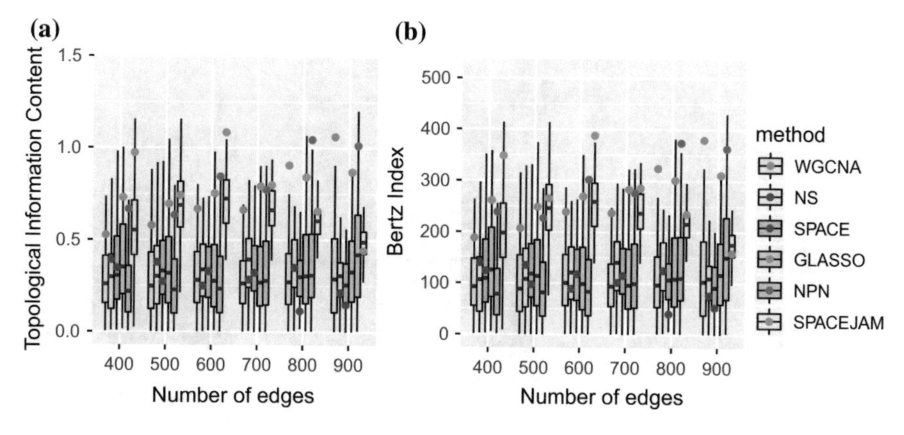

Fig. 10 Comparison of distribution of absolute differences of *symmetry* descriptors in estimated ER^+ and ER^- networks. Plots in (**a**) and (**b**) show the distribution of absolute differences of topological information (**a**) and Bertz index (**b**) in networks with different number of edges

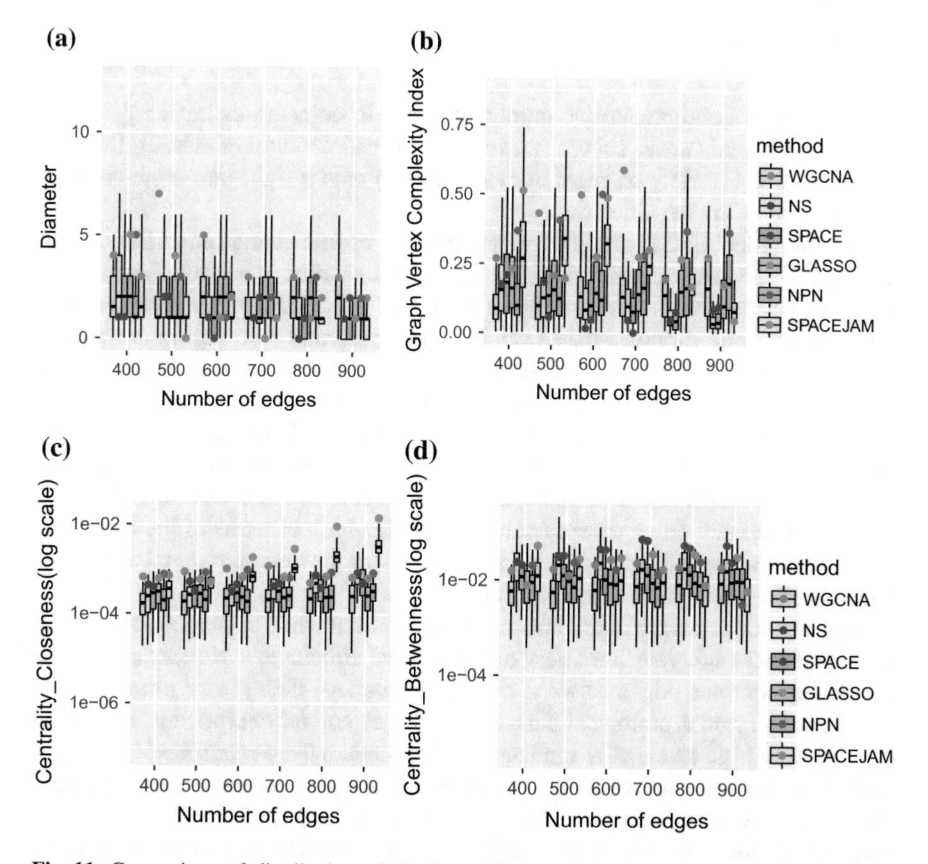

Fig. 11 Comparison of distribution of absolute differences of *spread* descriptors in estimated ER^+ and ER^- networks. Plots in (**a**)–(**d**) show the distribution of absolute differences of the diameter (**a**), vertex complexity (**b**), closeness centrality (**c**) and betweenness centrality (**d**) in networks with different number of edges

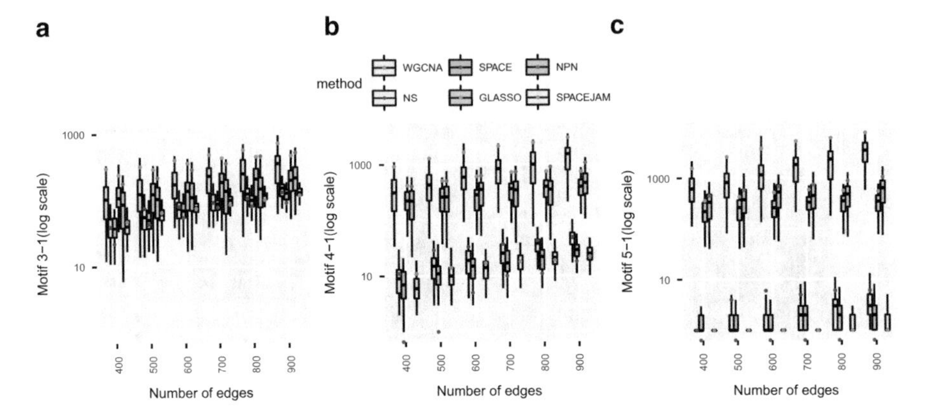

Fig. 12 Comparison of distributions of absolute differences of number of *network motifs* in estimated ER$^+$ and ER$^-$ networks: (a) Motif 3-1, (b) Motif 4-1, (c) Motif 5-1

6 Discussion

We conducted a comprehensive numerical study to compare estimated gene networks of different cancer subtypes using various estimation methods. To this end, we considered a variety of network descriptors to gain insight into more complex properties of estimated networks.

Our numerical investigation reveals a number of interesting properties of estimated gene networks across two different populations. First, our results suggest that the estimated networks from graphical lasso and its extension for handling non-Gaussian random variables based on the nonparanormal distribution are similar to simple (weighted) gene co-expression networks. The surprising aspect of this finding is that network estimates from the two former methods encode *conditional dependencies*, while the latter simply focuses on *marginal dependencies*. In theory, these two types of dependencies are very different. However, these findings corroborate with recent studies that have established interesting connections between graphical lasso and co-expression networks, particularly in terms of the connected components of the estimated networks. It seems that the nonparanormal estimation procedure further signifies these relations.

The second surprising finding from our study is that while estimated networks of different cancer subtypes have very different local structures—as measured by the number of common edges between the two networks—their global properties are less distinct. From a biological perspective, this is not very surprising. Biological systems pose high levels of redundancy, which renders them robustness to changes in the environment. This redundancy implies that changes in edges and local patterns of connectivity are less likely to affect the global properties of the networks. However, this finding can also be explained by differences among network estimation procedures. Specifically, one can argue that global properties of estimated networks

Table 1 *P*-values for testing equality of various descriptors for estimated networks of ER^+ and ER^- networks with $|E| = 500$ edges

Network descriptor	Network estimation methods					
	WGCNA	NS	SPACE	GLASSO	NPN	SPACEJAM
# Common edges	**0**	**0**	**0**	**0**	**0**	**0**
First quartile	1	0.164	0.338	1	1	0.998
Median	1	1	1	0.384	0.086	1
Third quartile	1	1	1	1	1	0.232
Max	0.26	1	0.882	0.914	0.252	0.558
IQR_deg	1	1	0.358	1	1	0.182
# deg one	**0.02**	0.53	0.284	0.202	**0.002**	**0.036**
Diameter	**0.006**	0.594	0.46	0.13	0.29	1
Cent.Degree	0.17	0.96	0.858	0.832	0.178	0.458
Cent.Betwenness	**0.052**	0.32	**0.076**	0.364	**0.068**	0.134
Cent.Closeness	**0**	0.106	0.426	0.112	**0**	0.504
Clusetr.Num	**0.094**	0.33	0.616	0.134	**0.038**	0.208
ZI	**0.072**	0.456	0.504	**0.094**	**0.018**	0.502
Topo_info	0.114	0.382	0.602	0.116	**0.064**	0.394
BI	0.114	0.382	0.602	0.116	**0.064**	0.394
GraphVertexComplexity	**0.004**	0.304	0.808	0.36	**0.014**	0.838
MA	0.742	0.502	0.678	0.214	0.13	0.328
Energy	**0.076**	0.904	0.822	0.224	**0.05**	0.368
Clust_coef	**0.04**	0.25	**0.026**	**0.006**	**0.022**	0.866
Motif.3_1	**0.04**	0.228	0.668	**0.032**	**0.064**	0.448
Motif.4_1	**0.004**	**0.06**	0.988	**0.048**	0.11	0.298
Motif.5_1	**0.002**	**0.04**	1	0.144	0.262	0.2

The *p*-values are calculated by comparing the observed values of descriptors with those obtained from $B = 500$ pairs of networks generated from randomly sampled observations; see text for details. *P*-values smaller than 0.1 are shown in bold.

are determined by the estimation procedure. In other words, while patterns of (conditional or marginal) dependency across estimated networks of cancer subtypes are clearly different, the global properties of these estimated networks seem to be driven, to a large degree, by the estimation procedure used to obtain these estimates. Our observations highlight the need for development of rigorous methodologies to (1) identify changes in local structures of gene networks in different biological conditions and (2) better understand the effect of these local changes on global network properties that explain the behavior of biological systems.

Acknowledgements This work was partially supported by grants from the US National Science Foundation (DMS-1161565) and the National Institute of Health (1K01HL124050-01A1).

References

1. Schadt, E.E.: Molecular networks as sensors and drivers of common human diseases. Nature **461**(7261), 218–223 (2009)
2. Janjić, V., Pržulj, N.: Biological function through network topology: a survey of the human diseasome. Brief. Funct. Genomics **11**(6), 522–532 (2012)
3. Coulson, J.M.: Transcriptional regulation: cancer, neurons and the rest. Curr. Biol. **15**(17), R665–R668 (2005)
4. Simpson, R.J., Dorow, D.S.: Cancer proteomics: from signaling networks to tumor markers. Trends Biotechnol. **19**, 40–48 (2001)
5. Osborn, O., Olefsky, J.M.: The cellular and signaling networks linking the immune system and metabolism in disease. Nat. Med. **18**(3), 363–374 (2012)
6. Horvath, S., Zhang, B., Carlson, M., Lu, K.V., Zhu, S., Felciano, R.M., Laurance, M.F., Zhao, W., Qi, S., Chen, Z., et al.: Analysis of oncogenic signaling networks in glioblastoma identifies ASPM as a molecular target. Proc. Natl. Acad. Sci. **103**(46), 17402–17407 (2006)
7. Ule, J., Jensen, K.B., Ruggiu, M., Mele, A., Ule, A., Darnell, R.B.: CLIP identifies Nova-regulated RNA networks in the brain. Science **302**(5648), 1212–1215 (2003)
8. Luscombe, N.M., Babu, M.M., Yu, H., Snyder, M., Teichmann, S.A., Gerstein, M.: Genomic analysis of regulatory network dynamics reveals large topological changes. Nature **431**(7006), 308–312 (2004)
9. Ideker, T., Krogan, N.J.: Differential network biology. Mol. Syst. Biol. **8**(1), 565 (2012)
10. Zhang, B., Li, H., Riggins, R.B., Zhan, M., Xuan, J., Zhang, Z., Hoffman, E.P., Clarke, R., Wang, Y.: Differential dependency network analysis to identify condition-specific topological changes in biological networks. Bioinformatics **25**(4), 526–532 (2009)
11. West, J., Bianconi, G., Severini, S., Teschendorff, A.E.: Differential network entropy reveals cancer system hallmarks. Sci. Rep. **2** (2012)
12. Henderson, J., Michailidis, G.: Network reconstruction using nonparametric additive ode models. PLoS One **9**(4), e94003 (2014)
13. Langfelder, P., Horvath, S.: WGCNA: an R package for weighted correlation network analysis. BMC Bioinf. **9**(1), 559 (2008)
14. Meinshausen, N., Bühlmann, P.: High-dimensional graphs and variable selection with the lasso. Ann. Stat. **34**(3), 1436–1462 (2006)
15. Friedman, J., Hastie, T., Tibshirani, R: Sparse inverse covariance estimation with the graphical lasso. Biostatistics **9**(3), 432–441 (2008)
16. Peng, J., Wang, P., Zhou, N., Zhu, J.: Partial correlation estimation by joint sparse regression models. J. Am. Stat. Assoc. **104**(486) (2009)
17. Zhao, T., Liu, H., Roeder, K., Lafferty, J., Wasserman, L.: The huge package for high-dimensional undirected graph estimation in R. J. Mach. Learn. Res. **13**(1), 1059–1062 (2012)
18. Voorman, A., Shojaie, A., Witten, D.: Graph estimation with joint additive models. Biometrika **101**(1), 85–101 (2014)
19. Lauritzen, S.L.: Graphical Models. Oxford University Press, Oxford (1996)
20. Koller, D., Friedman, N.: Probabilistic Graphical Models: Principles and Techniques. MIT, Cambridge (2009)
21. Friedman, N.: Inferring cellular networks using probabilistic graphical models. Science **303**(5659), 799–805 (2004)
22. Markowetz, F., Spang, R.: Inferring cellular networks–a review. BMC Bioinf. **8**(Suppl 6), S5 (2007)
23. Krämer, N., Schäfer, J., Boulesteix, A.-L.: Regularized estimation of large-scale gene association networks using graphical Gaussian models. BMC Bioinf. **10**(1), 384 (2009)
24. Sedaghat, N., Saegusa, T., Randolph, T., Shojaie, A.: Comparative study of computational methods for reconstructing genetic networks of cancer-related pathways. Cancer Informat. **13**(Suppl 2), 55 (2014)

25. Allen, J.D., Xie, Y., Chen, M., Girard, L., Xiao, G.: Comparing statistical methods for constructing large scale gene networks. PLoS One **7**(1), e29348 (2012)
26. Wille, A., Zimmermann, P., Vranová, E., Fürholz, A., Laule, A., Bleuler, S., Hennig, L., Prelic, A., von Rohr, P., Thiele, L., et al.: Sparse graphical Gaussian modeling of the isoprenoid gene network in Arabidopsis thaliana. Genome Biol. **5**(11), R92 (2004)
27. Chu, J.-H., Weiss, S.T., Carey, V.J., Raby, B.A.: A graphical model approach for inferring large-scale networks integrating gene expression and genetic polymorphism. BMC Syst. Biol. **3**(1), 55 (2009)
28. Strimmer, K., Moulton, V.: Likelihood analysis of phylogenetic networks using directed graphical models. Mol. Biol. Evol. **17**(6), 875–881 (2000)
29. Yu, J., Smith, V.A., Wang, P.P., Hartemink, A.J., Jarvis, E.D.: Advances to Bayesian network inference for generating causal networks from observational biological data. Bioinformatics **20**(18), 3594–3603 (2004)
30. Chickering, D.M.: Learning Bayesian networks is NP-complete. In: Learning From Data, pp. 121–130. Springer, Berlin (1996)
31. Shojaie, A., Jauhiainen, A., Kallitsis, M., Michailidis, G.: Inferring regulatory networks by combining perturbation screens and steady state gene expression profiles. PLoS One **9**(2), e82393 (2014)
32. Markowetz, F.: How to understand the cell by breaking it: network analysis of gene perturbation screens. PLoS Comput. Biol. **6**(2), e1000655 (2010)
33. Shojaie, A., Michailidis, G.: Discovering graphical granger causality using the truncating lasso penalty. Bioinformatics **26**(18), i517–i523 (2010)
34. Shojaie, A., Basu, S., Michailidis, G.: Adaptive thresholding for reconstructing regulatory networks from time-course gene expression data. Stat. Biosci. **4**(1), 66–83 (2012)
35. Pearson, K.: Note on regression and inheritance in the case of two parents. Proc. R. Soc. Lond. **58**(347–352), 240–242 (1895)
36. Cover, T.M., Thomas, J.A.: Elements of Information Theory. Wiley, New York (2012)
37. Reshef, D.N., Reshef, Y.A., Finucane, H.K., Grossman, S.R., McVean, G., Turnbaugh, P.J., Lander, E.S., Mitzenmacher, M., Sabeti, P.C.: Detecting novel associations in large data sets. Science **334**(6062), 1518–1524 (2011)
38. Margolin, A.A., Nemenman, I., Basso, K., Wiggins, C., Stolovitzky, G., Favera, R.D., Califano, A.: ARACNE: an algorithm for the reconstruction of gene regulatory networks in a mammalian cellular context. BMC Bioinf. **7**(Suppl 1), S7 (2006)
39. Montes, R.A., Coello, G., González-Aguilera, K.L., Marsch-Martínez, N., de Folter, S., Alvarez-Buylla, E.R.: ARACNe-based inference, using curated microarray data, of Arabidopsis thaliana root transcriptional regulatory networks. BMC Plant Biol. **14**(1), 97 (2014)
40. Ravikumar, P., Wainwright, M.J., Raskutti, G., Yu, B., et al.: High-dimensional covariance estimation by minimizing l1-penalized log-determinant divergence. Electron. J. Stat. **5**, 935–980 (2011)
41. Liu, H., Lafferty, J., Wasserman, L.: The nonparanormal: semiparametric estimation of high dimensional undirected graphs. J. Mach. Learn. Res. **10**, 2295–2328 (2009)
42. Li, A., Horvath, S.: Network neighborhood analysis with the multi-node topological overlap measure. Bioinformatics **23**(2), 222–231 (2007)
43. Yip, A.M., Horvath, S.: Gene network interconnectedness and the generalized topological overlap measure. BMC Bioinf. **8**(1), 22 (2007)
44. Xue, L., Zou, H., et al.: Regularized rank-based estimation of high-dimensional nonparanormal graphical models. Ann. Stat. **40**(5), 2541–2571 (2012)
45. Liu, H., Han, F., Yuan, M., Lafferty, J., Wasserman, L., et al.: High-dimensional semiparametric Gaussian copula graphical models. Ann. Stat. **40**(4), 2293–2326 (2012)
46. Jacob, L., Obozinski, G., Vert, J.-P..: Group lasso with overlap and graph lasso. In: Proceedings of the 26th Annual International Conference on Machine Learning, pp. 433–440. ACM, New York (2009)
47. Meier, L., Van De Geer, S., Bühlmann, P.: The group lasso for logistic regression. J. R. Stat. Soc. Ser. B Stat. Methodol. **70**(1), 53–71 (2008)

48. Newman, M.E.J.: Scientific collaboration networks. II. Shortest paths, weighted networks, and centrality. Phys. Rev. E **64**(1), 016132 (2001)
49. Nikolić, S., Kovačević, G., Miličević, A., Trinajstić, N.: The Zagreb indices 30 years after. Croat. Chem. Acta **76**(2), 113–124 (2003)
50. Diudea, M.V., Gutman, I., Jantschi, L.: Molecular Topology. Nova Science Publishers, Huntington, NY (2001)
51. Albert, R.: Scale-free networks in cell biology. J. Cell Sci. **118**(21), 4947–4957 (2005)
52. Gutman, I., Li, X., Zhang, J.: Graph energy. In: Analysis of Complex Networks. From Biology to Linguistics. Wiley–VCH, Weinheim (2009)
53. Pavlopoulos, G.A., Secrier, M., Moschopoulos, C.N., Soldatos, T.G., Kossida, S., Aerts, J., Schneider, R., Bagos, P.G., et al.: Using graph theory to analyze biological networks. BioData Min. **4**(1), 10 (2011)
54. Wilhelm, T., Hollunder, J.: Information theoretic description of networks. Phys. A Stat. Mech. Appl. **385**(1), 385–396 (2007)
55. Kim, J., Wilhelm, T.: What is a complex graph? Phys. A Stat. Mech. Appl. **387**(11), 2637–2652 (2008)
56. Pahl-Wostl, C.: The Dynamic Nature of Ecosystems: Chaos and Order Entwined. Wiley (1995)
57. Okamoto, K., Chen, W., Li, X.-Y.: Ranking of closeness centrality for large-scale social networks. In: Frontiers in Algorithmics, pp. 186–195. Springer, Berlin (2008)
58. Raychaudhury, C., Ray, S.K., Ghosh, J.J., Roy, A.B., Basak, S.C.: Discrimination of isomeric structures using information theoretic topological indices. J. Comput. Chem. **5**(6), 581–588 (1984)
59. MacArthur, B.D., Sánchez-García, R.J., Anderson, J.W.: Symmetry in complex networks. Discrete Appl. Math. **156**(18), 3525–3531 (2008)
60. Mowshowitz, A., Dehmer, M.: A symmetry index for graphs. J. Math. Biophys. **30**, 533–546 (2010)
61. Gross, J.L., Yellen, J.: Handbook of Graph Theory. CRC, Boca Raton, FL (2004)
62. Bonchev, D.G., Rouvray, D.H.: Complexity: Introduction and Fundamentals, vol. 7. CRC, Boca Raton, FL (2003)
63. Bertz, S.H.: The first general index of molecular complexity. J. Am. Chem. Soc. **103**(12), 3599–3601 (1981)
64. Devillers, J., Balaban, A.T.: Topological indices and related descriptors in QSAR and QSPAR. CRC, Boca Raton, FL (2000)
65. Mowshowitz, A.: Entropy and the complexity of graphs: I. an index of the relative complexity of a graph. Bull. Math. Biophys. **30**(1), 175–204 (1968)
66. Kim, W., Li, M., Wang, J., Pan, Y.: Biological network motif detection and evaluation. BMC Systems Biol. **5**(Suppl 3), S5 (2011)
67. Milo, R., Shen-Orr, S., Itzkovitz, S., Kashtan, N., Chklovskii, D., Alon, U.: Network motifs: simple building blocks of complex networks. Science **298**(5594), 824–827 (2002)
68. Middendorf, M., Ziv, E., Wiggins, C.H.: Inferring network mechanisms: the drosophila melanogaster protein interaction network. Proc. Natl. Acad. Sci. U. S. A. **102**(9), 3192–3197 (2005)
69. Albert, I., Albert, R.: Conserved network motifs allow protein–protein interaction prediction. Bioinformatics **20**(18), 3346–3352 (2004)
70. Butts, C.T., Carley, K.: Multivariate methods for interstructural analysis CASOS Working Paper. Carnegie Mellon University (2001)
71. Butts, C.T.: Social network analysis with sna. J. Stat. Softw. **24**(6), 1–51 (2008)
72. Witten, D.M., Friedman, J.H., Simon, N.: New insights and faster computations for the graphical lasso. J. Comput. Graph. Stat. **20**(4), 892–900 (2011)
73. Mazumder, R., Hastie, T.: Exact covariance thresholding into connected components for large-scale graphical lasso. J. Mach. Learn. Res. **13**(1), 781–794 (2012)
74. Luo, S., Song, R., Witten, D.: Sure screening for Gaussian graphical models (2014). arXiv preprint arXiv:1407.7819
75. Erdös, P., Renyi, A.: On random graphs I. Publ. Math. Debr. **6**, 290–297 (1959)

A Computationally Efficient Approach for Modeling Complex and Big Survival Data

Kevin He, Yanming Li, Qingyi Wei, and Yi Li

Abstract Modern data collection techniques have resulted in an increasing number of big clustered time-to-event data sets, wherein patients are often observed from a large number of healthcare providers. Semiparametric frailty models are a flexible and powerful tool for modeling clustered time-to-event data. In this manuscript, we first provide a computationally efficient approach based on a minimization–maximization algorithm to fit semiparametric frailty models in large-scale settings. We then extend the proposed method to incorporate complex data structures such as time-varying effects, for which many existing methods fail because of lack of computational power. The finite-sample properties and the utility of the proposed method are examined through an extensive simulation study and an analysis of the national kidney transplant data.

1 Introduction

In recent years, advancing technology has resulted in an increasing number of big time-to-event data sets, wherein patients are often observed from multiple clusters (e.g., healthcare providers). For multi-clusters analysis, fixed effects model with clusters as fixed effects is attractive if the sample sizes across clusters are large. However, as is often seen in multi-cluster studies, there are many clusters with relatively few patients. An alternative to a fixed effects approach is the random effects or frailty model, in which clusters-specific effects are treated as random samples from a specific probability distribution.

A wide variety of random effects models have been studied in survival analysis. Among them, the gamma frailty model [1–3] and the log-normal frailty model [4–6] are the most extensively studied approaches for time-to-event data. One reason for

K. He • Y. Li • Y. Li (✉)
Department of Biostatistics, University of Michigan, Ann Arbor, MI 48109, USA
e-mail: kevinhe@umich.edu; liyanmin@umich.edu; yili@umich.edu

Q. Wei
Duke University School of Medicine and Duke Cancer Institute, Duke University Medical Center, 27710 Durham, NC, USA
e-mail: qingyi.wei@duke.edu

© Springer International Publishing AG 2017

S.E. Ahmed (ed.), *Big and Complex Data Analysis*, Contributions to Statistics,
DOI 10.1007/978-3-319-41573-4_10

the popularity of the gamma frailty model is that it has a closed form Laplace transformation for the survival function. Although the log-normal frailty model has no explicit evaluation of the Laplace transform, it allows more flexibility and has been commonly used to fit clustered frailty models [6].

Despite their popularity, the computational complexity of random effects models have limited their use in big data. First, the numerical calculations may have tremendous costs when the dimensionality of predictors is large [7]. Second, when the number of subjects grows, the difficulty of model construction may also increases dramatically. For instance, big time-to-event data are usually complex, e.g., associations between disease outcomes and risk factors may involve complex functional forms such as time-varying effects [8]. In the context of survival analysis, time-varying effects have been studied for application with relatively small sample sizes [9–14]. To estimate such a model, the data set is typically expanded in a repeated measurement format (counting process style), e.g., the time is divided into small time intervals where one single event occurs in each time interval. The covariate values and outcome in the interval for each subject still under observation are stacked into a large data set. Even with a moderate sample size, such an expansion leads to a extremely large data which will be often infeasible to handle with existing computational capability. As an example, data set with 5000 event (assuming no ties) will lead to an expanded data set with records more than 12 millions, which easily out-powers a computer with 8G memory. To avoid the expansion of large-scale data, an alternative approach based on Kronecker product was suggested by Perperoglou et al. [15], with a Newton's method applied by iteratively updating the gradients and Hessian matrices. However, in large-scale survival analyses with massive sample size and large number of predictors, it is computationally expensive to calculate and invert the Hessian matrix. The commonly used Newton-type method may converge slowly or even fail. Finally, numerical problems may arise with skewed covariates (e.g., binary variables with extreme proportion). Extremely small at-risk sets in certain groups may lead to unstable estimations.

To improve the computation efficiency and fill the gap in the existing literature, we first develop an computationally efficient algorithm for estimating the Cox proportional hazards model in the presence of a large number of covariates. The proposed approach combines the strength of the quasi-Newton and minimization–maximization (MM) algorithm. To address the correlation due to clustering, we then extend the proposed algorithm to semiparametric frailty models. Finally, the proposed algorithm is generalized to estimate time-varying effects in complex and big survival data. The proposed method has a connection with coordinate descent which is widely used in high-dimensional data analysis. It should be noted, however, that our general aim is to estimate each predictor's effect instead of variable selection. This is different than a typical constrained optimization approach. In the latter approach, the dimensionality of the data is often much larger than the sample size and the estimated covariate effects are shrunken via penalization.

2 MM Algorithms for Cox Proportional Hazards Model

2.1 The Model

Let D_i denote the time to death and C_i be the censoring time for patient i, $i = 1, \ldots, n$. The observation time is denoted as $T_i = \min\{D_i, C_i\}$, and the death indicator is given by $\delta_i = I(D_i \le C_i)$. Let $\mathbf{X}_i = (X_{i1}, \ldots, X_{ip})^T$ be a p-dimensional covariate vector for the ith patient. We assume that, conditional on $\mathbf{X}_i$, D_i is independently censored by C_i. To model the death hazard, consider

$$\lambda_i(t|\mathbf{X}_i) = \lim_{dt \to 0} \frac{1}{dt} Pr(t \le D_i < t + dt | D_i \ge t, \mathbf{X}_i),$$

which we model by $\lambda_i(t|\mathbf{X}_i) = \lambda_0(t) \exp(\mathbf{X}_i^T \boldsymbol{\beta})$, where $\lambda_0(t)$ is the baseline hazard function and $\boldsymbol{\beta} = (\beta_1, \ldots, \beta_p)^T$ is a vector of parameters. The corresponding log-partial likelihood is given by

$$l(\boldsymbol{\beta}) = \sum_{i=1}^{n} \delta_i \left[\mathbf{X}_i^T \boldsymbol{\beta} - \log \left\{ \sum_{\ell \in R_i} \exp\left(\mathbf{X}_\ell^T \boldsymbol{\beta}\right) \right\} \right], \tag{1}$$

where $R_i = \{\ell : T_\ell \ge T_i\}$ is the at-risk set. Let $\nabla l(\boldsymbol{\beta})$ denote the first derivative of the log-partial likelihood with respect to $\boldsymbol{\beta}$. We have

$$\nabla l(\boldsymbol{\beta}) = \sum_{i=1}^{n} \delta_i \left\{ \mathbf{X}_i - \frac{\sum_{\ell \in R_i} \mathbf{X}_\ell \exp(\mathbf{X}_\ell^T \boldsymbol{\beta})}{\sum_{\ell \in R_i} \exp(\mathbf{X}_\ell^T \boldsymbol{\beta})} \right\},$$

Let $\nabla^2 l(\boldsymbol{\beta})$ denote the second derivative of the log-partial likelihood with respect to $\boldsymbol{\beta}$. We have

$$-\nabla^2 l(\boldsymbol{\beta}) = \sum_{i=1}^{n} \delta_i \left[\frac{\sum_{\ell \in R_i} \mathbf{X}_\ell^{\otimes 2} \exp(\mathbf{X}_\ell^T \boldsymbol{\beta})}{\sum_{\ell \in R_i} \exp(\mathbf{X}_\ell^T \boldsymbol{\beta})} - \left\{ \frac{\sum_{\ell \in R_i} \mathbf{X}_\ell \exp(\mathbf{X}_\ell^T \boldsymbol{\beta})}{\sum_{\ell \in R_i} \exp(\mathbf{X}_\ell^T \boldsymbol{\beta})} \right\}^{\otimes 2} \right],$$

where $\otimes$ is the Kronecker product.

2.2 Proposed Method

The proposed method is based on MM algorithm. For some good review on MM methods, the readers are referred to [16–19]. We first consider the Cox proportional hazards model. In a minorization step, we minorize the log-partial likelihood by a surrogate function, which is chosen to separate the parameters. We begin with the observation that the log-partial likelihood (1) is a concave function of $\boldsymbol{\beta}$. Given the mth step estimate $\hat{\boldsymbol{\beta}}^{(m)}$, an application of Jensen's inequality leads to the following minority surrogate function:

$$l(\boldsymbol{\beta}) \geq \sum_{j=1}^{p}\sum_{i=1}^{n} \alpha_j \delta_i \left[\frac{X_{ij}}{\alpha_j}(\beta_j - \hat{\beta}_j^{(m)}) + \mathbf{X}_i^T \hat{\boldsymbol{\beta}}^{(m)} - \log\left\{ \sum_{\ell \in R_i} \exp\left(\frac{X_{\ell j}}{\alpha_j}(\beta_j - \hat{\beta}_j^{(m)}) \right.\right.\right.$$

$$\left.\left.\left. + \mathbf{X}_\ell^T \hat{\boldsymbol{\beta}}^{(m)} \right)\right\}\right] = g(\boldsymbol{\beta}|\hat{\boldsymbol{\beta}}^{(m)}) = \sum_{j=1}^{p} g(\beta_j|\hat{\boldsymbol{\beta}}^{(m)}), \tag{2}$$

where $g(\beta_j|\hat{\boldsymbol{\beta}}^{(m)})$ is defined implicitly, all $\alpha_j \geq 0$, $\sum_j \alpha_j = 1$ and $\alpha_j > 0$ whenever $X_{ij} \neq 0$. A candidate for α_j is

$$\alpha_j = \frac{\sum_{i=1}^{n} |X_{ij}|}{\sum_{j=1}^{p}\sum_{i=1}^{n} |X_{ij}|}.$$

As we will show in the next paragraph, the choice of α_j is not crucial.

In the maximization step, we maximize (or monotonically increase) the surrogate function to produce the next iteration estimators. For instance, given the mth iteration estimate $\widehat{\boldsymbol{\beta}}^{(m)}$, for $j = 1, \ldots, p$, consider $g(\beta_j|\hat{\boldsymbol{\beta}}^{(m)})$ and update coordinate-wise directions β_j cyclically. Up to a constant, $v > 0$, such a procedure is equivalent to the approach based on coordinate descent; e.g., for $j = 1, \ldots, p$,

$$\hat{\beta}_j^{(m+1)} = \hat{\beta}_j^{(m)} - \alpha_j \{\nabla^2 g(\beta_j|\hat{\boldsymbol{\beta}}^{(m)})\}^{-1} \nabla g(\beta_j|\hat{\boldsymbol{\beta}}^{(m)})), \tag{3}$$

where $\mathbf{X}^T \hat{\boldsymbol{\beta}}^{(m)}$ is treated as an offset. The α_j in (5) and (3) can be considered as part of the step-size control. As long as the ascent property is achieved, the choice of α_j is not crucial.

2.3 Computational Issues

The proposed algorithm maximizes the original log-partial likelihood via the surrogate functions. Simplicity is obtained by separating the variables of optimization problem. That means, we replace the complicated objective functions with a sum of simpler functions, $g(\beta_j|\boldsymbol{\beta}^{(m)})$, each of which depends only on one component of parameter space. The computational speed for optimizing the surrogate functions is linear in p, which is much faster than $O(p^3)$ from inverting the original Hessian matrix. Furthermore, following the argument in Chap. 12 of [18], the ascent property in the MM algorithm depends only on increasing the surrogate function, not on maximizing it. Therefore, one-step Newton estimators (with step-size control) provide sufficient and rapid updates at each MM step, which further improves the computational efficiency.

To accelerate the convergence of the MM algorithm, we consider a strategy proposed by [18]. Denote the corresponding MM estimation in the $(m+1)$th iteration as $M(\hat{\boldsymbol{\beta}}^{(m)})$ and a composite function $M(M(\cdot))$ by $M \circ M(\cdot)$. Define vector

$$v = M \circ M(\widehat{\boldsymbol{\beta}}^{(m)}) - M(\widehat{\boldsymbol{\beta}}^{(m)})$$

and

$$u = M(\widehat{\boldsymbol{\beta}}^{(m)}) - \widehat{\boldsymbol{\beta}}^{(m)}.$$

Compute the accelerated MM updates as

$$\widehat{\boldsymbol{\beta}}^{(m+1)} = M(\widehat{\boldsymbol{\beta}}^{(m)}) - V(U^T U - U^V)^{-1} U^T \{\widehat{\boldsymbol{\beta}}^{(m)} - M(\widehat{\boldsymbol{\beta}}^{(m)})\}$$

Iterate $\widehat{\boldsymbol{\beta}}$ until converge.

3 MM Algorithms for Penalized Partial Likelihood Estimation of Semiparametric Frailty Model

3.1 The Model

One way to fit the log-normal frailty model is the penalized partial likelihood (PPL) approach developed by McGilchrist and Aisbett [5]. For completeness of exposure, we summarize the algorithm as follows. Let T_{hi} and C_{hi} represent the survival and censoring times, respectively, for the ith patient in the hth cluster. Observation times are denoted by $X_{hi} = T_{hi} \wedge C_{hi}$. The observed death indicators are denoted by $\delta_{hi} = I(T_{hi} \leq C_{hi})$. Let H be the number of clusters, and the total number of subjects be $n = \sum_{h=1}^{H} n_h$, where n_h is the number of subjects in cluster h.

We consider a hazard function

$$\lambda_h(t|\mathbf{X}_i) = \lambda_0(t) \exp(\mathbf{X}_i^T \boldsymbol{\beta} + w_h),$$

where $\mathbf{w} = (w_1, \ldots, w_H)$ is a vector of random effects with independent normal distribution $w_h \sim N(0, \sigma^2)$ for $h = 1, \ldots, H$. Considering the random effects as another set of parameters, the logarithm of the penalized partial likelihood can be written as the sum of the log-partial likelihood and the log of the density of the random effects

$$l_{\text{ppl}}(\boldsymbol{\beta}, \mathbf{w}, \sigma) = l(\boldsymbol{\beta}, \mathbf{w}) + l_{\text{pen}}(\mathbf{w}, \sigma),$$

where

$$l(\boldsymbol{\beta}, \mathbf{w}) = \sum_{h=1}^{H} \sum_{i=1}^{n_h} \delta_{hi} \left[\mathbf{X}_{hi}^T \boldsymbol{\beta} + w_h - \log \left\{ \sum_{q\ell \in R_{hi}} \exp\left(\mathbf{X}_{q\ell}^T \boldsymbol{\beta} + w_q \right) \right\} \right], \tag{4}$$

and

$$l_{\text{pen}}(\mathbf{w}, \sigma) = -\frac{1}{2} \sum_{h=1}^{H} \left\{ \frac{w_h^2}{\sigma^2} + \log(2\pi\sigma^2) \right\},$$

where R_{hi} contains all patients still at risk at time T_{hi} regardless the clusters.

The maximization of the penalized partial likelihood includes an inner and an outer loop. The inner loop estimates $\boldsymbol{\beta}$ and $\mathbf{w}$ by a Newton's procedure to maximize $l(\boldsymbol{\beta}, \mathbf{w})$ based on a provisional value of σ (best linear unbiased predictor—BLUP). The outer loop fits the restricted maximum likelihood estimator (REML) for σ^2 based on the BLUPs. Then the procedure is iterated until convergence. Specifically,

$$\begin{bmatrix} \hat{\boldsymbol{\beta}}^{(m+1)} \\ \widehat{\mathbf{w}}^{(m+1)} \end{bmatrix} = \begin{bmatrix} \hat{\boldsymbol{\beta}}^{(m)} \\ \widehat{\mathbf{w}}^{(m)} \end{bmatrix} - \boldsymbol{\Omega} \begin{bmatrix} \partial l_{\text{ppl}} / \partial \boldsymbol{\beta} \\ \partial l_{\text{ppl}} / \partial \mathbf{w} \end{bmatrix}_{\boldsymbol{\beta} = \hat{\boldsymbol{\beta}}^{(m)},\ \mathbf{w} = \widehat{\mathbf{w}}^{(m)}}$$

where

$$\boldsymbol{\Omega} = \begin{bmatrix} \boldsymbol{\Omega}_{11} & \boldsymbol{\Omega}_{12} \\ \boldsymbol{\Omega}_{21} & \boldsymbol{\Omega}_{22} \end{bmatrix}$$

is the inverse of the square $(p + H)$-dimensional Hessian matrix $\mathbf{A}$ with $\mathbf{A}$ given by

$$\mathbf{A} = \begin{bmatrix} \mathbf{A}_{11} & \mathbf{A}_{12} \\ \mathbf{A}_{21} & \mathbf{A}_{22} \end{bmatrix} = \begin{bmatrix} \partial^2 l_{\text{ppl}} / \partial \boldsymbol{\beta} \partial \boldsymbol{\beta}^T & \partial^2 l_{\text{ppl}} / \partial \boldsymbol{\beta} \partial \mathbf{w}^T \\ \partial^2 l_{\text{ppl}} / \partial \boldsymbol{\beta} \partial \mathbf{w}^T & \partial^2 l_{\text{ppl}} / \partial \mathbf{w} \partial \mathbf{w}^T \end{bmatrix}$$

More details of this algorithm can be found in Duchateau and Janssen [20].

3.2 Proposed Method

When the number of clusters or the number of covariates is large, it may be computationally expensive to evaluate or invert the square $(p + H)$-dimensional Hessian matrix, prohibiting its application to big data settings. To address this issue, we extend the MM algorithm to the semiparametric frailty models. Specifically, for a provisional value of σ, we consider the following minority surrogate function:

$$\begin{aligned}
l_{\text{ppl}}(\boldsymbol{\beta}, \mathbf{w}) \geq & \sum_{j=1}^{p}\sum_{h=1}^{H}\sum_{i=1}^{n_h} \alpha_j \delta_{hi} \left[\frac{X_{hij}}{\alpha_j}(\beta_j - \hat{\beta}_j^{(m)}) + \mathbf{X}_{hi}^T \hat{\boldsymbol{\beta}}^{(m)} + \hat{w}_h^{(m)} \right. \\
& \left. - \log\left\{ \sum_{q\ell \in R_{hi}} \exp\left(\frac{X_{q\ell j}}{\alpha_j}(\beta_j - \hat{\beta}_j^{(m)}) + \mathbf{X}_{q\ell}^T \hat{\boldsymbol{\beta}}^{(m)} + \hat{w}_q^{(m)} \right) \right\} \right] \\
& + \sum_{h=1}^{H}\sum_{i=1}^{n_h} \alpha_h \delta_{hi} \left[\frac{w_h - \hat{w}_h^{(m)}}{\alpha_h} + \mathbf{X}_{hi}^T \hat{\boldsymbol{\beta}}^{(m)} + \hat{w}_h^{(m)} \right. \\
& \left. - \sum_{h=1}^{H} \log\left\{ \sum_{q\ell \in R_{hi}} \exp\left(\frac{Z_{q\ell,h}(w_h - \hat{w}_h^{(m)})}{\alpha_h} + \mathbf{X}_{q\ell}^T \hat{\boldsymbol{\beta}}^{(m)} + \hat{w}_q^{(m)} \right) \right\} \right] \\
& - \frac{1}{2}\sum_{h=1}^{H} \left\{ \frac{w_h^2}{\sigma^2} + \log(2\pi\sigma^2) \right\} \\
= & \; g(\boldsymbol{\beta}, \mathbf{w} | \hat{\boldsymbol{\beta}}^{(m)}, \hat{\boldsymbol{w}}^{(m)}) = \sum_{j=1}^{p} g(\boldsymbol{\beta}_j | \hat{\boldsymbol{\beta}}^{(m)}, \hat{\boldsymbol{w}}^{(m)}) + \sum_{h=1}^{H} g(w_h | \hat{\boldsymbol{\beta}}^{(m)}, \hat{\boldsymbol{w}}^{(m)}),
\end{aligned}$$

where $Z_{q\ell,h} = 1$ if $q = h$ (i.e., the patient belongs to cluster h) and $Z_{q\ell,h} = 0$ otherwise. In the inner loop, we treat $\hat{w}_h^{(m)}$ as offsets and update coordinate-wise estimate of β_j cyclically: for $j = 1, \ldots, p$

$$\hat{\boldsymbol{\beta}}_j^{(m+1)} = \hat{\boldsymbol{\beta}}_j^{(m)} - \alpha \left\{ \nabla^2 g(\hat{\boldsymbol{\beta}}_j^{(m)} | \hat{\boldsymbol{\beta}}^{(m)}, \hat{\boldsymbol{w}}^{(m)}) \right\}^{-1} \nabla g(\hat{\boldsymbol{\beta}}_j^{(m)} | \hat{\boldsymbol{\beta}}^{(m)}, \hat{\boldsymbol{w}}^{(m)}).$$

Similarly, we treat $\hat{\boldsymbol{\beta}}^{(m)}$ as offsets and update coordinate-wise estimate of w_h cyclically: for $h = 1, \ldots, H$

$$\hat{w}_h^{(m+1)} = \hat{w}_h^{(m)} - \alpha \left\{ \nabla^2 g(\hat{w}_h^{(m)} | \hat{\boldsymbol{\theta}}^{(m)}, \hat{\boldsymbol{w}}^{(m)}) \right\}^{-1} \nabla g(\hat{w}_h^{(m)} | \hat{\boldsymbol{\theta}}^{(m)}, \hat{\boldsymbol{w}}^{(m)}).$$

Follows the approach based on [4], an approximated REML estimate for σ^2 is given by

$$(\hat{\sigma}^2)^{(m+1)} = \frac{\sum_{h=1}^{H} (\hat{w}_h^{(m)})^2}{H - r},$$

where $r = \alpha \sum_{h=1}^{H} \nabla^2 g(\hat{w}_h^{(m)} | \hat{\boldsymbol{\beta}}^{(m)}, \hat{\boldsymbol{w}}^{(m)}) / (\hat{\sigma}^2)^{(m)}$.

4 MM Algorithm for Semiparametric Frailty Model with Time-Varying Effects

We now extend the MM algorithm to semiparametric frailty models with time-varying effects. Let $\boldsymbol{\beta}(t) = (\beta_1(t), \ldots, \beta_p(t))$ be a p-dimensional vector of potentially time-varying effects. We consider a hazard function

$$\lambda_h(t|\mathbf{X}_i) = \lambda_0(t)\exp(\mathbf{X}_i^T\boldsymbol{\beta}(t) + \mathbf{w}_h).$$

The corresponding log-partial likelihood (4) described in Sect. 3 is replaced by

$$l(\boldsymbol{\beta}, \mathbf{w}) = \sum_{h=1}^{H}\sum_{i=1}^{n_h}\delta_{hi}\left[\mathbf{X}_{hi}^T\boldsymbol{\beta}(T_{hi}) + w_h - \log\left\{\sum_{\ell\in R_i}\exp\left(\mathbf{X}_{h\ell}^T\boldsymbol{\beta}(T_{hi}) + w_h\right)\right\}\right],$$

To estimate $\boldsymbol{\beta}$, a commonly applied approximation is to span $\boldsymbol{\beta}(\cdot)$ by a set of B-splines on a fixed grid of knots, usually taken to be equally spaced to cover the range of time or equal number of events within each interval. For instance, each $\beta_j(\cdot)$ is an expansion of the form

$$\beta_j(t) = \boldsymbol{\Theta}_j^T\mathbf{B}(t) = \sum_{k=1}^{K}\theta_{jk}B_k(t),\ \ j = 1, \ldots, p,$$

where K is the dimension of the basis functions, the $B(t) = (B_1(t), \ldots, B_K(t))^T$ form a basis for a finite-dimensional space, and $\boldsymbol{\Theta}_j = (\theta_{j1}, \ldots, \theta_{jK})$ is a vector of coefficients with θ_{jk} as the corresponding coefficient for the kth component of the jth covariate. Consider parameter vector $\boldsymbol{\theta} = vech(\boldsymbol{\Theta})$, the vectorization of $\boldsymbol{\Theta}$ by row, the log-partial likelihood function is

$$l(\boldsymbol{\theta}, \mathbf{w}) = \sum_{h=1}^{H}\sum_{i=1}^{n_h}\delta_{hi}\left[\mathbf{X}_{hi}^T\boldsymbol{\Theta}\mathbf{B}(T_{hi}) + w_h - \log\left\{\sum_{\ell\in R_i}\exp\left(\mathbf{X}_{h\ell}^T\boldsymbol{\Theta}\mathbf{B}(T_{hi}) + w_h\right)\right\}\right],$$

We consider the following minority surrogate function:

$$l_{\text{ppl}}(\boldsymbol{\theta}, \mathbf{w}) \geq \sum_{j=1}^{p}\sum_{h=1}^{H}\sum_{i=1}^{n_h}\alpha_j\delta_{hi}\left[\frac{X_{hij}}{\alpha_j}(\boldsymbol{\theta}_j - \hat{\boldsymbol{\theta}}_j^{(m)})\mathbf{B}(T_{hi}) + \mathbf{X}_{hi}^T\hat{\boldsymbol{\Theta}}^{(m)}\mathbf{B}(T_{hi}) + \hat{w}_h\right.$$
$$\left. - \log\left\{\sum_{q\ell\in R_{hi}}\exp\left(\frac{X_{q\ell j}}{\alpha_j}(\boldsymbol{\theta}_j - \hat{\boldsymbol{\theta}}_j^{(m)})\mathbf{B}(T_{hi}) + \mathbf{X}_{q\ell}^T\hat{\boldsymbol{\Theta}}^{(m)}\mathbf{B}(T_{hi}) + \hat{w}_q^{(m)}\right)\right\}\right]$$

$$
\begin{aligned}
&+\sum_{h=1}^{H}\sum_{i=1}^{n_h}\alpha_h\delta_{hi}\Bigg[\frac{w_h-\hat{w}_h^{(m)}}{\alpha_h}+\mathbf{X}_{hi}^T\hat{\boldsymbol{\Theta}}^{(m)}\mathbf{B}(T_{hi})+\hat{w}_h^{(m)}\\
&-\sum_{h=1}^{H}\log\left\{\sum_{q\ell\in R_{hi}}\exp\left(\frac{Z_{q\ell,h}(w_h-\hat{w}_h^{(m)})}{\alpha_h}+\mathbf{X}_{q\ell}^T\hat{\boldsymbol{\Theta}}^{(m)}\mathbf{B}(T_{hi})+\hat{w}_q^{(m)}\right)\right\}\Bigg]\\
&-\frac{1}{2}\sum_{h=1}^{H}\left\{\frac{w_h^2}{\sigma^2}+\log(2\pi\sigma^2)\right\}\\
&=g(\boldsymbol{\theta},\mathbf{w}|\hat{\boldsymbol{\theta}}^{(m)},\hat{\boldsymbol{w}}^{(m)})=\sum_{j=1}^{p}g(\boldsymbol{\theta}_j|\hat{\boldsymbol{\theta}}^{(m)},\hat{\boldsymbol{w}}^{(m)})+\sum_{h=1}^{H}g(w_h|\hat{\boldsymbol{\theta}}^{(m)},\hat{\boldsymbol{w}}^{(m)}).
\end{aligned}
$$

The remaining algorithms are the same as those in Sect. 3.

5 Convergence Properties

The numerical convergence of the MM algorithm can be described by the following proposition:

Proposition 1 *Any sequence of iterates* $\boldsymbol{\beta}^{(m+1)} = M(\boldsymbol{\beta}^{(m)})$ *generated by the iteration map* $M(\boldsymbol{\beta})$ *of the MM algorithm possesses a limit, and that limit is the optimal point.*

Proof of Proposition 1 The inequalities

$$
l(\boldsymbol{\beta}^{(m+1)})\geq g(\boldsymbol{\beta}^{(m+1)}|\boldsymbol{\beta}^{(m)})\geq g(\boldsymbol{\beta}^{(m)}|\boldsymbol{\beta}^{(m)})=l(\boldsymbol{\beta}^{(m)})
$$

follow from the choice of $\boldsymbol{\beta}^{(m+1)}$ and the minorization condition (5) described in Sect. 2.2. Given the fact that log-partial likelihood function is smooth, if the parameter space is bounded, then all super-level sets $\{\boldsymbol{\beta} : l(\boldsymbol{\beta}) \geq c\}$, for a constant c, are compact, and the maximum value of log-partial likelihood is attained (e.g., Weierstrass's theorem). Note that such a bounded assumption is applicable in most practical applications. Apply Proposition 12.4.4 of [18], then Proposition 1 follows.

6 Simulation Study

Finite-sample properties of the proposed method and their alternative were evaluated under three models: Cox proportional hazards model, semiparametric frailty models with time-independent effects or time-varying effects.

6.1 Setting 1: Cox Proportional Hazards Model

Death times were generated from an exponential model, $\lambda(t|\mathbf{X}_i) = 0.5\exp(\mathbf{X}_i^T\boldsymbol{\beta})$ for $i = 1, \ldots, n$. The sample size was $n = 1000$ and the number of covariates was $p = 100$, generated from independent standard normal distributions. The first five variables had coefficients $1, 1, -1, -1, 1$, while the rest had zero coefficients. Censoring times were generated from uniform distributions, with the percentage of censored subjects being approximately 20–30 %. Each data configuration was replicated 100 times. We compared the proposed MM algorithm described in Sect. 2.1. (termed MM), its accelerated modification described in Sect. 2.3 (termed MM2) and a "cocktail" algorithm proposed by Yang and Zou [21]. Specifically, instead of iteratively update $l_j''(\hat{\boldsymbol{\beta}}^{(m)})$ in formula (3) described in Sect. 2.2, the "cocktail" algorithm used an upper bound for the second derivative which is fixed across iteration

$$\Omega_{jj} = \sum_{i=1}^{n} \frac{\delta_i}{4} \left\{ \max_{\ell \in R_i}(X_{\ell j}) - \min_{\ell \in R_i}(X_{\ell j}) \right\}^2 .$$

Table 1 reports average bias (average over $p = 100$ and 100 simulation replications), average mean square error (MSE), empirical coverage probabilities (termed CP) based on 100 bootstraps, median number of iterations until convergence (termed Step), and average computation time (termed Time). Table 1 clearly indicates that the proposed MM algorithms provide better estimation in terms of both convergence speed and estimation accuracy. Moreover, the accelerated modification further reduced the number of iterations.

6.2 Setting 2: Log-Normal Frailty Model

Death times were generated from the log-normal frailty model with constant baseline hazards 0.5 and the random effects were generated from normal distribution with mean 0 and standard deviation 0.4. We considered 100 clusters with sample size within each cluster following a Poisson distribution with rate 50. The covariates were generated from the same distribution as those in Setting 1. We compared the proposed MM algorithm described in Sect. 3, its accelerated version (MM2) and the PPL based on the Newton's procedure (R package *coxme*). Table 2 reports average

Table 1 Setting 1: Cox proportional hazards model

Method	Bias	MSE	CP	Step	Time (s)
Coxtail	0.0410	0.0034	0.974	244.43	38.04
MM	0.0412	0.0028	0.967	18.03	2.69
MM2	0.0413	0.0028	0.967	9.01	2.07

Table 2 Setting 2: log-normal frailty model

Method	Bias of $\hat{\boldsymbol{\beta}}$	MSE of $\hat{\boldsymbol{\beta}}$	CP of $\hat{\boldsymbol{\beta}}$	Bias of $\hat{\sigma}$	MSE of $\hat{\sigma}$	CP of $\hat{\sigma}$	Step	Time (s)
PPL	0.0142	0.0003	0.952	0.0007	0.0008	0.735	NA	49.04
MM	0.0142	0.0003	0.952	0.0009	0.0008	0.735	39.38	42.41
MM2	0.0142	0.0003	0.952	0.0007	0.0008	0.735	21.94	39.89

bias, average mean square error (MSE) and empirical coverage probabilities (termed CP) for $\hat{\boldsymbol{\beta}}$ and $\hat{\sigma}$, median number of iterations until convergence (termed Step), and the average computation time (termed Time).

Note that the asymptotic variance for the estimates of the regression parameters and random effects variance estimate in PPL approach were provided by McGilchrist and Aisbett [5] and McGilchrist [4]. This issue, however, requires further investigation in our settings as the proposed method is an iterative profile likelihood-type of algorithm. A useful tool might be bootstrap. Specifically, the empirical coverage probabilities studied in this subsection were based on a nonparametric bootstrap algorithm proposed by Therneau and Grambsch [22]: (1) choose H clusters by sampling with replacement from the H clusters in the study; (2) let the bootstrap sample be the subjects from the selected clusters; and (3) fit the proposed procedure to this bootstrap sample. This procedure was repeated 100 times. The estimates $\hat{\boldsymbol{\beta}}^{\star}$ and $\hat{\sigma}^{\star}$ were stored for each bootstrap sample. The standard errors of the estimators $\hat{\boldsymbol{\beta}}$ and $\hat{\sigma}$ were calculated based on the variability of $\hat{\boldsymbol{\beta}}^{\star}$ and $\hat{\sigma}^{\star}$.

The proposed MM algorithm has comparable performances with the PPL in this setting. For all methods studied, the CPs of $\hat{\boldsymbol{\beta}}$ are closed to the nominal value, 0.95. However, the estimated standard error of the random effects variance estimate underestimates the standard error, and the corresponding CPs are substantially lower than the nominal value of 0.95. This corresponds to the conclusion drawn by Morris [23] for linear mixed models, e.g., the variances of the BLUPs are biased downwards. Due to this bias, bootstrapping BLUP's results in underestimated variation in the data. Further investigation of the properties will be necessary.

6.3 *Setting 3: Log-Normal Frailty Model with Time-Varying Effects*

The number of clusters and the covariate distribution were the same as those in setting 2. We let β_1 be a time-varying effect such that $\beta_1(t) = 3\sin(3\pi t/4)$. Other covariate effects were the same as previous settings. Ten basis functions were used for implementing B-spline based methods. Each data configuration was replicated 100 times. The average bias of $\hat{\sigma}$ is 0.002 and the median number of iterations until convergence is 33.9. Figure 1 depicts that the proposed MM estimators are sufficiently accurate.

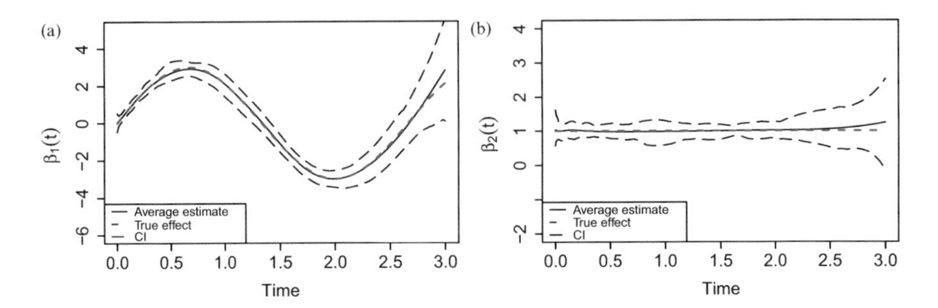

Fig. 1 Estimated coefficients in simulations. (**a**) Time-varying effect. (**b**) Time-independent effect

7 Analysis

The motivating data were obtained from the Organ Procurement and Transplantation Network (OPTN). The United Network for Organ Sharing (UNOS) administers the OPTN under contract with the US Department of Health and Human Services (HHS). The complete data set can be requested from the Organ Procurement and Transplantation Network (https://optn.transplant.hrsa.gov/). Included in the analysis were adult patients ($\geq$ 18 years of age at transplant) who underwent deceased-donor kidney transplantation between January 1990 and December 2008. Adjustment covariates in this study included age, race, gender, donation after cardiac death (DCD), expanded criteria donor (ECD), BMI, dialysis time, indicator of previous kidney transplant, cold ischemic time, and comorbidity conditions (e.g., glomerulonephritis, polycystic kidney disease, diabetes, hypertension). Graft failure was considered to occur when the transplanted kidney ceased to function. Failure time (recorded in years) was defined as the time from transplantation to graft failure or death, whichever occurred first. The final sample size was $n = 146,248$ from 282 transplant centers.

The proposed MM algorithm described in Sect. 4 was employed to investigate the potential time-varying effects. Figure 2 shows a fitted subset of the potential time-varying coefficients with the approximate 95 % point-wise confidence intervals. These results suggested that the effect of diabetes and black race varies over time, resulting in a strengthening of associations with death over time. However, the results for glomerulonephritis, polycystic kidney disease, and hypertension should be interpreted with caution. As shown in Fig. 2, their effects were minimal in the early stage of the follow-up period, but were amplified in the late stage. This may be due to the small at-risk sets at the late stage, resulting in very wide confidence intervals.

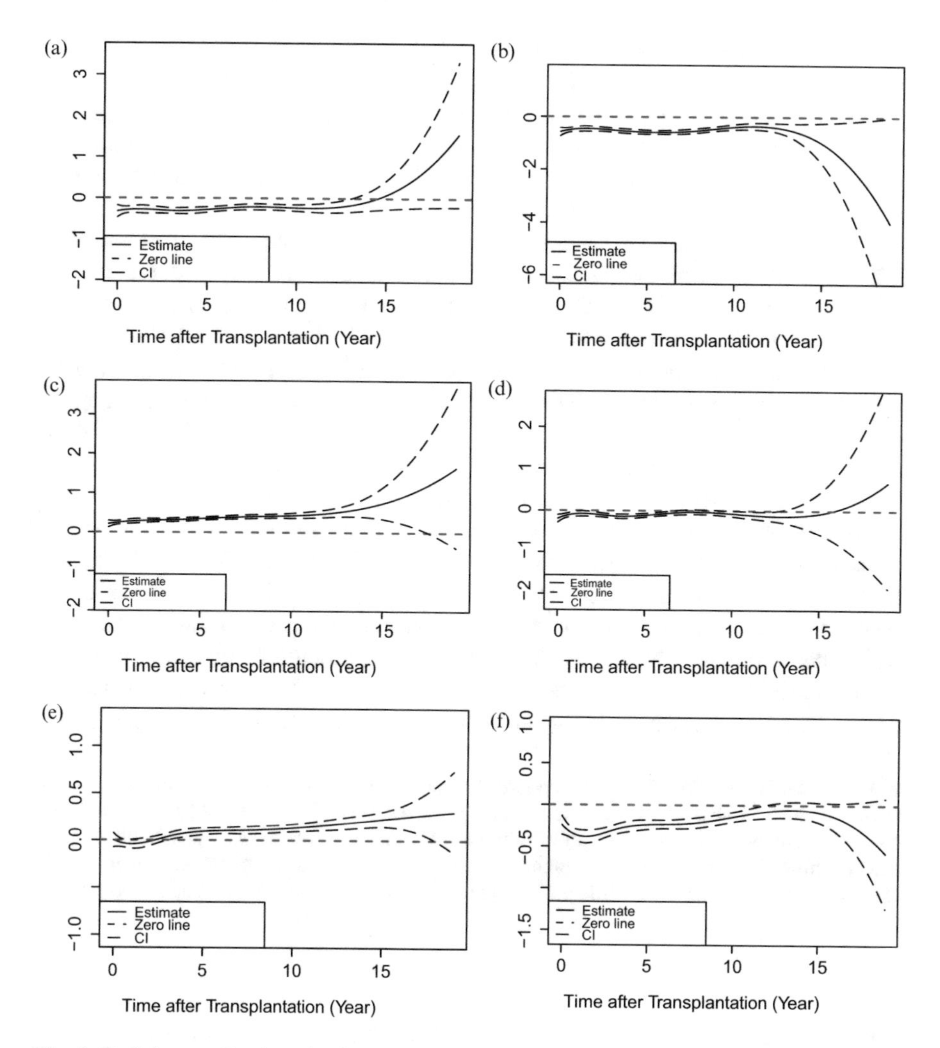

Fig. 2 Real data application: the data were obtained from the Organ Procurement and Transplantation Network (OPTN). (**a**) Glomerulonephritis. (**b**) Polycystic kidney disease (**c**) Diabetes (**d**) Hypertension (**e**) Race: Black (**f**) Race: Hispanic

8 Discussion

Statistical analysis of big clustered time-to-event data presents daunting statistical challenges as well as exciting opportunities. The computation and inversion of the Hessian matrix of the log-partial likelihood is very expensive and may exceed computation memory. To handle problems with large numbers of parameters, we propose a novel algorithm, which combines the strength of quasi-Newton, MM algorithm, and coordinate descent. The proposed algorithm improves upon the traditional semiparametric frailty models in several aspects. For instance, the proposed algorithms avoid calculation of high-dimensional second derivatives of the log-partial likelihood, and hence, are competitive in term of computation speed and memory usage. Simplicity is obtained by separating the variables of the optimization problem. The proposed methods also provide a useful tool for modeling complex data structures such as time-varying effects.

The overall C index [24] has been routinely used in the medical literature as a natural extension of the ROC curve to survival analysis. A key component in the assessment of model performance is its ability to distinguish subjects who will develop an event from those who will not. In large-scale multi-cluster time-to-event data, a within cluster strategy (e.g., only subjects within each cluster are compared) can greatly reduce the number of calculations. This advantage is especially important for large-scale data exemplified in our study. Risk prediction in time-varying effects model, however, is challenging as it is more complex than evaluating the performance of Cox proportional hazard models.

As suggested by the reviewer, the penalized partial likelihood (PPL) approach is closely connected with the hierarchical likelihood (H-likelihood) method [25, 26]. By treating the frailties as parameters, these approaches avoid integration of unobserved frailties over the frailty distribution. Instead, frailties are jointly estimated with other parameters of interest. This property is particularly appealing when the frailty distribution is not a conjugate prior. However, when the censoring rate is high, parameter estimates may be biased and further bias correction can be helpful [26].

Acknowledgements This work was supported in part by Health Resources and Services Administration contract 234-2005-37011C. The content is the responsibility of the authors alone and does not necessarily reflect the views or policies of the Department of Health and Human Services, nor does mention of trade names, commercial products, or organizations imply endorsement by the US Government. Yi Li's research is partly supported by the Chinese Natural Science Foundation (11528102).

References

1. Clayton, D.G.: A model for association in bivariate life table and its application in epidemiological studies of familiar tendency in chronic disease incidence. Biometrika **65**, 141–151 (1978)
2. Clayton, D.G., Cuzick, J.: Multivariate generalization of the proportional hazards model (with discussion). J. R. Stat. Soc. Ser. A **148**, 82–117 (1985)
3. Klein, J.P.: Semiparametric estimation of random effects using the Cox model based on the EM algorithm. Biometrics **48**, 795–806 (1992)
4. McGilchrist, C.A.: REML estimation for survival models with frailty. Biometrics **49**, 221–225 (1993)
5. McGilchrist, C.A., Aisbett, C.W.: Regression with frailty in survival analysis. Biometrics **47**, 461–466 (1991)
6. Yamaguchi, T., Ohashi, Y.: Investigating centre effects in a multi-centre clinical trial of superficial bladder cancer. Stat. Med. **18**, 1961–1971 (1999)

7. He, K., Kalbfleisch, J.D., Li, Y., Li, Y.J.: Evaluating readmission rates in dialysis facilities with or without adjustment for hospital effects. Lifetime Data Anal. **19**(4), 490–512 (2013)
8. Dekker, F.W., de Mutsert, R., van Dijk, P.C., Zoccali, C., Jager, K.J.: Survival analysis: time-dependent effects and time-varying risk factors. Kidney Int. **74**(8), 994–997 (2008)
9. Zucker, D.M., Karr, A.F.: Nonparametric survival analysis with time-dependent covariate effects: a penalized partial likelihood approach. Ann. Stat. **18**(1), 329–353 (1990)
10. Gray, R.J.: Flexible methods for analyzing survival data using splines, with applications to breast cancer prognosis. Am. J. Kidney Dis. **87**(420), 942–951 (1992)
11. Gray, R.J.: Spline-based tests in survival analysis. Biometrics **50**(3), 640–652 (1994)
12. Hastie, T., Tibshirani, R.: Varying-coefficient models. J. R. Stat. Soc. Ser. B **55**, 757–796 (1993)
13. Verweij, P.J.M., van Houwelingen, H.C.: Time-dependent effects of fixed covariates in cox regression. Biometrics **51**, 1550–1556 (1995)
14. Berger, U., Schäer, J., Ulm, K.: Dynamic Cox modelling based on fractional polynomials: time-variations in gastric cancer prognosis. Stat. Med. **22**(7), 1163–1180 (2003)
15. Perperoglou, A., le Cessie, S., van Houwelingen, H.C.: A fast routine for fitting Cox models with time varying effects of the covariates. Comput. Methods Prog. Biomed. **25**, 154–161 (2006)
16. Hunter, D.R., Lange, K.: A tutorial on MM algorithms. Am. Stat. **58**, 30–37 (2004)
17. Lange, K., Hunter, D.R., Yang, I.: Optimization transfer using surrogate objective functions (with discussion). J. Comput. Graph. Stat. **9**, 1–20 (2000)
18. Lange, K.: Optimization, 2nd edn. Springer Texts in Statistics. Springer, New York (2012)
19. Wu, T.T., Lange, K.: The MM alternative to EM. Stat. Sci. **29**, 492–505 (2010)
20. Duchateau, L., Janssen, P.: Springer Texts in Statistics. Springer, New York (2008)
21. Yang, Y., Zou, H.: A cocktail algorithm for solving the elastic net penalized cox's regression in high dimensions. Stat. Interface **6**, 167–173 (2013)
22. Therneau, T.M., Grambsch, P.M.: Modeling Survival Data, Extending the Cox Model. Springer, New York (2000)
23. Morris, J.S.: He BLUPs are not "best" when it comes to bootstrapping. Stat. Probab. Lett. **56**, 425–430 (2002)
24. Pencina, M.J., D'Agostino, R.B.: Overall C as a measure of discrimination in survival analysis: model specific population value and confidence interval estimation. Stat. Med. **23**(13), 2109–2023 (2004)
25. Lee, Y., Nelder, J.A.: Hierarchical generalized linear models. J. R. Stat. Soc. Ser. B **58**, 619–678 (1996)
26. Jeon, J., Hsu, L., Gorfine, M.: Bias correction in the hierarchical likelihood approach to the analysis of multivariate survival data. Biostatistics **13**(3), 384–97 (2012)

Tests of Concentration for Low-Dimensional and High-Dimensional Directional Data

Christine Cutting, Davy Paindaveine, and Thomas Verdebout

Abstract We consider asymptotic inference for the concentration of directional data. More precisely, we propose tests for concentration (1) in the low-dimensional case where the sample size n goes to infinity and the dimension p remains fixed, and (2) in the high-dimensional case where both n and p become arbitrarily large. To the best of our knowledge, the tests we provide are the first procedures for concentration that are valid in the (n, p)-asymptotic framework. Throughout, we consider parametric FvML tests, that are guaranteed to meet asymptotically the nominal level constraint under FvML distributions only, as well as "pseudo-FvML" versions of such tests, that meet asymptotically the nominal level constraint within the whole class of rotationally symmetric distributions. We conduct a Monte-Carlo study to check our asymptotic results and to investigate the finite-sample behavior of the proposed tests.

1 Introduction

The present paper deals with directional data, that is multivariate data for which only the directions (and not the magnitudes) are measured and which therefore belong to the unit sphere $\mathcal{S}^{p-1} := \{\mathbf{x} \in \mathbb{R}^p : \|\mathbf{x}\|^2 = \mathbf{x}'\mathbf{x} = 1\}$ of $\mathbb{R}^p$. Such data arise in many different disciplines and in particular are often encountered in earth sciences such as astrophysics [4] and meteorology [10]. Since the seminal paper of [9], they have been extensively studied; we refer to [16] for a general overview of the topic.

C. Cutting • T. Verdebout
Département de Mathématique - CP 210, Université libre de Bruxelles, Boulevard du Triomphe, B-1050 Brussels, Belgium
e-mail: chcutting@ulb.ac.be; tverdebo@ulb.ac.be

D. Paindaveine (✉)
Département de Mathématique and ECARES, Université libre de Bruxelles, Avenue F.D. Roosevelt, 50, CP 114/04, B-1050 Brussels, Belgium
e-mail: dpaindav@ulb.ac.be

© Springer International Publishing AG 2017

S.E. Ahmed (ed.), *Big and Complex Data Analysis*, Contributions to Statistics,
DOI 10.1007/978-3-319-41573-4_11

More and more applications involve data whose dimension can be large compared to the sample size. This is also the case for directional data : high-dimensional data can indeed be found in magnetic resonance (see [8]), gene-expression (see [2]), or in text mining (see [3]). Such data cannot be analyzed via standard statistical techniques and require developing new appropriate methods. In this vein, tests of hypotheses for high-dimensional directional data have been recently proposed in [5–7, 15] and [17]. While [5–7] and [17] focused on the null hypothesis of uniformity on high-dimensional unit spheres, [15] tackled the high-dimensional spherical location problem.

In this paper, we consider another testing problem in directional statistics, namely the problem of testing the null hypothesis that the underlying *concentration* is equal to some given value. A distributional setup where concentration has been classically considered is related to the celebrated *Fisher-von Mises-Langevin* (*FvML*) distributions, that have received a lot of attention in the literature; see, e.g., Sects. 10.4–10.6 in [16]. FvML distributions on $\mathcal{S}^{p-1}$ admit probability density functions (with respect to the surface area measure) that are of the form

$$\mathbf{x} \to f(\mathbf{x}) := c_{p,\kappa} \exp(\kappa\, \mathbf{x}'\boldsymbol{\theta}),$$

where $c_{p,\kappa}(> 0)$ is a normalization constant, $\boldsymbol{\theta} \in \mathcal{S}^{p-1}$ is a location parameter, and $\kappa(> 0)$ is a concentration parameter. The larger the value of κ, the more concentrated about $\boldsymbol{\theta}$ the distribution is. In the fixed-p case, the problem of developing inferential procedures on $\boldsymbol{\theta}$ and/or κ has been extensively studied in the literature. When testing $\mathcal{H}_0 : \boldsymbol{\theta} = \boldsymbol{\theta}_0$ against $\mathcal{H}_1 : \boldsymbol{\theta} \neq \boldsymbol{\theta}_0$, for instance, one of the most classical tests is the score test from Watson [23]. This test was shown in [18] to be locally and asymptotically optimal, and is furthermore robust to high-dimensionality (see [15]).

Besides the tests described in [16], tests of hypotheses that specifically address problems on the concentration parameter can mainly be found in [13, 20] and [22]. These tests are fixed-p FvML likelihood ratio or score tests. Such tests are asymptotically efficient in the FvML case, but are not robust to departures from FvML distributions (as we explain in Sect. 2, concentration can be defined away from the FvML case). Fixed-p robust procedures for concentration have therefore been proposed by [11] and [12] in the one-sample case and recently by [21] in the multi-sample case. In all cases, however, fixed-p tests for concentration fail to be robust to high-dimensionality. The objective of the present paper is therefore to provide high-dimensional tests for concentration.

The paper is organized as follows. In Sect. 2, we first define the problem of testing for concentration. Then we propose a new robust fixed-p test and investigate its asymptotic properties. In Sect. 3, we develop a high-dimensional test for concentration and we study its (n, p)-asymptotic properties under the null hypothesis. Finally, in Sect. 4, we conduct low-dimensional and high-dimensional Monte-Carlo simulations to confirm our theoretical results and investigate the finite-sample properties of the proposed tests.

2 Testing for Concentration in Low Dimensions

Let $\mathbf{X}_1, \ldots, \mathbf{X}_n$ be independent random p-vectors sharing an FvML distribution with location $\boldsymbol{\theta}$ and concentration κ. We consider the problem of testing the null hypothesis $\mathscr{H}_0 : \kappa = \kappa_0$ against $\mathscr{H}_1 : \kappa \neq \kappa_0$, where $\kappa_0 > 0$ is fixed. Of course, κ is then the parameter of interest, while $\boldsymbol{\theta}$ plays the role of a nuisance parameter. The null hypothesis $\mathscr{H}_0$ is clearly invariant with respect to the group of rotations, so that the invariance principle leads to resorting to tests that are invariant under this group. Since the group of rotations is actually generating the null hypothesis $\mathscr{H}_0$, invariant tests are distribution-free under $\mathscr{H}_0$. All tests we will consider in this paper are invariant, so that we may throughout, without any loss of generality, restrict to the case where $\boldsymbol{\theta}$ coincides with the first vector of the canonical basis of $\mathbb{R}^p$.

Denoting by $I_\nu(\cdot)$ the order-ν modified Bessel function of the first kind, it is easy to show that

$$e_1 := \mathrm{E}[\mathbf{X}_i'\boldsymbol{\theta}] = h_p(\kappa), \qquad i = 1, \ldots, n, \tag{1}$$

where the mapping

$$\begin{aligned} h_p : \mathbb{R}^+ &\to (0, 1) \\ z &\mapsto \frac{I_{p/2}(z)}{I_{p/2-1}(z)} \end{aligned} \tag{2}$$

is one-to-one. Consequently, concentration, for fixed-p, may equivalently be measured through e_1, and one may rephrase the null hypothesis $\mathscr{H}_0 : \kappa = \kappa_0$ as $\mathscr{H}_0 : e_1 = e_{10}$, with $e_{10} := h_p(\kappa_0)$. In the sequel, we rather adopt the latter formulation of the null hypothesis, since this formulation, unlike the former, makes sense away from the FvML case.

As mentioned in the introduction, the tests for concentration available in the literature are mainly of a likelihood ratio or score nature. The most classical test for the null hypothesis $\mathscr{H}_0 : e_1 = e_{10}$ is the Watamori and Jupp [22] score test $\phi_{\mathrm{WJ}}^{(n)}$ that rejects the null hypothesis at asymptotic level α whenever

$$T_{\mathrm{WJ}}^{(n)} := \frac{n(\|\bar{\mathbf{X}}_n\| - e_{10})^2}{1 - \frac{p-1}{\kappa_0} e_{10} - e_{10}^2} > \chi^2_{1,1-\alpha},$$

where $\bar{\mathbf{X}}_n := n^{-1}\sum_{i=1}^n \mathbf{X}_i$ and $\chi^2_{\ell,1-\alpha}$ stands for the α-upper quantile of the chi-square distribution with ℓ degrees of freedom. This test is asymptotically equivalent to the corresponding FvML likelihood ratio test, hence is locally and asymptotically optimal in the FvML case; see [14]. Because of its parametric nature, however, $\phi^{(n)}_{\mathrm{WJ}}$ relies crucially on the FvML assumption, in the sense that there is no guarantee that it meets the asymptotic level constraint away from the FvML case.

In this section, we show that an appropriate robustification of $\phi^{(n)}_{\mathrm{WJ}}$ is valid under the class of *rotationally symmetric* distributions. A random vector $\mathbf{X}$, taking values on the unit sphere $\mathscr{S}^{p-1}$ of $\mathbb{R}^p$, is said to be *rotationally symmetric* about $\boldsymbol{\theta}\,(\in \mathscr{S}^{p-1})$ if and only if, for all orthogonal $p \times p$ matrices $\mathbf{O}$ satisfying $\mathbf{O}\boldsymbol{\theta} = \boldsymbol{\theta}$, the random vectors $\mathbf{OX}$ and $\mathbf{X}$ are equal in distribution. If, further, $\mathbf{X}$ is absolutely continuous (still with respect to the surface area measure on $\mathscr{S}^{p-1}$), then the corresponding density is of the form

$$\mathbf{x} \to c_{p,f}\, f(\mathbf{x}'\boldsymbol{\theta}), \tag{3}$$

where $c_{p,f}(> 0)$ is a normalization constant and $f : [-1,1] \to \mathbb{R}$ is some nonnegative function. In the general (possibly non-absolutely continuous) case, rotationally symmetric distributions are characterized by the location parameter $\boldsymbol{\theta}$ and the cumulative distribution function F of $\mathbf{X}'\boldsymbol{\theta}$; such distributions are therefore of a semiparametric nature. The rotationally symmetric distribution associated with $\boldsymbol{\theta}$ and F will be denoted as $\mathscr{R}_p(\boldsymbol{\theta}, F)$. For identifiability purposes, it will be tacitly assumed throughout that F belongs to the collection $\mathscr{F}$ of cumulative distribution functions $F : [-1,1] \to [0,1]$ such that $e_1 = \mathrm{E}[\mathbf{X}'\boldsymbol{\theta}] > 0$ (the assumption that $e_1 \neq 0$ makes the pair $\{\pm\boldsymbol{\theta}\}$ identifiable and imposing further that $e_1 > 0$ makes $\boldsymbol{\theta}$ itself identifiable). When a null hypothesis of the form $\mathscr{H} : e_1 = e_{10}$ is considered, $\mathscr{F}_0$ will stand for the subset of $\mathscr{F}$ corresponding to the null hypothesis.

FvML distributions are (absolutely continuous) rotationally symmetric distributions, and correspond to $f(t) = \exp(\kappa t)$, or, equivalently, to

$$F_{p,\kappa}(t) = c_{p,\kappa} \int_{-1}^{t} (1 - s^2)^{(p-3)/2} \exp(\kappa s)\, ds \qquad (t \in [-1,1]),$$

where $c_{p,\kappa}$ is the same normalization constant as in the introduction. According to the equivalence between κ and e_1 in (1) and (2), the FvML cumulative distribution function $F_{p,\kappa}$ belongs to $\mathscr{F}$ (resp., to $\mathscr{F}_0$) if and only if $\kappa > 0$ (resp., if and only if $\kappa = \kappa_0 := h_p^{-1}(e_{10})$).

Assume now that a random sample $\mathbf{X}_1, \ldots, \mathbf{X}_n$ from a rotationally symmetric distribution is available. We then consider the robustified test $\phi^{(n)}_{\mathrm{WJm}}$ that rejects the null hypothesis $\mathscr{H}_0 : e_1 = e_{10}$ at asymptotic level α whenever

$$T^{(n)}_{\mathrm{WJm}} := \frac{n(\|\bar{\mathbf{X}}_n\| - e_{10})^2}{\hat{e}_{n2} - e_{10}^2} > \chi^2_{1,1-\alpha},$$

where we let $\hat{e}_{n2} := \bar{\mathbf{X}}_n' \mathbf{S}_n \bar{\mathbf{X}}_n / \|\bar{\mathbf{X}}_n\|^2$, with $\mathbf{S}_n := n^{-1} \sum_{i=1}^n \mathbf{X}_i \mathbf{X}_i'$. In the FvML case, $\phi_{\mathrm{WJm}}^{(n)}$ is asymptotically equivalent to $\phi_{\mathrm{WJ}}^{(n)}$ under the null hypothesis (hence also under sequences of contiguous alternatives), but $\phi_{\mathrm{WJm}}^{(n)}$ is further asymptotically valid (in the sense that it meets asymptotically the nominal level constraint) under any rotationally symmetric distribution. This is made precise in the following result (see Appendix for a proof).

Theorem 1 *Fix $p \in \{2, 3, \ldots\}$, $\boldsymbol{\theta} \in \mathcal{S}^{p-1}$, and $F \in \mathcal{F}_0$, and denote by $\mathcal{R}_p^{(n)}(\boldsymbol{\theta}, F)$ the hypothesis under which the random p-vectors $\mathbf{X}_1, \ldots, \mathbf{X}_n$ are mutually independent and share the distribution $\mathcal{R}_p(\boldsymbol{\theta}, F)$. Then,*

(i) under $\mathcal{R}_p^{(n)}(\boldsymbol{\theta}, F)$, $T_{\mathrm{WJm}}^{(n)}$ converges weakly to the χ_1^2 distribution as $n \to \infty$;
(ii) under $\mathcal{R}_p^{(n)}(\boldsymbol{\theta}, F_{p,\kappa_0})$, with $\kappa_0 = h_p^{-1}(e_{10})$, $T_{\mathrm{WJm}}^{(n)} - T_{\mathrm{WJ}}^{(n)} = o_{\mathrm{P}}(1)$ as $n \to \infty$, so that $\phi_{\mathrm{WJm}}^{(n)}$ is locally and asymptotically optimal in the FvML case.

This result shows that the robustified test $\phi_{\mathrm{WJm}}^{(n)}$ enjoys nice properties. Like any fixed-p test, however, it requires the sample size n to be large compared to the dimension p. Figure 1 below indeed confirms that, parallel to the classical test $\phi_{\mathrm{WJ}}^{(n)}$, the robustified test $\phi_{\mathrm{WJm}}^{(n)}$ fails to maintain the proper null size in high dimensions. In the next section, we therefore define high-dimensional tests for concentration.

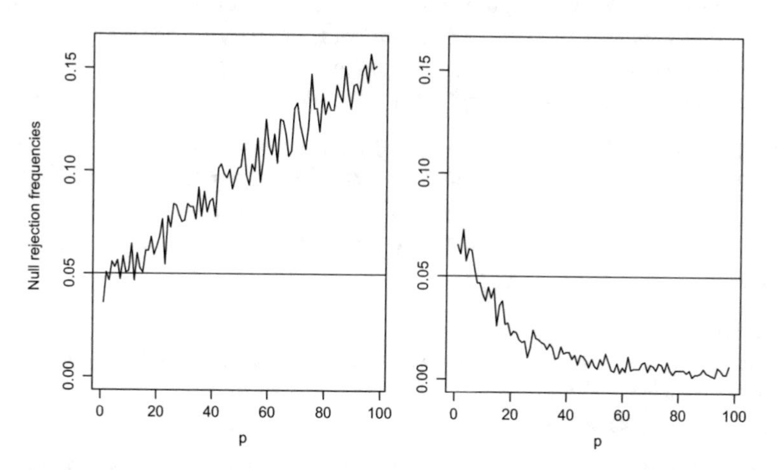

Fig. 1 For any $p = 2, 3, \ldots, 100$, the *left panel* reports null rejection frequencies of the fixed-p FvML test $\phi_{\mathrm{WJ}}^{(n)}$ for $\mathcal{H}_0 : \kappa = p$ (at nominal level 5 %), obtained from $M = 1500$ independent random samples of size $n = 100$ from the FvML distribution with a location $\boldsymbol{\theta}$ equal to the first vector of the canonical basis of $\mathbb{R}^p$. The right panel reports the corresponding rejection frequencies of the robustified test $\phi_{\mathrm{WJm}}^{(n)}$

3 Testing for Concentration in High Dimensions

3.1 The FvML Case

We start with the high-dimensional FvML case. To this end, it is natural to consider triangular arrays of observations $\mathbf{X}_{ni}$, $i = 1, \ldots, n$, $n = 1, 2, \ldots$ such that, for any n, the FvML random vectors $\mathbf{X}_{n1}, \mathbf{X}_{n2}, \ldots, \mathbf{X}_{nn}$ are mutually independent from $\mathscr{R}_{p_n}(\boldsymbol{\theta}_n, F_{p_n,\kappa})$, where the sequence (p_n) goes to infinity with n and where $\boldsymbol{\theta}_n \in \mathscr{S}^{p_n-1}$ for any n (we will denote the resulting hypothesis as $\mathscr{R}_{p_n}(\boldsymbol{\theta}_n, F_{p_n,\kappa})$). In the present high-dimensional framework, however, considering a fixed, that is p-independent, value of κ is not appropriate. Indeed, for any fixed $\kappa > 0$, Proposition 1(i) below shows that $\mathbf{X}'_{ni}\boldsymbol{\theta}_n$, under $\mathscr{R}^{(n)}_{p_n}(\boldsymbol{\theta}_n, F_{p_n,\kappa})$, converges in quadratic mean to zero. In other words, irrespective of the value of κ, the sequence of FvML distributions considered eventually puts mass on the "equator" $\{\mathbf{x} \in \mathscr{S}^{p_n-1} : \mathbf{x}'\boldsymbol{\theta}_n = 0\}$ only, which leads to a common concentration scheme across κ-values. For p-independent κ-values, the problem of testing $\mathscr{H}_0 : \kappa = \kappa_0$ versus $\mathscr{H}_1 : \kappa \neq \kappa_0$ for a given κ_0 is therefore ill-posed in high dimensions.

We then rather consider null hypotheses of the form $\mathscr{H}_0 : e_{n1} = e_{10}$, where we let $e_{n1} := \mathrm{E}[\mathbf{X}'_{n1}\boldsymbol{\theta}_n]$ and where $e_{10} \in (0, 1)$ is fixed. Such hypotheses, in the FvML case, are associated with triangular arrays as above but where the concentration parameter κ assumes a value that depends on n in an appropriate way. The following result makes precise the delicate relation between the resulting concentration sequence κ_n and the alternative concentration parameter e_{1n} in the high-dimensional case (see Appendix for a proof).

Proposition 1 *Let (p_n) be a sequence of positive integers diverging to ∞, $(\boldsymbol{\theta}_n)$ be an arbitrary sequence such that $\boldsymbol{\theta}_n \in \mathscr{S}^{p_n-1}$ for any n, and (κ_n) be a sequence in $(0, \infty)$. Under the resulting sequence of hypotheses $\mathscr{R}^{(n)}_{p_n}(\boldsymbol{\theta}_n, F_{p_n,\kappa_n})$, write $e_{n1} := \mathrm{E}[\mathbf{X}'_{n1}\boldsymbol{\theta}_n]$ and $\tilde{e}_{n2} := \mathrm{Var}[\mathbf{X}'_{n1}\boldsymbol{\theta}_n]$. Then we have the following (where all convergences are as $n \to \infty$):*

(i) $\kappa_n/p_n \to 0 \Leftrightarrow e_{n1} \to 0$;
(ii) $\kappa_n/p_n \to c \in (0, \infty) \Leftrightarrow e_{n1} \to g_1(c)$, *where* $g_1 : (0, \infty) \to (0, 1) : x \mapsto x/(\frac{1}{2} + (x^2 + \frac{1}{4})^{1/2})$;
(iii) $\kappa_n/p_n \to \infty \Leftrightarrow e_{n1} \to 1$.

In cases (i) and (iii), $\tilde{e}_{n2} \to 0$, whereas in case (ii), $\tilde{e}_{n2} \to g_2(c)$, for some function $g_2 : (0, \infty) \to (0, 1)$.

Parts (i) and (iii) of this proposition are associated with the null hypotheses $\mathscr{H}_0 : e_{n1} = 0$ and $\mathscr{H}_0 : e_{n1} = 1$, respectively. The former null hypothesis has already been addressed in [7], while the latter is extremely pathological since it corresponds to distributions that put mass on a single point on the sphere, namely $\boldsymbol{\theta}_n$. As already announced above, we therefore focus throughout on the null hypothesis $\mathscr{H}_0 : e_{n1} = e_{10}$, where $e_{10} \in (0, 1)$ is fixed. Part (ii) of Proposition 1 shows that, in the FvML case, this can be obtained only when κ_n goes to infinity at the same rate as p_n; more precisely, the null hypothesis $\mathscr{H}_0 : e_{n1} = e_{10}$ is associated with sequences (κ_n) such that $\kappa_n/p_n \to c_0$, with $c_0 = g_1^{-1}(e_{10})$.

As shown in Fig. 1, the fixed-p tests $\phi_{\rm WJ}^{(n)}/\phi_{\rm WJm}^{(n)}$ fail to be robust to high-dimensionality, which calls for corresponding high-dimensional tests. The following result, that is proved in Appendix, shows that, in the FvML case, such a high-dimensional test is the test $\phi_{\rm CPV}^{(n)}$ that rejects $\mathscr{H}_0 : e_{n1} = e_{10}$ whenever

$$|Q_{\rm CPV}^{(n)}| > z_{\alpha/2},$$

where

$$Q_{\rm CPV}^{(n)} := \frac{\sqrt{p_n}\big(n\|\bar{\mathbf{X}}_n\|^2 - 1 - (n-1)e_{10}^2\big)}{\sqrt{2}\Big(p_n\big(1 - \frac{e_{10}}{c_0} - e_{10}^2\big)^2 + 2np_n e_{10}^2\big(1 - \frac{e_{10}}{c_0} - e_{10}^2\big) + \big(\frac{e_{10}}{c_0}\big)^2\Big)^{1/2}},$$

with $c_0 = g_1^{-1}(e_{10})$, and where z_β stands for the β-upper quantile of the standard normal distribution.

Theorem 2 *Let (p_n) be a sequence of positive integers diverging to ∞, $(\boldsymbol{\theta}_n)$ be an arbitrary sequence such that $\boldsymbol{\theta}_n \in \mathscr{S}^{p_n-1}$ for any n, and (κ_n) be a sequence in $(0,\infty)$ such that, for any n, $e_{n1} = e_{10}$ under $\mathscr{R}_{p_n}^{(n)}(\boldsymbol{\theta}_n, F_{p_n,\kappa_n})$. Then, under the sequence of hypotheses $\mathscr{R}_{p_n}^{(n)}(\boldsymbol{\theta}_n, F_{p_n,\kappa_n})$, $Q_{\rm CPV}^{(n)}$ converges weakly to the standard normal distribution as $n \to \infty$.*

As in the fixed-p case, the test $\phi_{\rm CPV}^{(n)}$ is a parametric test whose (n,p)-asymptotic validity requires stringent FvML assumptions. In the next section, we therefore propose a robustified version of this test, that is robust to both high-dimensionality and departures from the FvML case.

3.2 The General Rotationally Symmetric Case

We intend to define a high-dimensional test for concentration that is valid in the general rotationally symmetric case. To this end, consider triangular arrays of observations $\mathbf{X}_{ni}$, $i = 1,\ldots,n$, $n = 1,2,\ldots$ such that, for any n, the random p_n-vectors $\mathbf{X}_{n1}, \mathbf{X}_{n2}, \ldots, \mathbf{X}_{nn}$ are mutually independent and share a rotationally symmetric distribution with location parameter $\boldsymbol{\theta}_n$ and cumulative distribution F_n, where the sequence (p_n) goes to infinity with n and where $\boldsymbol{\theta}_n \in \mathscr{S}^{p_n-1}$ for any n (in line with Sect. 2, F_n is the cumulative distribution function of $\mathbf{X}_{n1}'\boldsymbol{\theta}_n$). As above, the corresponding hypothesis will be denoted as $\mathscr{R}_{p_n}^{(n)}(\boldsymbol{\theta}_n, F_n)$.

As in the FvML case, we consider the problem of testing the null hypothesis $\mathcal{H}_0$: $e_{n1} = e_{10}$, where $e_{10} \in (0, 1)$ is fixed. In the present rotationally symmetric case, we propose a robustified version of the test $\phi^{(n)}_{\rm CPV}$ above. This robustified test, $\phi^{(n)}_{\rm CPVm}$ say, rejects the null hypothesis at asymptotic level α whenever

$$|Q^{(n)}_{\rm CPVm}| > z_{\alpha/2},$$

where

$$Q^{(n)}_{\rm CPVm} := \frac{\sqrt{p_n}\big(n\|\bar{\mathbf{X}}_n\|^2 - 1 - (n-1)e^2_{10}\big)}{\sqrt{2}\big(p_n\big(\hat{e}_{n2} - \|\bar{\mathbf{X}}_n\|^2\big)^2 + 2np_ne^2_{10}\big(\hat{e}_{n2} - \|\bar{\mathbf{X}}_n\|^2\big) + (1-\hat{e}_{n2})^2\big)^{1/2}};$$

recall from Sect. 2 that $\hat{e}_{n2} = \bar{\mathbf{X}}_n'\mathbf{S}_n\bar{\mathbf{X}}_n/\|\bar{\mathbf{X}}_n\|^2$, with $\mathbf{S}_n := n^{-1}\sum_{i=1}^n \mathbf{X}_i\mathbf{X}_i'$. The following result shows that, under mild assumptions, this test is asymptotically valid in the general rotationally symmetric case (see Appendix for a proof).

Theorem 3 *Let (p_n) be a sequence of positive integers diverging to ∞, and $(\boldsymbol{\theta}_n)$ be an arbitrary sequence such that $\boldsymbol{\theta}_n \in \mathcal{S}^{p_n-1}$ for any n. Let (F_n) be a sequence of cumulative distribution functions over $[-1, 1]$ such that, under $\mathcal{R}^{(n)}_{p_n}(\boldsymbol{\theta}_n, F_n)$, one has $e_{n1} = e_{10}$ for any n, and*

$$(i)\ n\tilde{e}_{n2} \to \infty, \quad (ii)\ \min\Big(\frac{p_n\tilde{e}^2_{n2}}{f^2_{n2}}, \frac{\tilde{e}_{n2}}{n}\Big) = o(1), \quad (iii)\ \tilde{e}_{n4}/\tilde{e}^2_{n2} = o(n),$$
$$\text{and}\ \ (iv)\ f_{n4}/f^2_{n2} = o(n), \tag{4}$$

where we let $\tilde{e}_{n\ell} := \mathrm{E}[(\mathbf{X}_{ni}'\boldsymbol{\theta}_n - e_{n1})^\ell]$ and $f_{n\ell} := \mathrm{E}[(1-(\mathbf{X}_{ni}'\boldsymbol{\theta}_n)^2)^{\ell/2}]$. Then, under the sequence of hypotheses $\mathcal{R}^{(n)}_{p_n}(\boldsymbol{\theta}_n, F_n)$, $Q^{(n)}_{\rm CPVm}$ converges weakly to the standard normal distribution as $n \to \infty$.

As explained in [7], Conditions (ii)–(iv) are extremely mild. In particular, they hold in the FvML case, irrespective of the sequences (κ_n) and (p_n) considered, provided, of course, that $p_n \to \infty$ as $n \to \infty$. Condition (i) is more restrictive. In the FvML case, for instance, it imposes that $p_n/n = o(1)$ as $n \to \infty$. Such a restriction originates in the need to estimate the quantity $\tilde{e}_{n2}$, which itself requires estimating $\boldsymbol{\theta}_n$ in an appropriate way.

4 Simulations

In this section, our objective is to study the small-sample behavior of the tests proposed in this paper. More precisely, we investigate whether or not the asymptotic critical values, for moderate-to-large sample sizes n (and dimensions p, in the high-dimensional case), lead to null rejection frequencies that are close to the nominal level.

4.1 The Low-Dimensional Case

We first consider the low-dimensional case. For each combination of $\kappa \in \{1, 3\}$ and $p \in \{3, 4, 5\}$, we generated $M = 2500$ independent random samples $\mathbf{X}_1, \ldots, \mathbf{X}_n$ of size $n = 50$ from the Purkayastha rotationally symmetric distribution $\mathcal{R}_p(\boldsymbol{\theta}, G_{p,\kappa})$, based on

$$G_{p,\kappa}(t) = d_{p,\kappa} \int_{-1}^{t} (1 - s^2)^{(p-3)/2} \exp(-\kappa \arccos(s))\, ds \qquad (t \in [-1, 1]),$$

where $d_{p,\kappa}$ is a normalizing constant; for $\boldsymbol{\theta}$, we took the first vector of the canonical basis of $\mathbb{R}^p$. In each case, we considered the testing problem $\mathcal{H}_0 : e_1 = e_{10}$ vs $\mathcal{H}_1 : e_1 \neq e_{10}$, where e_{10} is taken as the underlying value of $\mathrm{E}[\mathbf{X}_1'\boldsymbol{\theta}]$ (which depends on n and p). On each sample generated above, we then performed (1) the FvML test $\phi_{\mathrm{WJ}}^{(n)}$ and (2) its robustified version $\phi_{\mathrm{WJm}}^{(n)}$, both at nominal level 5%. Figure 2 provides the resulting empirical—by construction, null—rejection frequencies. Inspection of this figure reveals that, unlike the FvML test $\phi_{\mathrm{WJ}}^{(n)}$, the robustified test $\phi_{\mathrm{WJm}}^{(n)}$ meets the level constraint in all cases.

4.2 The High-Dimensional Case

To investigate the behavior of the proposed high-dimensional tests, we performed two simulations. In the first one, we generated, for every $(n, p) \in C_1 \times C_1$, with $C_1 = \{30, 100, 400\}$, $M = 2500$ independent random samples of size n from the FvML distributions $\mathcal{R}_p(\boldsymbol{\theta}, F_{p,\kappa})$, where $\boldsymbol{\theta}$ is the first vector of the canonical basis of $\mathbb{R}^p$ and where we took $\kappa = p$. In the second simulation, we generated, for every $(n, p) \in C_2 \times C_2$, with $C_2 = \{30, 100\}$, $M = 2{,}500$ independent random samples of size n from the Purkayastha distributions $\mathcal{R}_p(\boldsymbol{\theta}, G_{p,\kappa})$, still with $\kappa = p$ and the same $\boldsymbol{\theta}$ as above. The Purkayastha distribution is numerically hard to generate for dimensions larger than 150, which is the only reason why the dimensions considered in this second simulation are smaller than in the first one.

Parallel to the simulations conducted for fixed p, we considered the testing problem $\mathcal{H}_0 : e_1 = e_{10}$ vs $\mathcal{H}_1 : e_1 \neq e_{10}$, where e_{10} is the underlying value of $\mathrm{E}[\mathbf{X}_1'\boldsymbol{\theta}]$. On all samples that were generated, we then performed the four following tests at nominal level 5%: (1) the low-dimensional FvML test $\phi_{\mathrm{WJ}}^{(n)}$, (2) its robustified version $\phi_{\mathrm{WJm}}^{(n)}$, (3) the high-dimensional FvML test $\phi_{\mathrm{CPV}}^{(n)}$, and (4) its robustified version $\phi_{\mathrm{CPVm}}^{(n)}$. The resulting empirical (null) rejection frequencies are provided in Figs. 3 and 4, for the FvML and Purkayastha cases, respectively. The results show that

(a) the low-dimensional tests $\phi_{\mathrm{WJ}}^{(n)}$ and $\phi_{\mathrm{WJm}}^{(n)}$ clearly fail to be robust to high-dimensionality;

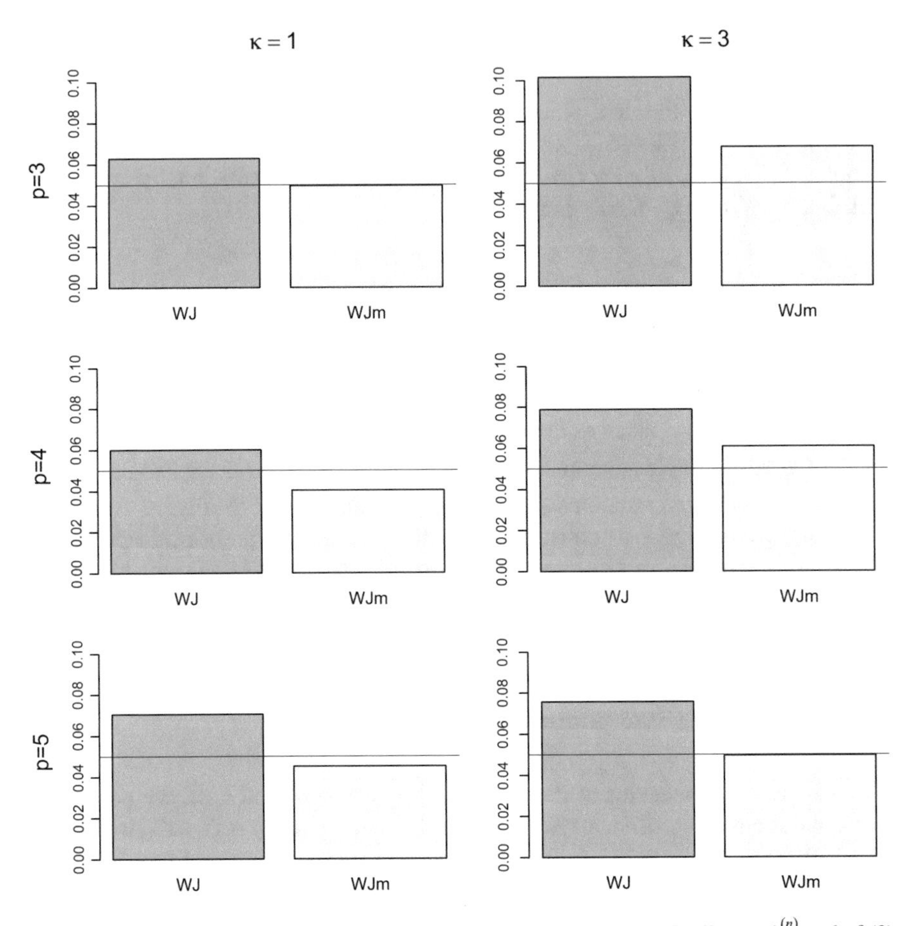

Fig. 2 Empirical null rejection frequencies of (1) the low-dimensional FvML test $\phi^{(n)}_{\mathrm{WJ}}$ and of (2) its robustified version $\phi^{(n)}_{\mathrm{WJm}}$, under various p-dimensional Purkayastha rotationally symmetric distributions involving two different concentrations κ. Rejection frequencies are obtained from 2500 independent samples of size 50, and all tests are performed at asymptotic level 5 %; see Sect. 4.1 for details

(b) at the FvML, $\phi^{(n)}_{\mathrm{CPV}}$ is asymptotically valid when n and p are moderate to large;
(c) away from the FvML, the high-dimensional test $\phi^{(n)}_{\mathrm{CPV}}$ is not valid, but its robustified version $Q^{(n)}_{\mathrm{CPVm}}$ is when $n \geq p$.

In order to illustrate the asymptotic normality result in Theorems 2 and 3, we computed, for each (n,p) configuration and each distribution considered (FvML or Purkayastha), kernel estimators for the densities of $Q^{(n)}_{\mathrm{CPV}}$ and $Q^{(n)}_{\mathrm{CPVm}}$, based on the various collections of 2500 values of these test statistics obtained above. In all cases, we used Gaussian kernels with a bandwidth obtained from the "rule of thumb" in [19]. The resulting kernel density estimators are plotted in Figs. 5 and 6, for FvML

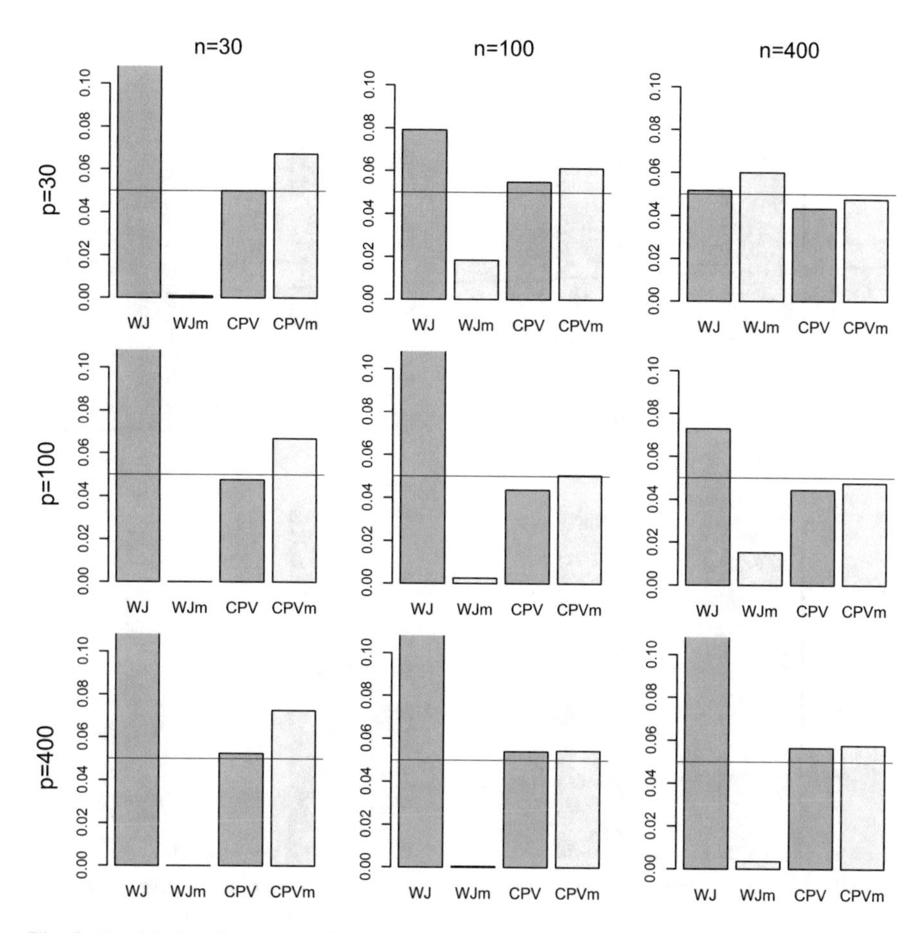

Fig. 3 Empirical null rejection frequencies, from 2500 independent samples, of (1) the low-dimensional FvML test $\phi_{\mathrm{WJ}}^{(n)}$, (2) its robustified version $\phi_{\mathrm{WJm}}^{(n)}$, (3) the high-dimensional FvML test $\phi_{\mathrm{CPV}}^{(n)}$, and (4) its robustified version $\phi_{\mathrm{CPVm}}^{(n)}$ (all performed at asymptotic level 5 %), under p-dimensional FvML distributions for various dimensions p and sample sizes n; see Sect. 4.2 for details

and Purkayastha distributions, respectively. Clearly, Fig. 5 supports the results that both test statistics are asymptotically standard normal under the null hypothesis, whereas Fig. 6 illustrates that this asymptotic behavior still holds for $Q_{\mathrm{CPVm}}^{(n)}$ (but not for $Q_{\mathrm{CPV}}^{(n)}$) away from the FvML case.

Acknowledgements D. Paindaveine's research supported by an A.R.C. contract from the Communauté Française de Belgique and by the IAP research network grant P7/06 of the Belgian government (Belgian Science Policy).

T. Verdebout's research is supported by a grant from the "Banque Nationale de Belgique".

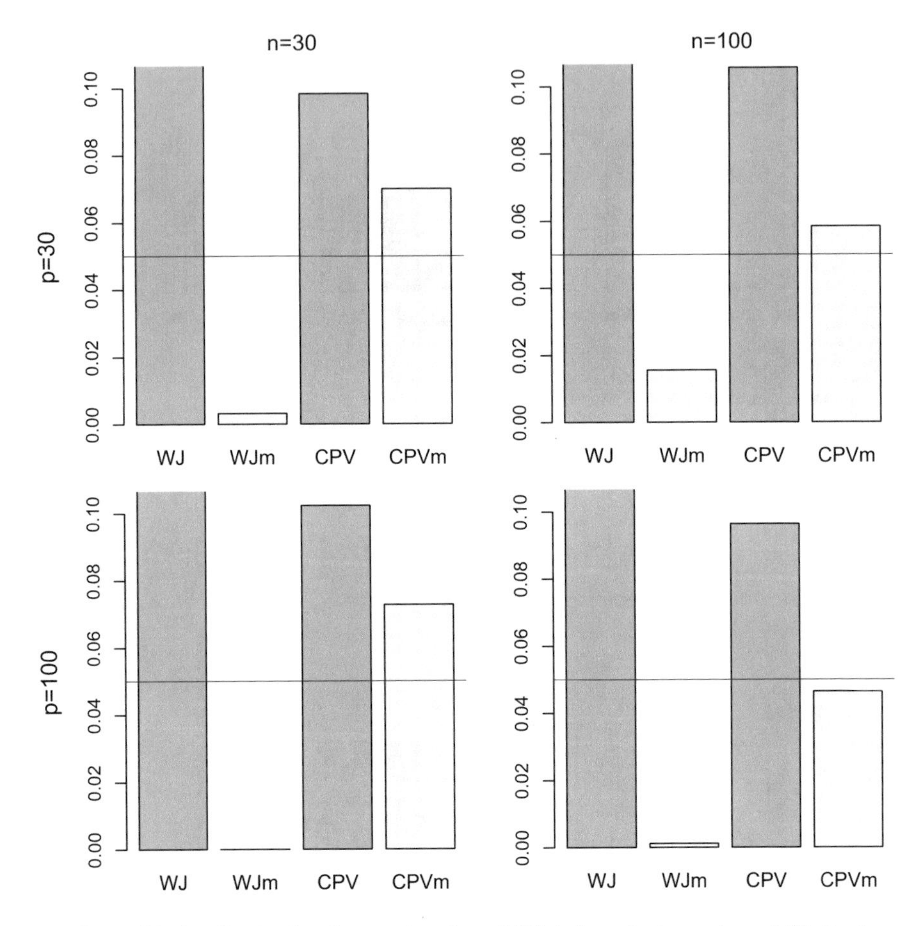

Fig. 4 Empirical null rejection frequencies, from 2500 independent samples, of (1) the low-dimensional FvML test $\phi^{(n)}_{\mathrm{WJ}}$, (2) its robustified version $\phi^{(n)}_{\mathrm{WJm}}$, (3) the high-dimensional FvML test $\phi^{(n)}_{\mathrm{CPV}}$, and (4) its robustified version $\phi^{(n)}_{\mathrm{CPVm}}$ (all performed at asymptotic level 5 %), under p-dimensional Purkayastha distributions for various dimensions p and sample sizes n; see Sect. 4.2 for details

Appendix

Proof of Theorem 1 (i) All expectations and variances when proving Part (i) of the theorem are taken under $\mathscr{R}_p^{(n)}(\boldsymbol{\theta}, F)$ and all stochastic convergences are taken as $n \to \infty$ under $\mathscr{R}_p^{(n)}(\boldsymbol{\theta}, F)$. Since

$$n^{1/2}(\bar{\mathbf{X}}_n - e_{10}\boldsymbol{\theta}) = O_{\mathrm{P}}(1), \tag{5}$$

the delta method (applied to the mapping $\mathbf{x} \mapsto \mathbf{x}/\|\mathbf{x}\|$) yields

$$n^{1/2}(\mathbf{Y}_n - \boldsymbol{\theta}) = e_{10}^{-1}[\mathbf{I}_p - \boldsymbol{\theta}\boldsymbol{\theta}']n^{1/2}(\bar{\mathbf{X}}_n - e_{10}\boldsymbol{\theta}) + o_{\mathrm{P}}(1), \tag{6}$$

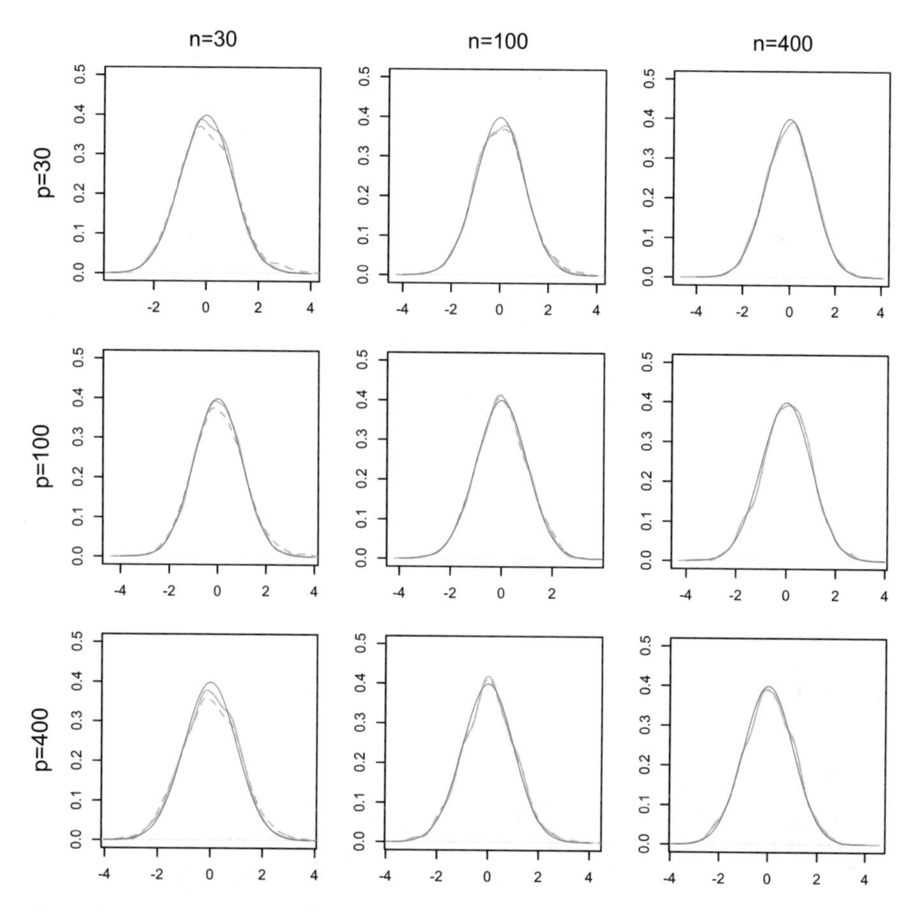

Fig. 5 Plots of kernel density estimators (based on Gaussian kernels and bandwidths resulting from the "rule of thumb" in [19]) of the (null) densities of $Q^{(n)}_{\mathrm{CPV}}$ (*thick solid line*) and $Q^{(n)}_{\mathrm{CPVm}}$ (*thick dashed line*) for various values of n and p, based on $M = 2500$ random samples of size n from the p-dimensional FvML distribution with concentration $\kappa = p$; see Sect. 4.2 for details. For the sake of comparison, the standard normal density is also plotted (*thin solid line*)

where we wrote $\mathbf{Y}_n := \bar{\mathbf{X}}_n / \|\bar{\mathbf{X}}_n\|$. This, and the fact that

$$\mathbf{S}_n \xrightarrow{\mathrm{P}} \mathrm{E}[\mathbf{X}_1\mathbf{X}_1'] = \mathrm{E}[(\mathbf{X}_1'\boldsymbol{\theta})^2]\boldsymbol{\theta}\boldsymbol{\theta}' + \frac{1 - \mathrm{E}[(\mathbf{X}_1'\boldsymbol{\theta})^2]}{p-1}(\mathbf{I}_p - \boldsymbol{\theta}\boldsymbol{\theta}'),$$

where $\mathbf{I}_p$ denotes the p-dimensional identity matrix, readily implies that

$$\hat{\sigma}_n^2 := \frac{\bar{\mathbf{X}}_n'\mathbf{S}_n\bar{\mathbf{X}}_n}{\|\bar{\mathbf{X}}_n\|^2} - e_{10}^2 = \mathbf{Y}_n'\mathbf{S}_n\mathbf{Y}_n - e_{10}^2 \xrightarrow{\mathrm{P}} \mathrm{E}[(\mathbf{X}_1'\boldsymbol{\theta})^2] - e_{10}^2 = \mathrm{Var}[\mathbf{X}_1'\boldsymbol{\theta}]. \quad (7)$$

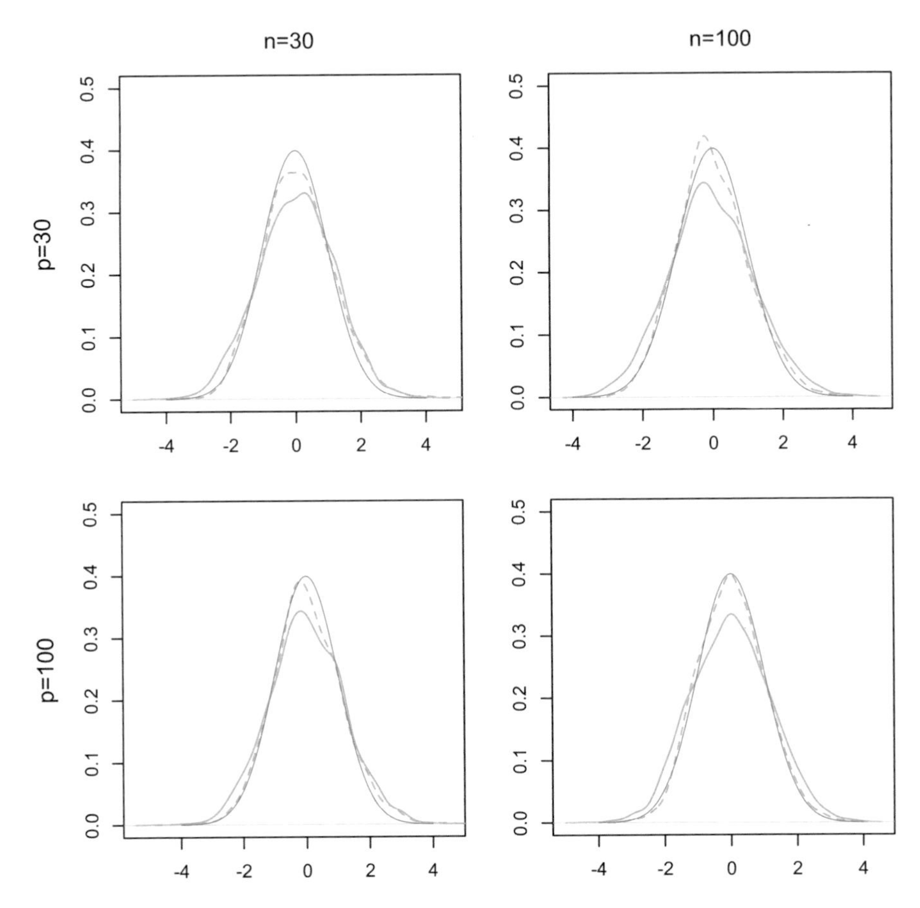

Fig. 6 Plots of kernel density estimators (based on Gaussian kernels and bandwidths resulting from the "rule of thumb" in [19]) of the (null) densities of $Q^{(n)}_{\mathrm{CPV}}$ (*thick solid line*) and $Q^{(n)}_{\mathrm{CPVm}}$ (*thick dashed line*) for various values of n and p, based on $M = 2500$ random samples of size n from the p-dimensional Purkayastha distribution with concentration $\kappa = p$; see Sect. 4.2 for details. For the sake of comparison, the standard normal density is also plotted (*thin solid line*)

Now, write

$$\frac{n^{1/2}(\|\bar{\mathbf{X}}_n\| - e_{10})}{\hat{\sigma}_n} = \frac{n^{1/2}\bar{\mathbf{X}}_n'(\mathbf{Y}_n - \boldsymbol{\theta})}{\hat{\sigma}_n} + \frac{n^{1/2}(\bar{\mathbf{X}}_n'\boldsymbol{\theta} - e_{10})}{\hat{\sigma}_n} =: S_{1n} + S_{2n}, \tag{8}$$

say. It directly follows from (5) to (7) that $S_{1n} = o_{\mathrm{P}}(1)$ as $n \to \infty$. As for S_{2n}, the central limit theorem and Slutsky's lemma yield that S_{2n} is asymptotically standard normal. This readily implies that

$$T^{(n)}_{\mathrm{WJm}} = \left(\frac{n^{1/2}(\|\bar{\mathbf{X}}_n\| - e_{10})}{\hat{\sigma}_n}\right)^2 \xrightarrow{\mathscr{L}} \chi^2_1.$$

(ii) In view of the derivations above, the continuous mapping theorem implies that, for any $\boldsymbol{\theta} \in \mathcal{S}^{p-1}$ and $F \in \mathcal{F}_0$,

$$T_{\mathrm{WJm}}^{(n)} = \frac{n(\|\bar{\mathbf{X}}_n\| - e_{10})^2}{\mathrm{Var}[\mathbf{X}_1'\boldsymbol{\theta}]} + o_{\mathrm{P}}(1)$$

as $n \to \infty$ under $\mathcal{R}_p^{(n)}(\boldsymbol{\theta}, F)$. The result then follows from the fact that, under $\mathcal{R}_p^{(n)}(\boldsymbol{\theta}, F_{p,\kappa_0})$, with $\kappa_0 = h_p^{-1}(e_{10})$, $\mathrm{Var}[\mathbf{X}_1'\boldsymbol{\theta}] = 1 - \frac{p-1}{\kappa_0} e_{10} - e_{10}^2$; see, e.g., Lemma S.2.1 from [7]. □

Proof of Proposition 1 From Lemma S.2.1 in [7], we have that, under $\mathcal{R}_{p_n}^{(n)}(\boldsymbol{\theta}_n, F_{p_n,\kappa_n})$,

$$e_{n1} = \frac{I_{p_n/2}(\kappa_n)}{I_{p_n/2-1}(\kappa_n)} \quad \text{and} \quad \tilde{e}_{n2} = 1 - \frac{p_n - 1}{\kappa_n} e_{n1} - e_{n1}^2.$$

The result then readily follows from

$$\frac{z}{\nu + 1 + \sqrt{z^2 + (\nu+1)^2}} \leq \frac{I_{\nu+1}(z)}{I_\nu(z)} \leq \frac{z}{\nu + \sqrt{z^2 + \nu^2}} \tag{9}$$

for any $\nu, z > 0$; see (9) in [1]. □

Proof of Theorem 2 Writing $e_{n2} := \mathrm{E}[(\mathbf{X}_{n1}'\boldsymbol{\theta}_n)^2]$, Theorem 5.1 in [7] entails that, under $\mathcal{R}_{p_n}^{(n)}(\boldsymbol{\theta}_n, F_{p_n,\kappa_n})$, where (κ_n) is an *arbitrary* sequence in $(0, \infty)$,

$$\frac{\sqrt{p_n}\big(n\|\bar{\mathbf{X}}_n\|^2 - 1 - (n-1)e_{n1}^2\big)}{\sqrt{2}\big(p_n\tilde{e}_{n2}^2 + 2np_n e_{n1}^2\tilde{e}_{n2} + (1 - e_{n2})^2\big)^{1/2}}$$

converges weakly to the standard normal distribution as $n \to \infty$. The result then follows from the fact that, under $\mathcal{R}_{p_n}^{(n)}(\boldsymbol{\theta}_n, F_{p_n,\kappa_n})$, where the sequence (κ_n) is such that, for any n, $e_{n1} = e_{10}$ under $\mathcal{R}_{p_n}^{(n)}(\boldsymbol{\theta}_n, F_{p_n,\kappa_n})$, one has

$$e_{n2} = 1 - \frac{p_n - 1}{\kappa_n} e_{10}, \quad \tilde{e}_{n2} = 1 - \frac{p_n - 1}{\kappa_n} e_{10} - e_{10}^2, \quad \text{and} \quad \kappa_n/p_n \to c_0 \text{ as } n \to \infty;$$

see Proposition 1(ii). □

The proof of Theorem 3 requires the three following preliminary results:

Lemma 1 *Let Z be a random variable such that* $\mathrm{P}[|Z| \leq 1] = 1$. *Then* $\mathrm{Var}[Z^2] \leq 4\,\mathrm{Var}[Z]$.

Lemma 2 *Let the assumptions of Theorem 3 hold. Write* $\hat{e}_{n1} = \|\bar{\mathbf{X}}_n\|$ *and* $\hat{e}_{n2} := \bar{\mathbf{X}}_n'\mathbf{S}_n\bar{\mathbf{X}}_n/\|\bar{\mathbf{X}}_n\|^2$. *Then, as* $n \to \infty$ *under* $\mathcal{R}_{p_n}^{(n)}(\boldsymbol{\theta}_n, F_{p_n,\kappa_n})$, *(i)* $(\hat{e}_{n1}^2 - e_{10}^2)/(e_{n2} - e_{10}^2) = o_{\mathrm{P}}(1)$ *and (ii)* $(\hat{e}_{2n} - e_{n2})/(e_{n2} - e_{10}^2) = o_{\mathrm{P}}(1)$.

Lemma 3 *Let the assumptions of Theorem 3 hold. Write* $\sigma_n^2 := p_n(e_{n2} - e_{10}^2)^2 + 2np_n e_{10}^2(e_{n2} - e_{10}^2) + (1 - e_{n2})^2$ *and* $\hat{\sigma}_n^2 := p_n(\hat{e}_{n2} - \hat{e}_{n1}^2)^2 + 2np_n e_{10}^2(\hat{e}_{n2} - \hat{e}_{n1}^2) + (1 - \hat{e}_{n2})^2$. *Then* $(\hat{\sigma}_n^2 - \sigma_n^2)/\sigma_n^2 = o_{\mathrm{P}}(1)$ *as* $n \to \infty$ *under* $\mathscr{R}_{p_n}^{(n)}(\boldsymbol{\theta}_n, F_{p_n,\kappa_n})$.

Proof of Lemma 1 Let Z_a and Z_b be mutually independent and identically distributed with the same distribution as Z. Since $|x^2 - y^2| \leq 2|x - y|$ for any $x, y \in [-1, 1]$, we have that

$$\mathrm{Var}[Z^2] = \frac{1}{2}\,\mathrm{E}[(Z_a^2 - Z_b^2)^2] \leq 2\,\mathrm{E}[(Z_a - Z_b)^2] = 4\,\mathrm{Var}[Z],$$

which proves the result. □

Proof of Lemma 2 All expectations and variances in this proof are taken under the sequence of hypotheses $\mathscr{R}_{p_n}^{(n)}(\boldsymbol{\theta}_n, F_n)$ considered in the statement of Theorem 3, and all stochastic convergences are taken as $n \to \infty$ under the same sequence of hypotheses. (i) Proposition 5.1 from [7] then yields

$$\mathrm{E}[\hat{e}_{n1}^2] = \mathrm{E}[\|\bar{\mathbf{X}}_n\|^2] = \frac{n-1}{n}\,e_{10}^2 + \frac{1}{n} \tag{10}$$

and

$$\begin{aligned}\mathrm{Var}[\hat{e}_{n1}^2] = \mathrm{Var}[\|\bar{\mathbf{X}}_n\|^2] &= \frac{2(n-1)}{n^3}\,\tilde{e}_{2n}^2 + \frac{4(n-1)^2}{n^3}\,e_{10}^2\tilde{e}_{n2} + \frac{2(n-1)}{n^3(p_n-1)}(1-e_{n2}^2)^2 \\ &= \frac{4}{n}\,e_{10}^2\tilde{e}_{n2} + O(n^{-2})\end{aligned} \tag{11}$$

as $n \to \infty$. In view of Condition (i) in Theorem 3, this readily implies

$$\begin{aligned}\mathrm{E}\Big[\Big(\frac{\hat{e}_{n1}^2 - e_{10}^2}{\tilde{e}_{n2}}\Big)^2\Big] &= \mathrm{Var}\Big[\frac{\hat{e}_{n1}^2 - e_{10}^2}{\tilde{e}_{n2}}\Big] + \Big(\mathrm{E}\Big[\frac{\hat{e}_{n1}^2 - e_{10}^2}{\tilde{e}_{n2}}\Big]\Big)^2 \\ &= \frac{4e_{10}^2}{n\tilde{e}_{n2}} + O\Big(\frac{1}{n^2\tilde{e}_{n2}^2}\Big) + \Big(\frac{1-e_{10}^2}{n\tilde{e}_{n2}}\Big)^2 = o(1)\end{aligned}$$

as $n \to \infty$, which establishes Part (i) of the result.

(ii) Write

$$\frac{\hat{e}_{n2} - e_{n2}}{\tilde{e}_{n2}} = \frac{1}{\tilde{e}_{n2}}\Big(\Big(\frac{1}{\hat{e}_{n1}^2} - \frac{1}{e_{10}^2}\Big)\bar{\mathbf{X}}_n'\mathbf{S}_n\bar{\mathbf{X}}_n + \frac{1}{e_{10}^2}\,\bar{\mathbf{X}}_n'\mathbf{S}_n\bar{\mathbf{X}}_n - e_{n2}\Big).$$

Part (i) of the result shows that $(\hat{e}_{n1}^2 - e_{10}^2)/\tilde{e}_{n2}$ is $o_{\mathrm{P}}(1)$ as $n \to \infty$. Since (10) and (11) yield that $\hat{e}_{n1}$ converges in probability to $e_{10}(\neq 0)$, this implies that $(\hat{e}_{n1}^{-2} - e_{10}^{-2})/\tilde{e}_{n2}$ is

$o_P(1)$ as $n \to \infty$. This, and the fact that $\bar{\mathbf{X}}_n' \mathbf{S}_n \bar{\mathbf{X}}_n = O_P(1)$ as $n \to \infty$, readily yields

$$\frac{\hat{e}_{n2} - e_{n2}}{\tilde{e}_{n2}} = \frac{1}{\tilde{e}_{n2}} \left(\frac{1}{e_{10}^2} \bar{\mathbf{X}}_n' \mathbf{S}_n \bar{\mathbf{X}}_n - e_{n2} \right) + o_P(1) \tag{12}$$

as $n \to \infty$. Since

$$\frac{1}{e_{10}^2} \bar{\mathbf{X}}_n' \mathbf{S}_n \bar{\mathbf{X}}_n = \frac{1}{e_{10}^2} (\bar{\mathbf{X}}_n - e_{10}\boldsymbol{\theta})' \mathbf{S}_n (\bar{\mathbf{X}}_n - e_{10}\boldsymbol{\theta}) + \frac{2}{e_{10}} (\bar{\mathbf{X}}_n - e_{10}\boldsymbol{\theta})' \mathbf{S}_n \boldsymbol{\theta} + \boldsymbol{\theta}' \mathbf{S}_n \boldsymbol{\theta},$$

the result follows if we can prove that

$$A_n := \frac{1}{\tilde{e}_{n2}} (\bar{\mathbf{X}}_n - e_{10}\boldsymbol{\theta})' \mathbf{S}_n (\bar{\mathbf{X}}_n - e_{10}\boldsymbol{\theta}), \;\; B_n := \frac{1}{\tilde{e}_{n2}} (\bar{\mathbf{X}}_n - e_{10}\boldsymbol{\theta})' \mathbf{S}_n \boldsymbol{\theta},$$
$$\text{and} \;\; C_n := \frac{1}{\tilde{e}_{n2}} (\boldsymbol{\theta}' \mathbf{S}_n \boldsymbol{\theta} - e_{n2})$$

all are $o_P(1)$ as $n \to \infty$.

Starting with A_n, (10) yields

$$\mathrm{E}[|A_n|] \leq \frac{1}{\tilde{e}_{n2}} \mathrm{E}[\|\bar{\mathbf{X}}_n - e_{10}\boldsymbol{\theta}\|^2] = \frac{1}{\tilde{e}_{n2}} \left(\frac{n-1}{n} e_{10}^2 + \frac{1}{n} - e_{10}^2 \right) = \frac{1 - e_{10}^2}{n \tilde{e}_{n2}} = o(1) \tag{13}$$

as $n \to \infty$. Since convergence in L_1 is stronger than convergence in probability, this implies that $A_n = o_P(1)$ as $n \to \infty$. Turning to B_n, the Cauchy–Schwarz inequality and (13) provide

$$\mathrm{E}[|B_n|] \leq \frac{1}{\tilde{e}_{n2}} \mathrm{E}[\|\bar{\mathbf{X}}_n - e_{10}\boldsymbol{\theta}\|^2] = o(1),$$

as $n \to \infty$, so that B_n is indeed $o_P(1)$ as $n \to \infty$. Finally, it follows from Lemma 1 that

$$\mathrm{E}[C_n^2] = \frac{1}{\tilde{e}_{n2}^2} \mathrm{E}[(\boldsymbol{\theta}' \mathbf{S}_n \boldsymbol{\theta} - e_{n2})^2] = \frac{1}{n \tilde{e}_{n2}^2} \mathrm{Var}[(\mathbf{X}_{n1}' \boldsymbol{\theta})^2] \leq \frac{4}{n \tilde{e}_{n2}} = o(1)$$

as $n \to \infty$, so that C_n is also $o_P(1)$ as $n \to \infty$. This establishes the result. □

Proof of Lemma 3 As in the proof of Lemma 2, all expectations and variances in this proof are taken under the sequence of hypotheses $\mathscr{R}_{p_n}^{(n)}(\boldsymbol{\theta}_n, F_n)$ considered in the statement of Theorem 3, and all stochastic convergences are taken as $n \to \infty$ under the same sequence of hypotheses.

Let then $\tilde{\sigma}_n^2 := 2np_n e_{10}^2 (e_{n2} - e_{10}^2)$. Since Condition (i) in Theorem 3 directly entails that $\sigma_n^2 / \tilde{\sigma}_n^2 \to 1$ as $n \to \infty$, it is sufficient to show that $(\hat{\sigma}_n^2 - \sigma_n^2)/\tilde{\sigma}_n^2$ is $o_P(1)$

as $n \to \infty$. To do so, write

$$\hat{\sigma}_n^2 - \sigma_n^2 = A_n + B_n + C_n, \tag{14}$$

where

$$A_n := p_n \left((\hat{e}_{n2} - \hat{e}_{n1}^2)^2 - (e_{n2} - e_{10}^2)^2 \right), \quad B_n := 2np_n e_{10}^2 \left(\hat{e}_{n2} - \hat{e}_{n1}^2 - e_{n2} + e_{10}^2 \right),$$

and

$$C_n := (1 - \hat{e}_{n2})^2 - (1 - e_{n2})^2.$$

Since

$$\frac{|A_n|}{\tilde{\sigma}_n^2} \leq \frac{p_n}{\tilde{\sigma}_n^2} = \frac{1}{2ne_{10}^2(e_{n2} - e_{10}^2)} \quad \text{and} \quad \frac{|C_n|}{\tilde{\sigma}_n^2} \leq \frac{1}{\tilde{\sigma}_n^2} = \frac{1}{2np_n e_{10}^2(e_{n2} - e_{10}^2)},$$

almost surely, Condition (i) in Theorem 3 implies that $A_n/\tilde{\sigma}_n^2$ and $C_n/\tilde{\sigma}_n^2$ are $o_{\mathrm{P}}(1)$ as $n \to \infty$. The result then follows from the fact that, in view of Lemma 2,

$$\frac{B_n}{\tilde{\sigma}_n^2} = \frac{(\hat{e}_{n2} - e_{n2}) - (\hat{e}_{n1}^2 - e_{10}^2)}{e_{n2} - e_{10}^2}$$

is also $o_{\mathrm{P}}(1)$ as $n \to \infty$. □

Proof of Theorem 3 Decompose $Q_{\mathrm{CPVm}}^{(n)}$ into

$$Q_{\mathrm{CPVm}}^{(n)} = \frac{\sigma_n}{\hat{\sigma}_n} \times \frac{\sqrt{p_n} \left(n\|\bar{\mathbf{X}}_n\|^2 - 1 - (n-1)e_{10}^2 \right)}{\sqrt{2}\, \sigma_n} =: \frac{\sigma_n}{\hat{\sigma}_n} \times V_n, \tag{15}$$

say. Theorem 5.1 in [7] entails that, under the sequence of hypotheses $\mathscr{R}_{p_n}^{(n)}(\boldsymbol{\theta}_n, F_n)$ considered in the statement of the theorem, V_n is asymptotically standard normal as $n \to \infty$. The result therefore follows from Lemma 3 and the Slutsky's lemma. □

References

1. Amos, D.E.: Computation of modified Bessel functions and their ratios. Math. Comput. **28**(125), 239–251 (1974)
2. Banerjee, A., Ghosh, J.: Frequency sensitive competitive learning for scalable balanced clustering on high-dimensional hyperspheres. IEEE Trans. Neural Netw. **15**, 702–719 (2004)
3. Banerjee, A., Dhillon, I.S., Ghosh, J., Sra, S.: Clustering on the unit hypersphere using von Mises-Fisher distributions. J. Mach. Learn. Res. **6**, 1345–1382 (2005)
4. Briggs, M.S.: Dipole and quadrupole tests of the isotropy of gamma-ray burst locations. Astrophys. J. **407**, 126–134 (1993)

5. Cai, T., Jiang, T.: Phase transition in limiting distributions of coherence of high-dimensional random matrices. J. Multivar. Anal. **107**, 24–39 (2012)
6. Cai, T., Fan, J., Jiang, T.: Distributions of angles in random packing on spheres. J. Mach. Learn. Res. **14**, 1837–1864 (2013)
7. Cutting, C., Paindaveine, D., Verdebout, T.: testing uniformity on high-dimensional spheres against monotone rotationally symmetric alternatives. Ann. Stat. (to appear)
8. Dryden, I.L.: Statistical analysis on high-dimensional spheres and shape spaces. Ann. Statist. **33**, 1643–1665 (2005)
9. Fisher, R.A.: Dispersion on a sphere. Proc. R. Soc. Lond. Ser. A **217**, 295–305 (1953)
10. Fisher, N.: Problems with the current definitions of the standard deviation of wind direction. J. Clim. Appl. Meteorol. **26**(11), 1522–1529 (1987)
11. Ko, D.: Robust estimation of the concentration parameter of the von Mises-Fisher distribution. Ann. Statist. **20**(2), 917–928 (1992)
12. Ko, D., Guttorp, P.: Robustness of estimators for directional data. Ann. Statist. **16**(2), 609–618 (1988)
13. Larsen, P., Blæsild, P., Sørensen, M.: Improved likelihood ratio tests on the von Mises–Fisher distribution. Biometrika **89**(4), 947–951 (2002)
14. Ley, C., Verdebout, T.: Local powers of optimal one-and multi-sample tests for the concentration of Fisher-von Mises-Langevin distributions. Int. Stat. Rev. **82**, 440–456 (2014)
15. Ley, C., Paindaveine, D., Verdebout, T.: High-dimensional tests for spherical location and spiked covariance. J. Multivar. Anal. **139**, 79–91 (2015)
16. Mardia, K.V., Jupp, P.E.: Directional Statistics, vol. 494. Wiley, New York (2009)
17. Paindaveine, D., Verdebout, T.: On high-dimensional sign tests. Bernoulli **22**, 1745–1769 (2016)
18. Paindaveine, D., Verdebout, T.: Optimal rank-based tests for the location parameter of a rotationally symmetric distribution on the hypersphere. In: Hallin, M., Mason, D., Pfeifer, D., Steinebach, J. (eds.) Mathematical Statistics and Limit Theorems: Festschrift in Honor of Paul Deheuvels, pp. 249-270. Springer (2015)
19. Silverman, B.W.: Density Estimation for Statistics and Data Analysis, vol. 26. CRC Press, London (1986)
20. Stephens, M.: Multi-sample tests for the fisher distribution for directions. Biometrika **56**(1), 169–181 (1969)
21. Verdebout, T.: On some validity-robust tests for the homogeneity of concentrations on spheres. J. Nonparametr. Stat. **27**, 372–383 (2015)
22. Watamori, Y., Jupp, P.E.: Improved likelihood ratio and score tests on concentration parameters of von Mises–Fisher distributions. Stat. Probabil. Lett. **72**(2), 93–102 (2005)
23. Watson, G.S.: Statistics on Spheres. Wiley, New York (1983)

Nonparametric Testing for Heterogeneous Correlation

Stephen Bamattre, Rex Hu, and Joseph S. Verducci

Abstract In the presence of weak overall correlation, it may be useful to investigate if the correlation is significantly and substantially more pronounced over a subpopulation. Two different testing procedures are compared. Both are based on the rankings of the values of two variables from a data set with a large number n of observations. The first maintains its level against Gaussian copulas; the second adapts to general alternatives in the sense that the number of parameters used in the test grows with n. An analysis of wine quality illustrates how the methods detect heterogeneity of association between chemical properties of the wine, which are attributable to a mix of different cultivars.

Keywords Absolute rank differences • Beta distribution • Frank copula • Gaussian copula • Kendall's tau • Mallows' model • Multistage ranking model • Permutations • Seriation

1 Introduction

The goal of this paper is to offer new methods for discovering association between two variables that is supported only in a subpopulation. For example, while higher counts of HDLs are generally associated with lower risk of myocardial infarction, researchers [10, 18] have found subpopulations that do not adhere to this trend. In marketing, subpopulations of designated marketing areas (DMAs) in the USA respond differentially to TV advertising campaigns, and the identification of DMAs that are sensitive to ad exposure enables efficient spending of ad dollars. In preclinical screening of potential drugs, various subpopulations of chemicals elicit concomitant responses from sets of hepatocyte genes, which can be used to discover gene networks that breakdown classes of drugs, without having to pre-specify how the classes are formed. The new methods thus lead to a whole new approach to analysis of large data sets.

S. Bamattre (✉) • R. Hu • J.S. Verducci
Department of Statistics, The Ohio State University, Columbus, Ohio 43210

© Springer International Publishing AG 2017

S.E. Ahmed (ed.), *Big and Complex Data Analysis*, Contributions to Statistics,
DOI 10.1007/978-3-319-41573-4_12

When covariates are available, regression analysis classically attempts to identify a supporting subpopulation via interaction effects, but these may be difficult to interpret properly. In the presence of overall correlation, it may be useful to investigate directly if the correlation is significantly and substantially more pronounced over a subpopulation. This becomes feasible when representatives of supporting subpopulations are embedded in large samples. The novel statistical tests described in this paper are designed to probe large samples to ascertain if there is such a subpopulation.

The general setting is this: A large number n of observations are sampled from a bivariate continuous distribution. The basic assumption is that the population consists of two subpopulations. In one, the two variables are positively (or negatively) associated; in the other, the two variables are independent. While some distributional assumptions are required even to define the notion of homogeneous association, the underlying intent is to make the tests robust to assumptions about the distributions governing both the null and alternative hypotheses.

Notation for the rest of the paper is as follows: Let $X \sim F$ and $Y \sim G$ have joint, continuous distribution H. For any sample $\{(x_i, y_i) \mid i = 1, \ldots, n\}$, the empirical marginal distributions are defined by

$$\hat{F}_n(x) = \frac{1}{n} \sum_{i=1}^{n} 1\{x_i \le x\} \text{ and } \hat{G}_n(y) = \frac{1}{n} \sum_{i=1}^{n} 1\{y_i \le y\}.$$

The ranking π of the sample $\{x_i \mid i = 1, \ldots, n\}$ is the function $\pi : \{x_i \mid i = 1, \ldots, n\} \to \{1, \ldots, n\}$ defined by

$$\pi(x_i) = \sum_{j=1}^{n} 1\{x_i \le x_j\}.$$

The corresponding ranking of $\{y_i \mid i = 1, \ldots, n\}$ is denoted by ν. Spearman's footrule distance with a sample $\{(x_i, y_i) \mid i = 1, \ldots, n\}$ is defined through the sample rankings as

$$d_S = \sum_{i=1}^{n} |\pi(x_i) - \nu(y_i)|.$$

The Kendall's distance associated with the sample is defined as

$$\begin{aligned} D_K([x_1, \ldots, x_n], [y_1, \ldots, y_n]) &= \sum_{i<j} 1\{(x_i - x_j)(y_i - y_j) < 0\} \\ &= \sum_{i<j} 1\{(\pi(x_i) - \pi(x_j))(\nu(y_i) - \nu(y_j)) < 0\} \\ &= d_K(\pi, \nu) \end{aligned}$$

which depends only on the rankings π and ν of the sample $\{x_i\}$ and $\{y_i\}$. Since H is continuous, Kendall's tau coefficient has the form

$$T_K\left([x_1, \ldots, x_n], [y_1, \ldots, y_n]\right) = 1 - \frac{4D_K(\pi, \nu)}{n(n-1)}.$$

Mallows (1957) model for rankings takes the form

$$P_\phi(\nu \mid \pi) = C(\phi)\, e^{-\phi d_K(\pi,\nu)}$$

where the normalizing constant $C(\phi)$ has a tractable form (Fligner and Verducci 1986) known as a Poincare polynomial [3]. Distributional forms for the data are in terms of copulas:

$$C_H(F(X), G(Y)) = H(X, Y)$$

which are distribution functions on the unit square, having uniform margins. Two copulas play a fundamental role in motivating the tests: the Gaussian copula and the Frank Copula. If (X, Y) has a bivariate normal distribution H with standardized margins and correlation ρ, then its corresponding copula is

$$C_\rho(u, v) = \Phi_2\left(\Phi^{-1}(u), \Phi^{-1}(v); \rho\right)$$

where Φ is the standard normal CDF. The bivariate distributions C_ρ and Φ_2 are indexed solely by the underlying correlation ρ. The Frank copula [6, 7] has the form

$$C_\theta(u, v) = -\frac{1}{\theta}\log\left(1 + \frac{\left(e^{-\theta u} - 1\right)\left(e^{-\theta v} - 1\right)}{\left(e^{-\theta} - 1\right)}\right).$$

The next two sections describe two new tests for detecting subpopulations that support association: the Components of Spearman's Footrule (CSF) test and the Components of Kendall's Tau (CKT) test. The CSF test is scaled according to a Gaussian copula and the CKT test is scaled according to a Frank copula. The CSF test is computationally fast, and the CKT test adapts to a large variety of alternatives. The following two sections cover their performance under simulations. Concluding remarks are in last section.

2 Components of Spearman's Footrule

While Spearman's footrule [2] measures the overall disarray in a sample, the distribution of individual absolute rank differences

$$d_i = |\pi(x_i) - \nu(y_i)|$$

proves to be very useful in detecting subsamples with distinctly less disarray than would be expected under homogeneous association. Because the rankings depend on the whole sample, the $\{d_i\}$ are not independent. Nevertheless, we loosely define their *empirical distribution* as

$$S_n(d) = \frac{1}{n}\sum_{i=1}^{n} 1\{d_i \leq d\}.$$

As a step toward determining asymptotic forms for this distribution, we offer the following lemmas:

Lemma 1 *For any sample* $\{(X_i, Y_i) \mid i = 1, \ldots, n\}$*, from a joint distribution H with compact support, let (X,Y) be a newly, independent sampled observation. Then, for rankings* π *and* ν *for the extended sample of* $n+1$ *observations,*

$$\left[\frac{\pi(X)}{n+1}, \frac{\nu(Y)}{n+1}\right] \underset{a.s.}{\rightarrow} [F(X), G(Y)]$$

and its asymptotic distribution is the underlying copula $C_H[F(X), G(Y)]$ *of H.*

Lemma 2 *Under independence, the asymptotic distribution of the scaled absolute rank differences*

$$S_n = \left|\frac{\pi(X)}{n+1} - \frac{\nu(Y)}{n+1}\right|$$

is Beta$(1, 2)$*.*

Proposition 3 *Under a Gaussian*(ρ) *copula,* S_n *converges to a Beta*$(1, \beta(\rho))$ *distribution.*

Although we do not have a formal proof for this proposition, many simulations with $n = 1000$ affirm the proposition and produce a smooth curve for $\beta(\rho)$. See Fig. 1 for one such example.

The null hypothesis is that (X, Y) have a Gaussian copula. The alternative is that (X, Y) come from a mixture of two subpopulations in which under one they are independent, and under the other they are positively associated. To test for negative association, simply replace Y by $-Y$. No particular form is assumed for the positively associated subpopulation, but it is informative to examine the case where this component is Gaussian. Figure 2 illustrates S_n and its histogram under such a mixture.

Because the differences in distributions under the null and alternative are small, large samples are required to distinguish the two. As noted from the histogram in Fig. 2, most of the distinguishing information is contained at the low end of the distribution. This makes sense because a subpopulation supporting positive association should have a surplus of points where the ranks of X and Y closely agree.

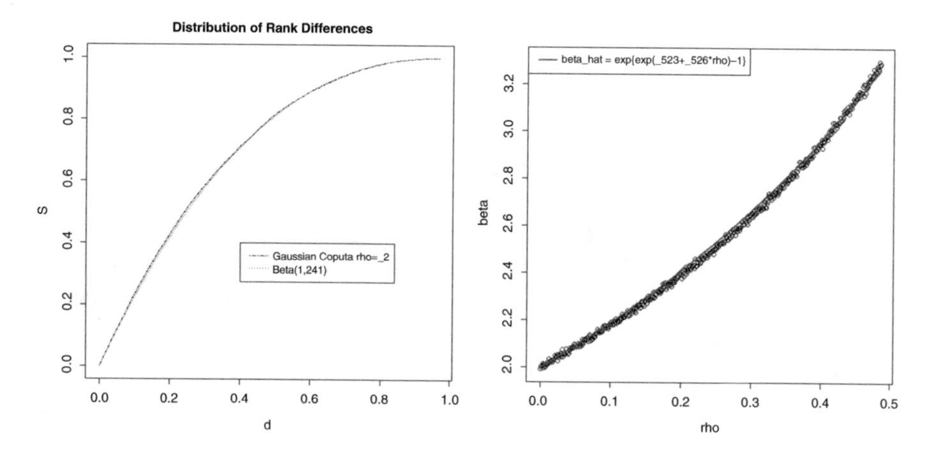

Fig. 1 *Left panel* shows the close agreement of S_n with Beta(1, β (ρ)) when sampling $n = 10,000$ observations from a Gaussian($\rho = 0.2$) copula. The *right panel* illustrates the ˛(j) curve for $0 < \rho < 0.5$

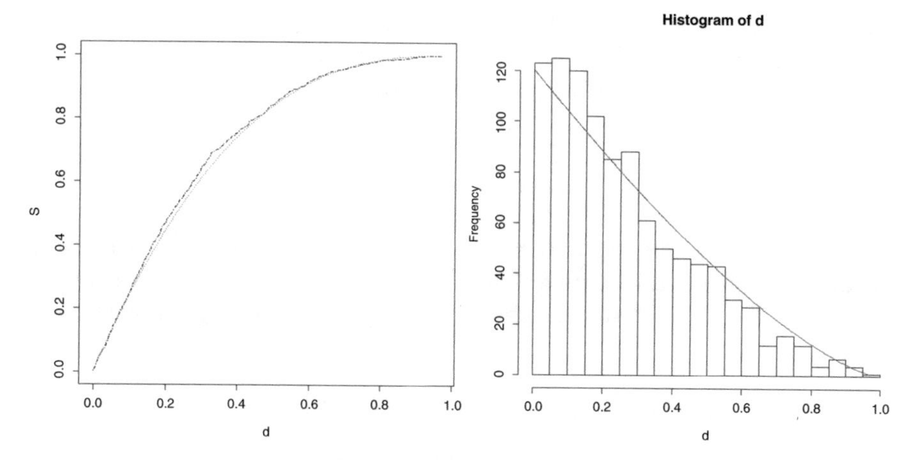

Fig. 2 (Standardized) distribution of rank differences under mixture of Gaussian(0.6) and independent copulas with overall correlation 0.3 compared to beta(1,2.65)

Thus a test statistic based on absolute ranked differences should emphasize the lower order statistics. Such statistics come under the heading of L-statistics. It is possible to tailor a test toward alternative features of interest such as proportionate size of the subpopulation and the strength of association within it. Exact distributions of partial or weighted sums of absolute rank differences are quite complicated due to dependencies [16], even under the null hypothesis of independence. A very simple general purpose test statistic is

$$T_S = \sum_{i=1}^{n} 1\left\{\frac{|\pi(x_i) - \nu(y_i)|}{n} < 0.2\right\}.$$

Using the observed overall correlation r in place of ρ, the null distribution of T_S may be simulated under the Gaussian copula or approximated as a Binomial test statistic using the probability from the Beta$(1, \beta)$ as in Proposition 3. In the latter case, ignoring weak dependencies, the 0.05 level test has power of 80 % of detecting a Gaussian subpopulation of 25 % with r =0.8 for $n = 1000$.

3 Components of Kendall's Tau

Although the CSF test is both simple and computationally efficient, it has a conceptual shortcoming arising from the use of Spearman's footrule distance to characterize association in a subpopulation. The issue is that the components of the footrule distance in the subpopulation depend on the encompassing population; that is, when the sample is a full population, with associated subpopulation Ω, the component set from the footrule from Ω

$$\{d_i \mid i \in \Omega\} = \{|\pi(x_i) - \nu(y_i)| \mid i \in \Omega\}$$

depends heavily on the rankings π and ν determined by the full population. In contrast, the component set from Kendall's distance depends only on the relative rankings within Ω, which may be constructed from just on the original values in Ω. That is,

$$\begin{aligned}&\left\{1\left[\left(\pi(x_i) - \pi(x_j)\right)\left(\nu(y_i) - \nu(y_j)\right) < 0\right] \mid i,j \in \Omega\right\}\\ &\quad = \left\{1\left[\left(x_i - x_j\right)\left(y_i - y_j\right) < 0\right] \mid i,j \in \Omega\right\}\end{aligned}$$

Thus the subpopulation discordances (components of Kendall's distance) do not depend upon the embedding population, whereas the subpopulation disarray (components of Spearman's footrule distance) do. This invariance has a number of beneficial properties, such as allowing the CKT test to retain power in situations where the ranges of the $\{X_i\}$ and $\{Y_i\}$ values in the subpopulation are more restricted than those in the full population.

The notion of homogeneous association based on Kendall's distance differs from that based on the Spearman's footrule used for the CSF test. In this case the natural null hypothesis should be a distribution depending only on Kendall's distance. Furthermore it should have the greatest entropy for a given value of Kendall's tau because this formulation would attribute as much variability as possible to the null distribution, making it a conservative (least favorable) test [11]. To construct a distribution that has this structure, simply sample from an arbitrary copula, and then reorder the Y-values according to a permutation $\nu(\mathbf{Y})$ sampled independently from a Mallows model centered at the ranking $\pi(\mathbf{X})$ of the X-values. Quite remarkably, any such process asymptotically leads to a Frank copula. Proposition 4, based on [17], gives a precise statement.

Proposition 4 *Let $\{(X_i, Y_i) \mid i = 1, \ldots, n\}$ be independent samples from a distribution H with continuous marginals F and G, and associated copula C with continuous partial derivatives. Let $\pi(\mathbf{X})$ be the ranking of $\pi(\mathbf{X}) = [X_1, \ldots, X_n]$ and $\nu(\mathbf{Y})$ be the ranking of $\nu(\mathbf{Y}) = [Y_1, \ldots, Y_n]$. Assume that for all n sufficiently large, the conditional distribution of $\nu(\mathbf{Y})$ given $\pi(\mathbf{X})$ is Mallows, with center at $\pi(\mathbf{X})$ and scale ϕ_n. If $\phi_n \to 0$, and there exists $\theta \neq 0$ such that*

$$n\left(1 - e^{-\phi_n}\right) \to \theta,$$

then C is the Frank Copula C_θ.

Proof First, we establish that if the conditional distribution of $\nu(\mathbf{Y})$ given $\pi(\mathbf{X})$ is a Mallows distribution, then the copula C is radially symmetric. The *pseudo-observations* for each pair (X_i, Y_i) are defined as functions of the pair and the empirical margins

$$\left(\hat{U}_i, \hat{V}_i\right) = \frac{n}{n+1}\left(\hat{F}_n(X_i), \hat{G}_n(Y_i)\right).$$

These are functions of the rankings $\pi(\mathbf{X})$ and $\nu(\mathbf{Y})$:

$$\hat{U}_i = 1 - \frac{\pi(X_i)}{n+1}, \quad \hat{V}_i = 1 - \frac{\nu(Y_i)}{n+1}.$$

By the symmetry of the Mallows model, the joint distribution of the pseudo-observations $\left(\hat{U}_1, \hat{V}_1\right), \ldots, \left(\hat{U}_n, \hat{V}_n\right)$ is identical to the joint distribution of $\left(1 - \hat{U}_1, 1 - \hat{V}_1\right), \ldots, \left(1 - \hat{U}_n, 1 - \hat{V}_n\right)$. Consider empirical distributions based on these observations [9]:

$$\hat{C}_n(u, v) = \frac{1}{n}\sum_{i=1}^{n} 1\left\{\hat{U}_i \leq u, \hat{V}_i \leq v\right\}$$

$$\hat{D}_n(u, v) = \frac{1}{n}\sum_{i=1}^{n} 1\left\{1 - \hat{U}_i \leq u, 1 - \hat{V}_i \leq v\right\}.$$

Since H has continuous marginals and C has continuous partial derivatives, then [4] established that $\hat{C}_n$ is a consistent estimator of the copula C, and likewise $\hat{D}_n$ is a consistent estimator of the survival copula $\bar{C}$, where

$$\bar{C}(u, v) = u + v - 1 + C(1 - u, 1 - v).$$

Hence, $\bar{C} = C$, which implies that the copula C is radially symmetric [13, p. 37]. Since C is radially symmetric, an asymptotically equivalent definition of the *empirical copula* is

$$\begin{aligned} \tilde{C}_n(u, v) &= \frac{1}{n} \sum_{i=1}^{n} 1 \left\{ \frac{\pi(X_i)}{n} \leq u, \frac{\nu(Y_i)}{n} \leq v \right\} \\ &= \frac{1}{n} \sum_{i=1}^{n} \delta_{(\pi(X_i)/n, \nu(Y_i)/n)} \end{aligned}$$

which places mass of $\frac{1}{n}$ on each random point $\left(\frac{\pi(X_i)}{n}, \frac{\nu(Y_i)}{n}\right) \in [0, 1]^2$. This empirical copula is expressed by the following point process [17]: For $n \in \mathbb{N}$,

$$\mu_n(B, \omega) = \frac{1}{n} \sum_{i=1}^{n} 1 \left\{ \left(\frac{\pi(X_i)}{n}, \frac{\nu(Y_i)}{n} \right) \in B \right\}$$

for each bounded Borel set $B \subseteq \mathbb{R}^2$.

By assumption, the regularity conditions on the Mallows scale are satisfied as $n \to \infty$:

$$\phi_n \to 0, \ \exists \theta \in \mathbb{R}/\{0\} \ni n\left(1 - e^{-\phi_n}\right) \to \theta.$$

Under these conditions, the primary result of [17] is applied: As $n \to \infty$, the random measures $\mu_n(\cdot, \omega)$ weakly converge to the measure μ_θ, defined by

$$\begin{aligned} d\mu_\theta(u, v) = &\frac{(\theta/2)\sinh(\theta/2)}{\left(e^{\theta/4}\cosh(\theta[u - v]/2) - e^{-\theta/4}\cosh(\theta[u + v - 1]/2)\right)^2} \\ &\times I_{[0,1]^2}(u, v)\, \partial u \partial v. \end{aligned}$$

Simply converting the trigonometric functions to exponential form and simplifying yields

$$d\mu_\theta(u, v) = \frac{\theta\left(1 - e^{-\theta}\right)e^{-\theta(u+v)}}{\left(1 - e^{-\theta} - \left(1 - e^{-\theta u}\right)\left(1 - e^{-\theta v}\right)\right)^2} I_{[0,1]^2}(u, v)\, \partial u \partial v.$$

By recognition, the limiting measure $d\mu_\theta$ is that of the (Frank) Copula C_θ. Recall, $\tilde{C}_n$ is a consistent estimator of the underlying copula C, and converges weakly to C_θ, so we conclude that $C = C_\theta$. □

Pursuing this result further allows for inspection of the adequacy of the asymptotic result for finite samples. A function $\phi(\theta)$ for matching the Mallows ϕ parameter to the Frank θ parameter may be obtained by equating expressions for τ_ϕ and τ_θ from these models. For any Archimedean copula, there is a relatively simple formula $\tau = 4\mathrm{E}[C(U,V) - 1]$ [8]; for the Frank copula, a specialized form [13, p. 171], [7] is

$$\tau_\theta = 1 - \frac{4}{\theta}[1 - D(\theta)] = 1 - \frac{4}{\theta}\left[1 - \frac{1}{\theta}\int_0^\theta \frac{t}{e^t - 1}\partial t\right]$$

where the scaled integral $D(\gamma)$ is known as the Debye-1 function, available in the "gsl" (Gnu Scientific Library) package of R. For the Mallows model,

$$\tau_\phi = \frac{2}{\pi}\arctan(0.18n\phi)$$

Equating τ_θ and τ_ϕ leads to the relationship (Fig. 3)

$$\phi = \frac{100}{18n}\tan\left[\frac{\pi}{2}\left\{1 - \frac{4}{\theta}[1 - D(\theta)]\right\}\right] \approx \frac{0.9694}{n}\theta.$$

Empirical evidence for the applicability of Proposition 4 comes in two stages: (1) The distribution of Kendall's distance under Frank(θ) and under Mallows($\phi(\theta)$) both converge to the same normal distribution; (2) As n gets large the product density of the sample under Frank(θ) converges to an increasing function of the Kendall's distance between $\pi(\mathbf{X})$ and $\nu(\mathbf{Y})$ of the sample. Figure 4 illustrates results from the following confirmatory experiment:

- Generate 1000 sets of 1000 points from a Frank($\theta = 3$) copula
- Compute the Kendall's distance D and the Frank density d for each set
- Plot d vs D on a log-log scale.

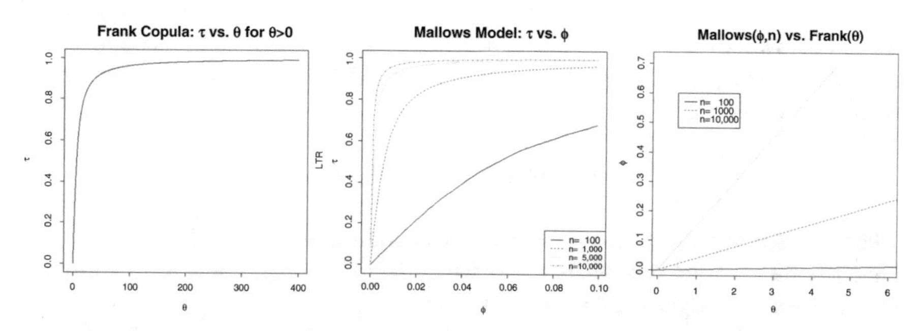

Fig. 3 Scale relationships. *Left*: Kendall's τ vs. the Frank scale θ; *center*: Kendall's τ vs. the Mallows scale ϕ for $n = 100, 1000, 5000, 10{,}000$; *right*: Mallows ϕ_n vs. Frankθ, for $n = 100, 1000, 5000$

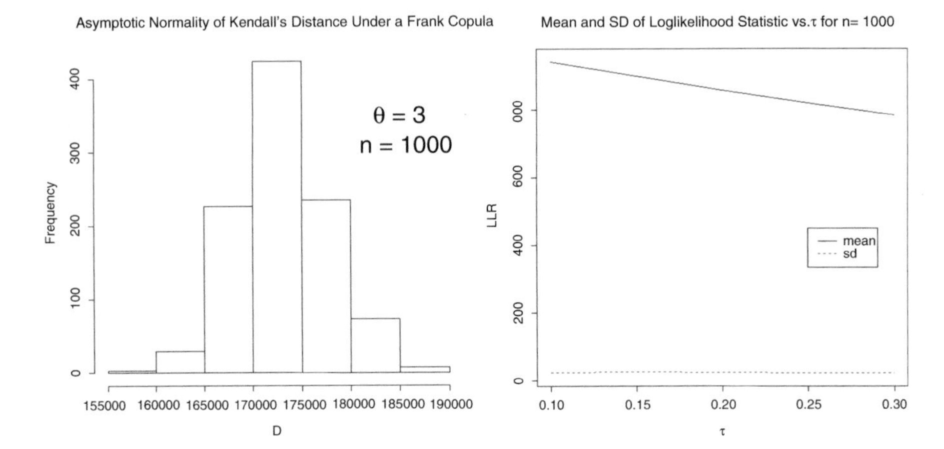

Fig. 4 Association between X and Y in a Frank copula approaches a Mallows model for the ranking $\nu(\mathbf{Y})$ in a large sample centered at $\pi(\mathbf{X})$. *Left*: approximate normality Kendall's distance D in samples of size $n = 1000$ from a Frank($\theta = 3$) copula; *right*: log-log plot of the density of each sample vs. its Kendall's distance D

Note also that the Frank copula is radially symmetric, $C(u, v) = u + v - 1 + C(1 - u, 1 - v)$, which is a necessary condition for the density of a sample to depend only on its Kendall's distance. With the assurance that there are copulas with the conditional distribution of $\nu(\mathbf{Y})$ given $\pi(\mathbf{X})$ well approximated by a Mallows model, this becomes the null hypothesis:

$$H_0 : \nu(\mathbf{Y}) \circ \pi^{-1}(\mathbf{X}) \sim \text{Mallows}(\theta), \text{ for some } \theta > 0.$$

In view of Proposition 4, for large samples, this is approximately the same as assuming that (X,Y) are governed by a Frank copula, in which case, it matters little if the roles of X and Y are exchanged. The general alternative against which we would like a test to be sensitive is that there is a subpopulation with high association with the remainder having (little or) no association. The test for heterogeneity should maintain power over a wide variety of alternative distributions for the subpopulation supporting strong association. With these considerations, the alternative hypothesis is formulated as

$$H_A : (F(X), G(Y)) \sim M$$

where M is a mixture of two homogeneous copulas: H_1 on which $(F(X), G(Y))$ have a common $\tau = \tau_1$, and H_2 under which $(F(X), G(Y))$ come from a mixture of homogeneous copulas, all of which have $\tau < \tau_1$.

To test against such a general alternative, the strategy is first to reorder the sample so that the tau measure of association is decreasing; then test if the pattern for the rate of decrease matches that under the null hypothesis. Specifically, an adaptive model encompassing the Mallows model is adopted, with the number of free parameters in the model increasing with sample size. This component of Kendall's tau (CKT) test proceeds in four steps:

(1) Fit a Mallows model centered at π (**X**) to ν (**Y**) and compute the likelihood.
(2) Reorder the data points $\{(X_i, Y_i) \mid i = 1, \ldots, n\}$, so that Kendall's tau coefficient is decreasing. Here we use the Fast BCS algorithm of [19], which has computational complexity n^3, but may be implemented [15] to perform in n^2 time. Call the reordering σ.
(3) Use moving average maximum average maximum likelihood estimators to smoothly fit a multistage ranking model to the relative rankings of $\left[Y_{\sigma(1)}, \ldots, Y_{\sigma(k)}\right]$ to $\left[X_{\sigma(1)}, \ldots, X_{\sigma(k)}\right]$ at each stage k. See [14]. Compute the likelihood under this (encompassing) model.
(4) Use the (Generalized) Likelihood Ratio statistic to test H_0.

Comments on the four steps:

(1) Since Kendall's tau distance is invariant to reordering of observations, this is the same as fitting a Mallows model, centered at ranking (σX), to the ranking (σY), where σ is the taupath reordering.
(2) The idea of reordering is to put the points displaying the highest amount of association earlier in the sequence in order to identify the subpopulation with highest empirical association. The reordering is not unique. Yu et al. [19] discuss various algorithms.
(3) The multistage ranking model decomposes the number of discordances [up to (n choose 2)] between ranking (σY) and ranking (σX), as a sum of $n-1$ variables $\{V_k\}$ with ranges $\{0, \ldots, k\}$, $k = 1, \ldots, n-1$. The model has likelihood $L = c(\theta)\, e^{-\sum \theta_k V_k}$ which reduces to the likelihood of Mallows model when all component parameters are equal.
(4) The conditions needed to justify an asymptotic chi-square distribution for this statistic do not hold in this setting. Currently, we simulate the distribution under the Frank copula to get an appropriate reference. We are working to find a more precise characterization of the LR in this setting.

The null distribution of this likelihood ratio appears to be close to normal, with its mean decreasing with the common correlation τ, and standard deviation constant. See Fig. 5. Note that, for $n = 1000$, the variance of $2 \cdot \text{LLR} \approx 2500$ is clearly less than its $2 \cdot \text{mean}(2 \cdot \text{LLR})$ theoretical value for a chi-square distribution, which is in the range $(3100, 3800)$ when $\tau \in (0.10, 0.30)$.

Instead of fixed n and varying τ, Fig. 5 depicts the relationship between *LLR* and n with fixed τ. The overall relationship between the moments of *LLR* and the parameters τ and n is not yet known, but using a practical additive approximation in the range $0.1 < \tau < 0.3$ and $500 < n < 3000$, the basic asymptotic α-level CKT test has the form: Reject H_0 if

$$Z = \frac{\text{LLR} - (n + 20 - 797\hat{\tau})}{0.02n + 7} > z_{1-\alpha},$$

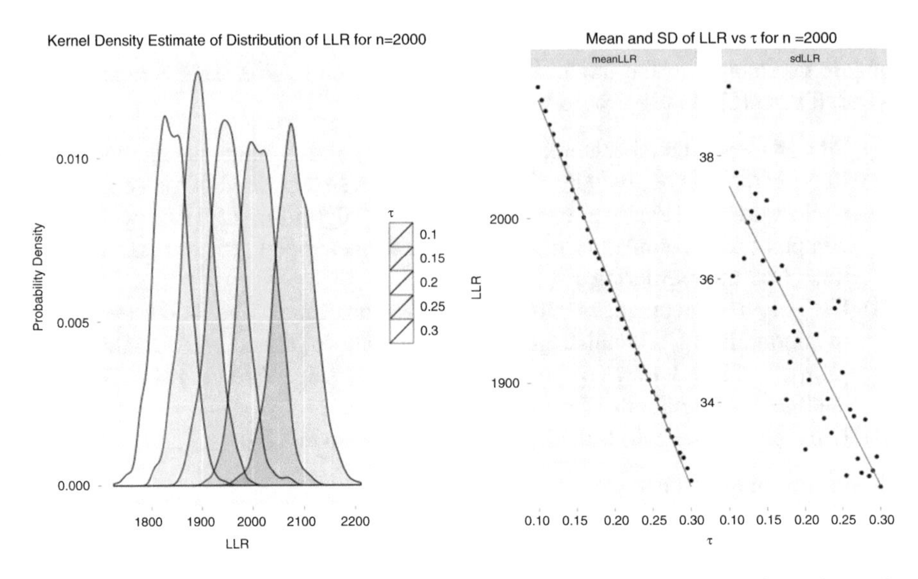

Fig. 5 Simulation of log-likelihood ratio (LLR) statistic for CKT test under Frank copulas. *Left*: Kernel density estimate of the distribution of LLR, based on 5000 simulations of size $n = 2000$, for fixed τ. *Right*: decreasing pattern of mean and constancy of standard deviation for LLR under Frank copulas at different levels of τ for $n = 2000$

where $\hat{\tau}$ is Kendall's correlation coefficient and $z_{1-\alpha}$ is the $(1 - \alpha)$ th quantile of the standard normal.

4 Simulations for Robustness and Power

First, performance of the tests is checked by maintenance of levels under various Gaussian and Frank copulas; subsequently power is examined. The CSF test is based on the number of absolute rank differences less than 0.2. Figure 6 shows the null distributions of p-values for the CSF test applied to samples of size $n = 1000$ generated 100,000 times under the Gaussian(ρ) models. These distributions start to become stochastically smaller than uniform for $\rho > 0.45$. Otherwise the test is conservative in the range $0 < \rho < 0.45$ and $0 < \alpha < 0.05$ as illustrated by the observed number of type 1 errors at the $\alpha = 0.05$ level.

Under similar Gaussian copulas, the adjustment of the mean of the log-likelihood for the estimated overall τ makes the CKT test behave conservatively for large values of ρ, but gives highly significant values for ρ values near 0. See Fig. 7, in which, due to computational limitations, lowess-smoothed curves describe the p-distribution based on only 100 simulations. In the presence of very low overall correlation, it is advisable to use the CSF test as a screen for the CKT, which will protect the CKT from finding uneven levels of τ association when ρ association

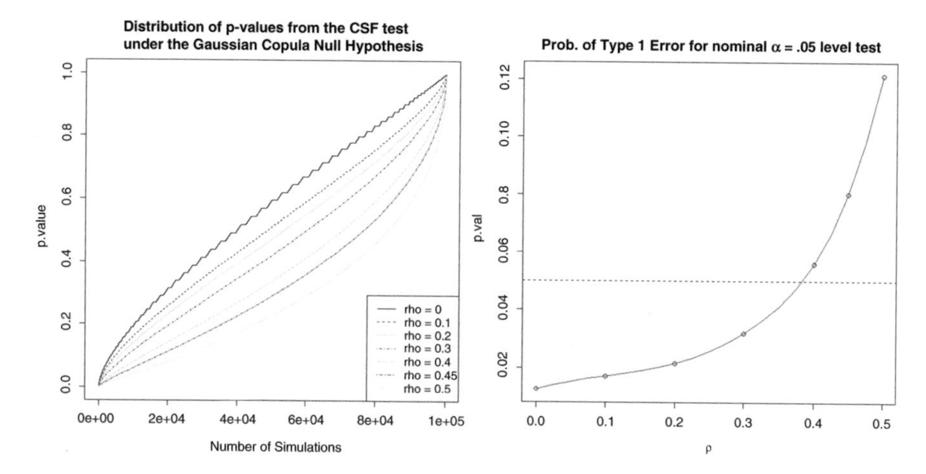

Fig. 6 CSF results from 100,000 simulation experiments of size $n = 1000$ for values of ρ in a Gaussian copula. *Left*: distribution of *p*-values for seven values of null correlation; *Right*: observed probabilities of Type I error for a nominal $\alpha = 0.05$ test. The test is conservative for values of $\rho < 0.45$

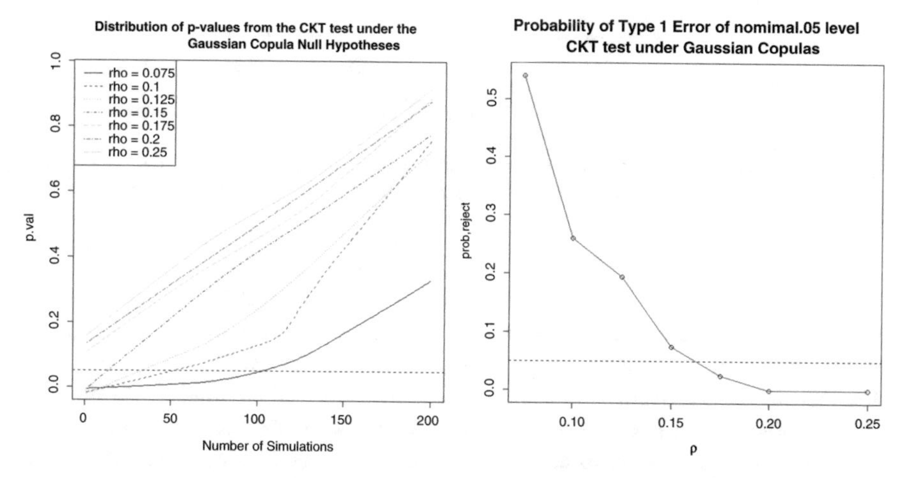

Fig. 7 CKT results from 200 simulation experiments of size $n = 1000$ for values of ρ in a Gaussian copula; *Left*: distribution of *p*-values for seven values of the null correlation; *Right*: observed probabilities of Type I error for a nominal $\alpha = 0.05$ test. The test is conservative for values of $\rho > 0.16$

is homogeneous. Again, this tendency toward excess false positives happens only when the overall ρ association is close to 0. In this case a special test [14] is available for the null hypothesis of independence. Under a Frank copula, the CSF test behaves properly near independence, but loses its level when τ gets large. See Fig. 7.

Several factors affect the power curves of both the CSF and CKT tests: *sample size* (n is fixed at 500 or 1000); *proportionate size of the subpopulation* (fixed at

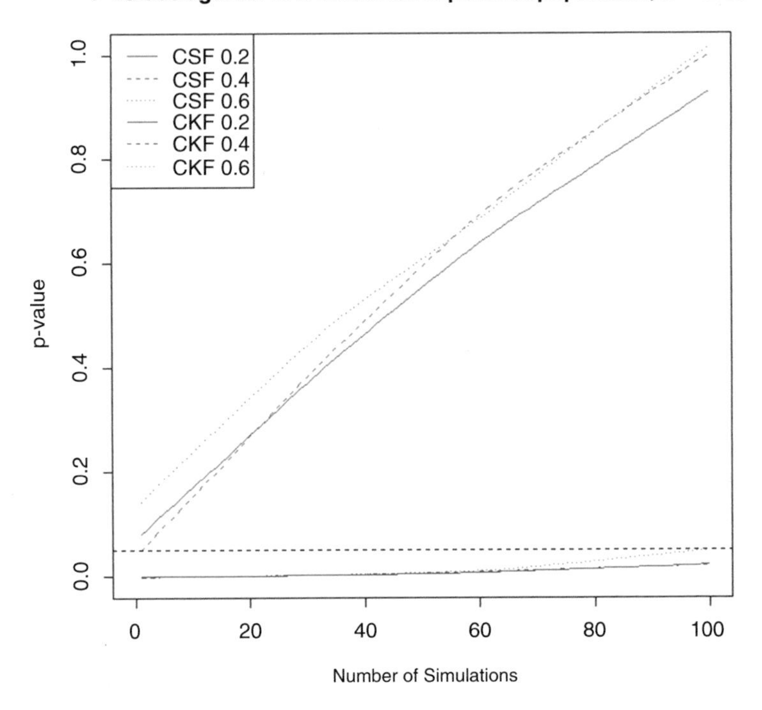

Fig. 8 *P*-values against alternative mixture of Gaussian copulas with sample size $n = 1000$ and subpopulation proportion $= 40\,\%$. *Dashed horizontal lines* at $\alpha = 0.05$ indicate the power of a level 0.05 test

$40\,\%$); *strength of association in the subpopulation* ($\rho, \tau \in \{0.7, 0.8, 0.9\}$); and, most importantly, the *form of the subpopulation*. Against the null hypothesis of a Gaussian copula, the alternative is a mixture of copulas, where the variables are assumed to be independent in the complement of the subpopulation. Against the null hypothesis of a Frank copula, the subpopulation is selected at random and its conditional distribution is forced into a stronger Mallows model. This allows the population margins to remain uniform while possibly restricting the range of the subpopulation.

Figure 8 shows the distribution of p-values of both CSF and CKT tests against $40\,\%$ Gaussian with $0.12 \leq \rho \leq 0.13$. For this range of overall correlation the CKT test holds its level and is conservative for overall correlation $\rho < 0.12$, which is the case here. Nevertheless, it achieves perfect power when the subpopulation $\rho \geq 0.125$, even though its power quickly diminishes to $10\,\%$ for $\rho = 0.12$ in the subpopulation. It also performs better than CSF in this range.

Under the Mallows alternative, $n = 1000$ points are generated from a uniform distribution, 400 points are then sampled from a quantile range of x values and the y values resorted according to a random draw from a Mallow($\phi\,(\tau)$) model.

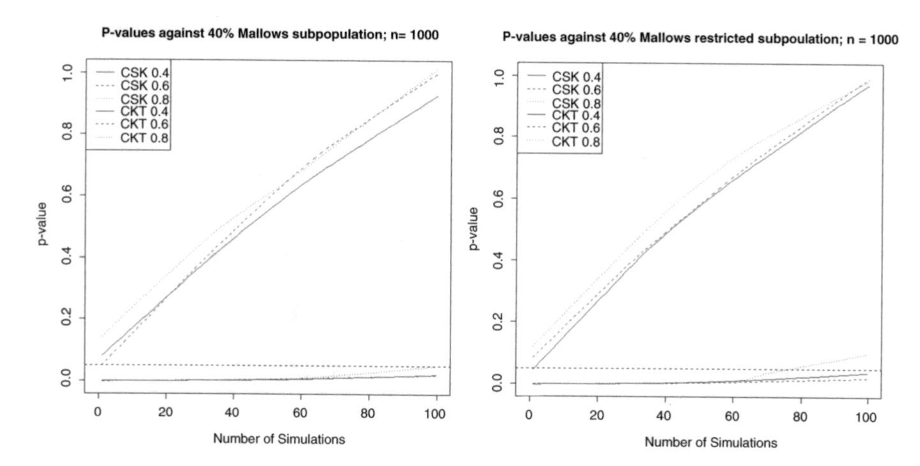

Fig. 9 Distribution of p-values for Mallows alternatives, based on 100 simulations of sample size $n = 1000$. *Left*: associated subgroup spans the full range of x-values. *Right*: span is restricted to the 20-to-80th percentiles region of x-values in the larger population

Values of τ used are 0.4, 0.5, and 0.6. Figure 9 shows the distributions of p-values from the $\alpha = 0.05$ level CSF and CKT tests over 100 simulations. The left panel corresponds to the subpopulation being sampled from the full range, while the right panel corresponds to samples between the 20th and 80th percentiles of x-values. The CKT test performs much better than the CSF test against these alternatives. The CKT has essentially perfect detection when the subpopulation spans the whole range, and at least 70 % power in the 20–80 percentile range. The CSF has no power in either scenario.

5 Example

Wine cultivars are varieties of grapes that have been cultivated through selective breeding. Different varieties may be characterized by certain chemical properties of the wine they produce. Early work in supervised learning has been used to classify wine cultivars using chemical measurements of wine sample [1]. These data, available at (http://archive.ics.uci.edu/ml/machine-learning-databases/wine), are reanalyzed here using the CKT and CSF tests as unsupervised methods of detecting different association structures that might help characterize different cultivated varieties.

Figure 10 shows the relationship between flavonoids and phenols in the data set consisting of 13 measurements from 178 wine samples derived from three different cultivars. To the untrained eye, the overall plot looks typical of homogeneous association, but both the CKT ($p = 0.0002$) and CSF (p=0.027) indicate heterogeneity. Identification of cultivars in the plot shows separation of cultivar 1

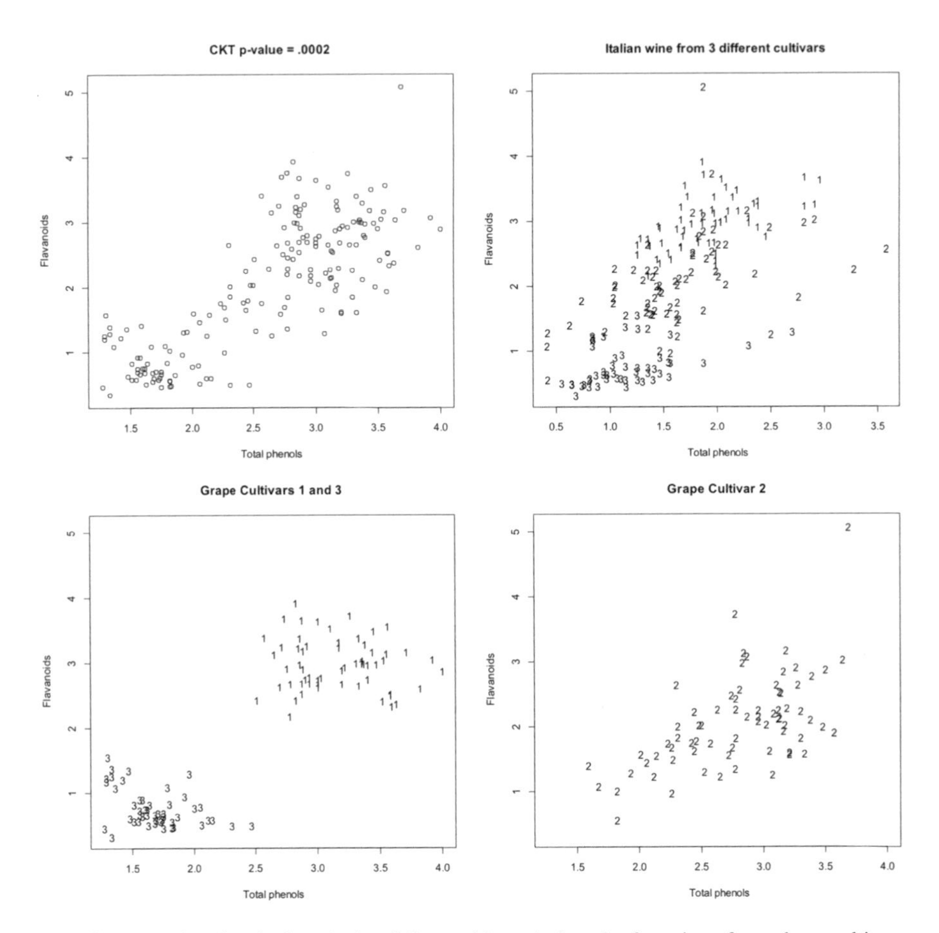

Fig. 10 Example: chemical analysis of flavonoids and phenols, for wines from three cultivars (varieties)

and 3 samples from each other, with slightly negative association within each of these groups; however, their positioning contributes a kind of ecological correlation to the overall sample. In contrast, samples from cultivar 2 show a strong positive association between flavonoid and phenol content. This suggests an underlying genetic difference.

It is impressive that CKT can detect this heterogeneity of association from the unlabelled data, which looks like an overall positive association, part of which is ecological correlation. Although the CSF test does also indicate association, it is not as sensitive at detecting it in this situation, and its p-value would not present a strong case for heterogeneity if any correction is attempted for multiple comparisons over the 13 choose 2 (78) pairs of variables available.

6 Concluding Remarks

The ability to detect subpopulations that drive association has the potential of changing the way statistics are used to unveil structures in "Big Data." Instead of employing extensive model searching with complex interaction, now methods with fewer model assumptions are available to ascertain with precision is there is any simple mixture that better explains monotone association between variables. The CSF and CKT tests achieve this, either working together to screen and confirm or separately to find different forms of the subpopulation that most strongly supports the association.

These tests, however, are formally restricted to different forms of the meaning of "homogeneous association." Strict legitimacy of the CSF test depends on the assumption of a Gaussian copula underlying the null distribution, whereas the CKT test depends on the assumption of a Frank copula underlying the null distribution. Although there is some evidence of limited robustness, much more work should be done to explore the behavior of these tests under general conditions. For example, both the Gaussian and Frank copulas are radially symmetric; it is unclear how sensitive the tests would be to asymmetric notions of homogeneous association.

The computationally efficiency of the CSF test is important because the sample size n needs to be in the thousands before there is much hope of reliably detecting these subtle but important differences. In contrast with the CSF test, the justification of CKT is a bit more compelling, based on intrinsic association within the subpopulation. We have been using CSF at a liberal $\alpha = 0.05$ level as a screening devise to reduce the number of pairs of variables to be tested at a more stringent level.

Detecting heterogeneity of association is a difficult task. Such detection is practical only when the overall association is not too strong, the association in the subpopulation is strong, and the sample size is large. Nevertheless, such scenarios abound. We believe that these new methods will make statistics ever more relevant in making good sense from Big Data.

Acknowledgement We thank the referee for their thoughtful and helpful review.

References

1. Aeberhard, S., Coomans, D., de Vel, O.: Improvements to the classification performance of RDA. J. Chemometr. **7**(2), 99–115 (1993)
2. Diaconis, P., Graham, R.L.: Spearman's footrule as a measure of disarray. J. R. Stat. Soc. Ser. B - Stat. Methodol. **39**, 262–268 (1977)
3. Diaconis, P., Ram, A.: Analysis of systematic scan metropolis algorithms using Iwahori-Hecke algebra techniques. Mich. Math. J. **48**, 157–190 (2000)
4. Fermanian, J.D., Radulovic, D., Wegkamp, M.: Weak convergence of empirical copula processes. Bernoulli **10**, 847–860 (2004)

5. Fligner, M.A., Verducci, J.S.: Distance based ranking models. Journal of the Royal Statistical Society B, **48**, 359–369 (1986)
6. Frank, M.J.: On the simultaneous associativity of F(x, y) and x + y − F(x, y). Aequationes Math. **19**, 194–226 (1979)
7. Genest, C.: Frank's family of bivariate distributions. Biometrika **74**(3), 549–555 (1987)
8. Genest, C., MacKay, J.: The joy of copulas: bivariate distributions with uniform marginals. Am. Stat. **40**, 280–283 (1986)
9. Genest, C., Nešlehová, J.: On tests of radial symmetry for bivariate copulas. Stat. Pap. **55**, 1107–1119 (2014)
10. Katz, G.: How much do we know about HDL cholesterol? Clin. Correlat. (2014) (http://www.clinicalcorrelations.org/?p=7298)
11. Lehmann, E.L., Romano, J.P.: Testing Statistical Hypotheses, 3rd edn. Springer, New York (2006).
12. Mallows, C.: Non-Null Ranking Models. Biometrika, **44**(1), 114–130 (1957)
13. Nelsen, R.B.: An Introduction to Copulas, 2nd edn. Springer, New York (2006)
14. Sampath, S., Verducci, J.: Detecting the end of agreement between two long ranked lists. Stat. Anal. Data Min. **6**(6), 458–471 (2013)
15. Sampath, S., Caloiaro, A., Johnson, W., Verducci, J.: The top-K tau-path screen for monotone association in subpopulations. WIREs Comput. Stat. (2016). doi:10.1002/wics.1382
16. Sen, P.K., Salama, I.A., Quade, D.: Spearman's footrule: asymptotics in applications. Chil. J. Stat. **2**, 3–20 (2011)
17. Starr, S.: Thermodynamic limit for the Mallows model on S_n. J. Math. Phys. **50**, 195–208 (2009)
18. Voight, B.F., et al.: Plasma HDL cholesterol and risk of myocardial infarction: a Mendelian randomisation study. Lancet **380**(9841), 572–580 (2012)
19. Yu, L., Verducci, J., Blower, P.: The tau-path test for monotone association in an unspecified subpopulation: applications to chemogenomic data mining. Stat. Methodol. **8**, 97–111 (2011)

Part III
Statistics Learning and Applications

Optimal Shrinkage Estimation in Heteroscedastic Hierarchical Linear Models

S.C. Kou and Justin J. Yang

Abstract Shrinkage estimators have profound impacts in statistics and in scientific and engineering applications. In this article, we consider shrinkage estimation in the presence of linear predictors. We formulate two heteroscedastic hierarchical regression models and study optimal shrinkage estimators in each model. A class of shrinkage estimators, both parametric and semiparametric, based on unbiased risk estimate (URE) is proposed and is shown to be (asymptotically) optimal under mean squared error loss in each model. Simulation study is conducted to compare the performance of the proposed methods with existing shrinkage estimators. We also apply the method to real data and obtain encouraging and interesting results.

1 Introduction

Shrinkage estimators, hierarchical models and empirical Bayes methods, dating back to the groundbreaking works of [24] and [21], have profound impacts in statistics and in scientific and engineering applications. They provide effective tools to pool information from (scientifically) related populations for simultaneous inference—the data on each population alone often do not lead to the most effective estimation, but by pooling information from the related populations together (for example, by shrinking toward their consensus "center"), one could often obtain more accurate estimate for each individual population. Ever since the seminal works of [24] and [10], an impressive list of articles has been devoted to the study of shrinkage estimators in normal models, including [1, 2, 4–6, 8, 12, 14, 16, 22, 25], among others.

In this article, we consider shrinkage estimation in the presence of linear predictors. In particular, we study *optimal* shrinkage estimators for *heteroscedastic* data under *linear* models. Our study is motivated by three main considerations. First, in many practical problems, one often encounters heteroscedastic (unequal variance) data; for example, the sample sizes for different groups are not all equal. Second, in many statistical applications, in addition to the heteroscedastic response variable,

S.C. Kou (✉) • J.J. Yang
Department of Statistics, Harvard University, 1 Oxford Street, Cambridge, MA 02138, USA
e-mail: kou@stat.harvard.edu; juchenjustinyang@fas.harvard.edu

© Springer International Publishing AG 2017

S.E. Ahmed (ed.), *Big and Complex Data Analysis*, Contributions to Statistics,
DOI 10.1007/978-3-319-41573-4_13

one often has predictors. For example, the predictors could represent longitudinal patterns [7, 9, 27], exam scores [22], characteristics of hospital patients [18], etc. Third, in applying shrinkage estimators to real data, it is quite natural to ask for the *optimal* way of shrinkage.

The (risk) optimality is not addressed by the conventional estimators, such as the empirical Bayes ones. One might wonder if such an optimal shrinkage estimator exists in the first place. We shall see shortly that in fact (asymptotically) optimal shrinkage estimators do exist and that the optimal estimators are *not* empirical Bayes ones but are characterized by an unbiased risk estimate (URE).

The study of optimal shrinkage estimators under the heteroscedastic normal model was first considered in [29], where the (asymptotic) optimal shrinkage estimator was identified for both the parametric and semiparametric cases. Xie et al. [30] extends the (asymptotic) optimal shrinkage estimators to exponential families and heteroscedastic location-scale families. The current article can be viewed as an extension of the idea of optimal shrinkage estimators to heteroscedastic linear models.

We want to emphasize that this article works on a theoretical setting somewhat different from [30] but can still cover its main results. Our theoretical results show that the optimality of the proposed URE shrinkage estimators does not rely on normality nor on the tail behavior of the sampling distribution. What we require here are the symmetry and the existence of the fourth moment for the standardized variable.

This article is organized as follows. We first formulate the heteroscedastic linear models in Sect. 2. Interestingly, there are two parallel ways to do so, and both are natural extensions of the heteroscedastic normal model. After reviewing the conventional empirical Bayes methods, we introduce the construction of our optimal shrinkage estimators for heteroscedastic linear models in Sect. 3. The optimal shrinkage estimators are based on an unbiased risk estimate (URE). We show in Sect. 4 that the URE shrinkage estimators are asymptotically optimal in risk. In Sect. 5 we extend the shrinkage estimators to a semiparametric family. Simulation studies are conducted in Sect. 6. We apply the URE shrinkage estimators in Sect. 7 to the baseball data set of [2] and observe quite interesting and encouraging results. We conclude in Sect. 8 with some discussion and extension. The appendix details the proofs and derivations for the theoretical results.

2 Heteroscedastic Hierarchical Linear Models

Consider the heteroscedastic estimation problem

$$Y_i|\boldsymbol{\theta} \overset{\text{indep.}}{\sim} \mathcal{N}(\theta_i, A_i), \quad i = 1, \ldots, p, \tag{1}$$

where $\boldsymbol{\theta} = (\theta_1, \ldots, \theta_p)^T$ is the unknown mean vector, which is to be estimated, and the variances $A_i > 0$ are unequal, which are assumed to be known. In many statistical applications, in addition to the heteroscedastic $\boldsymbol{Y} = (Y_1, \ldots, Y_p)^T$, one often has predictors $\boldsymbol{X}$. A natural question is to consider a heteroscedastic linear model that incorporates these covariates. Notation-wise, let $\{Y_i, \boldsymbol{X}_i\}_{i=1}^p$ denote the p independent statistical units, where Y_i is the response variable of the i-th unit, and $\boldsymbol{X}_i = (X_{1i}, \ldots, X_{ki})^T$ is a k-dimensional column vector that corresponds to the k covariates of the i-th unit. The $k \times p$ matrix

$$\boldsymbol{X} = \left[\boldsymbol{X}_1 | \cdots | \boldsymbol{X}_p\right], \quad \boldsymbol{X}_1, .., \boldsymbol{X}_p \in \mathbb{R}^k,$$

where $\boldsymbol{X}_i$ is the i-th column of $\boldsymbol{X}$, then contains the covariates for all the units. Throughout this article we assume that $\boldsymbol{X}$ has full rank, i.e., rank$(\boldsymbol{X}) = k$.

To include the predictors, we note that, interestingly, there are *two* different ways to build up a heteroscedastic hierarchical linear model, which lead to different structure for shrinkage estimation.

Model I: Hierarchical linear model. On top of (1), the θ_i's are $\theta_i \overset{\text{indep.}}{\sim} \mathcal{N}\left(\boldsymbol{X}_i^T \boldsymbol{\beta}, \lambda\right)$, where $\boldsymbol{\beta}$ and λ are both *unknown* hyper-parameters. Model I has been suggested as early as [26]. See [16] and [17] for more discussions. The special case of no covariates (i.e., $k = 1$ and $\boldsymbol{X} = [1| \cdots |1]$) is studied in depth in [29].

Model II: Bayesian linear regression model. Together with (1), one assumes $\boldsymbol{\theta} = \boldsymbol{X}^T \boldsymbol{\beta}$ with $\boldsymbol{\beta}$ following a conjugate prior distribution $\boldsymbol{\beta} \sim \mathcal{N}_k(\boldsymbol{\beta}_0, \lambda \boldsymbol{W})$, where $\boldsymbol{W}$ is a *known* $k \times k$ positive definite matrix and $\boldsymbol{\beta}_0$ and λ are *unknown* hyper-parameters. Model II has been considered in [3, 15, 20] among others; it includes ridge regression as a special case when $\boldsymbol{\beta}_0 = \boldsymbol{0}_k$ and $\boldsymbol{W} = \boldsymbol{I}_k$.

Figure 1 illustrates these two hierarchical linear models. Under Model I, the posterior mean of $\boldsymbol{\theta}$ is $\hat{\theta}_i^{\lambda,\boldsymbol{\beta}} = \lambda(\lambda + A_i)^{-1} Y_i + A_i(\lambda + A_i)^{-1} \boldsymbol{X}_i^T \boldsymbol{\beta}$ for $i = 1, \ldots, p$, so the shrinkage estimation is formed by directly shrinking the raw observation Y_i toward a linear combination of the k covariates $\boldsymbol{X}_i$. If we denote $\mu_i = \boldsymbol{X}_i^T \boldsymbol{\beta}$,

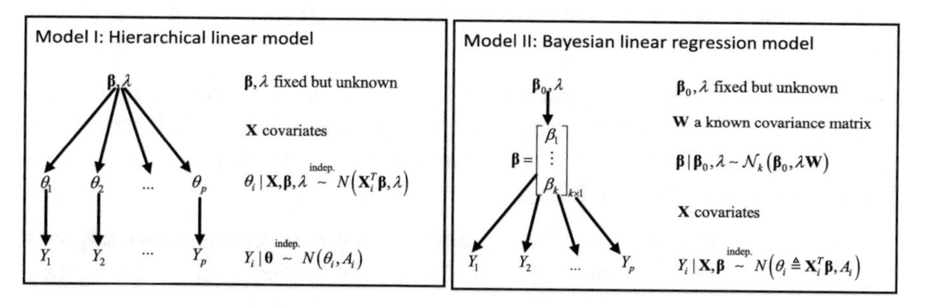

Fig. 1 Graphical illustration of the two heteroscedastic hierarchical linear models

and $\boldsymbol{\mu} = (\mu_1, \ldots, \mu_p)^T \in \mathscr{L}_{\text{row}}(\boldsymbol{X})$, the row space of $\boldsymbol{X}$, then we can rewrite the posterior mean of $\boldsymbol{\theta}$ under Model I as

$$\hat{\theta}^{\lambda,\boldsymbol{\mu}} = \frac{\lambda}{\lambda + A_i} Y_i + \frac{A_i}{\lambda + A_i} \mu_i, \quad \text{with } \boldsymbol{\mu} \in \mathscr{L}_{\text{row}}(\boldsymbol{X}). \tag{2}$$

Under Model II, the posterior mean of $\boldsymbol{\theta}$ is

$$\hat{\boldsymbol{\theta}}^{\lambda,\boldsymbol{\beta}_0} = \boldsymbol{X}^T \hat{\boldsymbol{\beta}}^{\lambda,\boldsymbol{\beta}_0}, \quad \text{with } \hat{\boldsymbol{\beta}}^{\lambda,\boldsymbol{\beta}_0} = \lambda \boldsymbol{W}(\lambda \boldsymbol{W} + \boldsymbol{V})^{-1} \hat{\boldsymbol{\beta}}^{\text{WLS}} + \boldsymbol{V}(\lambda \boldsymbol{W} + \boldsymbol{V})^{-1} \boldsymbol{\beta}_0, \tag{3}$$

where $\hat{\boldsymbol{\beta}}^{\text{WLS}} = \left(\boldsymbol{X}\boldsymbol{A}^{-1}\boldsymbol{X}^T\right)^{-1} \boldsymbol{X}\boldsymbol{A}^{-1}\boldsymbol{Y}$ is the weighted least squares estimate of the regression coefficient, $\boldsymbol{A}$ is the diagonal matrix $\boldsymbol{A} = \operatorname{diag}(A_1, \ldots, A_p)$, and $\boldsymbol{V} = (\boldsymbol{X}\boldsymbol{A}^{-1}\boldsymbol{X}^T)^{-1}$. Thus, the estimate for θ_i is linear in $\boldsymbol{X}_i$, and the "shrinkage" is achieved by shrinking the regression coefficient from the weighted least squares estimate $\hat{\boldsymbol{\beta}}^{\text{WLS}}$ toward the prior coefficient $\boldsymbol{\beta}_0$.

As both Models I and II are natural generalizations of the heteroscedastic normal model (1), we want to investigate if there is an optimal choice of the hyper-parameters in each case. Specifically, we want to investigate the best empirical choice of the hyper-parameters in each case under the mean squared error loss

$$l_p(\boldsymbol{\theta}, \hat{\boldsymbol{\theta}}) = \frac{1}{p} \left\| \boldsymbol{\theta} - \hat{\boldsymbol{\theta}} \right\|^2 = \frac{1}{p} \sum_{i=1}^{p} \left(\theta_i - \hat{\theta}_i\right)^2 \tag{4}$$

with the associated risk of $\hat{\boldsymbol{\theta}}$ defined by

$$R_p(\boldsymbol{\theta}, \hat{\boldsymbol{\theta}}) = \mathbb{E}_{\boldsymbol{Y}|\boldsymbol{\theta}} \left(l_p(\boldsymbol{\theta}, \hat{\boldsymbol{\theta}}) \right),$$

where the expectation is taken with respect to $\boldsymbol{Y}$ given $\boldsymbol{\theta}$.

Remark 1 Even though we start from the Bayesian setting to motivate the form of shrinkage estimators, our discussion will be all based on the frequentist setting. Hence all probabilities and expectations throughout this article are fixed at the unknown true $\boldsymbol{\theta}$, which is free in $\mathbb{R}^p$ for Model I and confined in $\mathscr{L}_{\text{row}}(\boldsymbol{X})$ for Model II.

Remark 2 The diagonal assumption of $\boldsymbol{A}$ is quite important for Model I but not so for Model II, as in Model II we can always apply some linear transformations to obtain a diagonal covariance matrix. Without loss of generality, we will keep the diagonal assumption for $\boldsymbol{A}$ in Model II.

For the ease of exposition, we will next overview the conventional empirical Bayes estimates in a general two-level hierarchical model, which includes both

Models I and II:

$$\boldsymbol{Y}|\boldsymbol{\theta} \sim \mathcal{N}_p(\boldsymbol{\theta}, \boldsymbol{A}) \text{ and } \boldsymbol{\theta} \sim \mathcal{N}_p(\boldsymbol{\mu}, \boldsymbol{B}), \tag{5}$$

where $\boldsymbol{B}$ is a non-negative definite symmetric matrix that is restricted in an allowable set $\mathscr{B}$, and $\boldsymbol{\mu}$ is in the row space $\mathscr{L}_{\text{row}}(\boldsymbol{X})$ of $\boldsymbol{X}$.

Remark 3 Under Model I, $\boldsymbol{\mu}$ and $\boldsymbol{B}$ take the form of $\boldsymbol{\mu} = \boldsymbol{X}^T\boldsymbol{\beta}$ and $\boldsymbol{B} \in \mathscr{B} = \{\lambda \boldsymbol{I}_p : \lambda > 0\}$, whereas under Model II, $\boldsymbol{\mu}$ and $\boldsymbol{B}$ take the form of $\boldsymbol{\mu} = \boldsymbol{X}^T\boldsymbol{\beta}_0$ and $\boldsymbol{B} \in \mathscr{B} = \{\lambda \boldsymbol{X}^T\boldsymbol{W}\boldsymbol{X} : \lambda > 0\}$. It is interesting to observe that in Model I, $\boldsymbol{B}$ is of full rank, while in Model II, $\boldsymbol{B}$ is of rank k. As we shall see, this distinction will have interesting theoretical implications for the optimal shrinkage estimators.

Lemma 1 *Under the two-level hierarchical model (5), the posterior distribution is*

$$\boldsymbol{\theta}|\boldsymbol{Y} \sim \mathcal{N}_p\left(\boldsymbol{B}(\boldsymbol{A}+\boldsymbol{B})^{-1}\boldsymbol{Y} + \boldsymbol{A}(\boldsymbol{A}+\boldsymbol{B})^{-1}\boldsymbol{\mu}, \boldsymbol{A}(\boldsymbol{A}+\boldsymbol{B})^{-1}\boldsymbol{B}\right),$$

and the marginal distribution of $\boldsymbol{Y}$ *is* $\boldsymbol{Y} \sim \mathcal{N}_p(\boldsymbol{\mu}, \boldsymbol{A}+\boldsymbol{B})$.

For given values of $\boldsymbol{B}$ and $\boldsymbol{\mu}$, the posterior mean of the parameter $\boldsymbol{\theta}$ leads to the Bayes estimate

$$\hat{\boldsymbol{\theta}}^{\boldsymbol{B},\boldsymbol{\mu}} = \boldsymbol{B}(\boldsymbol{A}+\boldsymbol{B})^{-1}\boldsymbol{Y} + \boldsymbol{A}(\boldsymbol{A}+\boldsymbol{B})^{-1}\boldsymbol{\mu}. \tag{6}$$

To use the Bayes estimate in practice, one has to specify the hyper-parameters in $\boldsymbol{B}$ and $\boldsymbol{\mu}$. The conventional empirical Bayes method uses the marginal distribution of $\boldsymbol{Y}$ to estimate the hyper-parameters. For instance, the empirical Bayes maximum likelihood estimates (EBMLE) $\hat{\boldsymbol{B}}^{\text{EBMLE}}$ and $\hat{\boldsymbol{\mu}}^{\text{EBMLE}}$ are obtained by maximizing the marginal likelihood of $\boldsymbol{Y}$:

$$\left(\hat{\boldsymbol{B}}^{\text{EBMLE}}, \hat{\boldsymbol{\mu}}^{\text{EBMLE}}\right) = \underset{\substack{\boldsymbol{B}\in\mathscr{B} \\ \boldsymbol{\mu}\in\mathscr{L}_{\text{row}}(\boldsymbol{X})}}{\text{argmax}} -(\boldsymbol{Y}-\boldsymbol{\mu})^T(\boldsymbol{A}+\boldsymbol{B})^{-1}(\boldsymbol{Y}-\boldsymbol{\mu}) - \log(\det(\boldsymbol{A}+\boldsymbol{B})).$$

Alternatively, the empirical Bayes method-of-moment estimates (EBMOM) $\hat{\boldsymbol{B}}^{\text{EBMOM}}$ and $\hat{\boldsymbol{\mu}}^{\text{EBMOM}}$ are obtained by solving the following moment equations for $\boldsymbol{B} \in \mathscr{B}$ and $\boldsymbol{\mu} \in \mathscr{L}_{\text{row}}(\boldsymbol{X})$:

$$\boldsymbol{\mu} = \boldsymbol{X}^T\left(\boldsymbol{X}(\boldsymbol{A}+\boldsymbol{B})^{-1}\boldsymbol{X}^T\right)^{-1}\boldsymbol{X}(\boldsymbol{A}+\boldsymbol{B})^{-1}\boldsymbol{Y},$$

$$\boldsymbol{B} = (\boldsymbol{Y}-\boldsymbol{\mu})(\boldsymbol{Y}-\boldsymbol{\mu})^T - \boldsymbol{A}.$$

If no solutions of $\boldsymbol{B}$ can be found in $\mathscr{B}$, we then set $\hat{\boldsymbol{B}}^{\text{EBMOM}} = \boldsymbol{0}_{p\times p}$. Adjustment for the loss of k degrees of freedom from the estimation of $\boldsymbol{\mu}$ might be applicable for $\boldsymbol{B} = \lambda\boldsymbol{C}$ ($\boldsymbol{C} = \boldsymbol{I}_p$ for Model I and $\boldsymbol{X}^T\boldsymbol{W}\boldsymbol{X}$ for Model II): we can replace the second moment equation by

$$\lambda = \left(\frac{p}{p-k} \frac{\|\boldsymbol{Y} - \boldsymbol{\mu}\|^2}{\mathrm{tr}\,(\boldsymbol{C})} - \frac{\mathrm{tr}\,(\boldsymbol{A})}{\mathrm{tr}\,(\boldsymbol{C})} \right)^+ .$$

The corresponding empirical Bayes shrinkage estimator $\hat{\boldsymbol{\theta}}^{\mathrm{EBMLE}}$ or $\hat{\boldsymbol{\theta}}^{\mathrm{EBMOM}}$ is then formed by plugging $(\hat{\boldsymbol{B}}^{\mathrm{EBMLE}}, \hat{\boldsymbol{\mu}}^{\mathrm{EBMLE}})$ or $(\hat{\boldsymbol{B}}^{\mathrm{EBMOM}}, \hat{\boldsymbol{\mu}}^{\mathrm{EBMOM}})$ into Eq. (6).

3 URE Estimates

The formulation of the empirical Bayes estimates raises a natural question: which one is preferred $\hat{\boldsymbol{\theta}}^{\mathrm{EBMLE}}$ or $\hat{\boldsymbol{\theta}}^{\mathrm{EBMOM}}$? More generally, is there an optimal way to choose the hyper-parameters? It turns out that neither $\hat{\boldsymbol{\theta}}^{\mathrm{EBMLE}}$ nor $\hat{\boldsymbol{\theta}}^{\mathrm{EBMOM}}$ is optimal. The (asymptotically) optimal estimate, instead of relying on the marginal distribution of $\boldsymbol{Y}$, is characterized by an unbiased risk estimate (URE). The idea of forming a shrinkage estimate through URE for heteroscedastic models is first suggested in [29]. We shall see that in our context of hierarchical linear models (both Models I and II) the URE estimators that we are about to introduce have (asymptotically) optimal risk properties.

The basic idea behind URE estimators is the following. Ideally we want to find the hyper-parameters that give the smallest risk. However, since the risk function depends on the unknown $\boldsymbol{\theta}$, we cannot directly minimize the risk function in practice. If we can find a good estimate of the risk function instead, then minimizing this proxy of the risk will lead to a competitive estimator.

To formally introduce the URE estimators, we start from the observation that, under the mean squared error loss (4), the risk of the Bayes estimator $\hat{\boldsymbol{\theta}}^{\boldsymbol{B},\boldsymbol{\mu}}$ for fixed $\boldsymbol{B}$ and $\boldsymbol{\mu}$ is

$$R_p(\boldsymbol{\theta}, \hat{\boldsymbol{\theta}}^{\boldsymbol{B},\boldsymbol{\mu}}) = \frac{1}{p} \left\| \boldsymbol{A} \left(\boldsymbol{A} + \boldsymbol{B}\right)^{-1} (\boldsymbol{\mu} - \boldsymbol{\theta}) \right\|^2 + \frac{1}{p} \mathrm{tr} \left(\boldsymbol{B} \left(\boldsymbol{A} + \boldsymbol{B}\right)^{-1} \boldsymbol{A} \left(\boldsymbol{A} + \boldsymbol{B}\right)^{-1} \boldsymbol{B} \right), \tag{7}$$

which can be easily shown using the bias-variance decomposition of the mean squared error. As the risk function involves the unknown $\boldsymbol{\theta}$, we cannot directly minimize it. However, an unbiased estimate of the risk is available:

$$\mathrm{URE}\,(\boldsymbol{B}, \boldsymbol{\mu}) = \frac{1}{p} \left\| \boldsymbol{A} \left(\boldsymbol{A} + \boldsymbol{B}\right)^{-1} (\boldsymbol{Y} - \boldsymbol{\mu}) \right\|^2 + \frac{1}{p} \mathrm{tr} \left(\boldsymbol{A} - 2\boldsymbol{A} \left(\boldsymbol{A} + \boldsymbol{B}\right)^{-1} \boldsymbol{A} \right), \tag{8}$$

which again can be easily shown using the bias-variance decomposition of the mean squared error. Intuitively, if $\mathrm{URE}\,(\boldsymbol{B}, \boldsymbol{\mu})$ is a good approximation of the actual risk, then we would expect the estimator obtained by minimizing the URE to have good properties. This leads to the URE estimator $\hat{\boldsymbol{\theta}}^{\mathrm{URE}}$, defined by

$$\hat{\boldsymbol{\theta}}^{\mathrm{URE}} = \hat{\boldsymbol{B}}^{\mathrm{URE}}(\boldsymbol{A} + \hat{\boldsymbol{B}}^{\mathrm{URE}})^{-1}\boldsymbol{Y} + \boldsymbol{A}(\boldsymbol{A} + \hat{\boldsymbol{B}}^{\mathrm{URE}})^{-1}\hat{\boldsymbol{\mu}}^{\mathrm{URE}}, \tag{9}$$

where

$$\left(\hat{\boldsymbol{B}}^{\mathrm{URE}}, \hat{\boldsymbol{\mu}}^{\mathrm{URE}}\right) = \underset{\boldsymbol{B}\in\mathscr{B},\ \boldsymbol{\mu}\in\mathscr{L}_{\mathrm{row}}(\boldsymbol{X})}{\operatorname{argmin}} \ \mathrm{URE}\,(\boldsymbol{B}, \boldsymbol{\mu}).$$

It is worth noting that the value of $\boldsymbol{\mu}$ that minimizes (8) for a given $\boldsymbol{B}$ is neither the ordinary least squares (OLS) nor the weighted least squares (WLS) regression estimate, echoing similar observation as in [29].

In the URE estimator (9), $\hat{\boldsymbol{B}}^{\mathrm{URE}}$ and $\hat{\boldsymbol{\mu}}^{\mathrm{URE}}$ are jointly determined by minimizing the URE. When the number of independent statistical units p is small or moderate, joint minimization of $\boldsymbol{B}$ and the vector $\boldsymbol{\mu}$, however, may be too ambitious. In this setting, it might be beneficial to set $\boldsymbol{\mu}$ by a predetermined rule and only optimize $\boldsymbol{B}$, as it might reduce the variability of the resulting estimate. In particular, we can consider shrinking toward a generalized least squares (GLS) regression estimate

$$\hat{\boldsymbol{\mu}}^{\boldsymbol{M}} = \boldsymbol{X}^T\left(\boldsymbol{X}\boldsymbol{M}\boldsymbol{X}^T\right)^{-1}\boldsymbol{X}\boldsymbol{M}\boldsymbol{Y} = \boldsymbol{P}_{\boldsymbol{M},\boldsymbol{X}}\boldsymbol{Y},$$

where $\boldsymbol{M}$ is a *prespecified* symmetric positive definite matrix. This use of $\hat{\boldsymbol{\mu}}^{\boldsymbol{M}}$ gives the shrinkage estimate $\hat{\boldsymbol{\theta}}^{\boldsymbol{B},\hat{\boldsymbol{\mu}}^{\boldsymbol{M}}} = \boldsymbol{B}(\boldsymbol{A}+\boldsymbol{B})^{-1}\boldsymbol{Y} + \boldsymbol{A}(\boldsymbol{A}+\boldsymbol{B})^{-1}\hat{\boldsymbol{\mu}}^{\boldsymbol{M}}$, where one only needs to determine $\boldsymbol{B}$. We can construct another URE estimate for this purpose. Similar to the previous construction, we note that $\hat{\boldsymbol{\theta}}^{\boldsymbol{B},\hat{\boldsymbol{\mu}}^{\boldsymbol{M}}}$ has risk

$$\begin{aligned} R_p(\boldsymbol{\theta}, \hat{\boldsymbol{\theta}}^{\boldsymbol{B},\hat{\boldsymbol{\mu}}^{\boldsymbol{M}}}) =& \frac{1}{p}\left\|\boldsymbol{A}\left(\boldsymbol{A}+\boldsymbol{B}\right)^{-1}\left(\boldsymbol{I}_p - \boldsymbol{P}_{\boldsymbol{M},\boldsymbol{X}}\right)\boldsymbol{\theta}\right\|^2 \\ &+ \frac{1}{p}\mathrm{tr}\left(\left(\boldsymbol{I}_p - \boldsymbol{A}\left(\boldsymbol{A}+\boldsymbol{B}\right)^{-1}\left(\boldsymbol{I}_p - \boldsymbol{P}_{\boldsymbol{M},\boldsymbol{X}}\right)\right)\boldsymbol{A}\right. \\ &\times \left.\left(\boldsymbol{I}_p - \boldsymbol{A}\left(\boldsymbol{A}+\boldsymbol{B}\right)^{-1}\left(\boldsymbol{I}_p - \boldsymbol{P}_{\boldsymbol{M},\boldsymbol{X}}\right)\right)^T\right). \end{aligned} \tag{10}$$

An unbiased risk estimate of it is

$$\mathrm{URE}_{\boldsymbol{M}}\left(\boldsymbol{B}\right) = \frac{1}{p}\left\|\boldsymbol{A}\left(\boldsymbol{A}+\boldsymbol{B}\right)^{-1}\left(\boldsymbol{Y} - \hat{\boldsymbol{\mu}}^{\boldsymbol{M}}\right)\right\|^2 + \frac{1}{p}\mathrm{tr}\left(\boldsymbol{A} - 2\boldsymbol{A}\left(\boldsymbol{A}+\boldsymbol{B}\right)^{-1}\left(\boldsymbol{I}_p - \boldsymbol{P}_{\boldsymbol{M},\boldsymbol{X}}\right)\boldsymbol{A}\right). \tag{11}$$

Both (10) and (11) can be easily proved by the bias-variance decomposition of mean squared error. Minimizing $\mathrm{URE}_{\boldsymbol{M}}\left(\boldsymbol{B}\right)$ over $\boldsymbol{B}$ gives the URE GLS shrinkage estimator (which shrinks toward $\hat{\boldsymbol{\mu}}^{\boldsymbol{M}}$):

$$\hat{\boldsymbol{\theta}}_{\boldsymbol{M}}^{\mathrm{URE}} = \hat{\boldsymbol{B}}_{\boldsymbol{M}}^{\mathrm{URE}} \left(\boldsymbol{A} + \hat{\boldsymbol{B}}_{\boldsymbol{M}}^{\mathrm{URE}}\right)^{-1} \boldsymbol{Y} + \boldsymbol{A} \left(\boldsymbol{A} + \hat{\boldsymbol{B}}_{\boldsymbol{M}}^{\mathrm{URE}}\right)^{-1} \hat{\boldsymbol{\mu}}^{\boldsymbol{M}}, \tag{12}$$

where

$$\hat{\boldsymbol{B}}_{\boldsymbol{M}}^{\mathrm{URE}} = \underset{\boldsymbol{B} \in \mathscr{B}}{\operatorname{argmin}}\, \mathrm{URE}_{\boldsymbol{M}}(\boldsymbol{B}).$$

Remark 4 When $\boldsymbol{M} = \boldsymbol{I}_p$, clearly $\hat{\boldsymbol{\mu}}^{\boldsymbol{M}} = \hat{\boldsymbol{\mu}}^{\mathrm{OLS}}$, the ordinary least squares regression estimate. When $\boldsymbol{M} = \boldsymbol{A}^{-1}$, then $\hat{\boldsymbol{\mu}}^{\boldsymbol{M}} = \hat{\boldsymbol{\mu}}^{\mathrm{WLS}}$, the weighted least squares regression estimate.

Remark 5 Tan [28] briefly discussed the URE minimization approach for Model I without the covariates in [29] in relation to [11], where Model I is assumed but an unbiased estimate of the mean prediction error (rather than the mean squared error) is used to form a predictor (rather than an estimator).

Remark 6 In the homoscedastic case, (12) reduces to standard shrinkage toward a subspace $\mathscr{L}_{\mathrm{row}}(\boldsymbol{X})$, as discussed, for instance, in [23] and [19].

4 Theoretical Properties of URE Estimates

This section is devoted to the risk properties of the URE estimators. Our core theoretical result is to show that the risk estimate URE is not only unbiased for the risk but, more importantly, uniformly close to the actual loss. We therefore expect that minimizing URE would lead to an estimate with competitive risk properties.

4.1 Uniform Convergence of URE

To present our theoretical result, we first define $\mathscr{L}$ to be a subset of $\mathscr{L}_{\mathrm{row}}(\boldsymbol{X})$:

$$\mathscr{L} = \{\boldsymbol{\mu} \in \mathscr{L}_{\mathrm{row}}(\boldsymbol{X}) : \|\boldsymbol{\mu}\| \le M p^{\kappa} \|\boldsymbol{Y}\|\},$$

where M is a large and fixed constant and $\kappa \in [0, 1/2)$ is a constant. Next, we introduce the following regularity conditions:

(A) $\sum_{i=1}^{p} A_i^2 = O(p)$; (B) $\sum_{i=1}^{p} A_i \theta_i^2 = O(p)$; (C) $\sum_{i=1}^{p} \theta_i^2 = O(p)$;
(D) $p^{-1}\boldsymbol{X}\boldsymbol{A}\boldsymbol{X}^T \to \boldsymbol{\Omega}_D$; (E) $p^{-1}\boldsymbol{X}\boldsymbol{X}^T \to \boldsymbol{\Omega}_E > 0$;
(F) $p^{-1}\boldsymbol{X}\boldsymbol{A}^{-1}\boldsymbol{X}^T \to \boldsymbol{\Omega}_F > 0$; (G) $p^{-1}\boldsymbol{X}\boldsymbol{A}^{-2}\boldsymbol{X}^T \to \boldsymbol{\Omega}_G$.

The theorem below shows that URE $(\boldsymbol{B}, \boldsymbol{\mu})$ not only unbiasedly estimates the risk but also is (asymptotically) uniformly close to the actual loss.

Theorem 1 *Assume conditions (A)–(E) for Model I or assume conditions (A) and (D)–(G) for Model II. In either case, we have*

$$\sup_{\boldsymbol{B}\in\mathscr{B},\ \boldsymbol{\mu}\in\mathscr{L}} \left|\mathrm{URE}\left(\boldsymbol{B},\boldsymbol{\mu}\right) - l_p\left(\boldsymbol{\theta}, \hat{\boldsymbol{\theta}}^{\boldsymbol{B},\boldsymbol{\mu}}\right)\right| \to 0 \text{ in } L^1, \text{ as } p \to \infty.$$

We want to remark here that the set $\mathscr{L}$ gives the allowable range of $\boldsymbol{\mu}$: the norm of $\boldsymbol{\mu}$ is up to an $o\left(p^{1/2}\right)$ multiple of the norm of $\boldsymbol{Y}$. This choice of $\mathscr{L}$ does not lead to any difficulty in practice because, given a large enough constant M, it will cover the shrinkage location of any sensible shrinkage estimator. We note that it is possible to define the range of sensible shrinkage locations in other ways (e.g., one might want to define it by ∞-norm in $\mathbb{R}^p$), but we find our setting more theoretically appealing and easy to work with. In particular, our assumption of the exponent $\kappa < 1/2$ is flexible enough to cover most interesting cases, including $\hat{\boldsymbol{\mu}}^{\mathrm{OLS}}$, the ordinary least squares regression estimate, and $\hat{\boldsymbol{\mu}}^{\mathrm{WLS}}$, the weighted least squares regression estimate (as in Remark 4) as shown in the following lemma.

Lemma 2 *(i)* $\hat{\boldsymbol{\mu}}^{\mathrm{OLS}} \in \mathscr{L}$. *(ii) Assume* (A) *and* (A′) $\sum_{i=1}^{p} A_i^{-2-\delta} = O(p)$ *for some* $\delta > 0$*; then* $\hat{\boldsymbol{\mu}}^{\mathrm{WLS}} \in \mathscr{L}$ *for* $\kappa = 4^{-1} + (4+2\delta)^{-1}$ *and a large enough M.*

Remark 7 We want to mention here that Theorem 1 in the case of Model I covers Theorem 5.1 of [29] (which is the special case of $k = 1$ and $\boldsymbol{X} = [1|1|\ldots|1]$) because the restriction of $|\mu| \le \max_{1\le i\le p} |Y_i|$ in [29] is contained in $\mathscr{L}$ as

$$\max_{1\le i\le p} |Y_i| = (\max_{1\le i\le p} Y_i^2)^{1/2} \le (\sum_{i=1}^{p} Y_i^2)^{1/2} = \|\boldsymbol{Y}\|.$$

Furthermore, we do not require the stronger assumption of $\sum_{i=1}^{p} |\theta_i|^{2+\delta} = O(p)$ for some $\delta > 0$ made in [29]. Note that in this case ($k = 1$ and $\boldsymbol{X} = [1|1|\ldots|1]$) we do not even require conditions (D) and (E), as condition (A) directly implies $\mathrm{tr}((\boldsymbol{X}\boldsymbol{X}^T)^{-1}\boldsymbol{X}\boldsymbol{A}\boldsymbol{X}^T) = O(1)$, the result we need in the proof of Theorem 1 for Model I.

Remark 8 In the proof of Theorem 1, the sampling distribution of $\boldsymbol{Y}$ is involved only through the moment calculations, such as $\mathbb{E}(\mathrm{tr}(\boldsymbol{Y}\boldsymbol{Y}^T - \boldsymbol{A} - \boldsymbol{\theta}\boldsymbol{\theta}^T)^2)$ and $\mathbb{E}(\|\boldsymbol{Y}\|^2)$. It is therefore straightforward to generalize Theorem 1 to the case of

$$Y_i = \theta_i + \sqrt{A_i} Z_i,$$

where Z_i follows *any* distribution with mean 0, variance 1, $\mathbb{E}\left(Z_i^3\right) = 0$, and $\mathbb{E}\left(Z_i^4\right) < \infty$. This is noteworthy as our result also covers that of [30] but the methodology we employ here does not require to control the tail behavior of Z_i as in [29, 30].

4.2 Risk Optimality

In this section, we consider the risk properties of the URE estimators. We will show that, under the hierarchical linear models, the URE estimators have (asymptotically) optimal risk, whereas it is not necessarily so for other shrinkage estimators such as the empirical Bayes ones.

A direct consequence of the uniform convergence of URE is that the URE estimator has a loss/risk that is asymptotically no larger than that of any other shrinkage estimators. Furthermore, the URE estimator is asymptotically as good as the oracle loss estimator. To be precise, let $\tilde{\boldsymbol{\theta}}^{\mathrm{OL}}$ be the oracle loss (OL) estimator defined by plugging

$$\left(\tilde{\boldsymbol{B}}^{\mathrm{OL}}, \tilde{\boldsymbol{\mu}}^{\mathrm{OL}}\right) = \underset{\boldsymbol{B}\in\mathscr{B},\ \boldsymbol{\mu}\in\mathscr{L}}{\operatorname{argmin}}\ l_p\left(\boldsymbol{\theta}, \hat{\boldsymbol{\theta}}^{\boldsymbol{B},\boldsymbol{\mu}}\right)$$

$$= \underset{\boldsymbol{B}\in\mathscr{B},\ \boldsymbol{\mu}\in\mathscr{L}}{\operatorname{argmin}} \left\| \boldsymbol{B}(\boldsymbol{A}+\boldsymbol{B})^{-1}\boldsymbol{Y} + \boldsymbol{A}(\boldsymbol{A}+\boldsymbol{B})^{-1}\boldsymbol{\mu} - \boldsymbol{\theta} \right\|^2$$

into (6). Of course, $\tilde{\boldsymbol{\theta}}^{\mathrm{OL}}$ is not really an estimator, since it depends on the unknown $\boldsymbol{\theta}$ (hence we use the notation $\tilde{\boldsymbol{\theta}}^{\mathrm{OL}}$ rather than $\hat{\boldsymbol{\theta}}^{\mathrm{OL}}$). Although not obtainable in practice, $\tilde{\boldsymbol{\theta}}^{\mathrm{OL}}$ lays down the theoretical limit that one can ever hope to reach. The next theorem shows that the URE estimator $\hat{\boldsymbol{\theta}}^{\mathrm{URE}}$ is asymptotically as good as the oracle loss estimator, and, consequently, it is asymptotically at least as good as any other shrinkage estimator.

Theorem 2 *Assume the conditions of Theorem 1 and that $\hat{\boldsymbol{\mu}}^{\mathrm{URE}} \in \mathscr{L}$. Then*

$$\lim_{p\to\infty} \mathbb{P}\left(l_p\left(\boldsymbol{\theta}, \hat{\boldsymbol{\theta}}^{\mathrm{URE}}\right) \geq l_p\left(\boldsymbol{\theta}, \tilde{\boldsymbol{\theta}}^{\mathrm{OL}}\right) + \epsilon\right) = 0 \quad \forall \epsilon > 0,$$

$$\limsup_{p\to\infty} \left(R_p\left(\boldsymbol{\theta}, \hat{\boldsymbol{\theta}}^{\mathrm{URE}}\right) - R_p\left(\boldsymbol{\theta}, \tilde{\boldsymbol{\theta}}^{\mathrm{OL}}\right)\right) = 0.$$

Corollary 1 *Assume the conditions of Theorem 1 and that $\hat{\boldsymbol{\mu}}^{\mathrm{URE}} \in \mathscr{L}$. Then for any estimator $\hat{\boldsymbol{\theta}}^{\hat{\boldsymbol{B}}_p,\hat{\boldsymbol{\mu}}_p} = \hat{\boldsymbol{B}}_p\left(\boldsymbol{A}+\hat{\boldsymbol{B}}_p\right)^{-1}\boldsymbol{Y} + \boldsymbol{A}\left(\boldsymbol{A}+\hat{\boldsymbol{B}}_p\right)^{-1}\hat{\boldsymbol{\mu}}_p$ with $\hat{\boldsymbol{B}}_p \in \mathscr{B}$ and $\hat{\boldsymbol{\mu}}_p \in \mathscr{L}$, we always have*

$$\lim_{p\to\infty} \mathbb{P}\left(l_p\left(\boldsymbol{\theta}, \hat{\boldsymbol{\theta}}^{\mathrm{URE}}\right) \geq l_p\left(\boldsymbol{\theta}, \hat{\boldsymbol{\theta}}^{\hat{\boldsymbol{B}}_p,\hat{\boldsymbol{\mu}}_p}\right) + \epsilon\right) = 0 \quad \forall \epsilon > 0,$$

$$\limsup_{p\to\infty} \left(R_p\left(\boldsymbol{\theta}, \hat{\boldsymbol{\theta}}^{\mathrm{URE}}\right) - R_p\left(\boldsymbol{\theta}, \hat{\boldsymbol{\theta}}^{\hat{\boldsymbol{B}}_p,\hat{\boldsymbol{\mu}}_p}\right)\right) \leq 0.$$

Corollary 1 tells us that the URE estimator in either Model I or II is asymptotically optimal: it has (asymptotically) the smallest loss and risk among all shrinkage estimators of the form (6).

4.3 Shrinkage Toward the Generalized Least Squares Estimate

The risk optimality also holds when we consider the URE estimator $\hat{\boldsymbol{\theta}}_M^{\text{URE}}$ that shrinks toward the GLS regression estimate $\hat{\boldsymbol{\mu}}^M = \boldsymbol{P}_{M,X}\boldsymbol{Y}$ as introduced in Sect. 3.

Theorem 3 *Assume the conditions of Theorem 1, $\hat{\boldsymbol{\mu}}^M \in \mathscr{L}$, and*

$$p^{-1}\boldsymbol{X}\boldsymbol{M}\boldsymbol{X}^T \to \boldsymbol{\Omega}_1 > 0, \quad p^{-1}\boldsymbol{X}\boldsymbol{A}\boldsymbol{M}\boldsymbol{X}^T \to \boldsymbol{\Omega}_2, \quad p^{-1}\boldsymbol{X}\boldsymbol{M}\boldsymbol{A}^2\boldsymbol{M}\boldsymbol{X}^T \to \boldsymbol{\Omega}_3, \tag{13}$$

where only the first and third conditions above are assumed for Model I and only the first and the second are assumed for Model II. Then we have

$$\sup_{\boldsymbol{B}\in\mathscr{B}} \left| \text{URE}_M(\boldsymbol{B}) - l_p\left(\boldsymbol{\theta}, \hat{\boldsymbol{\theta}}^{\boldsymbol{B},\hat{\boldsymbol{\mu}}^M}\right)\right| \to 0 \text{ in } L^1 \text{ as } p \to \infty. \tag{14}$$

As a corollary, for any estimator $\hat{\boldsymbol{\theta}}^{\hat{\boldsymbol{B}}_p,\hat{\boldsymbol{\mu}}^M} = \hat{\boldsymbol{B}}_p\left(\boldsymbol{A}+\hat{\boldsymbol{B}}_p\right)^{-1}\boldsymbol{Y} + \boldsymbol{A}\left(\boldsymbol{A}+\hat{\boldsymbol{B}}_p\right)^{-1}\hat{\boldsymbol{\mu}}^M$ with $\hat{\boldsymbol{B}}_p \in \mathscr{B}$, we always have

$$\lim_{p\to\infty} \mathbb{P}\left(l_p\left(\boldsymbol{\theta}, \hat{\boldsymbol{\theta}}_M^{\text{URE}}\right) \geq l_p\left(\boldsymbol{\theta}, \hat{\boldsymbol{\theta}}^{\hat{\boldsymbol{B}}_p,\hat{\boldsymbol{\mu}}^M}\right) + \epsilon\right) = 0 \quad \forall \epsilon > 0,$$

$$\limsup_{p\to\infty}\left(R_p\left(\boldsymbol{\theta}, \hat{\boldsymbol{\theta}}_M^{\text{URE}}\right) - R_p\left(\boldsymbol{\theta}, \hat{\boldsymbol{\theta}}^{\hat{\boldsymbol{B}}_p,\hat{\boldsymbol{\mu}}^M}\right)\right) \leq 0.$$

Remark 9 For shrinking toward $\hat{\boldsymbol{\mu}}^{\text{OLS}}$, where $\boldsymbol{M} = \boldsymbol{I}_p$, we know from Lemma 2 that $\hat{\boldsymbol{\mu}}^{\text{OLS}}$ is automatically in $\mathscr{L}$, so we only need one more condition $p^{-1}\boldsymbol{X}\boldsymbol{A}^2\boldsymbol{X}^T \to \boldsymbol{\Omega}_3$ for Model I. For shrinking toward $\hat{\boldsymbol{\mu}}^{\text{WLS}}$, where $\boldsymbol{M} = \boldsymbol{A}^{-1}$, (13) is the same as the conditions (E) and (F) of Theorem 1, so additionally we only need to assume (A′) of Lemma 2 and (F) for Model I.

5 Semiparametric URE Estimators

We have established the (asymptotic) optimality of the URE estimators $\hat{\boldsymbol{\theta}}^{\text{URE}}$ and $\hat{\boldsymbol{\theta}}_M^{\text{URE}}$ in the previous section. One limitation of the result is that the class over which the URE estimators are optimal is specified by a parametric form: $\boldsymbol{B} = \lambda\boldsymbol{C}$ $(0 \leq \lambda \leq$

∞) in Eq. (6), where $\boldsymbol{C} = \boldsymbol{I}_p$ for Model I and $\boldsymbol{C} = \boldsymbol{X}^T\boldsymbol{W}\boldsymbol{X}$ for Model II. Aiming to provide a more flexible and, at the same time, efficient estimation procedure, we consider in this section a class of semiparametric shrinkage estimators. Our consideration is inspired by Xie et al. [29].

5.1 Semiparametric URE Estimator Under Model I

To motivate the semiparametric shrinkage estimators, let us first revisit the Bayes estimator $\hat{\boldsymbol{\theta}}^{\lambda,\boldsymbol{\mu}}$ under Model I, as given in (2). It is seen that the Bayes estimate of each mean parameter θ_i is obtained by shrinking Y_i toward the linear estimate $\mu_i = \boldsymbol{X}_i^T\boldsymbol{\beta}$, and that the amount of shrinkage is governed by A_i, the variance: the larger the variance, the stronger is the shrinkage. This feature makes intuitive sense.

With this observation in mind, we consider the following shrinkage estimators under Model I:

$$\hat{\theta}_i^{\boldsymbol{b},\boldsymbol{\mu}} = (1 - b_i)\, Y_i + b_i\mu_i, \quad \text{with } \boldsymbol{\mu} \in \mathscr{L}_{\text{row}}(\boldsymbol{X}),$$

where $\boldsymbol{b}$ satisfies the monotonic constraint

$$\text{MON}(\boldsymbol{A}) : b_i \in [0, 1],\ b_i \leq b_j \text{ whenever } A_i \leq A_j.$$

MON ($\boldsymbol{A}$) asks the estimator to shrink more for an observation with a larger variance. Since other than this intuitive requirement, we do not post any parametric restriction on b_i, this class of estimators is semiparametric in nature.

Following the optimality result for the parametric case, we want to investigate, for such a general estimator $\hat{\boldsymbol{\theta}}^{\boldsymbol{b},\boldsymbol{\mu}}$ with $\boldsymbol{b} \in \text{MON}(\boldsymbol{A})$ and $\boldsymbol{\mu} \in \mathscr{L}_{\text{row}}(\boldsymbol{X})$, whether there exists an optimal choice of $\boldsymbol{b}$ and $\boldsymbol{\mu}$. In fact, we will see shortly that such an optimal choice exists, and this asymptotically optimal choice is again characterized by an unbiased risk estimate (URE). For a general estimator $\hat{\boldsymbol{\theta}}^{\boldsymbol{b},\boldsymbol{\mu}}$ with *fixed* $\boldsymbol{b}$ and $\boldsymbol{\mu} \in \mathscr{L}_{\text{row}}(\boldsymbol{X})$, an unbiased estimate of its risk $R_p(\boldsymbol{\theta}, \hat{\boldsymbol{\theta}}^{\boldsymbol{b},\boldsymbol{\mu}})$ is

$$\text{URE}^{SP}(\boldsymbol{b}, \boldsymbol{\mu}) = \frac{1}{p}\left\|\text{diag}(\boldsymbol{b})(\boldsymbol{Y} - \boldsymbol{\mu})\right\|^2 + \frac{1}{p}\text{tr}\left(\boldsymbol{A} - 2\text{diag}(\boldsymbol{b})\boldsymbol{A}\right),$$

which can be easily seen by taking $\boldsymbol{B} = \boldsymbol{A}(\text{diag}(\boldsymbol{b})^{-1} - \boldsymbol{I}_p)$ in (8). Note that we use the superscript "*SP*" (semiparametric) to denote it. Minimizing over $\boldsymbol{b}$ and $\boldsymbol{\mu}$ leads to the semiparametric URE estimator $\hat{\boldsymbol{\theta}}_{SP}^{\text{URE}}$, defined by

$$\hat{\boldsymbol{\theta}}_{SP}^{\text{URE}} = (\boldsymbol{I}_p - \text{diag}(\hat{\boldsymbol{b}}_{SP}^{\text{URE}}))\boldsymbol{Y} + \text{diag}(\hat{\boldsymbol{b}}_{SP}^{\text{URE}})\hat{\boldsymbol{\mu}}_{SP}^{\text{URE}}, \tag{15}$$

where

$$\left(\hat{\boldsymbol{b}}_{SP}^{\mathrm{URE}}, \hat{\boldsymbol{\mu}}_{SP}^{\mathrm{URE}}\right) = \underset{\boldsymbol{b} \in \mathrm{MON}(\boldsymbol{A}),\ \boldsymbol{\mu} \in \mathscr{L}_{\mathrm{row}}(\boldsymbol{X})}{\operatorname{argmin}} \mathrm{URE}^{SP}(\boldsymbol{b}, \boldsymbol{\mu}).$$

Theorem 4 *Assume conditions (A)–(E). Then under Model I we have*

$$\sup_{\boldsymbol{b} \in \mathrm{MON}(\boldsymbol{A}),\ \boldsymbol{\mu} \in \mathscr{L}} \left| \mathrm{URE}^{SP}(\boldsymbol{b}, \boldsymbol{\mu}) - l_p\left(\boldsymbol{\theta}, \hat{\boldsymbol{\theta}}^{\boldsymbol{b}, \boldsymbol{\mu}}\right) \right| \to 0 \text{ in } L^1 \text{ as } p \to \infty.$$

As a corollary, for any estimator $\hat{\boldsymbol{\theta}}^{\hat{\boldsymbol{b}}_p, \hat{\boldsymbol{\mu}}_p} = (\boldsymbol{I}_p - \mathrm{diag}(\hat{\boldsymbol{b}}_p))\boldsymbol{Y} + \mathrm{diag}(\hat{\boldsymbol{b}}_p)\hat{\boldsymbol{\mu}}_p$ *with* $\hat{\boldsymbol{b}}_p \in \mathrm{MON}(\boldsymbol{A})$ *and* $\hat{\boldsymbol{\mu}}_p \in \mathscr{L}$, *we always have*

$$\lim_{p \to \infty} \mathbb{P}\left(l_p\left(\boldsymbol{\theta}, \hat{\boldsymbol{\theta}}_{SP}^{\mathrm{URE}}\right) \geq l_p\left(\boldsymbol{\theta}, \hat{\boldsymbol{\theta}}^{\hat{\boldsymbol{b}}_p, \hat{\boldsymbol{\mu}}_p}\right) + \epsilon \right) = 0 \quad \forall \epsilon > 0,$$

$$\limsup_{p \to \infty} \left(R_p\left(\boldsymbol{\theta}, \hat{\boldsymbol{\theta}}_{SP}^{\mathrm{URE}}\right) - R_p\left(\boldsymbol{\theta}, \hat{\boldsymbol{\theta}}^{\hat{\boldsymbol{b}}_p, \hat{\boldsymbol{\mu}}_p}\right)\right) \leq 0.$$

The proof is the same as the proofs of Theorem 1 and Corollary 1 for the case of Model I except that we replace each term of $A_i/(\lambda + A_i)$ by b_i.

5.2 Semiparametric URE Estimator Under Model II

We saw in Sect. 2 that, under Model II, shrinkage is achieved by shrinking the regression coefficient from the weighted least squares estimate $\hat{\boldsymbol{\beta}}^{\mathrm{WLS}}$ toward the prior coefficient $\boldsymbol{\beta}_0$. This suggests us to formulate the semiparametric estimators through the regression coefficient. The Bayes estimate of the regression coefficient is

$$\hat{\boldsymbol{\beta}}^{\lambda, \boldsymbol{\beta}_0} = \lambda \boldsymbol{W}(\lambda \boldsymbol{W} + \boldsymbol{V})^{-1}\hat{\boldsymbol{\beta}}^{\mathrm{WLS}} + \boldsymbol{V}(\lambda \boldsymbol{W} + \boldsymbol{V})^{-1}\boldsymbol{\beta}_0, \quad \text{with } \boldsymbol{V} = (\boldsymbol{X}\boldsymbol{A}^{-1}\boldsymbol{X}^T)^{-1}$$

as shown in (3). Applying the spectral decomposition on $\boldsymbol{W}^{-1/2}\boldsymbol{V}\boldsymbol{W}^{-1/2}$ gives $\boldsymbol{W}^{-1/2}\boldsymbol{V}\boldsymbol{W}^{-1/2} = \boldsymbol{U}\boldsymbol{\Lambda}\boldsymbol{U}^T$, where $\boldsymbol{\Lambda} = \mathrm{diag}(d_1, \ldots, d_k)$ with $d_1 \leq \cdots \leq d_k$. Using this decomposition, we can rewrite the regression coefficient as

$$\hat{\boldsymbol{\beta}}^{\lambda, \boldsymbol{\beta}_0} = \lambda \boldsymbol{W}^{1/2}\boldsymbol{U}(\lambda \boldsymbol{I}_k + \boldsymbol{\Lambda})^{-1}\boldsymbol{U}^T\boldsymbol{W}^{-1/2}\hat{\boldsymbol{\beta}}^{\mathrm{WLS}} + \boldsymbol{W}^{1/2}\boldsymbol{U}\boldsymbol{\Lambda}(\lambda \boldsymbol{I}_k + \boldsymbol{\Lambda})^{-1}\boldsymbol{U}^T\boldsymbol{W}^{-1/2}\boldsymbol{\beta}_0.$$

If we denote $\boldsymbol{Z} = \boldsymbol{U}^T \boldsymbol{W}^{1/2} \boldsymbol{X}$ as the transformed covariate matrix, the estimate $\hat{\boldsymbol{\theta}}^{\lambda,\boldsymbol{\beta}_0} = \boldsymbol{X}^T \hat{\boldsymbol{\beta}}^{\lambda,\boldsymbol{\beta}_0}$ of $\boldsymbol{\theta}$ can be rewritten as

$$\hat{\boldsymbol{\theta}}^{\lambda,\boldsymbol{\beta}_0} = \boldsymbol{Z}^T \left(\lambda \left(\lambda \boldsymbol{I}_k + \boldsymbol{\Lambda} \right)^{-1} \boldsymbol{U}^T \boldsymbol{W}^{-1/2} \hat{\boldsymbol{\beta}}^{\mathrm{WLS}} + \boldsymbol{\Lambda} \left(\lambda \boldsymbol{I}_k + \boldsymbol{\Lambda} \right)^{-1} \boldsymbol{U}^T \boldsymbol{W}^{-1/2} \boldsymbol{\beta}_0 \right).$$

Now we see that $\lambda \left(\lambda \boldsymbol{I}_k + \boldsymbol{\Lambda} \right)^{-1} = \mathrm{diag}(\lambda / (\lambda + d_i))$ plays the role as the shrinkage factor. The larger the value of d_i, the smaller $\lambda / (\lambda + d_i)$, i.e., the stronger the shrinkage toward $\boldsymbol{\beta}_0$. Thus, d_i can be viewed as the effective "variance" component for the i-th regression coefficient (under the transformation). This observation motivates us to consider semiparametric shrinkage estimators of the following form

$$\begin{aligned} \hat{\boldsymbol{\theta}}^{\boldsymbol{b},\boldsymbol{\beta}_0} &= \boldsymbol{Z}^T \left(\left(\boldsymbol{I}_k - \mathrm{diag}\left(\boldsymbol{b}\right) \right) \boldsymbol{U}^T \boldsymbol{W}^{-1/2} \hat{\boldsymbol{\beta}}^{\mathrm{WLS}} + \mathrm{diag}\left(\boldsymbol{b}\right) \boldsymbol{U}^T \boldsymbol{W}^{-1/2} \boldsymbol{\beta}_0 \right) \\ &= \boldsymbol{Z}^T \left(\left(\boldsymbol{I}_k - \mathrm{diag}\left(\boldsymbol{b}\right) \right) \boldsymbol{\Lambda} \boldsymbol{Z} \boldsymbol{A}^{-1} \boldsymbol{Y} + \mathrm{diag}\left(\boldsymbol{b}\right) \boldsymbol{U}^T \boldsymbol{W}^{-1/2} \boldsymbol{\beta}_0 \right), \end{aligned} \tag{16}$$

where $\boldsymbol{b}$ satisfies the following monotonic constraint

$$\mathrm{MON}\left(\boldsymbol{D}\right) : b_i \in [0,1]\,,\ b_i \le b_j \text{ whenever } d_i \le d_j.$$

This constraint captures the intuition that, the larger the effective variance, the stronger is the shrinkage.

For *fixed* $\boldsymbol{b}$ and $\boldsymbol{\beta}_0$, an unbiased estimate of the risk $R_p(\boldsymbol{\theta}, \hat{\boldsymbol{\theta}}^{\boldsymbol{b},\boldsymbol{\beta}_0})$ is

$$\begin{aligned} \mathrm{URE}^{SP}\left(\boldsymbol{b}, \boldsymbol{\beta}_0\right) = &\frac{1}{p} \left\| \boldsymbol{Z}^T \left(\boldsymbol{I}_k - \mathrm{diag}\left(\boldsymbol{b}\right) \right) \boldsymbol{\Lambda} \boldsymbol{Z} \boldsymbol{A}^{-1} \boldsymbol{Y} + \boldsymbol{Z}^T \mathrm{diag}\left(\boldsymbol{b}\right) \boldsymbol{U}^T \boldsymbol{W}^{-1/2} \boldsymbol{\beta}_0 - \boldsymbol{Y} \right\|^2 \\ &+ \frac{1}{p} \mathrm{tr}\left(2\boldsymbol{Z}^T \left(\boldsymbol{I}_k - \mathrm{diag}\left(\boldsymbol{b}\right) \right) \boldsymbol{\Lambda} \boldsymbol{Z} - \boldsymbol{A} \right), \end{aligned}$$

which can be shown using the bias-variance decomposition of the mean squared error. Minimizing it gives the URE estimate of $(\boldsymbol{b}, \boldsymbol{\beta}_0)$:

$$\left(\hat{\boldsymbol{b}}_{SP}^{\mathrm{URE}}, \left(\hat{\boldsymbol{\beta}}_0 \right)_{SP}^{\mathrm{URE}} \right) = \underset{\boldsymbol{b} \in \mathrm{MON}(\boldsymbol{D}),\ \boldsymbol{\beta}_0 \in \mathbb{R}^k}{\mathrm{argmin}} \mathrm{URE}^{SP}\left(\boldsymbol{b}, \boldsymbol{\beta}_0\right),$$

which upon plugging into (16) yields the semiparametric URE estimator $\hat{\boldsymbol{\theta}}_{SP}^{\mathrm{URE}}$ under Model II.

Theorem 5 *Assume conditions (A), (D)–(G). Then under Model II we have*

$$\sup_{\boldsymbol{b} \in \mathrm{MON}(\boldsymbol{D}),\ \boldsymbol{X}^T \boldsymbol{\beta}_0 \in \mathcal{L}} \left| \mathrm{URE}^{SP}\left(\boldsymbol{b}, \boldsymbol{\beta}_0\right) - l_p\left(\boldsymbol{\theta}, \hat{\boldsymbol{\theta}}^{\boldsymbol{b},\boldsymbol{\beta}_0} \right) \right| \to 0 \text{ in } L^1 \text{ as } p \to \infty.$$

As a corollary, for any estimator $\hat{\boldsymbol{\theta}}^{\hat{\boldsymbol{b}}_p, \hat{\boldsymbol{\beta}}_{0,p}}$ *obtained from (16) with* $\hat{\boldsymbol{b}}_p \in \text{MON}(\boldsymbol{D})$ *and* $\boldsymbol{X}^T \hat{\boldsymbol{\beta}}_0 \in \mathscr{L}$*, we always have*

$$\lim_{p\to\infty} \mathbb{P}\left(l_p\left(\boldsymbol{\theta}, \hat{\boldsymbol{\theta}}_{SP}^{\text{URE}}\right) \geq l_p\left(\boldsymbol{\theta}, \hat{\boldsymbol{\theta}}^{\hat{\boldsymbol{b}}_p, \hat{\boldsymbol{\beta}}_{0,p}}\right) + \epsilon\right) = 0 \quad \forall \epsilon > 0,$$

$$\limsup_{p\to\infty} \left(R_p\left(\boldsymbol{\theta}, \hat{\boldsymbol{\theta}}_{SP}^{\text{URE}}\right) - R_p\left(\boldsymbol{\theta}, \hat{\boldsymbol{\theta}}^{\hat{\boldsymbol{b}}_p, \hat{\boldsymbol{\beta}}_{0,p}}\right)\right) \leq 0.$$

The proof of the theorem is essentially identical to those of Theorem 1 and Corollary 1 for the case of Model II except that we replace each $d_i/(\lambda + d_i)$ by b_i.

6 Simulation Study

In this section, we conduct simulations to study the performance of the URE estimators. For the sake of space, we will focus on Model I. The four URE estimators are the parametric $\hat{\boldsymbol{\theta}}^{\text{URE}}$ of Eq. (9), the parametric $\hat{\boldsymbol{\theta}}_{\boldsymbol{M}}^{\text{URE}}$ of Eq. (12) that shrinks toward the OLS estimate $\hat{\boldsymbol{\mu}}^{\text{OLS}}$ (i.e., the matrix $\boldsymbol{M} = \boldsymbol{I}_p$), the semiparametric $\hat{\boldsymbol{\theta}}_{SP}^{\text{URE}}$ of Eq. (15), and the semiparametric $\hat{\boldsymbol{\theta}}_{SP}^{\text{URE, OLS}}$ that shrinks toward $\hat{\boldsymbol{\mu}}^{\text{OLS}}$, which is formed similarly to $\hat{\boldsymbol{\theta}}_{\boldsymbol{M}}^{\text{URE}}$ by replacing $A_i/(\lambda + A_i)$ with a sequence $\boldsymbol{b} \in \text{MON}(\boldsymbol{A})$. The competitors here are the two empirical Bayes estimators $\hat{\boldsymbol{\theta}}^{\text{EBMLE}}$ and $\hat{\boldsymbol{\theta}}^{\text{EBMOM}}$, and the positive part James-Stein estimator $\hat{\boldsymbol{\theta}}^{\text{JS+}}$ as described in [2, 17]:

$$\hat{\theta}_i^{\text{JS+}} = \hat{\mu}_i^{\text{WLS}} + \left(1 - \frac{p-k-2}{\sum_{i=1}^p \left(Y_i - \hat{\mu}_i^{\text{WLS}}\right)^2 / A_i}\right)^+ \left(Y_i - \hat{\mu}_i^{\text{WLS}}\right).$$

As a reference, we also compare these shrinkage estimators with $\tilde{\boldsymbol{\theta}}^{\text{OR}}$, the parametric oracle risk (OR) estimator, defined as plugging $\tilde{\lambda}^{\text{OR}} \boldsymbol{I}_p$ and $\tilde{\boldsymbol{\mu}}^{\text{OR}}$ into Eq. (6), where

$$\left(\tilde{\lambda}^{\text{OR}}, \tilde{\boldsymbol{\mu}}^{\text{OR}}\right) = \underset{0 \leq \lambda \leq \infty,\ \boldsymbol{\mu} \in \mathscr{L}_{\text{row}}(\boldsymbol{X})}{\text{argmin}} R_p\left(\boldsymbol{\theta}, \hat{\boldsymbol{\theta}}^{\lambda, \boldsymbol{\mu}}\right)$$

and the expression of $R_p(\boldsymbol{\theta}, \hat{\boldsymbol{\theta}}^{\lambda, \boldsymbol{\mu}})$ is given in (7) with $\boldsymbol{B} = \lambda \boldsymbol{I}_p$. The oracle risk estimator $\tilde{\boldsymbol{\theta}}^{\text{OR}}$ cannot be used without the knowledge of $\boldsymbol{\theta}$, but it does provide a sensible lower bound of the risk achievable by any shrinkage estimator with the given parametric form.

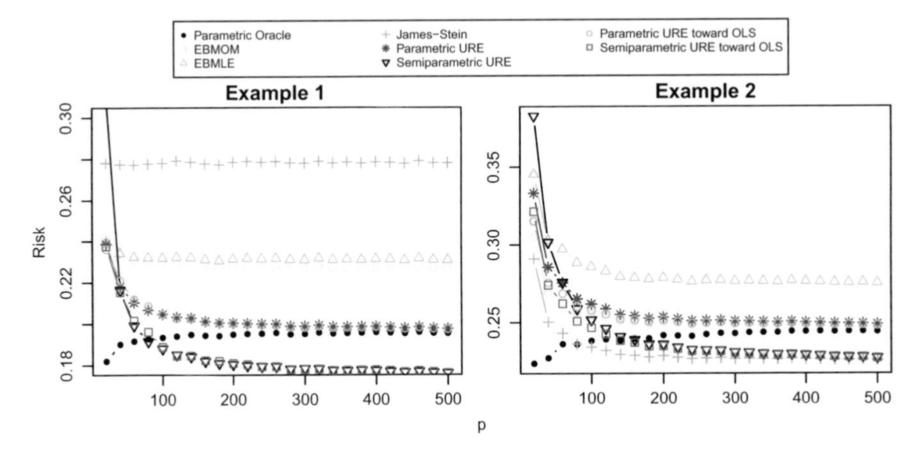

Fig. 2 Comparison of the risks of different shrinkage estimators for the two simulation examples

For each simulation, we draw (A_i, θ_i) $(i = 1, 2, \ldots, p)$ independently from a distribution $\pi\,(A_i, \theta_i|\boldsymbol{X}_i, \boldsymbol{\beta})$ and then draw Y_i given (A_i, θ_i). The shrinkage estimators are then applied to the generated data. This process is repeated 5000 times. The sample size p is chosen to vary from 20 to 500 with an increment of length 20. In the simulation, we fix a true but unknown $\boldsymbol{\beta} = (-1.5, 4, -3)^T$ and a known covariates $\boldsymbol{X}$, whose each element is randomly generated from Unif $(-10, 10)$. The risk performance of the different shrinkage estimators is given in Fig. 2.

Example 1 The setting in this example is chosen in such a way that it reflects grouping in the data:

$$A_i \sim 0.5 \cdot 1_{\{A_i=0.1\}} + 0.5 \cdot 1_{\{A_i=0.5\}};$$

$$\theta_i|A_i \sim N\left(2 \cdot 1_{\{A_i=0.1\}} + \boldsymbol{X}_i^T\boldsymbol{\beta}, 0.5^2\right);\; Y_i \sim N\left(\theta_i, A_i\right).$$

Here the normality for the sampling distribution of Y_i's is asserted. We can see that the four URE estimators perform much better than the two empirical Bayes ones and the James-Stein estimator. Also notice that both of the two (parametric and semiparametric) URE estimators that shrink towards $\hat{\boldsymbol{\mu}}^{\text{OLS}}$ is almost as good as the other two with general data-driven shrinkage location—largely due to the existence of covariate information. We note that this is quite different from the case of [29], where without the covariate information the estimator that shrinks toward the grand mean of the data performs significantly worse than the URE estimator with general data-driven shrinkage location.

Example 2 In this example, we allow Y_i to depart from the normal distribution to illustrate that the performance of those URE estimators does not rely on the normality assumption:

$$A_i \sim \text{Unif}\,(0.1, 1)\,;\ \theta_i = A_i + \boldsymbol{X}_i^T \boldsymbol{\beta};$$
$$Y_i \sim \text{Unif}(\theta_i - \sqrt{3}A_i, \theta_i + \sqrt{3}A_i).$$

As expected, the four URE estimators perform better or at least as good as the empirical Bayes estimators. The EBMLE estimator performs the worst due to its sensitivity on the normality assumption. We notice that the EBMOM estimator in this example has comparable performance with the two parametric URE estimators, which makes sense as moment estimates are more robust to the sampling distribution. An interesting feature that we find in this example is that the positive part James-Stein estimator can beat the parametric oracle risk estimator and perform better than all the other shrinkage estimators for small or moderate p, even though the semiparametric URE estimators will eventually surpass the James-Stein estimator, as dictated by the asymptotic theory for large p. This feature of the James-Stein estimate is again quite different from the non-regression setting discussed in [29], where the James-Stein estimate performs the worst throughout all of their examples. In both of our examples only the semiparametric URE estimators are robust to the different levels of heteroscedasticity.

We can conclude from these two simulation examples that the semiparametric URE estimators give competitive performance and are robust to the misspecification of the sampling distribution and the different levels of the heteroscedasticity. They thus could be useful tools in analyzing large-scale data for applied researchers.

7 Empirical Analysis

In this section, we study the baseball data set of [2]. This data set consists of the batting records for all the Major League Baseball players in the 2005 season. As in [2] and [29], we build a given shrinkage estimator based on the data in the first half season and use it to predict the second half season, which can then be checked against the true record of the second half season. For each player, let the number of at-bats be N and the successful number of batting be H, then we have $H_{ij} \sim Binomial(N_{ij}, p_j)$, where $i = 1, 2$ is the season indicator and $j = 1, \cdots, p$ is the player indicator. We use the following variance-stabilizing transformation [2] before applying the shrinkage estimators

$$Y_{ij} = \arcsin \sqrt{\frac{H_{ij} + 1/4}{N_{ij} + 1/2}},$$

which gives $Y_{ij} \dot{\sim} N(\theta_j, (4N_{ij})^{-1})$, $\theta_j = \arcsin \sqrt{p_j}$. We use

$$\mathrm{TSE}(\hat{\boldsymbol{\theta}}) = \sum_j (Y_{2j} - \hat{\theta}_j)^2 - \sum_j \frac{1}{4N_{2j}}.$$

as the error measurement for the prediction [2].

7.1 Shrinkage Estimation with Covariates

As indicated in [29], there exists a significant positive correlation between the player's batting ability and his total number of at-bats. Intuitively, a better player will be called for batting more frequently; thus, the total number of at-bats will serve as the main covariate in our analysis. The other covariate in the data set is the categorical variable of a player being a pitcher or not.

Table 1 summarizes the result, where the shrinkage estimators are applied three times—to all the players, the pitchers only, and the non-pitchers only. We use all the covariate information (number of at-bats in the first half season and being a pitcher or not) in the first analysis, whereas in the second and the third analyses we only use the number of at-bats as the covariate. The values reported are ratios of the error of a given estimator to that of the benchmark naive estimator, which simply uses the first half season Y_{1j} to predict the second half Y_{2j}. Note that in Table 1, if no covariate is involved (i.e., when $\boldsymbol{X} = [1|\cdots|1]$), the OLS reduces to the grand mean of the training data as in [29].

Table 1 Prediction errors of batting averages using different shrinkage estimators

	All		Pitchers		Non-pitchers	
p for estimation	567		81		486	
p for validation	499		64		435	
Covariates?	No	Yes	No	Yes	No	Yes
Naive	1	NA	1	NA	1	NA
Ordinary least squares (OLS)	0.852	0.242	0.127	0.115	0.378	0.333
Weighted least squares (WLS)	1.074	0.219	0.127	0.087	0.468	0.290
Parametric EBMOM	0.593	0.194	0.129	0.117	0.387	**0.256**
Parametric EBMLE	0.902	0.207	0.117	0.096	0.398	0.277
James-Stein	0.525	**0.184**	0.164	0.142	0.359	0.262
Parametric URE toward OLS	0.505	0.203	0.123	0.124	0.278	0.300
Parametric URE toward WLS	0.629	0.188	0.127	0.112	0.385	0.268
Parametric URE	0.422	0.215	0.123	0.130	0.282	0.310
Semiparametric URE toward OLS	0.409	0.197	0.081	0.097	0.261	0.299
Semiparametric URE toward WLS	0.499	**0.184**	0.098	**0.083**	0.336	**0.256**
Semiparametric URE	0.419	0.201	0.077	0.126	0.278	0.314

Bold numbers highlight the best performance with covariate(s) in each case

7.2 *Discussion of the Numerical Result*

There are several interesting observations from Table 1.

1. A quick glimpse shows that including the covariate information improves the performance of essentially all shrinkage estimators. This suggests that in practice incorporating good covariates would significantly improve the estimation and prediction.
2. In general, shrinking towards WLS provides much better performance than shrinking toward OLS or a general data-driven location. This indicates the importance of a good choice of the shrinkage location in a practical problem. An improperly chosen shrinkage location might even negatively impact the performance. The reason that shrinking towards a general data-driven location is not as good as shrinking toward WLS is probably due to that the sample size is not large enough for the asymptotics to take effect.
3. Table 1 also shows the advantage of semiparametric URE estimates. For each fixed shrinkage location type (toward OLS, WLS, or general), the semiparametric URE estimator performs almost always better than their parametric counterparts. The only one exception is in the non-pitchers only case with the general data-driven location, but even there the performance difference is ignorable.
4. The best performance in all three cases (all the players, the pitchers only, and the non-pitchers only) comes from the semiparametric URE estimator that shrinks toward WLS.
5. The James-Stein estimator *with* covariates performs quite well except in the pitchers only case, which is in sharp contrast with the performance of the James-Stein estimator *without* covariates. This again highlights the importance of covariate information. In the pitchers only case, the James-Stein performs the worst no matter one includes the covariates or not. This can be attributed to the fact that the covariate information (the total number of at-bats) is very weak for the pitchers only case; in the case of weak covariate information, how to properly estimate the shrinkage factors becomes the dominating issue, and the fact that the James-Stein estimator has only *one* uniform shrinkage factor makes it not competitive.

7.3 *Shrinkage Factors*

Figure 3 shows the shrinkage factors of all the shrinkage estimators with or without the covariates for the all-players case of Table 1. We see that the shrinkage factors are all reduced after including the covariates. This makes intuitive sense because the shrinkage location now contains the covariate information, and each shrinkage estimator uses this information by shrinking more toward it, resulting in smaller shrinkage factors.

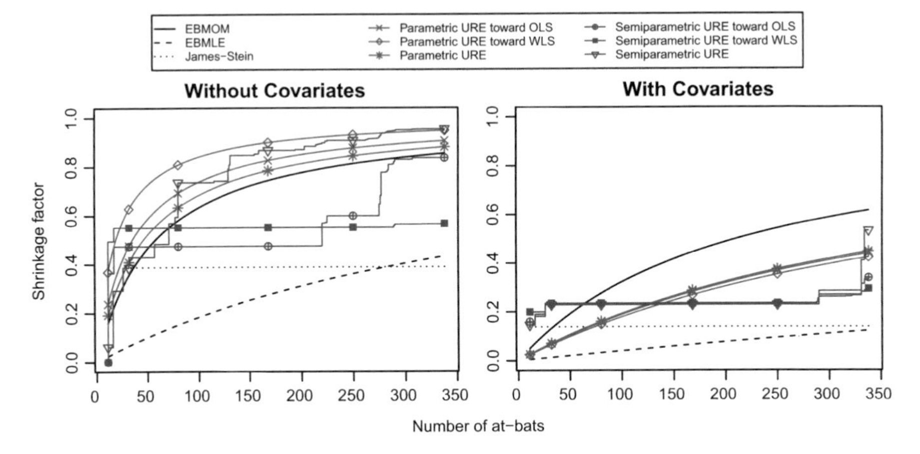

Fig. 3 Plot of the shrinkage factors $\hat{\lambda}/\left(\hat{\lambda}+A_i\right)$ or $1-\hat{b}_i$ of all the shrinkage estimators for the case of all players

8 Conclusion and Discussion

Inspired by the idea of unbiased risk estimate (URE) proposed in [29], we extend the URE framework to multivariate heteroscedastic linear models, which are more realistic in practical applications, especially for regression data that exhibits heteroscedasticity. Several parallel URE shrinkage estimators in the regression case are proposed, and these URE shrinkage estimators are all asymptotically optimal in risk compared to other shrinkage estimators, including the classical empirical Bayes ones. We also propose semiparametric estimators and conduct simulation to assess their performance under both normal and non-normal data. For data sets that exhibit a good linear relationship between the covariates and the response, a semiparametric URE estimator is expected to provide good estimation result, as we saw in the baseball data. It is also worth emphasizing that the risk optimality for the parametric and semiparametric URE estimators does not depend on the normality assumption of the sampling distribution of Y_i. Possible future work includes extending this URE minimization approach to simultaneous estimation in generalized linear models (GLMs) with canonical or more general link functions.

We conclude this article by extending the main results to the case of weighted mean squared error loss.

Weighted Mean Squared Error Loss One might want to consider the more general *weighted mean squared error* as the loss function:

$$l_p\left(\boldsymbol{\theta},\hat{\boldsymbol{\theta}};\boldsymbol{\psi}\right)=\frac{1}{p}\sum_{i=1}^{p}\psi_i\left(\theta_i-\hat{\theta}_i\right)^2,$$

where $\psi_i > 0$ are known weights such that $\sum_{i=1}^{p} \psi_i = p$. The framework proposed in this article is straightforward to generalize to this case.

For Model II, we only need to study the equivalent problem by the following transformation

$$Y_i \to \sqrt{\psi_i} Y_i, \ \theta_i \to \sqrt{\psi_i}\theta_i, \ \boldsymbol{X}_i \to \sqrt{\psi_i}\boldsymbol{X}_i, \ A_i \to \psi_i A_i, \tag{17}$$

and restate the corresponding regularity conditions in Theorem 1 by the transformed data and parameters. We then reduce the weighted mean square error problem back to the same setting we study in this article under the classical loss function (4).

Model I is more sophisticated than Model II to generalize. In addition to the transformation in Eq. (17), we also need $\lambda \to \psi_i \lambda$ in every term related to the individual unit i. Thus,

$$\sqrt{\psi_i}\theta_i | \boldsymbol{X}, \boldsymbol{\beta}, \lambda \overset{\text{indep.}}{\sim} N\left(\sqrt{\psi_i}\boldsymbol{X}_i^T \boldsymbol{\beta}, \lambda\psi_i\right),$$

so these transformed parameters $\sqrt{\psi_i}\theta_i$ are also heteroscedastic in the sense that they have different weights, while the setting we study before assumes all the weights on the θ_i are one. However, if we carefully examine the proof of Theorem 1 for the case of Model I, we can see that actually we do not much require the equal weights on the θ_i's. What is important in the proof is that the shrinkage factor for unit i is always of the form $A_i / (A_i + \lambda)$, which is *invariant* under the transformation $A_i \to \psi_i A_i$ and $\lambda \to \psi_i \lambda$. Thus, after reformulating the regularity conditions in Theorem 1 by the transformed data and parameters, we can still follow the same proof to conclude the risk optimality of URE estimators (parametric or semiparametric) even under the consideration of weighted mean squared error loss.

For completeness, here we state the most general result under the semiparametric setting for Model I. Let

$$\hat{\boldsymbol{\theta}}^{\text{URE}}_{SP,\boldsymbol{\psi}} = \left(\boldsymbol{I}_p - \text{diag}\left(\hat{\boldsymbol{b}}^{\text{URE}}_{\boldsymbol{\psi}}\right)\right) \boldsymbol{Y} + \text{diag}\left(\hat{\boldsymbol{b}}^{\text{URE}}_{\boldsymbol{\psi}}\right) \hat{\boldsymbol{\mu}}^{\text{URE}}_{\boldsymbol{\psi}},$$

$$\text{URE}(\boldsymbol{b}, \boldsymbol{\mu}; \boldsymbol{\psi}) = \frac{1}{p}\sum_{i=1}^{p} \psi_i \left(b_i^2 (Y_i - \mu_i)^2 + (1 - 2b_i) A_i\right),$$

$$\left(\hat{\boldsymbol{b}}^{\text{URE}}_{\boldsymbol{\psi}}, \hat{\boldsymbol{\mu}}^{\text{URE}}_{\boldsymbol{\psi}}\right) = \underset{\boldsymbol{b} \in \text{MON}(\boldsymbol{A}),\ \boldsymbol{\mu} \in \mathcal{L}_{\text{row}}(\boldsymbol{X})}{\text{argmin}} \text{URE}(\boldsymbol{b}, \boldsymbol{\mu}; \boldsymbol{\psi}).$$

Theorem 6 *Assume the following five conditions* (ψ-A) $\sum_{i=1}^{p} \psi_i^2 A_i^2 = O(p)$, ($\psi$-B) $\sum_{i=1}^{p} \psi_i^2 A_i \theta_i^2 = O(p)$, ($\psi$-C) $\sum_{i=1}^{p} \psi_i \theta_i^2 = O(p)$, ($\psi$-D) $p^{-1}\sum_{i=1}^{p} \psi_i^2 A_i \boldsymbol{X}_i \boldsymbol{X}_i^T$ *converges, and* (ψ-E) $p^{-1}\sum_{i=1}^{p} \psi_i \boldsymbol{X}_i \boldsymbol{X}_i^T \to \boldsymbol{\Omega}_{\boldsymbol{\psi}} > 0$. *Then we have*

$$\sup_{\boldsymbol{b} \in \text{MON}(\boldsymbol{A}),\ \boldsymbol{\mu} \in \mathcal{L}_{\boldsymbol{\psi}}} \left| \text{URE}(\boldsymbol{b}, \boldsymbol{\mu}; \boldsymbol{\psi}) - l_p\left(\boldsymbol{\theta}, \hat{\boldsymbol{\theta}}^{\boldsymbol{b},\boldsymbol{\mu}}; \boldsymbol{\psi}\right)\right| \underset{p\to\infty}{\to} 0 \text{ in } L^1,$$

where $\boldsymbol{\mu} \in \mathscr{L}_{\psi}$ if and only if $\boldsymbol{\mu} \in \mathscr{L}_{\text{row}}(\boldsymbol{X})$ and

$$\sum_{i=1}^{p} \psi_i \mu_i^2 \leq M p^{\kappa} \sum_{i=1}^{p} \psi_i Y_i^2$$

for a large and fixed constant M and a fixed exponent $\kappa \in [0, 1/2)$. As a corollary, for any estimator $\hat{\boldsymbol{\theta}}^{\hat{\boldsymbol{b}}_p, \hat{\boldsymbol{\mu}}_p} = (\boldsymbol{I}_p - \text{diag}(\hat{\boldsymbol{b}}_p))\boldsymbol{Y} + \text{diag}(\hat{\boldsymbol{b}}_p)\hat{\boldsymbol{\mu}}_p$ with $\hat{\boldsymbol{b}}_p \in \text{MON}(\boldsymbol{A})$ and $\hat{\boldsymbol{\mu}}_p \in \mathscr{L}_{\psi}$, we have

$$\lim_{p\to\infty} \mathbb{P}\left(l_p\left(\boldsymbol{\theta}, \hat{\boldsymbol{\theta}}_{SP,\psi}^{\text{URE}}\right) \geq l_p\left(\boldsymbol{\theta}, \hat{\boldsymbol{\theta}}^{\hat{\boldsymbol{b}}_p, \hat{\boldsymbol{\mu}}_p}\right) + \epsilon \right) = 0 \quad \forall \epsilon > 0,$$

$$\limsup_{p\to\infty} \left(R_p\left(\boldsymbol{\theta}, \hat{\boldsymbol{\theta}}_{SP,\psi}^{\text{URE}}\right) - R_p\left(\boldsymbol{\theta}, \hat{\boldsymbol{\theta}}^{\hat{\boldsymbol{b}}_p, \hat{\boldsymbol{\mu}}_p}\right)\right) \leq 0.$$

Acknowledgements S. C. Kou's research is supported in part by US National Science Foundation Grant DMS-1510446.

Appendix: Proofs and Derivations

Proof of Lemma 1 We can write $\boldsymbol{\theta} = \boldsymbol{\mu} + \boldsymbol{Z}_1$ and $\boldsymbol{Y} = \boldsymbol{\theta} + \boldsymbol{Z}_2$, where $\boldsymbol{Z}_1 \sim \mathscr{N}_p(\boldsymbol{0}, \boldsymbol{B})$ and $\boldsymbol{Z}_2 \sim \mathscr{N}_p(\boldsymbol{0}, \boldsymbol{A})$ are independent. Jointly $\begin{pmatrix} \boldsymbol{Y} \\ \boldsymbol{\theta} \end{pmatrix}$ is still multivariate normal with mean vector $\begin{pmatrix} \boldsymbol{\mu} \\ \boldsymbol{\mu} \end{pmatrix}$ and covariance matrix $\begin{pmatrix} \boldsymbol{A}+\boldsymbol{B} & \boldsymbol{B} \\ \boldsymbol{B} & \boldsymbol{B} \end{pmatrix}$. The result follows immediately from the conditional distribution of a multivariate normal distribution.

Proof of Theorem 1 We start from decomposing the difference between the URE and the actual loss as

$$\begin{aligned}
&\text{URE}(\boldsymbol{B}, \boldsymbol{\mu}) - l_p\left(\boldsymbol{\theta}, \hat{\boldsymbol{\theta}}^{\boldsymbol{B}, \boldsymbol{\mu}}\right) \\
=&\text{URE}(\boldsymbol{B}, \boldsymbol{0}_p) - l_p\left(\boldsymbol{\theta}, \hat{\boldsymbol{\theta}}^{\boldsymbol{B}, \boldsymbol{0}_p}\right) - \frac{2}{p}\text{tr}\left(\boldsymbol{A}(\boldsymbol{A}+\boldsymbol{B})^{-1}\boldsymbol{\mu}(\boldsymbol{Y}-\boldsymbol{\theta})^T\right) \qquad (18) \\
=&\frac{1}{p}\text{tr}\left(\boldsymbol{Y}\boldsymbol{Y}^T - \boldsymbol{A} - \boldsymbol{\theta}\boldsymbol{\theta}^T\right) - \frac{2}{p}\text{tr}\left(\boldsymbol{B}(\boldsymbol{A}+\boldsymbol{B})^{-1}\left(\boldsymbol{Y}\boldsymbol{Y}^T - \boldsymbol{Y}\boldsymbol{\theta}^T - \boldsymbol{A}\right)\right) \\
&- \frac{2}{p}\text{tr}\left(\boldsymbol{A}(\boldsymbol{A}+\boldsymbol{B})^{-1}\boldsymbol{\mu}(\boldsymbol{Y}-\boldsymbol{\theta})^T\right) \qquad (19) \\
=&\,(\text{I}) + (\text{II}) + (\text{III}).
\end{aligned}$$

To verify the first equality (18), note that

$$\begin{aligned}
&\text{URE}\,(\boldsymbol{B}, \boldsymbol{\mu}) - \text{URE}\,(\boldsymbol{B}, \boldsymbol{0}_p) \\
&= \frac{1}{p}\left\| \boldsymbol{A}\,(\boldsymbol{A}+\boldsymbol{B})^{-1}\,(\boldsymbol{Y}-\boldsymbol{\mu}) \right\|^2 - \frac{1}{p}\left\| \boldsymbol{A}\,(\boldsymbol{A}+\boldsymbol{B})^{-1}\,\boldsymbol{Y} \right\|^2 \\
&= -\frac{1}{p}\text{tr}\left(\boldsymbol{\mu}^T \left(\boldsymbol{A}\,(\boldsymbol{A}+\boldsymbol{B})^{-1}\right)^T \boldsymbol{A}\,(\boldsymbol{A}+\boldsymbol{B})^{-1}\,(2\boldsymbol{Y}-\boldsymbol{\mu}) \right), \\
&l_p\left(\boldsymbol{\theta}, \hat{\boldsymbol{\theta}}^{\boldsymbol{B},\boldsymbol{\mu}}\right) - l_p\left(\boldsymbol{\theta}, \hat{\boldsymbol{\theta}}^{\boldsymbol{B},\boldsymbol{0}_p}\right) \\
&= \frac{1}{p}\left\| \left(\boldsymbol{I}_p - \boldsymbol{A}\,(\boldsymbol{A}+\boldsymbol{B})^{-1}\right)\boldsymbol{Y} + \boldsymbol{A}\,(\boldsymbol{A}+\boldsymbol{B})^{-1}\,\boldsymbol{\mu} - \boldsymbol{\theta} \right\|^2 \\
&\quad - \frac{1}{p}\left\| \left(\boldsymbol{I}_p - \boldsymbol{A}\,(\boldsymbol{A}+\boldsymbol{B})^{-1}\right)\boldsymbol{Y} - \boldsymbol{\theta} \right\|^2 \\
&= \frac{1}{p}\text{tr}\left(\boldsymbol{\mu}^T \left(\boldsymbol{A}\,(\boldsymbol{A}+\boldsymbol{B})^{-1}\right)^T \left(2\left(\left(\boldsymbol{I}_p - \boldsymbol{A}\,(\boldsymbol{A}+\boldsymbol{B})^{-1}\right)\boldsymbol{Y} - \boldsymbol{\theta} \right) + \boldsymbol{A}\,(\boldsymbol{A}+\boldsymbol{B})^{-1}\,\boldsymbol{\mu} \right) \right).
\end{aligned}$$

Equation (18) then follows by rearranging the terms. To verify the second equality (19), note

$$\begin{aligned}
&\text{URE}\,(\boldsymbol{B}, \boldsymbol{0}_p) - l_p\left(\boldsymbol{\theta}, \hat{\boldsymbol{\theta}}^{\boldsymbol{B},\boldsymbol{0}_p}\right) \\
&= \frac{1}{p}\left\| \boldsymbol{A}\,(\boldsymbol{A}+\boldsymbol{B})^{-1}\,\boldsymbol{Y} \right\|^2 - \frac{1}{p}\left\| \left(\boldsymbol{I}_p - \boldsymbol{A}\,(\boldsymbol{A}+\boldsymbol{B})^{-1}\right)\boldsymbol{Y} - \boldsymbol{\theta} \right\|^2 \\
&\quad + \frac{1}{p}\text{tr}\left(\boldsymbol{A} - 2\boldsymbol{A}\,(\boldsymbol{A}+\boldsymbol{B})^{-1}\,\boldsymbol{A}\right) \\
&= \frac{1}{p}\text{tr}\left(\left(\boldsymbol{Y} - 2\left(\boldsymbol{I}_p - \boldsymbol{A}\,(\boldsymbol{A}+\boldsymbol{B})^{-1}\right)\boldsymbol{Y} + \boldsymbol{\theta} \right)^T (\boldsymbol{Y}-\boldsymbol{\theta}) \right) \\
&\quad + \frac{1}{p}\text{tr}\left(\boldsymbol{A} - 2\boldsymbol{A}\,(\boldsymbol{A}+\boldsymbol{B})^{-1}\,\boldsymbol{A}\right) \\
&= \frac{1}{p}\text{tr}\left(\boldsymbol{Y}\boldsymbol{Y}^T - \boldsymbol{A} - \boldsymbol{\theta}\boldsymbol{\theta}^T\right) - \frac{2}{p}\text{tr}\left(\boldsymbol{B}\,(\boldsymbol{A}+\boldsymbol{B})^{-1}\left(\boldsymbol{Y}\,(\boldsymbol{Y}-\boldsymbol{\theta})^T - \boldsymbol{A}\right) \right).
\end{aligned}$$

With the decomposition, we want to prove separately the uniform L^1 convergence of the three terms (I), (II), and (III).

Proof for the case of Model I.

The uniform L^2 convergence of (I) and (II) has been shown in Theorem 3.1 of [29] under our assumptions (A) and (B), so we focus on (III), i.e., we want to show that $\sup_{0 \le \lambda \le \infty,\ \boldsymbol{\mu} \in \mathscr{L}} |(\text{III})| \to 0$ in L^1 as $p \to \infty$.

Without loss of generality, let us assume $A_1 \leq A_2 \leq \cdots \leq A_p$. We have

$$\begin{aligned}\sup_{0\leq\lambda\leq\infty,\ \mu\in\mathscr{L}} |(\mathrm{III})| &= \frac{2}{p} \sup_{0\leq\lambda\leq\infty,\ \mu\in\mathscr{L}} \left| \sum_{i=1}^{p} \frac{A_i}{A_i+\lambda}\mu_i (Y_i - \theta_i) \right| \\ &\leq \frac{2}{p} \sup_{\mu\in\mathscr{L}} \sup_{0\leq c_1\leq\cdots\leq c_p\leq 1} \left| \sum_{i=1}^{p} c_i \mu_i (Y_i - \theta_i) \right| \\ &= \frac{2}{p} \sup_{\mu\in\mathscr{L}} \max_{1\leq j\leq p} \left| \sum_{i=j}^{p} \mu_i (Y_i - \theta_i) \right|,\end{aligned}$$

where the last equality follows from Lemma 2.1 of [13]. For a generic p-dimensional vector $\boldsymbol{v}$, we denote $[\boldsymbol{v}]_{j:p} = (0, \ldots 0, v_j, v_{j+1}, \ldots, v_p)$. Let $\boldsymbol{P}_X = \boldsymbol{X}^T \left(\boldsymbol{X}\boldsymbol{X}^T\right)^{-1} \boldsymbol{X}$ be the projection matrix onto $\mathscr{L}_{\text{row}}(\boldsymbol{X})$. Then since $\mathscr{L} \subset \mathscr{L}_{\text{row}}(\boldsymbol{X})$, we have

$$\begin{aligned}&\frac{2}{p} \sup_{\mu\in\mathscr{L}} \max_{1\leq j\leq p} \left| \sum_{i=j}^{p} \mu_i (Y_i - \theta_i) \right| = \frac{2}{p} \max_{1\leq j\leq p} \sup_{\mu\in\mathscr{L}} \left| \boldsymbol{\mu}^T [\boldsymbol{Y} - \boldsymbol{\theta}]_{j:p} \right| \\ =& \frac{2}{p} \max_{1\leq j\leq p} \sup_{\mu\in\mathscr{L}} \left| \boldsymbol{\mu}^T \boldsymbol{P}_X [\boldsymbol{Y} - \boldsymbol{\theta}]_{j:p} \right| \leq \frac{2}{p} \max_{1\leq j\leq p} \sup_{\mu\in\mathscr{L}} \|\boldsymbol{\mu}\| \times \left\| \boldsymbol{P}_X [\boldsymbol{Y} - \boldsymbol{\theta}]_{j:p} \right\| \\ =& \frac{2}{p} \max_{1\leq j\leq p} M p^{\kappa} \|\boldsymbol{Y}\| \times \left\| \boldsymbol{P}_X [\boldsymbol{Y} - \boldsymbol{\theta}]_{j:p} \right\|.\end{aligned}$$

Cauchy-Schwarz inequality thus gives

$$\mathbb{E}\left(\sup_{0\leq\lambda\leq\infty,\mu\in\mathscr{L}} |(\mathrm{III})| \right) \leq 2Mp^{\kappa-1} \sqrt{\mathbb{E}\left(\|\boldsymbol{Y}\|^2\right)} \times \sqrt{\mathbb{E}\left(\max_{1\leq j\leq p} \left\| \boldsymbol{P}_X [\boldsymbol{Y} - \boldsymbol{\theta}]_{j:p} \right\|^2 \right)}. \tag{20}$$

It is straightforward to see that, by conditions (A) and (C),

$$\sqrt{\mathbb{E}\left(\|\boldsymbol{Y}\|^2\right)} = \sqrt{\mathbb{E}(\textstyle\sum_{i=1}^{p} Y_i^2)} = \sqrt{\textstyle\sum_{i=1}^{p} \left(\theta_i^2 + A_i\right)} = O\left(p^{1/2}\right).$$

For the second term on the right-hand side of (20), let $\boldsymbol{P}_X = \boldsymbol{\Gamma}\boldsymbol{D}\boldsymbol{\Gamma}^T$ denote the spectral decomposition. Clearly,

$$\boldsymbol{D} = \operatorname{diag}\left(\underbrace{1, \ldots, 1}_{k \text{ copies}}, \underbrace{0, \ldots, 0}_{p-k \text{ copies}} \right).$$

It follows that

$$\mathbb{E}\left(\max_{1\le j\le p}\left\|\boldsymbol{P}_X[\boldsymbol{Y}-\boldsymbol{\theta}]_{j:p}\right\|^2\right)=\mathbb{E}\left(\max_{1\le j\le p}[\boldsymbol{Y}-\boldsymbol{\theta}]_{j:p}^T\boldsymbol{P}_X[\boldsymbol{Y}-\boldsymbol{\theta}]_{j:p}\right)$$

$$=\mathbb{E}\left(\max_{1\le j\le p}\operatorname{tr}\left(\boldsymbol{D}\boldsymbol{\Gamma}^T[\boldsymbol{Y}-\boldsymbol{\theta}]_{j:p}\left(\boldsymbol{\Gamma}^T[\boldsymbol{Y}-\boldsymbol{\theta}]_{j:p}\right)^T\right)\right)$$

$$=\mathbb{E}\left(\max_{1\le j\le p}\sum_{l=1}^{k}\left[\boldsymbol{\Gamma}^T[\boldsymbol{Y}-\boldsymbol{\theta}]_{j:p}\right]_l^2\right)$$

$$=\mathbb{E}\left(\max_{1\le j\le p}\sum_{l=1}^{k}\left(\sum_{m=j}^{p}\left[\boldsymbol{\Gamma}^T\right]_{lm}(Y_m-\theta_m)\right)^2\right)$$

$$\le\mathbb{E}\left(\sum_{l=1}^{k}\max_{1\le j\le p}\left(\sum_{m=j}^{p}\left[\boldsymbol{\Gamma}^T\right]_{lm}(Y_m-\theta_m)\right)^2\right)$$

$$=\sum_{l=1}^{k}\mathbb{E}\left(\max_{1\le j\le p}\left(\sum_{m=j}^{p}\left[\boldsymbol{\Gamma}^T\right]_{lm}(Y_m-\theta_m)\right)^2\right).$$

For each l, $M_j^{(l)}=\sum_{m=p-j+1}^{p}\left[\boldsymbol{\Gamma}^T\right]_{lm}(Y_m-\theta_m)$ forms a martingale, so by Doob's L^p maximum inequality,

$$\mathbb{E}\left(\max_{1\le j\le p}\left(M_j^{(l)}\right)^2\right)\le 4\mathbb{E}\left(M_p^{(l)}\right)^2=4\mathbb{E}\left(\sum_{m=1}^{p}\left[\boldsymbol{\Gamma}^T\right]_{lm}(Y_m-\theta_m)\right)^2$$

$$=4\sum_{m=1}^{p}\left[\boldsymbol{\Gamma}^T\right]_{lm}^2A_m=4\left[\boldsymbol{\Gamma}^T\boldsymbol{A}\boldsymbol{\Gamma}\right]_{ll}.$$

Therefore,

$$\mathbb{E}\left(\max_{1\le j\le p}\left\|\boldsymbol{P}_X[\boldsymbol{Y}-\boldsymbol{\theta}]_{j:p}\right\|^2\right)\le\sum_{l=1}^{k}4\left[\boldsymbol{\Gamma}^T\boldsymbol{A}\boldsymbol{\Gamma}\right]_{ll}$$

$$=4\sum_{l=1}^{p}[\boldsymbol{D}]_{ll}\left[\boldsymbol{\Gamma}^T\boldsymbol{A}\boldsymbol{\Gamma}\right]_{ll}=4\operatorname{tr}\left(\boldsymbol{D}\boldsymbol{\Gamma}^T\boldsymbol{A}\boldsymbol{\Gamma}\right)=4\operatorname{tr}\left(\boldsymbol{P}_X\boldsymbol{A}\right)$$

$$=4\operatorname{tr}\left(\boldsymbol{X}^T\left(\boldsymbol{X}\boldsymbol{X}^T\right)^{-1}\boldsymbol{X}\boldsymbol{A}\right)=4\operatorname{tr}\left(\left(\boldsymbol{X}\boldsymbol{X}^T\right)^{-1}\boldsymbol{X}\boldsymbol{A}\boldsymbol{X}^T\right)=O(1),$$

where the last equality uses conditions (D) and (E). We finally obtain

$$\mathbb{E}\left(\sup_{0\le\lambda\le\infty,\ \mu\in\mathcal{L}} |(\mathrm{III})|\right) \le o\left(p^{-1/2}\right) \times O\left(p^{1/2}\right) \times O(1) = o(1).$$

Proof for the case of Model II.
Under Model II, we know that

$$\sum_{i=1}^{p} A_i\theta_i^2 = \boldsymbol{\theta}^T \boldsymbol{A}\boldsymbol{\theta} = \boldsymbol{\beta}^T(\boldsymbol{X}\boldsymbol{A}\boldsymbol{X}^T)\boldsymbol{\beta} = O(p)$$

by condition (D). In other words, condition (D) implies condition (B). Therefore, we know that the term (I) $\to 0$ in L^2 as shown in Theorem 3.1 of [29], and we only need to show the uniform L^1 convergence of the other two terms, (II) and (III).

Recall that $\boldsymbol{B} \in \mathscr{B} = \left\{\lambda \boldsymbol{X}^T \boldsymbol{W}\boldsymbol{X} : \lambda > 0\right\}$ has only rank k under Model II. We can reexpress (II) and (III) in terms of low rank matrices. Let $\boldsymbol{V} = \left(\boldsymbol{X}\boldsymbol{A}^{-1}\boldsymbol{X}^T\right)^{-1}$. Woodbury formula gives

$$\begin{aligned}(\boldsymbol{A}+\boldsymbol{B})^{-1} &= \left(\boldsymbol{A}+\lambda\boldsymbol{X}^T\boldsymbol{W}\boldsymbol{X}\right)^{-1} = \boldsymbol{A}^{-1} - \boldsymbol{A}^{-1}\lambda\boldsymbol{X}^T\left(\boldsymbol{W}^{-1}+\lambda\boldsymbol{V}^{-1}\right)^{-1}\boldsymbol{X}\boldsymbol{A}^{-1} \\ &= \boldsymbol{A}^{-1} - \boldsymbol{A}^{-1}\lambda\boldsymbol{X}^T\boldsymbol{W}(\lambda\boldsymbol{W}+\boldsymbol{V})^{-1}\boldsymbol{V}\boldsymbol{X}\boldsymbol{A}^{-1},\end{aligned}$$

which tells us

$$\boldsymbol{B}(\boldsymbol{A}+\boldsymbol{B})^{-1} = \boldsymbol{I}_p - \boldsymbol{A}(\boldsymbol{A}+\boldsymbol{B})^{-1} = \lambda\boldsymbol{X}^T\boldsymbol{W}(\lambda\boldsymbol{W}+\boldsymbol{V})^{-1}\boldsymbol{V}\boldsymbol{X}\boldsymbol{A}^{-1}.$$

Let $\boldsymbol{U}\boldsymbol{\Lambda}\boldsymbol{U}^T$ be the spectral decomposition of $\boldsymbol{W}^{-1/2}\boldsymbol{V}\boldsymbol{W}^{-1/2}$, i.e., $\boldsymbol{W}^{-1/2}\boldsymbol{V}\boldsymbol{W}^{-1/2} = \boldsymbol{U}\boldsymbol{\Lambda}\boldsymbol{U}^T$, where $\boldsymbol{\Lambda} = \mathrm{diag}(d_1,\ldots,d_k)$ with $d_1 \le \cdots \le d_k$. Then $(\lambda\boldsymbol{W}+\boldsymbol{V})^{-1} = \boldsymbol{W}^{-1/2}\left(\lambda\boldsymbol{I}_k + \boldsymbol{W}^{-1/2}\boldsymbol{V}\boldsymbol{W}^{-1/2}\right)^{-1}\boldsymbol{W}^{-1/2} = \boldsymbol{W}^{-1/2}\boldsymbol{U}(\lambda\boldsymbol{I}_k+\boldsymbol{\Lambda})^{-1}\boldsymbol{U}^T\boldsymbol{W}^{-1/2}$, from which we obtain

$$\boldsymbol{B}(\boldsymbol{A}+\boldsymbol{B})^{-1} = \lambda\boldsymbol{X}^T\boldsymbol{W}(\lambda\boldsymbol{W}+\boldsymbol{V})^{-1}\boldsymbol{V}\boldsymbol{X}\boldsymbol{A}^{-1} = \lambda\boldsymbol{X}^T\boldsymbol{W}^{1/2}\boldsymbol{U}(\lambda\boldsymbol{I}_k+\boldsymbol{\Lambda})^{-1}\boldsymbol{\Lambda}\boldsymbol{U}^T\boldsymbol{W}^{1/2}\boldsymbol{X}\boldsymbol{A}^{-1}.$$

If we denote $\boldsymbol{Z} = \boldsymbol{U}^T\boldsymbol{W}^{1/2}\boldsymbol{X}$, i.e., $\boldsymbol{Z}$ is the transformed covariate matrix, then $\boldsymbol{B}(\boldsymbol{A}+\boldsymbol{B})^{-1} = \lambda\boldsymbol{Z}^T(\lambda\boldsymbol{I}_k+\boldsymbol{\Lambda})^{-1}\boldsymbol{\Lambda}\boldsymbol{Z}\boldsymbol{A}^{-1}$. It follows that

$$\begin{aligned}(\mathrm{II}) &= -\frac{2}{p}\mathrm{tr}\left(\boldsymbol{B}(\boldsymbol{A}+\boldsymbol{B})^{-1}\left(\boldsymbol{Y}\boldsymbol{Y}^T - \boldsymbol{Y}\boldsymbol{\theta}^T - \boldsymbol{A}\right)\right) \\ &= -\frac{2}{p}\mathrm{tr}\left(\lambda\boldsymbol{Z}^T(\lambda\boldsymbol{I}_k+\boldsymbol{\Lambda})^{-1}\boldsymbol{\Lambda}\boldsymbol{Z}\boldsymbol{A}^{-1}\left(\boldsymbol{Y}\boldsymbol{Y}^T - \boldsymbol{Y}\boldsymbol{\theta}^T - \boldsymbol{A}\right)\right) \\ &= -\frac{2}{p}\mathrm{tr}\left(\lambda(\lambda\boldsymbol{I}_k+\boldsymbol{\Lambda})^{-1}\boldsymbol{\Lambda}\boldsymbol{Z}\boldsymbol{A}^{-1}\left(\boldsymbol{Y}\boldsymbol{Y}^T - \boldsymbol{Y}\boldsymbol{\theta}^T - \boldsymbol{A}\right)\boldsymbol{Z}^T\right),\end{aligned}$$

$$
\begin{aligned}
\text{(III)} &= -\frac{2}{p}\operatorname{tr}\left(\boldsymbol{A}\left(\boldsymbol{A}+\boldsymbol{B}\right)^{-1}\boldsymbol{\mu}\left(\boldsymbol{Y}-\boldsymbol{\theta}\right)^{T}\right) \\
&= -\frac{2}{p}\operatorname{tr}\left(\left(\boldsymbol{I}_p-\lambda\boldsymbol{Z}^{T}\left(\lambda\boldsymbol{I}_k+\boldsymbol{\Lambda}\right)^{-1}\boldsymbol{\Lambda}\boldsymbol{Z}\boldsymbol{A}^{-1}\right)\boldsymbol{\mu}\left(\boldsymbol{Y}-\boldsymbol{\theta}\right)^{T}\right) \\
&= -\frac{2}{p}\operatorname{tr}\left(\boldsymbol{\mu}\left(\boldsymbol{Y}-\boldsymbol{\theta}\right)^{T}\right)+\frac{2}{p}\operatorname{tr}\left(\lambda\left(\lambda\boldsymbol{I}_k+\boldsymbol{\Lambda}\right)^{-1}\boldsymbol{\Lambda}\boldsymbol{Z}\boldsymbol{A}^{-1}\boldsymbol{\mu}\left(\boldsymbol{Y}-\boldsymbol{\theta}\right)^{T}\boldsymbol{Z}^{T}\right) \\
&= \text{(III)}_1+\text{(III)}_2 .
\end{aligned}
$$

We will next show that (II), (III)_1, and (III)_2 all uniformly converge to zero in L^1, which will then complete our proof.

Let $\boldsymbol{\Xi} = \boldsymbol{Z}\boldsymbol{A}^{-1}\left(\boldsymbol{Y}\boldsymbol{Y}^{T}-\boldsymbol{Y}\boldsymbol{\theta}^{T}-\boldsymbol{A}\right)\boldsymbol{Z}^{T}$. Then

$$
\begin{aligned}
\sup_{0\le\lambda\le\infty}|\text{(II)}| &= \frac{2}{p}\sup_{0\le\lambda\le\infty}\left|\sum_{i=1}^{k}\frac{\lambda d_i}{\lambda+d_i}\left[\boldsymbol{\Xi}\right]_{ii}\right| \\
&\le \frac{2}{p}\sup_{0\le c_1\le\cdots\le c_k\le d_k}\left|\sum_{i=1}^{k}c_i\left[\boldsymbol{\Xi}\right]_{ii}\right| = \frac{2}{p}\max_{1\le j\le k}\left|\sum_{i=j}^{k}d_k\left[\boldsymbol{\Xi}\right]_{ii}\right|,
\end{aligned}
$$

where the last equality follows as in Lemma 2.1 of [13]. As there are finite number of terms in the summation and the maximization, it suffices to show that

$$
d_k\left[\boldsymbol{\Xi}\right]_{ii}/p \to 0 \text{ in } L^2 \quad \text{for all } 1\le i\le k.
$$

To establish this, we note that $\left[\boldsymbol{\Xi}\right]_{ii} = \sum_{n=1}^{p}\sum_{m=1}^{p}\left(A_n^{-1}Y_n\left(Y_m-\theta_m\right)-\delta_{nm}\right)\left[\boldsymbol{Z}\right]_{in}\left[\boldsymbol{Z}\right]_{im}$,

$$
\begin{aligned}
\mathbb{E}\left(\left[\boldsymbol{\Xi}\right]_{ii}^{2}\right) = &\sum_{n,m,n',m'}\mathbb{E}\left(\left(A_n^{-1}Y_n\left(Y_m-\theta_m\right)-\delta_{nm}\right)\left(A_{n'}^{-1}Y_{n'}\left(Y_{m'}-\theta_{m'}\right)-\delta_{n'm'}\right)\right) \\
&\times\left[\boldsymbol{Z}\right]_{in}\left[\boldsymbol{Z}\right]_{im}\left[\boldsymbol{Z}\right]_{in'}\left[\boldsymbol{Z}\right]_{im'} .
\end{aligned}
$$

Depending on n, m, n', m' taking the same or distinct values, we can break the summation into 15 disjoint cases:

$$
\begin{aligned}
&\sum_{\text{all distinct}}+\sum_{\text{three distinct, } n=m}+\sum_{\text{three distinct, } n=n'}+\sum_{\text{three distinct, } n=m'} \\
&+\sum_{\text{three distinct, } m=n'}+\sum_{\text{three distinct, } m=m'}+\sum_{\text{three distinct, } n'=m'}+\sum_{\text{two distinct, } n=m,\, n'=m'}
\end{aligned}
$$

$$+ \sum_{\text{two distinct, } n=n',\, m=m'} + \sum_{\text{two distinct, } n=m',\, n'=m} + \sum_{\text{two distinct, } n=m=n'} + \sum_{\text{two distinct, } n=m=m'}$$

$$+ \sum_{\text{two distinct, } n=n'=m'} + \sum_{\text{two distinct, } m=n'=m'} + \sum_{n=m=n'=m'} .$$

Many terms are zero. Straightforward evaluation of each summation gives

$$\begin{aligned}
\mathbb{E}\left([\boldsymbol{\Xi}]_{ii}^2\right) &= \sum_{n=1}^{p} \mathbb{E}\left(\left(A_n^{-1} Y_n (Y_n - \theta_n) - 1\right)^2\right) [\mathbf{Z}]_{in}^4 \\
&\quad + \sum_{n=1}^{p} \sum_{m \neq n} \mathbb{E}\left(\left(A_n^{-1} Y_n (Y_m - \theta_m)\right)^2\right) [\mathbf{Z}]_{in}^2 [\mathbf{Z}]_{im}^2 \\
&\quad + \sum_{n=1}^{p} \sum_{m \neq n} \mathbb{E}\left(\left(A_n^{-1} Y_n (Y_m - \theta_m)\right)\left(A_m^{-1} Y_m (Y_n - \theta_n)\right)\right) [\mathbf{Z}]_{in}^2 [\mathbf{Z}]_{im}^2 \\
&\quad + 2 \sum_{n=1}^{p} \sum_{m \neq n} \mathbb{E}\left(\left(A_n^{-1} Y_n (Y_n - \theta_n) - 1\right)\left(A_m^{-1} Y_m (Y_n - \theta_n)\right)\right) [\mathbf{Z}]_{in}^3 [\mathbf{Z}]_{im} \\
&\quad + \sum_{n=1}^{p} \sum_{m \neq n',\, n' \neq n,\, m \neq n} \mathbb{E}\left(\left(A_m^{-1} Y_m (Y_n - \theta_n)\right)\left(A_{n'}^{-1} Y_{n'} (Y_n - \theta_n)\right)\right) [\mathbf{Z}]_{in}^2 [\mathbf{Z}]_{im} [\mathbf{Z}]_{in'} \\
&= \sum_{n=1}^{p} \frac{2A_n + \theta_n^2}{A_n} [\mathbf{Z}]_{in}^4 + \sum_{n=1}^{p} \sum_{m \neq n} \frac{A_n A_m + A_n \theta_m^2}{A_m^2} [\mathbf{Z}]_{in}^2 [\mathbf{Z}]_{im}^2 + \sum_{n=1}^{p} \sum_{m \neq n} [\mathbf{Z}]_{in}^2 [\mathbf{Z}]_{im}^2 \\
&\quad + 2 \sum_{n=1}^{p} \sum_{m \neq n} \frac{\theta_n \theta_m}{A_m} [\mathbf{Z}]_{in}^3 [\mathbf{Z}]_{im} + \sum_{n=1}^{p} \sum_{m \neq n',\, n' \neq n,\, m \neq n} \frac{A_n \theta_m \theta_{n'}}{A_m A_{n'}} [\mathbf{Z}]_{in}^2 [\mathbf{Z}]_{im} [\mathbf{Z}]_{in'} \\
&= \sum_{n,m=1}^{p} \frac{A_n}{A_m} [\mathbf{Z}]_{in}^2 [\mathbf{Z}]_{im}^2 + \sum_{n,m=1}^{p} [\mathbf{Z}]_{in}^2 [\mathbf{Z}]_{im}^2 + \sum_{n,m,n'=1}^{p} \frac{A_n \theta_m \theta_{n'}}{A_m A_{n'}} [\mathbf{Z}]_{in}^2 [\mathbf{Z}]_{im} [\mathbf{Z}]_{in'} .
\end{aligned}$$

Using matrix notation, we can reexpress the above equation as

$$\begin{aligned}
\mathbb{E}\left([\boldsymbol{\Xi}]_{ii}^2\right) &= \left[\boldsymbol{ZAZ}^T\right]_{ii} \left[\boldsymbol{ZA}^{-1}\boldsymbol{Z}^T\right]_{ii} + \left[\boldsymbol{ZZ}^T\right]_{ii}^2 + \left[\boldsymbol{ZAZ}^T\right]_{ii} \left[\boldsymbol{ZA}^{-1}\boldsymbol{\theta}\right]_i^2 \\
&\le \operatorname{tr}\left(\boldsymbol{ZAZ}^T\right) \operatorname{tr}\left(\boldsymbol{ZA}^{-1}\boldsymbol{Z}^T\right) + \operatorname{tr}\left(\boldsymbol{ZZ}^T\right)^2 + \operatorname{tr}\left(\boldsymbol{ZAZ}^T\right) \operatorname{tr}\left(\boldsymbol{\theta}^T \boldsymbol{A}^{-1}\boldsymbol{Z}^T\boldsymbol{ZA}^{-1}\boldsymbol{\theta}\right) \\
&= \operatorname{tr}\left(\boldsymbol{WXAX}^T\right) \operatorname{tr}\left(\boldsymbol{WXA}^{-1}\boldsymbol{X}^T\right) + \operatorname{tr}\left(\boldsymbol{WXX}^T\right)^2 \\
&\quad + \operatorname{tr}\left(\boldsymbol{WXAX}^T\right) \operatorname{tr}\left(\boldsymbol{\beta}^T \left(\boldsymbol{XA}^{-1}\boldsymbol{X}^T\right) \boldsymbol{W} \left(\boldsymbol{XA}^{-1}\boldsymbol{X}^T\right) \boldsymbol{\beta}\right),
\end{aligned}$$

which is $O(p)\,O(p) + O(p)^2 + O(p)\,O\left(p^2\right) = O\left(p^3\right)$ by conditions (D)-(F). Note also that condition (F) implies

$$d_k \leq \sum_{i=1}^{k} d_i = \operatorname{tr}\left(\boldsymbol{W}^{-1/2}\boldsymbol{V}\boldsymbol{W}^{-1/2}\right) = \operatorname{tr}\left(\boldsymbol{W}^{-1}\boldsymbol{V}\right) = \operatorname{tr}\left(\boldsymbol{W}^{-1}(\boldsymbol{X}\boldsymbol{A}^{-1}\boldsymbol{X}^T)^{-1}\right) = O\left(p^{-1}\right).$$

Therefore, we have

$$\mathbb{E}\left(d_k^2\,[\boldsymbol{\Xi}]_{ii}^2/p^2\right) = O\left(p^{-2}\right)O\left(p^3\right)/p^2 = O\left(p^{-1}\right) \to 0,$$

which proves

$$\sup_{0\leq\lambda\leq\infty} |(\mathrm{II})| \to 0 \text{ in } L^2, \quad \text{as } p \to \infty.$$

To prove the uniform convergence of $(\mathrm{III})_1$ to zero in L^1, we note that

$$\begin{aligned}\sup_{\mu\in\mathscr{L}} |(\mathrm{III})_1| &= \frac{2}{p}\sup_{\mu\in\mathscr{L}} \left|\boldsymbol{\mu}^T(\boldsymbol{Y}-\boldsymbol{\theta})\right| = \frac{2}{p}\sup_{\mu\in\mathscr{L}} \left|\boldsymbol{\mu}^T\boldsymbol{P}_X(\boldsymbol{Y}-\boldsymbol{\theta})\right| \\ &\leq \frac{2}{p}\sup_{\mu\in\mathscr{L}} \|\boldsymbol{\mu}\| \times \|\boldsymbol{P}_X(\boldsymbol{Y}-\boldsymbol{\theta})\| = \frac{2}{p}Mp^{\kappa}\,\|\boldsymbol{Y}\| \times \|\boldsymbol{P}_X(\boldsymbol{Y}-\boldsymbol{\theta})\|,\end{aligned}$$

so by Cauchy-Schwarz inequality

$$\mathbb{E}\left(\sup_{\mu\in\mathscr{L}} |(\mathrm{III})_1|\right) \leq 2Mp^{\kappa-1}\sqrt{\mathbb{E}\left(\|\boldsymbol{Y}\|^2\right)}\sqrt{\mathbb{E}\left(\|\boldsymbol{P}_X(\boldsymbol{Y}-\boldsymbol{\theta})\|^2\right)}. \tag{21}$$

Under Model II, $\boldsymbol{\theta} = \boldsymbol{X}^T\boldsymbol{\beta}$, so it follows that $\sum_{i=1}^p \theta_i^2 = \|\boldsymbol{\theta}\|^2 = \operatorname{tr}\left(\boldsymbol{\beta}\boldsymbol{\beta}^T\boldsymbol{X}\boldsymbol{X}^T\right) = O(p)$ by condition (E). Hence $\sqrt{\mathbb{E}\left(\|\boldsymbol{Y}\|^2\right)} = \sqrt{\sum_{i=1}^p\left(\theta_i^2 + A_i\right)} = O\left(p^{1/2}\right)$. For the second term on the right-hand side of (21), note that

$$\begin{aligned}\mathbb{E}\left(\|\boldsymbol{P}_X(\boldsymbol{Y}-\boldsymbol{\theta})\|^2\right) &= \mathbb{E}\left(\operatorname{tr}\left(\boldsymbol{P}_X(\boldsymbol{Y}-\boldsymbol{\theta})(\boldsymbol{Y}-\boldsymbol{\theta})^T\right)\right) \\ &= \operatorname{tr}\left(\boldsymbol{P}_X\boldsymbol{A}\right) = \operatorname{tr}\left(\left(\boldsymbol{X}\boldsymbol{X}^T\right)^{-1}\boldsymbol{X}\boldsymbol{A}\boldsymbol{X}^T\right) = O(1)\end{aligned}$$

by conditions (D) and (E). Thus, in aggregate, we have

$$\mathbb{E}\left(\sup_{\mu\in\mathscr{L}} |(\mathrm{III})_1|\right) \leq 2Mp^{\kappa-1}O\left(p^{1/2}\right)O(1) = o(1).$$

We finally consider the $(\mathrm{III})_2$ term. We have

$$\sup_{0\le\lambda\le\infty,\ \mu\in\mathscr{L}} |(\mathrm{III})_2| = \frac{2}{p}\sup_{\mu\in\mathscr{L}}\sup_{0\le\lambda\le\infty}\left|\sum_{i=1}^{k}\frac{\lambda d_i}{\lambda+d_i}\left[\mathbf{Z}\mathbf{A}^{-1}\boldsymbol{\mu}\left(\boldsymbol{Y}-\boldsymbol{\theta}\right)^T\mathbf{Z}^T\right]_{ii}\right|$$

$$\le \frac{2}{p}\sup_{\mu\in\mathscr{L}}\max_{1\le j\le k}\left|\sum_{i=j}^{k} d_k\left[\mathbf{Z}\mathbf{A}^{-1}\boldsymbol{\mu}\left(\boldsymbol{Y}-\boldsymbol{\theta}\right)^T\mathbf{Z}^T\right]_{ii}\right|$$

$$\le \frac{2d_k}{p}\sup_{\mu\in\mathscr{L}}\sum_{i=1}^{k}\left|\left[\mathbf{Z}\mathbf{A}^{-1}\boldsymbol{\mu}\left(\boldsymbol{Y}-\boldsymbol{\theta}\right)^T\mathbf{Z}^T\right]_{ii}\right|$$

$$= \frac{2d_k}{p}\sup_{\mu\in\mathscr{L}}\sum_{i=1}^{k}\left|\left[\mathbf{Z}\mathbf{A}^{-1}\boldsymbol{\mu}\right]_i\left[\mathbf{Z}\left(\boldsymbol{Y}-\boldsymbol{\theta}\right)\right]_i\right|$$

$$\le \frac{2d_k}{p}\sup_{\mu\in\mathscr{L}}\sqrt{\sum_{i=1}^{k}\left[\mathbf{Z}\mathbf{A}^{-1}\boldsymbol{\mu}\right]_i^2}\times\sqrt{\sum_{i=1}^{k}\left[\mathbf{Z}\left(\boldsymbol{Y}-\boldsymbol{\theta}\right)\right]_i^2}.$$

Thus, by Cauchy-Schwarz inequality

$$\mathbb{E}\left(\sup_{0\le\lambda\le\infty,\ \mu\in\mathscr{L}}|(\mathrm{III})_2|\right)\le\frac{2d_k}{p}\sqrt{\mathbb{E}\left(\sup_{\mu\in\mathscr{L}}\sum_{i=1}^{k}\left[\mathbf{Z}\mathbf{A}^{-1}\boldsymbol{\mu}\right]_i^2\right)}\times\sqrt{\mathbb{E}\left(\sum_{i=1}^{k}\left[\mathbf{Z}\left(\boldsymbol{Y}-\boldsymbol{\theta}\right)\right]_i^2\right)}.$$

Note that

$$\sup_{\mu\in\mathscr{L}}\sum_{i=1}^{k}\left[\mathbf{Z}\mathbf{A}^{-1}\boldsymbol{\mu}\right]_i^2 = \sup_{\mu\in\mathscr{L}}\sum_{i=1}^{k}\left(\sum_{m=1}^{p}\left[\mathbf{Z}\mathbf{A}^{-1}\right]_{im}\left[\boldsymbol{\mu}\right]_m\right)^2$$

$$\le \sup_{\mu\in\mathscr{L}}\sum_{i=1}^{k}\left(\sum_{m=1}^{p}\left[\mathbf{Z}\mathbf{A}^{-1}\right]_{im}^2\times\sum_{m=1}^{p}\left[\boldsymbol{\mu}\right]_m^2\right) = \sup_{\mu\in\mathscr{L}}\sum_{i=1}^{k}\left(\left[\mathbf{Z}\mathbf{A}^{-2}\mathbf{Z}^T\right]_{ii}\|\boldsymbol{\mu}\|^2\right)$$

$$= \mathrm{tr}\left(\mathbf{Z}\mathbf{A}^{-2}\mathbf{Z}^T\right)\sup_{\mu\in\mathscr{L}}\|\boldsymbol{\mu}\|^2 = \mathrm{tr}\left(\boldsymbol{W}\boldsymbol{X}\boldsymbol{A}^{-2}\boldsymbol{X}^T\right)\left(Mp^{\kappa}\|\boldsymbol{Y}\|\right)^2 = o\left(p^2\right)\|\boldsymbol{Y}\|^2,$$

where the last equality uses condition (G). Thus,

$$\mathbb{E}\left(\sup_{\mu\in\mathscr{L}}\sum_{i=1}^{k}\left[\mathbf{Z}\mathbf{A}^{-1}\boldsymbol{\mu}\right]_i^2\right) = o\left(p^3\right).$$

Also note that

$$\mathbb{E}\left(\sum_{i=1}^{k}[\boldsymbol{Z}(\boldsymbol{Y}-\boldsymbol{\theta})]_i^2\right)=\mathbb{E}\left(\operatorname{tr}\left(\boldsymbol{Z}^T\boldsymbol{Z}(\boldsymbol{Y}-\boldsymbol{\theta})(\boldsymbol{Y}-\boldsymbol{\theta})^T\right)\right)$$

$$=\operatorname{tr}\left(\boldsymbol{Z}^T\boldsymbol{Z}\boldsymbol{A}\right)=\operatorname{tr}\left(\boldsymbol{W}\boldsymbol{X}\boldsymbol{A}\boldsymbol{X}^T\right)=O(p)$$

by condition (D). Recall that $d_k = O\left(p^{-1}\right)$ by condition (F). It follows that

$$\mathbb{E}\left(\sup_{0\le\lambda\le\infty,\ \mu\in\mathscr{L}}|(\text{III})_2|\right)\le\frac{2}{p}O\left(p^{-1}\right)o\left(p^{3/2}\right)O\left(p^{1/2}\right)=o(1),$$

which completes our proof.

Proof of Lemma 2 The fact that $\hat{\boldsymbol{\mu}}^{\text{OLS}}\in\mathscr{L}$ is trivial as

$$\hat{\boldsymbol{\mu}}^{\text{OLS}}=\boldsymbol{X}^T\left(\boldsymbol{X}\boldsymbol{X}^T\right)^{-1}\boldsymbol{X}\boldsymbol{Y}=\boldsymbol{P_X}\boldsymbol{Y},$$

while the projection matrix $\boldsymbol{P_X}$ has induced matrix 2-norm $\|\boldsymbol{P_X}\|_2 = 1$. Thus, $\left\|\hat{\boldsymbol{\mu}}^{\text{OLS}}\right\|\le\|\boldsymbol{P_X}\|_2\|\boldsymbol{Y}\|=\|\boldsymbol{Y}\|$. For $\hat{\boldsymbol{\mu}}^{\text{WLS}}$, note that

$$\begin{aligned}\hat{\boldsymbol{\mu}}^{\text{WLS}}&=\boldsymbol{X}^T\left(\boldsymbol{X}\boldsymbol{A}^{-1}\boldsymbol{X}^T\right)^{-1}\boldsymbol{X}\boldsymbol{A}^{-1}\boldsymbol{Y}\\&=\boldsymbol{A}^{1/2}\left(\boldsymbol{X}\boldsymbol{A}^{-1/2}\right)^T\left(\boldsymbol{X}\boldsymbol{A}^{-1/2}\left(\boldsymbol{X}\boldsymbol{A}^{-1/2}\right)^T\right)^{-1}\left(\boldsymbol{X}\boldsymbol{A}^{-1/2}\right)\boldsymbol{A}^{-1/2}\boldsymbol{Y}\\&=\boldsymbol{A}^{1/2}\left(\boldsymbol{P}_{\boldsymbol{X}\boldsymbol{A}^{-1/2}}\right)\boldsymbol{A}^{-1/2}\boldsymbol{Y},\end{aligned}$$

where $\boldsymbol{P}_{\boldsymbol{X}\boldsymbol{A}^{-1/2}}$ is the ordinary projection matrix onto the row space of $\boldsymbol{X}\boldsymbol{A}^{-1/2}$ and has induced matrix 2-norm 1. It follows

$$\left\|\hat{\boldsymbol{\mu}}^{\text{WLS}}\right\|\le\left\|\boldsymbol{A}^{1/2}\right\|_2\left\|\boldsymbol{P}_{\boldsymbol{A}^{-1/2}\boldsymbol{X}}\right\|_2\left\|\boldsymbol{A}^{-1/2}\right\|_2\|\boldsymbol{Y}\|=\max_{1\le i\le p}A_i^{1/2}\times\max_{1\le i\le p}A_i^{-1/2}\times\|\boldsymbol{Y}\|.$$

Condition (A) gives

$$\max_{1\le i\le p}A_i^{1/2}=(\max_{1\le i\le p}A_i^2)^{1/4}\le(\sum_{i=1}^{p}A_i^2)^{1/4}=O\left(p^{1/4}\right).$$

Similarly, condition (A′) gives

$$\max_{1\le i\le p}A_i^{-1/2}=(\max_{1\le i\le p}A_i^{-2-\delta})^{1/(4+2\delta)}\le(\sum_{i=1}^{p}A_i^{-2-\delta})^{1/(4+2\delta)}=O\left(p^{1/(4+2\delta)}\right).$$

We then have proved that

$$\left\| \hat{\boldsymbol{\mu}}^{\mathrm{WLS}} \right\| \leq O\left(p^{1/4}\right) O\left(p^{1/(4+2\delta)}\right) \|\boldsymbol{Y}\| = O\left(p^{\kappa}\right) \|\boldsymbol{Y}\| .$$

Proof of Theorem 2 To prove the first assertion, note that

$$\mathrm{URE}\left(\hat{\boldsymbol{B}}^{\mathrm{URE}}, \hat{\boldsymbol{\mu}}^{\mathrm{URE}}\right) \leq \mathrm{URE}\left(\tilde{\boldsymbol{B}}^{\mathrm{OL}}, \tilde{\boldsymbol{\mu}}^{\mathrm{OL}}\right)$$

by the definition of $\hat{\boldsymbol{B}}^{\mathrm{URE}}$ and $\hat{\boldsymbol{\mu}}^{\mathrm{URE}}$, so Theorem 1 implies that

$$\begin{aligned}
& l_p\left(\boldsymbol{\theta}, \hat{\boldsymbol{\theta}}^{\mathrm{URE}}\right) - l_p\left(\boldsymbol{\theta}, \tilde{\boldsymbol{\theta}}^{\mathrm{OL}}\right) \\
& \leq l_p\left(\boldsymbol{\theta}, \hat{\boldsymbol{\theta}}^{\mathrm{URE}}\right) - \mathrm{URE}\left(\hat{\boldsymbol{B}}^{\mathrm{URE}}, \hat{\boldsymbol{\mu}}^{\mathrm{URE}}\right) + \mathrm{URE}\left(\tilde{\boldsymbol{B}}^{\mathrm{OL}}, \tilde{\boldsymbol{\mu}}^{\mathrm{OL}}\right) - l_p\left(\boldsymbol{\theta}, \tilde{\boldsymbol{\theta}}^{\mathrm{OL}}\right) \\
& \leq 2 \sup_{\boldsymbol{B} \in \mathscr{B},\ \boldsymbol{\mu} \in \mathscr{L}} \left| \mathrm{URE}\left(\boldsymbol{B}, \boldsymbol{\mu}\right) - l_p\left(\boldsymbol{\theta}, \hat{\boldsymbol{\theta}}^{\boldsymbol{B}, \boldsymbol{\mu}}\right) \right| \underset{p \to \infty}{\to} 0 \text{ in } L^1 \text{ and in probability,}
\end{aligned} \tag{22}$$

where the second inequality uses the condition that $\hat{\boldsymbol{\mu}}^{\mathrm{URE}} \in \mathscr{L}$. Thus, for any $\epsilon > 0$,

$$\begin{aligned}
& \mathbb{P}\left(l_p\left(\boldsymbol{\theta}, \hat{\boldsymbol{\theta}}^{\mathrm{URE}}\right) \geq l_p\left(\boldsymbol{\theta}, \tilde{\boldsymbol{\theta}}^{\mathrm{OL}}\right) + \epsilon\right) \\
& \leq \mathbb{P}\left(2 \sup_{\boldsymbol{B} \in \mathscr{B},\ \boldsymbol{\mu} \in \mathscr{L}} \left| \mathrm{URE}\left(\boldsymbol{B}, \boldsymbol{\mu}\right) - l_p\left(\boldsymbol{\theta}, \hat{\boldsymbol{\theta}}^{\boldsymbol{B}, \boldsymbol{\mu}}\right) \right| \geq \epsilon\right) \to 0.
\end{aligned}$$

To prove the second assertion, note that

$$l_p\left(\boldsymbol{\theta}, \tilde{\boldsymbol{\theta}}^{\mathrm{OL}}\right) \leq l_p\left(\boldsymbol{\theta}, \hat{\boldsymbol{\theta}}^{\mathrm{URE}}\right)$$

by the definition of $\tilde{\boldsymbol{\theta}}^{\mathrm{OL}}$ and the condition $\hat{\boldsymbol{\mu}}^{\mathrm{URE}} \in \mathscr{L}$. Thus, taking expectations on Eq. (22) easily gives the second assertion.

Proof of Corollary 1 Simply note that

$$l_p\left(\boldsymbol{\theta}, \tilde{\boldsymbol{\theta}}^{\mathrm{OL}}\right) \leq l_p\left(\boldsymbol{\theta}, \hat{\boldsymbol{\theta}}^{\hat{\boldsymbol{B}}_p, \hat{\boldsymbol{\mu}}_p}\right)$$

by the definition of $\tilde{\boldsymbol{\theta}}^{\mathrm{OL}}$. Thus,

$$l_p\left(\boldsymbol{\theta}, \hat{\boldsymbol{\theta}}^{\mathrm{URE}}\right) - l_p\left(\boldsymbol{\theta}, \hat{\boldsymbol{\theta}}^{\hat{\boldsymbol{B}}_p, \hat{\boldsymbol{\mu}}_p}\right) \leq l_p\left(\boldsymbol{\theta}, \hat{\boldsymbol{\theta}}^{\mathrm{URE}}\right) - l_p\left(\boldsymbol{\theta}, \tilde{\boldsymbol{\theta}}^{\mathrm{OL}}\right).$$

Then Theorem 2 clearly implies the desired result.

Proof of Theorem 3 We observe that

$$\mathrm{URE}_M(\boldsymbol{B}) - l_p\left(\boldsymbol{\theta}, \hat{\boldsymbol{\theta}}^{\boldsymbol{B},\hat{\boldsymbol{\mu}}^M}\right) = \mathrm{URE}\left(\boldsymbol{B}, \hat{\boldsymbol{\mu}}^M\right) - l_p\left(\boldsymbol{\theta}, \hat{\boldsymbol{\theta}}^{\boldsymbol{B},\hat{\boldsymbol{\mu}}^M}\right) + \frac{2}{p}\mathrm{tr}\left(\boldsymbol{A}(\boldsymbol{A}+\boldsymbol{B})^{-1}\boldsymbol{P}_{M,X}\boldsymbol{A}\right).$$

Since

$$\sup_{\boldsymbol{B}\in\mathscr{B}}\left|\mathrm{URE}\left(\boldsymbol{B}, \hat{\boldsymbol{\mu}}^M\right) - l_p\left(\boldsymbol{\theta}, \hat{\boldsymbol{\theta}}^{\boldsymbol{B},\hat{\boldsymbol{\mu}}^M}\right)\right| \le \sup_{\boldsymbol{B}\in\mathscr{B},\ \boldsymbol{\mu}\in\mathscr{L}}\left|\mathrm{URE}(\boldsymbol{B}, \boldsymbol{\mu}) - l_p\left(\boldsymbol{\theta}, \hat{\boldsymbol{\theta}}^{\boldsymbol{B},\boldsymbol{\mu}}\right)\right| \to 0 \text{ in } L^1$$

by Theorem 1, we only need to show that

$$\sup_{\boldsymbol{B}\in\mathscr{B}}\left|\frac{1}{p}\mathrm{tr}\left(\boldsymbol{A}(\boldsymbol{A}+\boldsymbol{B})^{-1}\boldsymbol{P}_{M,X}\boldsymbol{A}\right)\right| \to 0 \quad \text{as } p\to\infty.$$

Under Model I,

$$\begin{aligned}\mathrm{tr}\left(\boldsymbol{A}(\boldsymbol{A}+\boldsymbol{B})^{-1}\boldsymbol{P}_{M,X}\boldsymbol{A}\right) &= \sum_{i=1}^{p}\frac{A_i}{A_i+\lambda}[\boldsymbol{P}_{M,X}\boldsymbol{A}]_{ii}\\ &\le \left(\sum_{i=1}^{p}(\frac{A_i}{A_i+\lambda})^2 \times \sum_{i=1}^{p}[\boldsymbol{P}_{M,X}\boldsymbol{A}]_{ii}^2\right)^{1/2}\\ &\le \left(p\times\sum_{i=1}^{p}[\boldsymbol{P}_{M,X}\boldsymbol{A}]_{ii}^2\right)^{1/2}\\ &= p^{1/2}\sqrt{\mathrm{tr}\,(\boldsymbol{P}_{M,X}\boldsymbol{A}(\boldsymbol{P}_{M,X}\boldsymbol{A})^T)}, \quad \text{for all } \lambda\ge 0,\end{aligned}$$

but $\mathrm{tr}\,(\boldsymbol{P}_{M,X}\boldsymbol{A}\boldsymbol{A}\boldsymbol{P}_{M,X}^T) = \mathrm{tr}\left(\boldsymbol{X}^T(\boldsymbol{XMX}^T)^{-1}\boldsymbol{XMA}^2\boldsymbol{MX}^T(\boldsymbol{XMX}^T)^{-1}\boldsymbol{X}\right)$ $= \mathrm{tr}\left((\boldsymbol{XMX}^T)^{-1}(\boldsymbol{XMA}^2\boldsymbol{MX}^T)(\boldsymbol{XMX}^T)^{-1}(\boldsymbol{XX}^T)\right) = O(1)$ by (13) and condition (E). Therefore,

$$\sup_{\boldsymbol{B}\in\mathscr{B}}\left|\frac{1}{p}\mathrm{tr}\left(\boldsymbol{A}(\boldsymbol{A}+\boldsymbol{B})^{-1}\boldsymbol{P}_{M,X}\boldsymbol{A}\right)\right| = \frac{1}{p}O\left(p^{1/2}\right)O(1) = O(p^{-1/2}) \to 0.$$

Under Model II, $\boldsymbol{A}(\boldsymbol{A}+\boldsymbol{B})^{-1}=\boldsymbol{I}_p-\lambda\boldsymbol{Z}^T(\lambda\boldsymbol{I}_k+\boldsymbol{\Lambda})^{-1}\boldsymbol{\Lambda}\boldsymbol{Z}\boldsymbol{A}^{-1}$, where $\boldsymbol{W}^{-1/2}\boldsymbol{V}\boldsymbol{W}^{-1/2}=\boldsymbol{U}\boldsymbol{\Lambda}\boldsymbol{U}^T$, $\boldsymbol{\Lambda}=\operatorname{diag}(d_1,\ldots,d_k)$ with $d_1\leq\cdots\leq d_k$, and $\boldsymbol{Z}=\boldsymbol{U}^T\boldsymbol{W}^{1/2}\boldsymbol{X}$ as defined in the proof of Theorem 1. Thus,

$$\operatorname{tr}\left(\boldsymbol{A}(\boldsymbol{A}+\boldsymbol{B})^{-1}\boldsymbol{P}_{M,X}\boldsymbol{A}\right)=\operatorname{tr}(\boldsymbol{P}_{M,X}\boldsymbol{A})-\operatorname{tr}\left(\lambda\boldsymbol{Z}^T(\lambda\boldsymbol{I}_k+\boldsymbol{\Lambda})^{-1}\boldsymbol{\Lambda}\boldsymbol{Z}\boldsymbol{A}^{-1}\boldsymbol{P}_{M,X}\boldsymbol{A}\right).$$

We know that $\operatorname{tr}(\boldsymbol{P}_{M,X}\boldsymbol{A})=\operatorname{tr}\left(\left(\boldsymbol{X}\boldsymbol{M}\boldsymbol{X}^T\right)^{-1}(\boldsymbol{X}\boldsymbol{M}\boldsymbol{A}\boldsymbol{X}^T)\right)=O(1)$ by the assumption (13). $\operatorname{tr}\left(\lambda\boldsymbol{Z}^T(\lambda\boldsymbol{I}_k+\boldsymbol{\Lambda})^{-1}\boldsymbol{\Lambda}\boldsymbol{Z}\boldsymbol{A}^{-1}\boldsymbol{P}_{M,X}\boldsymbol{A}\right)=\operatorname{tr}\left(\lambda(\lambda\boldsymbol{I}_k+\boldsymbol{\Lambda})^{-1}\boldsymbol{\Lambda}\boldsymbol{Z}\boldsymbol{A}^{-1}\boldsymbol{P}_{M,X}\right.$ $\left.\boldsymbol{A}\boldsymbol{Z}^T\right)=\operatorname{tr}\left(\lambda(\lambda\boldsymbol{I}_k+\boldsymbol{\Lambda})^{-1}\boldsymbol{\Lambda}\boldsymbol{Z}\boldsymbol{A}^{-1}\boldsymbol{X}^T\left(\boldsymbol{X}\boldsymbol{M}\boldsymbol{X}^T\right)^{-1}\boldsymbol{X}\boldsymbol{M}\boldsymbol{A}\boldsymbol{Z}^T\right)$. The Cauchy-Schwarz inequality for matrix trace gives

$$\begin{aligned}
&\left|\operatorname{tr}\left(\left(\lambda(\lambda\boldsymbol{I}_k+\boldsymbol{\Lambda})^{-1}\boldsymbol{\Lambda}\right)\left(\boldsymbol{Z}\boldsymbol{A}^{-1}\boldsymbol{X}^T\left(\boldsymbol{X}\boldsymbol{M}\boldsymbol{X}^T\right)^{-1}\boldsymbol{X}\boldsymbol{M}\boldsymbol{A}\boldsymbol{Z}^T\right)\right)\right|\\
&\leq\operatorname{tr}^{1/2}\left(\left(\lambda(\lambda\boldsymbol{I}_k+\boldsymbol{\Lambda})^{-1}\boldsymbol{\Lambda}\right)^2\right)\\
&\quad\times\operatorname{tr}^{1/2}\left(\boldsymbol{Z}\boldsymbol{A}^{-1}\boldsymbol{X}^T\left(\boldsymbol{X}\boldsymbol{M}\boldsymbol{X}^T\right)^{-1}\boldsymbol{X}\boldsymbol{M}\boldsymbol{A}\boldsymbol{Z}^T\boldsymbol{Z}\boldsymbol{A}\boldsymbol{M}\boldsymbol{X}^T\left(\boldsymbol{X}\boldsymbol{M}\boldsymbol{X}^T\right)^{-1}\boldsymbol{X}\boldsymbol{A}^{-1}\boldsymbol{Z}^T\right).
\end{aligned}$$

Since

$$\operatorname{tr}\left(\left(\lambda(\lambda\boldsymbol{I}_k+\boldsymbol{\Lambda})^{-1}\boldsymbol{\Lambda}\right)^2\right)=\sum_{i=1}^{k}\left(\frac{\lambda d_i}{\lambda+d_i}\right)^2\leq kd_k^2=O\left(p^{-2}\right)\quad\text{for all }\lambda\geq 0$$

as shown in the proof of Theorem 1 and

$$\begin{aligned}
&\operatorname{tr}\left(\boldsymbol{Z}\boldsymbol{A}^{-1}\boldsymbol{X}^T\left(\boldsymbol{X}\boldsymbol{M}\boldsymbol{X}^T\right)^{-1}\boldsymbol{X}\boldsymbol{M}\boldsymbol{A}\boldsymbol{Z}^T\boldsymbol{Z}\boldsymbol{A}\boldsymbol{M}\boldsymbol{X}^T\left(\boldsymbol{X}\boldsymbol{M}\boldsymbol{X}^T\right)^{-1}\boldsymbol{X}\boldsymbol{A}^{-1}\boldsymbol{Z}^T\right)\\
&=\operatorname{tr}\left(\left(\boldsymbol{X}\boldsymbol{M}\boldsymbol{X}^T\right)^{-1}\boldsymbol{X}\boldsymbol{M}\boldsymbol{A}\boldsymbol{Z}^T\boldsymbol{Z}\boldsymbol{A}\boldsymbol{M}\boldsymbol{X}^T\left(\boldsymbol{X}\boldsymbol{M}\boldsymbol{X}^T\right)^{-1}\boldsymbol{X}\boldsymbol{A}^{-1}\boldsymbol{Z}^T\boldsymbol{Z}\boldsymbol{A}^{-1}\boldsymbol{X}^T\right)\\
&=\operatorname{tr}\left(\left(\boldsymbol{X}\boldsymbol{M}\boldsymbol{X}^T\right)^{-1}(\boldsymbol{X}\boldsymbol{M}\boldsymbol{A}\boldsymbol{X}^T)\boldsymbol{W}(\boldsymbol{X}\boldsymbol{A}\boldsymbol{M}\boldsymbol{X}^T)\left(\boldsymbol{X}\boldsymbol{M}\boldsymbol{X}^T\right)^{-1}(\boldsymbol{X}\boldsymbol{A}^{-1}\boldsymbol{X}^T)\boldsymbol{W}(\boldsymbol{X}\boldsymbol{A}^{-1}\boldsymbol{X}^T)\right)\\
&=O(p^2)
\end{aligned}$$

from (13) and condition (F), we have

$$\sup_{\boldsymbol{B}\in\mathscr{B}}\left|\frac{1}{p}\operatorname{tr}\left(\boldsymbol{A}(\boldsymbol{A}+\boldsymbol{B})^{-1}\boldsymbol{P}_{M,X}\boldsymbol{A}\right)\right|=\frac{1}{p}\left(O(1)+\sqrt{O\left(p^{-2}\right)\times O(p^2)}\right)=O(p^{-1})\to 0.$$

This completes our proof of (14). With this established, the rest of the proof is identical to that of Theorem 2 and Corollary 1.

References

1. Berger, J.O., Strawderman, W.E.: Choice of hierarchical priors: admissibility in estimation of normal means. Ann. Stat. **24**(3), 931–951 (1996)
2. Brown, L.D.: In-season prediction of batting averages: a field test of empirical Bayes and Bayes methodologies. Ann. Appl. Stat. **2**(1), 113–152 (2008)
3. Copas, J.B.: Regression, prediction and shrinkage. J. R. Stat. Soc. Ser. B Methodol. **45**(3), 311–354 (1983)
4. Efron, B., Morris, C.: Empirical Bayes on vector observations: an extension of Stein's method. Biometrika **59**(2), 335–347 (1972)
5. Efron, B., Morris, C.: Stein's estimation rule and its competitors—an empirical Bayes approach. J. Am. Stat. Assoc. **68**(341), 117–130 (1973)
6. Efron, B., Morris, C.: Data analysis using Stein's estimator and its generalizations. J. Am. Stat. Assoc. **70**(350), 311–319 (1975)
7. Fearn, T.: A Bayesian approach to growth curves. Biometrika **62**(1), 89–100 (1975)
8. Green, E.J., Strawderman, W.E.: The use of Bayes/empirical Bayes estimation in individual tree volume equation development. For. Sci. **31**(4), 975–990 (1985)
9. Hui, S.L., Berger, J.O.: Empirical Bayes estimation of rates in longitudinal studies. J. Am. Stat. Assoc. **78**(384), 753–760 (1983)
10. James, W., Stein, C.: Estimation with quadratic loss. In: Proceedings of the Fourth Berkeley Symposium on Mathematical Statistics and Probability, vol. 1, pp. 361–379. University of California Press, Berkeley (1961)
11. Jiang, J., Nguyen, T., Rao, J.S.: Best predictive small area estimation. J. Am. Stat. Assoc. **106**(494), 732–745 (2011)
12. Jones, K.: Specifying and estimating multi-level models for geographical research. Trans. Inst. Br. Geogr. **16**(2), 148–159 (1991)
13. Li, K.C.: Asymptotic optimality of C_L and generalized cross-validation in ridge regression with application to spline smoothing. Ann. Stat. **14(3)**, 1101–1102 (1986)
14. Lindley, D.V.: Discussion of a paper by C. Stein. J. R. Stat. Soc. Ser. B Methodol. **24**, 285–287 (1962)
15. Lindley, D.V.V., Smith, A.F.M.: Bayes estimates for the linear model. J. R. Stat. Soc. Ser. B Methodol. **34**(1), 1–41 (1972)
16. Morris, C.N.: Parametric empirical Bayes inference: theory and applications. J. Am. Stat. Assoc. **78**(381), 47–55 (1983)
17. Morris, C.N., Lysy, M.: Shrinkage estimation in multilevel normal models. Stat. Sci. **27**(1), 115–134 (2012)
18. Normand, S.L.T., Glickman, M.E., Gatsonis, C.A.: Statistical methods for profiling providers of medical care: issues and applications. J. Am. Stat. Assoc. **92**(439), 803–814 (1997)
19. Omen, S.D.: Shrinking towards subspaces in multiple linear regression. Technometrics **24**(4), 307–311 (1982). 1982
20. Raftery, A.E., Madigan, D., Hoeting, J.A.: Bayesian model averaging for linear regression models. J. Am. Stat. Assoc. **92**(437), 179–191 (1997)
21. Robbins, H.: An empirical Bayes approach to statistics. In: Proceedings of the Third Berkeley Symposium on Mathematical Statistics and Probability. Contributions to the Theory of Statistics, vol. 1, pp. 157–163. University of California Press, Berkeley (1956)
22. Rubin, D.B.: Using empirical Bayes techniques in the law school validity studies. J. Am. Stat. Assoc. **75**(372), 801–816 (1980)
23. Sclove, S.L., Morris, C., Radhakrishnan, R.: Non-optimality of preliminary-test estimators for the mean of a multivariate normal distribution. Ann. Math. Stat. **43**(5), 1481–1490 (1972)
24. Stein, C.: Inadmissibility of the usual estimator for the mean of a multivariate normal distribution. In: Proceedings of the Third Berkeley Symposium on Mathematical Statistics and Probability. Contributions to the Theory of Statistics, vol. 1, pp. 197–206. University of California Press, Berkeley (1956)

25. Stein, C.M.: Confidence sets for the mean of a multivariate normal distribution (with discussion). J. R. Stat. Soc. Ser. B Stat Methodol. **24**, 265–296 (1962)
26. Stein, C.: An approach to the recovery of inter-block information in balanced incomplete block designs. In: Neyman, F.J. (ed.) Research Papers in Statistics, pp. 351–366. Wiley, London (1966)
27. Strenio, J.F., Weisberg, H.I., Bryk, A.S.: Empirical Bayes estimation of individual growth-curve parameters and their relationship to covariates. Biometrics **39**(1), 71–86 (1983)
28. Tan, Z.: Steinized empirical Bayes estimation for heteroscedastic data. Stat. Sin. **26**, 1219–1248 (2016)
29. Xie, X., Kou, S.C., Brown, L.D.: SURE estimates for a heteroscedastic hierarchical model. J. Am. Stat. Assoc. **107**(500), 1465–1479 (2012)
30. Xie, X., Kou, S.C., Brown, L.D.: Optimal shrinkage estimation of mean parameters in family of distributions with quadratic variance. Ann. Stat. **44**, 564–597 (2016)

High Dimensional Data Analysis: Integrating Submodels

Syed Ejaz Ahmed and Bahadır Yüzbaşı

Abstract We consider an efficient prediction in sparse high dimensional data. In high dimensional data settings where $d \gg n$, many penalized regularization strategies are suggested for simultaneous variable selection and estimation. However, different strategies yield a different submodel with $d_i < n$, where d_i represents the number of predictors included in ith submodel. Some procedures may select a submodel with a larger number of predictors than others. Due to the trade-off between model complexity and model prediction accuracy, the statistical inference of model selection becomes extremely important and challenging in high dimensional data analysis. For this reason we suggest shrinkage and pretest strategies to improve the prediction performance of two selected submodels. Such a pretest and shrinkage strategy is constructed by shrinking an overfitted model estimator in the direction of an underfitted model estimator. The numerical studies indicate that our post-selection pretest and shrinkage strategy improved the prediction performance of selected submodels.

Keywords Monte Carlo simulation • Pretest, penalty and shrinkage strategies • Sparse regression models

1 Introduction

There are a host of buzzwords in today's data-centric world, and especially in digital and print media. We encounter data in every walk of life, and for analytically and objectively minded people, data is everything. However, making sense of the data and extracting meaningful information from it may not be an easy task. We come across buzzwords such as Big Data, high dimensional data, data visualization, data science, and open data without a proper definition of such words. The rapid

S. Ejaz Ahmed (✉)
Department of Mathematics and Statistics, Brock University, St. Catherines, Ontario, Canada
e-mail: sahmed5@brocku.ca

B. Yüzbaşı
Department of Econometrics, Inonu University, Malatya, Turkey
e-mail: b.yzb@hotmail.com

© Springer International Publishing AG 2017

S.E. Ahmed (ed.), *Big and Complex Data Analysis*, Contributions to Statistics,
DOI 10.1007/978-3-319-41573-4_14

growth in the size and scope of data sets in a host of disciplines has created a need for innovative statistical strategies analyzing such data. A variety of statistical and computational tools are needed to overcome such types of the data and to reveal the data story. However, in this paper, we focus on estimation of model parameters and prediction based on high dimensional data (HDD). In classical regression context we define HDD where number of predictors (d) are larger than the sample size (n). More importantly, the number of predictors are in millions and sample size maybe in hundreds. The modeling of HDD is an important feature in a host of research fields such as social sciences, bio-informatics, medical, environmental, engineering, and financial studies among others. A number of the classical techniques are available when $d < n$ to tell the data story. However, the existing classical strategies are not capable of yielding solutions for HDD. On the other hand, the buzzword "Big Data" is not very well defined, but its problems are real and statisticians need to play a vital role in this data world. The Big Data or Data Science is an emerging field stemming equally from research enterprise and public and private sectors. Undoubtedly, Big Data is the future of research in a host fields, and trans-disciplinary programs are required to develop the skills for Data Scientists. For example, many private and public agencies are using sophisticated number-crunching, data mining, or Big Data analytics to reveal patterns based on collected information. Clearly, there is an increasing demand for efficient prediction strategies for analyzing such data. Some examples of Big Data that have prompted demand are gene expression arrays, social network modeling, clinical, genetics, and phenotypic data.

Due to the trade-off between model prediction and model complexity, the model selection is an extremely important and challenging problem in high dimensional data analysis (HDDA). Over the past two decades, many penalized regularization approaches have been developed to perform variable selection and estimation simultaneously. These techniques, which deal with HDDA, generally rely on various L_1 penalty regularizes. The least absolute shrinkage and selection operator (Lasso) is one of the widely used approaches, Tibshirani [20]. It is a good strategy due to its convexity and computation efficiency. The Lasso is based on squared error and a penalty proportional to regression parameters. Schelldorfer et al. [19] provide a comprehensive summary of the consistency properties of the Lasso. Efron et al. [12] introduced the least angle regression algorithm which is a very fast way to draw the entire regularization path for aLasso estimate of the regression parameters. The penalized likelihood methods have been extensively studied in the literature, see, for example, Tran [22], Huang et al. [15], Kim et al. [16], Wang and Leng [23], Yuan and Lin [24], Leng et al. [17], and Tibshirani et al. [21]. Interestingly, the penalized likelihood methods are closely connected to Bayesian procedures. The Lasso estimate corresponds to a Bayes method that puts a Laplacian (double exponential) prior on the regression coefficients. Armagan et al. [5], Bhattacharya et al. [8], and Carvalho et al. [11] have shown that improvements can be achieved by using priors with heavier tails than the double exponential prior in particular, priors with polynomial tails.

In this paper, we focus on the Lasso, the Elastic-Net, the adaptive Lasso (aLasso), the minimax concave penalty (MCP), and the smoothly clipped absolute deviation method (SCAD). We blend these methods with the decades old method of "pretesting: variable section and post-estimation" to improve the prediction accuracy of penalty methods. The important contribution here is to incorporate the pretesting strategy after selecting the "overfitted (OF)" and "underfitted (UF)" models. Generally speaking, both Lasso and Elastic-Net strategies select OF models. On the other hand, aLasso, MCP, and SCAD produces yield UF models. Our goal is to combine an OF model (OFM) with a UF model (UFM) via pretesting to improve the model prediction and complexity simultaneously. We have the estimation problem of regression parameters when the model is sparse that there are many potential predictors in the model at-hand may not have any influence on the response of interest. Further, some of the predictors may have strong influence (strong signals), and some of them may have weak-moderate influence (weak-moderate signals) on the response of interest, respectively. It is possible that there may be extraneous predictors in the OFM. Consider if the main concern is treatment effect, or the effect of biomarkers: extraneous nuisance variables may be lab effects when several labs are involved, or the age and sex of patients. The analysis will be more meaningful if "nuisance variables" can be deleted from the OFM. Further, it is exceedingly important that we do not automatically remove all the predictors with weak/moderate signals from the model. This may result in selecting a biased UFM. A logical way to deal with this framework is to apply a pretest strategy that tests whether the coefficients with weak/moderate effects are zero and then estimates parameters in the model that include coefficients that are rejected by the test. Another strategy is to use estimators based on Stein-rule, where the estimated regression coefficient vector is shrunk in the direction of the candidate subspace. This "soft threshold" modification of the pretest method has been shown to be efficient in various frameworks. Ahmed et al. [4] and Ahmed and Yüzbaşı [3], among others, have investigated the properties of shrinkage and pretest methodologies for host models. In Sect. 2 we describe the model and review some penalty strategies. In Sect. 3 we introduce pretest and shrinkage strategies. The results of a simulation study are showcased in Sect. 4. Application to two real data sets are given in Sect. 5. Finally, we offer concluding remarks in Sect. 6.

2 Model Section and Penalty Estimation

We consider a high dimensional linear regression sparse model:

$$\mathbf{Y} = \mathbf{X}\boldsymbol{\beta} + \boldsymbol{\varepsilon}, \tag{1}$$

where $\mathbf{Y} = (y_1, \ldots, y_n)'$ is a vector of responses, $\mathbf{X} = (\mathbf{x}_1, \ldots, \mathbf{x}_n)'$ an $n \times d$ fixed design matrix, where $\mathbf{x}_i = (x_{i1}, \ldots, x_{id})'$, $\boldsymbol{\beta} = (\beta_1, \ldots, \beta_d)'$ is an unknown vector of parameters, $\boldsymbol{\varepsilon} = (\varepsilon_1, \ldots, \varepsilon_n)'$ is the vector of unobservable random errors, and the superscript ($'$) denotes the transpose of a vector or matrix. We do not make any distributional assumption about the errors except that $\boldsymbol{\varepsilon}$ has a cumulative distribution function $F(\cdot)$ with $E(\boldsymbol{\varepsilon}) = \mathbf{0}$, and $E(\boldsymbol{\varepsilon}\boldsymbol{\varepsilon}') = \sigma^2\mathbf{I}_n$, $\sigma^2 < \infty$.

For $n > d$ the least squares estimator (LSE) of $\boldsymbol{\beta}$ is obtained by minimizing the following function:

$$\hat{\boldsymbol{\beta}}^{\text{LSE}} = (\mathbf{X}'\mathbf{X})^{-1}\mathbf{X}'\mathbf{Y}.$$

However, when $n < d$ then $(\mathbf{X}'\mathbf{X})^{-1}$ will not exist and thus no solution. In this situation, we can use ridge regression to achieve a solution. On the other hand, to avoid the model complexity, penalized likelihood methods are popular nowadays. These methods involve penalizing the regression coefficients, and shrinking a subset of them towards zero. In other words, the penalized procedure produces a submodel and subsequently estimates the submodel parameters, as seen in [2]. However, in an effort to achieve meaningful estimation and selection properties, most penalized strategies make the following assumptions:

- Most of regression coefficients are zeros except for a few ones
- All nonzero β_j's are larger than noise level, $c\sigma\sqrt{(2/n)\log(d)}$ with $c \geq 1/2$.

Further, additional assumptions made regarding the designed covariates include the adaptive irrepresentable condition and the restricted eigenvalue condition. We refer to Zhao and Yu [27], Huang et al. [15], and Bickel et al. [9] for some insights.

Generally speaking, the Lasso and Elastic-Net (Enet) methods tend to select OFM, we refer to Leng et al. [17]. In reviewed literature, several modifications and methodologies have been suggested to improve the prediction accuracy for the Lasso strategy. For example, the SCAD [13], adaptive Lasso [28], MCP [25], and several others. Like Lasso, these methods select a submodel by shrinking a number of regression coefficients to zero and provide shrinkage estimators of the remaining coefficients. However, these methods may force the relatively a large number of weaker coefficients towards zeros as compared to Lasso, resulting in UFM, and are subject to a larger selection bias in the presence of a significant number of weak/moderate signals. This leads to the consideration of two models: the OFM that includes all predictors with strong signals and possible variables with weak and moderate signals, and a UFM that includes the predictors with strong signals while leaving out variables with weak signals. An appealing way to deal with this uncertainty about regression parameters is to use a pretest strategy that test whether the coefficients of the variables with weak/moderate signals are zero and then estimate parameters in the model that include coefficients that are rejected by the test.

Now, we briefly describe some penalized strategies. An important member of the penalized least squares family is the L_1 penalized least squares estimator, commonly known as the Lasso.

2.1 Lasso

This method was proposed by [20], it performs variable selection and parameter estimation simultaneously. The Lasso estimator is obtained by

$$\hat{\boldsymbol{\beta}}^{\text{Lasso}} = \arg\min_{\beta} \left\{ \sum_{i=1}^{n} (y_i - \sum_{j=1}^{d} x_{ij}\beta_j)^2 + \lambda \sum_{j=1}^{d} |\beta_j| \right\}. \tag{2}$$

Originally, Lasso solutions were obtained via quadratic programming. Later, [12] proposed Least Angle Regression (LARS), a type of stepwise regression, with which the Lasso estimates can be obtained at the same computational cost as that of an ordinary least squares estimation. Further, the Lasso estimator remains numerically feasible for dimensions of d that are much higher than the sample size n. Usually, Lasso will produce an OFM when there are many predictors with weak signals are in the initial model.

2.2 Elastic-Net

The Elastic-Net was proposed by Zou and Hastie [29] to overcome the limitations of the Lasso and Ridge methods.

$$\hat{\boldsymbol{\beta}}^{\text{Enet}} = (1+\frac{\lambda_2}{n})\arg\min_{\beta} \left\{ \sum_{i=1}^{n} (y_i - \sum_{j=1}^{d} x_{ij}\beta_j)^2 + \lambda_1 \sum_{j=1}^{d} |\beta_j| + \lambda_2 \sum_{j=1}^{d} \beta_j^2 \right\}, \tag{3}$$

where λ_2 is the ridge penalty parameter, penalizing the sum of the squared regression coefficients and λ_1 is the Lasso penalty, penalizing the sum of the absolute values of the regression coefficients, respectively.

2.3 SCAD

Fan and Li [13] proposed a non-concave penalty function referred to as SCAD. The SCAD method is given by

$$\hat{\boldsymbol{\beta}}^{\text{SCAD}} = \arg\min_{\beta} \left\{ \sum_{i=1}^{n} (y_i - \sum_{j=1}^{d} x_{ij}\beta_j)^2 + \lambda \sum_{j=1}^{d} p_{\alpha,\lambda}|\beta_j| \right\}.$$

Here $p_{\alpha,\lambda}(\cdot)$ is the smoothly clipped absolute deviation penalty. SCAD penalty is a symmetric and a quadratic spline on $[0, \infty)$ with knots at λ and $\alpha\lambda$, whose first order derivative is given by

$$p_{\alpha,\lambda}(x) = \lambda \left\{ I(|x| \leq \lambda) + \frac{(\alpha\lambda - |x|)^+}{(\alpha - 1)\lambda} I(|x| > \lambda) \right\}, \quad x \geq 0. \tag{4}$$

Here $\lambda > 0$ and $\alpha > 2$ are the tuning parameters. For $\alpha = \infty$, the expression (4) is equivalent to the L_1 penalty.

2.4 Adaptive Lasso

Zou [28] modified the Lasso penalty by using adaptive weights on L_1 penalties on the regression coefficients.

The aLasso estimator is obtained by

$$\hat{\boldsymbol{\beta}}^{\text{aLasso}} = \arg\min_{\beta} \left\{ \sum_{i=1}^{n} (y_i - \sum_{j=1}^{d} x_{ij}\beta_j)^2 + \lambda \sum_{j=1}^{d} \hat{w}_j |\beta_j| \right\}, \tag{5}$$

where the weight function is

$$\hat{w}_j = \frac{1}{|\hat{\beta}_j^*|^\gamma}; \quad \gamma > 0,$$

and $\hat{\beta}_j^*$ is a root-n consistent estimator of β. Equation (5) is a convex optimization problem and its global minimizer can be efficiently solved by [28].

2.5 MCP

Zhang [25] suggested an MCP method which is given by

$$\hat{\boldsymbol{\beta}}^{\text{MCP}} = \arg\min \left\{ \sum_{i=1}^{n} \left(y_i - \sum_{j=1}^{d} x_{ij}\beta_j \right)^2 + \sum_{j=1}^{d} \rho_\lambda(|\beta_j|, \gamma) \right\},$$

where $\rho_\lambda(\gamma)$ is the MCP penalty given by

$$\rho_\lambda(\gamma) = \int_0^t (\lambda - x/\gamma)^+ dx,$$

where $\gamma > 0$ is a regularization parameter.

These regularization techniques have been extensively used in a host of applications, and much research is still being conducted, making keeping track of all relevant research a difficult task. It has been widely recognized that penalty estimators are not efficient when the dimension d becomes extremely large compared with sample size n. There are still remaining challenging problems when d grows at a non-polynomial rate with n. Further, non-polynomial dimensionality brings forward substantial computational challenges. The main objective of this paper is about improving the estimation and/or prediction accuracy of the important set of the regression parameters by combining overfitted and underfitted models. As stated earlier, the Enet and Lasso produce an overfitted model as compared with aLasso, SCAD, and MCP methods. By design, the Enet and Lasso strategy retains some regression coefficients with weak effects in the resulted model. On the other hand, aggressive variable selection strategies may force moderate and weak effects coefficients towards zero, resulting in underfitted models with only variables of strong effect. The idea here is to combine estimators from an underfitted model with an overfitted model.

3 Integrating Overfitted and Underfitted Models

In this section we showcase how to combine two competing submodels to improve the estimation and prediction accuracy on both models.

3.1 *Working Model*

Let us consider a high dimensional sparse regression model with all possible predictors, including strong and weak-to-moderate signals.

$$\mathbf{Y} = \mathbf{X}\boldsymbol{\beta} + \boldsymbol{\varepsilon}, \quad d > n \tag{6}$$

where $\boldsymbol{\varepsilon}$'s are random errors distributed to be independent and identically distributed. Let us rewrite the model as follows:

$$\mathbf{Y} = \mathbf{X}_1\boldsymbol{\beta}_1 + \mathbf{X}_2\boldsymbol{\beta}_2 + \mathbf{X}_3\boldsymbol{\beta}_3 + \boldsymbol{\varepsilon}, \quad d = d_1 + d_2 + d_3 > n. \tag{7}$$

Further, the model is sparse, so it is expected that $d_1 + d_2 < n$ and $d_3 > n$, where d_1 is the dimension of strong signals, d_2 is for weak-moderate signals, and d_3 is associated with no signals. By assuming sparsity, the coefficients with no signals can be discarded by existing variable selection approaches. However, it is possible that some weak-moderate signals may be forced out from the model by an aggressive variable selection method. It is possible that the method at hand may not be able to separate weak signals from sparse signals, we refer to Zhang and Zhang [26] and others. Further, Hansen [14] has showed using simulation studies that post-selection least squares estimate can do better than penalty estimators under such scenarios. For some improved strategies, we refer to Belloni and Chernozhukov [7] and Liu and Yu [18].

In the current investigation, we are interested in estimation and prediction problems in a sparse model including weak-moderate signals. It is possible that one less aggressive variable selection strategy may yield an overfitted model, in the sense, that it is retaining predictors of strong and weak-moderate signals. On the other hand, other aggressive methods may give an underfitted model keeping only predictors of strong influence. Thus, the predictors with weak-moderate influence should be subject to further scrutiny to improve the prediction error.

We partition the design matrix such that $\mathbf{X} = (\mathbf{X}_1|\mathbf{X}_2|\mathbf{X}_3)$, where $\mathbf{X}_1$ is $n \times d_1$, $\mathbf{X}_2$ is $n \times d_2$, and $\mathbf{X}_3$ is $n \times d_3$ sub-matrix of predictors, respectively. Here we make the usual assumption that $d_1 \leq d_2 < n$ and $d_3 > n$.

Thus, our sparse model can be rewritten as:

$$\mathbf{Y} = \mathbf{X}_1\boldsymbol{\beta}_1 + \mathbf{X}_2\boldsymbol{\beta}_2 + \mathbf{X}_3\boldsymbol{\beta}_3 + \boldsymbol{\varepsilon}, \quad d > n, \ d_1 + d_2 < n. \tag{8}$$

3.2 Overfitted Model

We apply a less aggressive variable selection method which keeps both strong and weak-moderate signals in the resulting model as follows:

$$\mathbf{Y} = \mathbf{X}_1\boldsymbol{\beta}_1 + \mathbf{X}_2\boldsymbol{\beta}_2 + \boldsymbol{\varepsilon}, \quad d_1 \leq d_2 < n, \quad d_1 + d_2 < n. \tag{9}$$

Generally speaking, both Enet and Lasso strategies which usually eliminate the sparse signals and keep predictors with weak-moderate and strong signals in the resulting model. For brevity sake, we characterize such models as an overfitted model.

3.3 Underfitted Model

Suppose an aggressive variable selection method which keeps only predictors with strong signals and removes all other predictors, we call it an underfitted model. Thus, we have

$$\mathbf{Y} = \mathbf{X}_1\boldsymbol{\beta}_1 + \boldsymbol{\varepsilon}, \quad d_1 < n. \tag{10}$$

One can use aLasso, SCAD, or MCP strategy which usually keeps predictors only with the strong signals, and may yield a lower dimensional model as compared with Enet or Lasso.

Once again, we are interested in estimating $\boldsymbol{\beta}_1$ when $\boldsymbol{\beta}_2$ may be a null vector, but we are not certain that this is the case. We suggest pretest and shrinkage strategies for estimating $\boldsymbol{\beta}_1$ when model is sparse and $\boldsymbol{\beta}_2$ may be a null vector. It is natural to combine estimates of the overfitted model with the estimates of an underfitted model to improve the performance of an underfitted model.

3.4 Integrating Data

Now, we consider some shrinkage and pretest strategies to combine the information from overfitted and underfitted models.

First, we define the Linear Shrinkage (LS) estimator of $\boldsymbol{\beta}_1$ as follows:

$$\hat{\boldsymbol{\beta}}_1^{\mathrm{LS}} = \omega \hat{\boldsymbol{\beta}}_1^{\mathrm{UF}} + (1-\omega)\,\hat{\boldsymbol{\beta}}_1^{\mathrm{OF}}, \tag{11}$$

where $\omega \in [0, 1]$ denotes the shrinkage intensity. Ideally, the coefficient ω is chosen to minimize the mean squared error.

The pretest estimator (PT) of $\boldsymbol{\beta}_1$ defined by

$$\hat{\boldsymbol{\beta}}_1^{\mathrm{PT}} = \hat{\boldsymbol{\beta}}_1^{\mathrm{UF}} \mathrm{I}\left(W_n < \chi^2_{d_2,\alpha}\right) + \hat{\boldsymbol{\beta}}_1^{\mathrm{OF}} \mathrm{I}\left(W_n \geq \chi^2_{d_2,\alpha}\right),$$

or, equivalently,

$$\hat{\boldsymbol{\beta}}_1^{\mathrm{PT}} = \hat{\boldsymbol{\beta}}_1^{\mathrm{OF}} - \left(\hat{\boldsymbol{\beta}}_1^{\mathrm{OF}} - \hat{\boldsymbol{\beta}}_1^{\mathrm{UF}}\right) \mathrm{I}\left(W_n < \chi^2_{d_2,\alpha}\right),$$

where the weight function W_n is defined by

$$W_n = \frac{n}{\hat{\sigma}^2} (\hat{\boldsymbol{\beta}}_2^{\mathrm{LSE}})' (\mathbf{X}_2' \boldsymbol{M}_1 \mathbf{X}_2) \hat{\boldsymbol{\beta}}_2^{\mathrm{LSE}},$$

and $\boldsymbol{M}_1 = \mathbf{I}_n - \mathbf{X}_1 \left(\mathbf{X}_1'\mathbf{X}_1\right)^{-1} \mathbf{X}_1'$, $\hat{\boldsymbol{\beta}}_2^{\mathrm{LSE}} = \left(\mathbf{X}_2' \boldsymbol{M}_1 \mathbf{X}_2\right)^{-1} \mathbf{X}_2' \boldsymbol{M}_1 \mathbf{Y}$ and

$$\hat{\sigma}^2 = \frac{1}{n-1} (\mathbf{Y} - \mathbf{X}_1 \hat{\boldsymbol{\beta}}_1^{\mathrm{UF}})' (\mathbf{Y} - \mathbf{X}_1 \hat{\boldsymbol{\beta}}_1^{\mathrm{UF}}).$$

The $\hat{\boldsymbol{\beta}}_1^{\mathrm{UF}}$ may be aLasso, SCAD, or MCP estimator and the $\hat{\boldsymbol{\beta}}_1^{\mathrm{OF}}$ may be Enet or Lasso estimator.

Ahmed [1] proposed a shrinkage pretest estimation (SPT) strategy replacing $\hat{\boldsymbol{\beta}}_1^{\mathrm{UF}}$ by $\hat{\boldsymbol{\beta}}_1^{\mathrm{LS}}$ in (11) as follows:

$$\hat{\boldsymbol{\beta}}_1^{\mathrm{SPT}} = \left(\omega\hat{\boldsymbol{\beta}}_1^{\mathrm{UF}} + (1-\omega)\,\hat{\boldsymbol{\beta}}_1^{\mathrm{OF}}\right)\mathrm{I}\left(W_n < \chi^2_{d_2,\alpha}\right) + \hat{\boldsymbol{\beta}}_1^{\mathrm{OF}}\mathrm{I}\left(W_n \geq \chi^2_{d_2,\alpha}\right),$$

or, equivalently,

$$\hat{\boldsymbol{\beta}}_1^{\mathrm{SPT}} = \hat{\boldsymbol{\beta}}_1^{\mathrm{OF}} - \omega\left(\hat{\boldsymbol{\beta}}_1^{\mathrm{OF}} - \hat{\boldsymbol{\beta}}_1^{\mathrm{UF}}\right)\mathrm{I}\left(W_n < \chi^2_{d_2,\alpha}\right).$$

In the sprit of [2], the Stein-type shrinkage estimator of $\boldsymbol{\beta}_1$ is defined by combining overfitted model estimator $\hat{\boldsymbol{\beta}}_1^{\mathrm{OF}}$ with the underfitted $\hat{\boldsymbol{\beta}}_1^{\mathrm{UF}}$ as follows:

$$\hat{\boldsymbol{\beta}}_1^{\mathrm{S}} = \hat{\boldsymbol{\beta}}_1^{\mathrm{UF}} + \left(\hat{\boldsymbol{\beta}}_1^{\mathrm{OF}} - \hat{\boldsymbol{\beta}}_1^{\mathrm{UF}}\right)\left(1-(d_2-2)W_n^{-1}\right),\ d_2 \geq 3,$$

In an effort to avoid the over-shrinking problem inherited by $\hat{\boldsymbol{\beta}}_1^{\mathrm{S}}$ we suggest using the positive part of the shrinkage estimator of $\boldsymbol{\beta}_1$ defined by

$$\hat{\boldsymbol{\beta}}_1^{\mathrm{S+}} = \hat{\boldsymbol{\beta}}_1^{\mathrm{UF}} + \left(\hat{\boldsymbol{\beta}}_1^{\mathrm{OF}} - \hat{\boldsymbol{\beta}}_1^{\mathrm{UF}}\right)\left(1-(d_2-2)W_n^{-1}\right)^+,$$

where $z^+ = \max(0, z)$.

If we replace $\hat{\boldsymbol{\beta}}_1^{\mathrm{OF}}$ by $\hat{\boldsymbol{\beta}}_1^{\mathrm{S+}}$ in $\hat{\boldsymbol{\beta}}_1^{\mathrm{PT}}$, we obtain the improved pretest estimator (IPT) of $\boldsymbol{\beta}_1$ defined by

$$\hat{\boldsymbol{\beta}}_1^{\mathrm{IPT1}} = \hat{\boldsymbol{\beta}}_1^{\mathrm{S+}} - \left(\hat{\boldsymbol{\beta}}_1^{\mathrm{S+}} - \hat{\boldsymbol{\beta}}_1^{\mathrm{UF}}\right)\mathrm{I}\left(W_n < \chi^2_{d_2,\alpha}\right).$$

If we replace $\hat{\boldsymbol{\beta}}_1^{\mathrm{UF}}$ by $\hat{\boldsymbol{\beta}}_1^{\mathrm{LS}}$ in $\hat{\boldsymbol{\beta}}_1^{\mathrm{S+}}$, we obtain the improved pretest estimator of $\boldsymbol{\beta}_1$ defined by

$$\hat{\boldsymbol{\beta}}_1^{\mathrm{IPT2}} = \hat{\boldsymbol{\beta}}_1^{\mathrm{LS}} + \left(\hat{\boldsymbol{\beta}}_1^{\mathrm{OF}} - \hat{\boldsymbol{\beta}}_1^{\mathrm{LS}}\right)\left(1-(d_2-2)W_n^{-1}\right)^+.$$

In the following two sections we conduct numerical studies to appraise the relative performance of the above listed estimators.

4 Simulation Study

We conduct Monte-Carlo simulation experiments to study the relative performances of the proposed estimators under various practical settings.

We focus on large d small n and data generated from a high dimensional sparse linear model as follows:

$$y_i = x_{1i}\beta_1 + x_{2i}\beta_2 + \ldots + x_{di}\beta_d + \varepsilon_i, \; i = 1, 2, \ldots, n, \tag{12}$$

where ε_i's are independent and identically distributed standard normal and $x_{ij} = (\xi^1_{(ij)})^2 + \xi^2_{(ij)}$ with $\xi^1_{(ij)} \sim \mathcal{N}(0,1)$ and $\xi^2_{(ij)} \sim \mathcal{N}(0,1)$ for all $i = 1, 2, \ldots, n$, $j = 1, 2, \ldots, d$. We consider $\boldsymbol{\beta} = (\boldsymbol{\delta}^{(1)}_{d_1}, \boldsymbol{\delta}^{(2)}_{d_2}, \boldsymbol{\delta}^{(3)}_{d_3})'$, where $\boldsymbol{\delta}^{(1)}_{d_1}$ is the vector of strong signals, $\boldsymbol{\delta}^{(2)}_{d_2}$ represents weak-moderate signals, and $\boldsymbol{\delta}^{(3)}_{d_2}$ is the vector of no signals, that is, $\boldsymbol{\delta}^{(3)}_{d_3} = \mathbf{0}'_{d_3}$. We initially generate the data with $\boldsymbol{\delta}^{(1)}_{d_1} = \underbrace{(1, 1, \ldots, 1)'}_{d_1}$ and $\boldsymbol{\delta}^{(2)}_{d_2} = \mathbf{0}'_{d_2}, \boldsymbol{\delta}^{(3)}_{d_3} = \mathbf{0}'_{d_3}$, then we gradually increase the weak signals to examine the relative performance of the estimators in the presence of weak signals. Thus, we define $\Delta = \|\boldsymbol{\beta} - \boldsymbol{\beta}_0\|^2 \geq 0$, where $\boldsymbol{\beta}_0 = (\boldsymbol{\delta}^{(1)}_{d_1}, \boldsymbol{\delta}^{(2)}_{d_2}, \mathbf{0}_{d_3})'$. Data were generated by changing the values of $\boldsymbol{\beta}_2$ from zero vector such that $\Delta > 0$.

For brevity sake, we first examine the variable selection consistency for listed strategies for $(d_1, d_2, d_3, n) = (7, 30, 63, 50)$ in Figs. 1 and 2. In Fig. 1 OFM is defined based on Enet, and Lasso is an OFM in Fig. 2. The figures show that the percentage of predictors selected for each methods, respectively. For example, if the percentage of any one predictor is 100, then this predictor is selected always for all simulation steps. Similarly, if the percentage of any one predictor is 0, then this predictor is never selected in the simulation steps.

Figures 3 and 4 show that the number of selected coefficients via listed estimators when $\Delta = 0$. Figures 1, 2, 3, and 4 reveal that Enet and Lasso selected more variables than aLasso, SCAD, and MCP. The IPT2 selects more variables than the others after Enet and Lasso. On the other hand, PT and IPT1 select less predictors than LS, SPT, and IPT.

The relative performance of estimators are evaluated by using relative mean squared error (RMSE) criterion. The RMSE of an estimator $\boldsymbol{\beta}^*_1$ with respect to $\hat{\boldsymbol{\beta}}^{\text{OF}}_1$ is defined as follows:

$$\text{RMSE}\left(\boldsymbol{\beta}^*_1\right) = \frac{\text{MSE}\left(\hat{\boldsymbol{\beta}}^{\text{OF}}_1\right)}{\text{MSE}\left(\boldsymbol{\beta}^*_1\right)}, \tag{13}$$

where $\boldsymbol{\beta}^*_1$ is one of the listed estimators. The results are reported in Tables 1 and 2.

In Table 1, we use Enet is an overfitted model. We observed that MCP yields a much larger RMSE than both aLasso and SCAD at $\Delta = 0$. However, as expected, RMSE of all penalty estimators converge to zero for larger values of Δ. However, the performance pretest and linear shrinkage estimators are relatively good. More importantly, the RMSEs of the estimators based on pretest principle are bounded in Δ. Also, linear shrinkage estimators outperform the penalty estimators for all

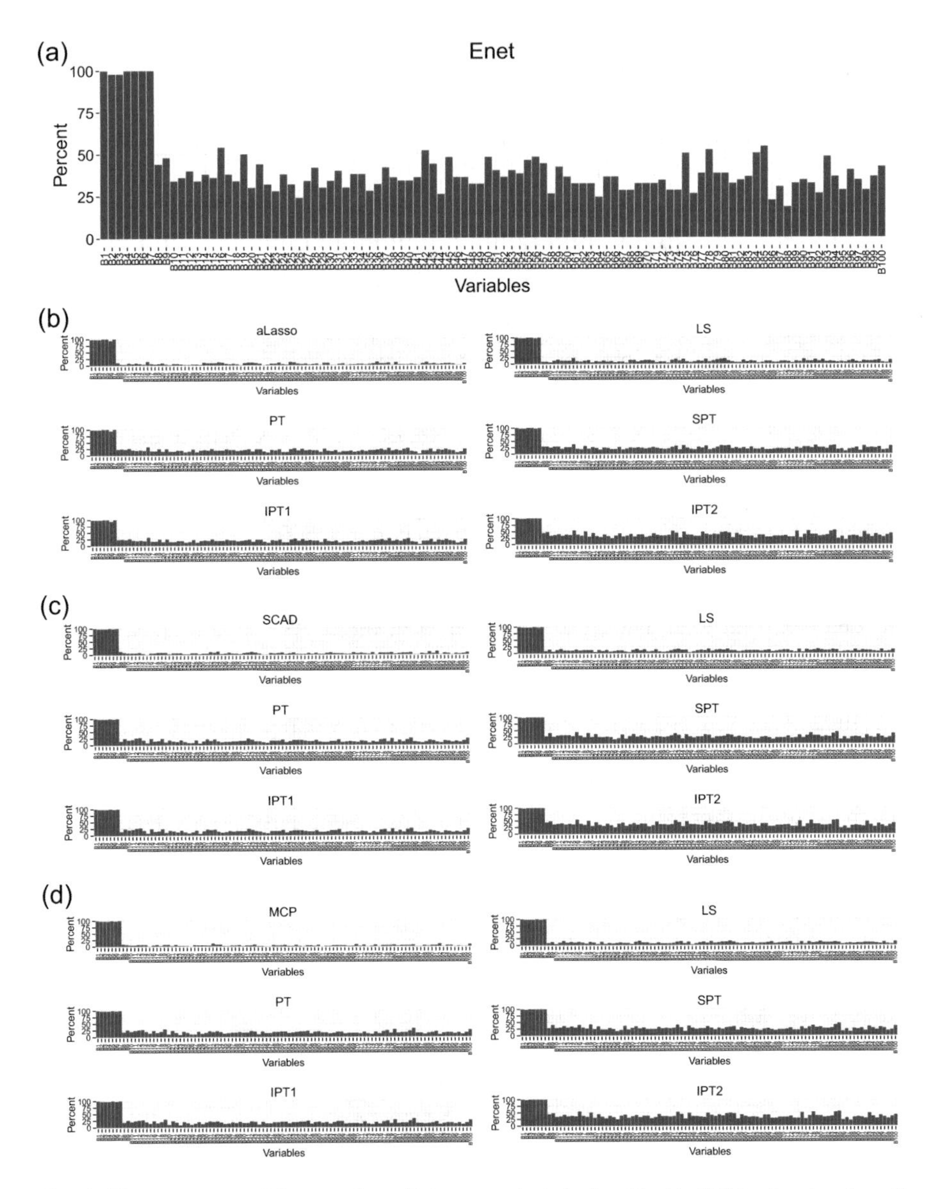

Fig. 1 The percentage of times each predictor was selected when Enet is OFM estimator, $\Delta = 0$ and $(d_1, d_2, d_3, n) = (7, 30, 63, 50)$. (**a**) Enet. (**b**) aLasso. (**c**) SCAD. (**d**) MCP

values Δ. The pretest estimator works well for small values of Δ. However, for intermediate values of Δ, the RMSE of penalty estimators outperform the pretest estimator. Table 2 also reveals similar results.

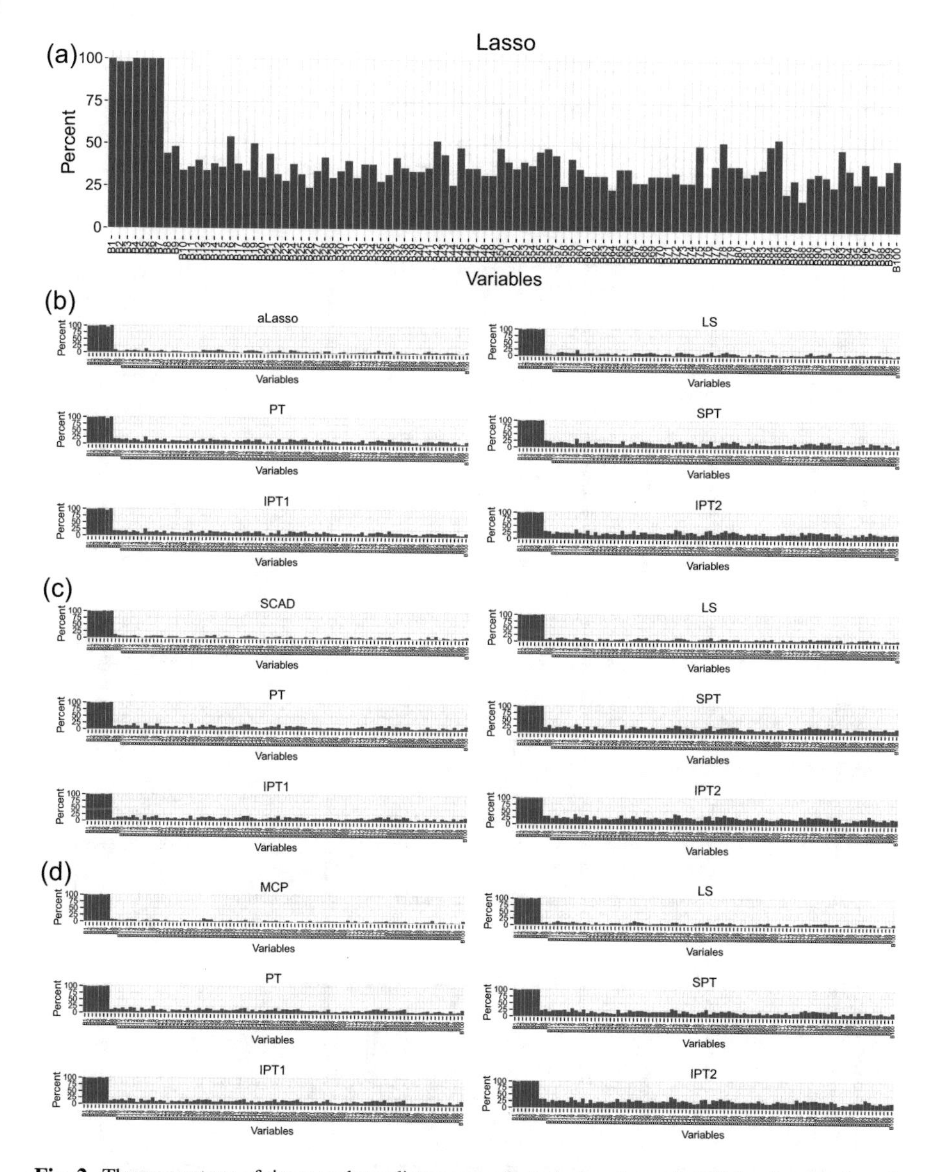

Fig. 2 The percentage of times each predictor was selected when Lasso is OFM estimator, $\Delta = 0$ and $(d_1, d_2, d_3, n) = (7, 30, 63, 50)$. (**a**) Lasso. (**b**) aLasso. (**c**) SCAD. (**d**) MCP

5 Real Data Analyses

Finally, in this section, we apply the proposed post-selection pretest and shrinkage strategies to the two data sets, of which the data descriptions are given below.

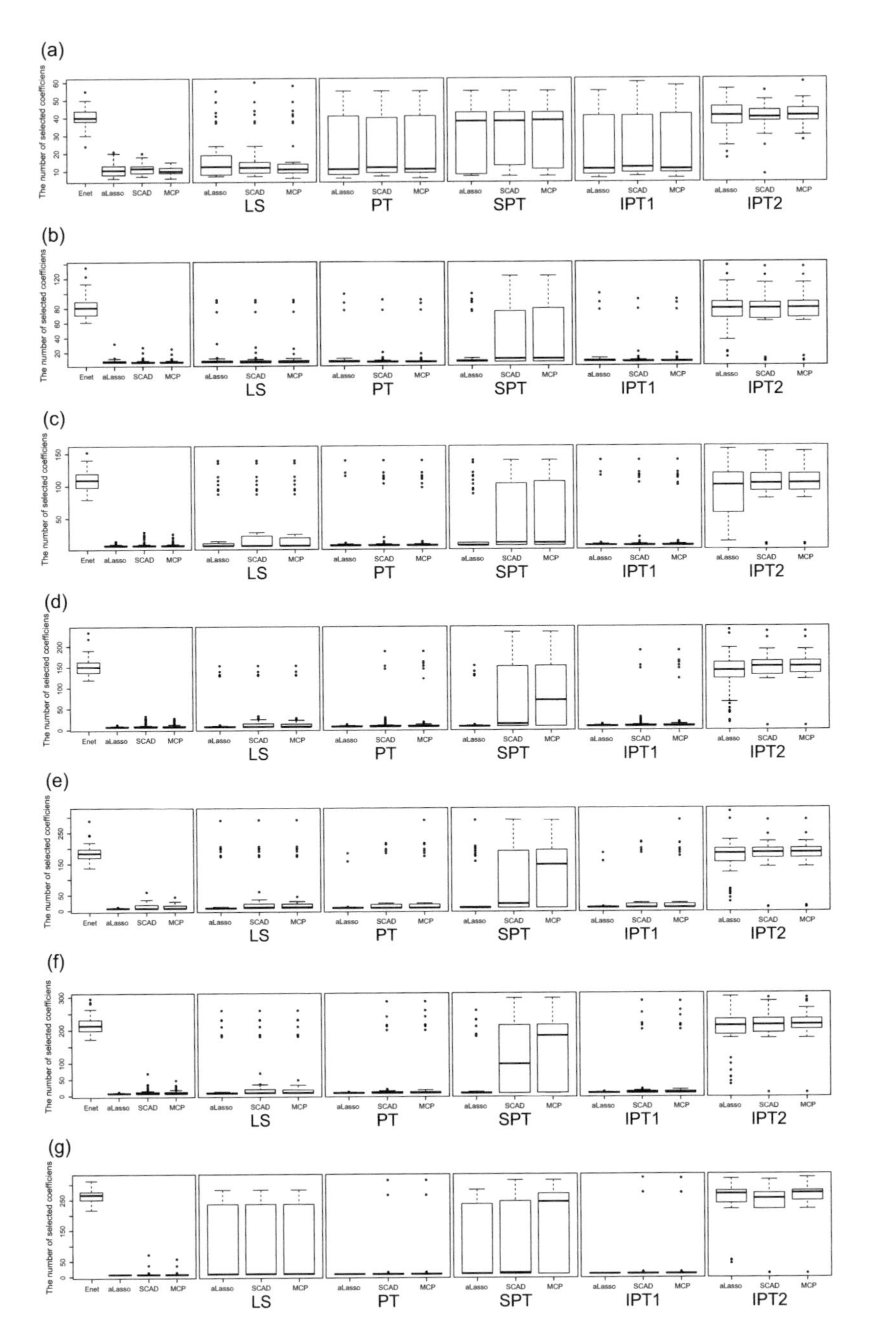

Fig. 3 The number of selected coefficients when Enet is OFM estimator and $\Delta = 0$. (**a**) $(d_1, d_2, d_3, n) = (7, 30, 63, 50)$. (**b**) $(d_1, d_2, d_3, n) = (7, 93, 300, 150)$. (**c**) $(d_1, d_2, d_3, n) = (7, 143, 600, 200)$. (**d**) $(d_1, d_2, d_3, n) = (7, 243, 1250, 300)$. (**e**) $(d_1, d_2, d_3, n) = (7, 293, 2700, 350)$. (**f**) $(d_1, d_2, d_3, n) = (7, 343, 5650, 400)$. (**g**) $(d_1, d_2, d_3, n) = (7, 443, 9550, 500)$

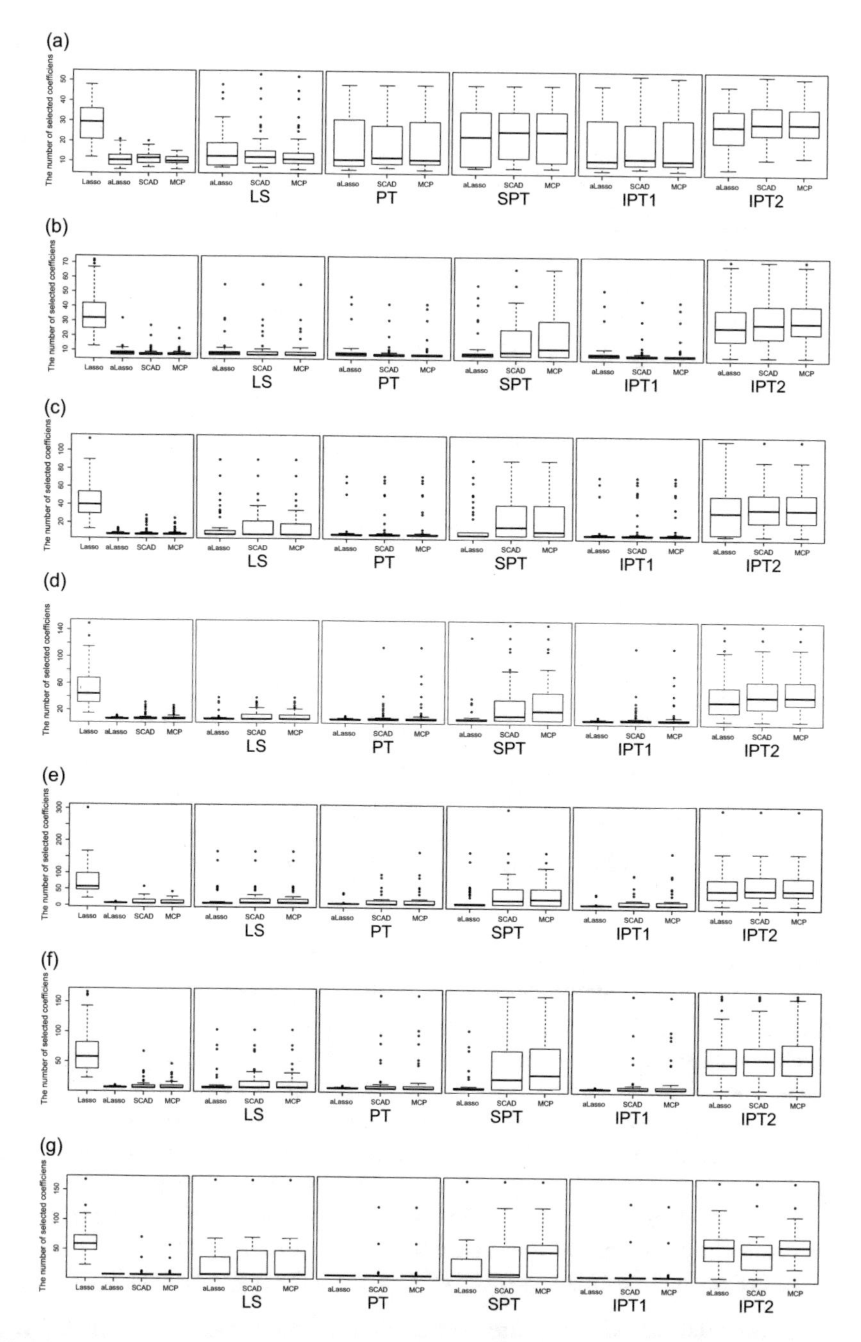

Fig. 4 The number of selected coefficients when Lasso is OFM estimator and $\Delta = 0$. (**a**) $(d_1, d_2, d_3, n) = (7, 30, 63, 50)$, (**b**) $(d_1, d_2, d_3, n) = (7, 93, 300, 150)$, (**c**) $(d_1, d_2, d_3, n) = (7, 143, 600, 200)$, (**d**) $(d_1, d_2, d_3, n) = (7, 243, 1250, 300)$, (**e**) $(d_1, d_2, d_3, n) = (7, 293, 2700, 350)$, (**f**) $(d_1, d_2, d_3, n) = (7, 343, 5650, 400)$, (**g**) $(d_1, d_2, d_3, n) = (7, 443, 9550, 500)$

Table 1 RMSE of the estimators when the OFM is Enet and $(d_1, d_2, d_3, n) = (7, 443, 9550, 500)$

UFM	Δ	$\hat{\beta}_1^{UF}$	$\hat{\beta}_1^{LS}$	$\hat{\beta}_1^{PT}$	$\hat{\beta}_1^{SPT}$	$\hat{\beta}_1^{IPT1}$	$\hat{\beta}_1^{IPT2}$
aLasso	0.0	13.305	3.115	13.305	3.115	13.305	1.497
	0.1	11.366	2.973	11.366	2.973	11.366	1.502
	0.2	7.059	2.774	5.231	2.555	6.958	1.451
	0.6	1.359	1.819	1.000	1.000	1.823	1.322
	0.7	0.910	1.476	1.000	1.000	1.382	1.304
	2.0	0.127	0.382	1.000	1.000	0.855	1.081
	4.0	0.031	0.107	1.000	1.000	0.853	1.024
	8.0	0.006	0.022	1.000	1.000	0.866	1.004
SCAD	0.0	7.427	2.860	4.045	2.372	7.267	2.978
	0.1	9.264	2.963	9.264	2.963	9.264	2.862
	0.2	6.067	2.712	2.801	2.036	5.884	2.575
	0.6	1.363	1.864	1.000	1.000	1.863	1.605
	0.7	0.909	1.500	1.000	1.000	1.412	1.403
	2.0	0.126	0.380	1.000	1.000	0.856	0.977
	4.0	0.031	0.107	1.000	1.000	0.853	0.939
	8.0	0.006	0.021	1.000	1.000	0.782	0.901
MCP	0.0	12.418	3.218	4.155	2.434	11.672	2.707
	0.1	11.816	3.130	7.782	2.881	11.815	2.823
	0.2	6.537	2.808	2.398	1.900	6.271	2.487
	0.6	1.348	1.847	1.000	1.000	1.846	1.631
	0.7	0.901	1.485	1.000	1.000	1.401	1.419
	2.0	0.127	0.384	1.000	1.000	0.870	0.976
	4.0	0.031	0.108	1.000	1.000	0.863	0.940
	8.0	0.006	0.022	1.000	1.000	0.863	0.928

- **Lung Adenocarcinoma (LA):** This data set was first analyzed by Beer et al. [6] using Affymetrix hu6800 microarrays. In this experiment there are $d = 7129$ gene expressions for $n = 86$, patients were collected from the University of Michigan Hospital. For numerical purpose, we draw 250 bootstrap samples with replacement from the corresponding data matrix. Further, we partitioned the data into a training set of 65 patients and a test set of 21 patients, respectively.
- **Acute Myeloid Leukemia (AML):** This data of AML patients was analyzed by Bullinger et al. [10]. For this data set, we have $d = 6283$ genes, and $n = 116$ patients. Again, we draw 250 bootstrap samples with replacement from the corresponding data matrix, and partitioned it into a training set of 100 patients, and a test set of 16 patients, respectively, to apply the suggested methods.

First, we obtain UFMs from three variable selection techniques: aLasso, SCAD, and MCP, respectively. On the other hand, OFMs are selected based on Enet and Lasso, respectively. Finally, we combine two selected submodels at a time to construct the suggested shrinkage and pretest post-selection estimators.

Table 2 RMSE of the estimators when the OFM is Lasso and $(d_1, d_2, d_3, n) = (7, 443, 9550, 500)$

UFM	Δ	$\hat{\boldsymbol{\beta}}_1^{\mathrm{UF}}$	$\hat{\boldsymbol{\beta}}_1^{\mathrm{LS}}$	$\hat{\boldsymbol{\beta}}_1^{\mathrm{PT}}$	$\hat{\boldsymbol{\beta}}_1^{\mathrm{SPT}}$	$\hat{\boldsymbol{\beta}}_1^{\mathrm{IPT1}}$	$\hat{\boldsymbol{\beta}}_1^{\mathrm{IPT2}}$
aLasso	0.0	6.145	6.264	6.145	6.325	6.145	6.149
	0.1	5.861	5.938	5.861	5.971	5.861	5.826
	0.2	3.168	3.239	3.168	3.260	3.168	3.221
	0.6	0.634	1.114	1.000	1.000	0.911	1.136
	0.7	0.490	1.101	1.000	1.000	0.839	1.108
	2.0	0.063	1.008	1.000	1.000	0.631	1.001
	4.0	0.015	1.002	1.000	1.000	0.747	1.000
	8.0	0.004	1.000	1.000	1.000	0.858	1.000
SCAD	0.0	3.456	3.509	2.498	2.626	3.358	3.570
	0.1	4.223	4.255	2.894	2.970	4.186	4.262
	0.2	2.922	3.013	1.809	1.918	2.908	2.994
	0.6	0.642	1.163	1.000	1.000	0.946	1.174
	0.7	0.490	1.129	1.000	1.000	0.867	1.127
	2.0	0.063	1.005	1.000	1.000	0.630	1.001
	4.0	0.015	1.002	1.000	1.000	0.751	1.000
	8.0	0.004	1.000	1.000	1.000	0.753	1.000
MCP	0.0	5.216	5.358	3.355	3.612	5.041	5.343
	0.1	5.597	5.700	2.905	3.009	5.489	5.551
	0.2	2.933	3.025	1.845	1.932	2.962	2.985
	0.6	0.640	1.161	1.000	1.000	0.943	1.172
	0.7	0.488	1.122	1.000	1.000	0.862	1.124
	2.0	0.063	1.006	1.000	1.000	0.645	1.001
	4.0	0.015	1.002	1.000	1.000	0.759	1.000
	8.0	0.004	1.000	1.000	1.000	0.773	1.000

To asses the performance of the post-selection estimators, we calculate relative prediction error (RPE) of an estimator $\boldsymbol{\beta}_{\vartheta}^{*}$ with respect to $\hat{\boldsymbol{\beta}}_{\vartheta}^{\mathrm{OF}}$ as follows:

$$\mathrm{RPE}\left(\boldsymbol{\beta}_{\vartheta}^{*}\right) = \frac{\sum_{i=1}^{250}\left[\mathbf{Y} - \mathbf{X}_{\vartheta}\boldsymbol{\beta}_{\vartheta}^{\mathrm{OF}(i)}\right]'\left[\mathbf{Y} - \mathbf{X}_{\vartheta}\boldsymbol{\beta}_{\vartheta}^{\mathrm{OF}(i)}\right]}{\sum_{i=1}^{250}\left[\mathbf{Y} - \mathbf{X}_{\vartheta}\boldsymbol{\beta}_{\vartheta}^{*(i)}\right]'\left[\mathbf{Y} - \mathbf{X}_{\vartheta}\boldsymbol{\beta}_{\vartheta}^{*(i)}\right]},$$

where "$^{(i)}$" indicates that the estimator is at ith sample of bootstrapping and "$_{\vartheta}$" is the index of the model selected by a given method.

First, we report the average number of selected predictors for both data sets in Tables 3 and 4.

The values of RPE are reported in Tables 5 and 6.

The results which are given in Tables 3 and 4 are consistent with the findings of our simulation study. Table 5 reports analysis of LA data. We observe that suggested

Table 3 The average number of selected predictors by UFMs and OFMs

Data	n	d	# of predictors		Data	n	d	# of predictors	
LA	86	7129	Enet	58	AML	116	6283	Enet	75
			Lasso	25				Lasso	32
			aLasso	6				aLasso	20
			SCAD	10				SCAD	14
			MCP	5				MCP	7

Table 4 The average number of selected predictors by post-selection methods

Data	OFM	UFM	LS	PT	SPT	IPT1	IPT2
LA	Enet	aLasso	52	19	52	19	54
		SCAD	44	10	44	10	41
		MCP	40	5	40	5	47
	Lasso	aLasso	23	9	24	7	24
		SCAD	22	12	20	12	20
		MCP	20	9	22	8	22
AML	Enet	aLasso	70	57	70	57	70
		SCAD	48	14	48	14	66
		MCP	45	7	56	7	58
	Lasso	aLasso	27	26	28	26	28
		SCAD	12	18	23	22	24
		MCP	9	18	18	17	23

Table 5 RPE of estimators for LA

OFM	UFM	$\hat{\boldsymbol{\beta}}_1^{\mathrm{UF}}$	$\hat{\boldsymbol{\beta}}_1^{\mathrm{LS}}$	$\hat{\boldsymbol{\beta}}_1^{\mathrm{PT}}$	$\hat{\boldsymbol{\beta}}_1^{\mathrm{SPT}}$	$\hat{\boldsymbol{\beta}}_1^{\mathrm{IPT1}}$	$\hat{\boldsymbol{\beta}}_1^{\mathrm{IPT2}}$
Enet	aLasso	1.1310	1.1622	1.0895	1.1061	1.1300	1.0850
	SCAD	1.1365	1.1474	1.1365	1.1474	1.1365	1.1398
	MCP	1.1592	1.1799	1.1592	1.1799	1.1592	1.1345
Lasso	aLasso	1.0884	1.1185	1.0540	1.0540	1.0833	1.0871
	SCAD	1.0937	1.1003	1.0752	1.0752	1.0916	1.0868
	MCP	1.1155	1.1344	1.0752	1.0752	1.1184	1.1054

post-selection estimators outperform both OFMs and UFMs. Further, for this data UFMs are relatively more efficient than OFMs. Table 6 provides analysis for AML data. Interestingly, for this data, overfitted models Enet and Lasso estimators are relatively efficient than underfitted estimators based on aLasso, SCAD, and MCP, respectively. The results of AML data also demonstrate that the suggested post-selection estimators are superior, with some exceptions.

Table 6 RPE of estimators for AML

OFM	UFM	$\hat{\beta}_1^{UF}$	$\hat{\beta}_1^{LS}$	$\hat{\beta}_1^{PT}$	$\hat{\beta}_1^{SPT}$	$\hat{\beta}_1^{IPT1}$	$\hat{\beta}_1^{IPT2}$
Enet	aLasso	0.7930	1.1713	0.8450	1.1484	0.8209	1.1423
	SCAD	1.1599	1.1915	1.1599	1.1915	1.1599	1.1302
	MCP	1.1798	1.2265	1.1798	1.2265	1.1798	1.1814
Lasso	aLasso	0.7707	1.1251	0.9873	1.0944	0.8201	1.0993
	SCAD	1.1260	1.1262	1.1428	1.1511	1.1412	1.1439
	MCP	1.1453	1.1739	1.1408	1.1408	1.1755	1.0949

6 Conclusions and Outlooks

In this study, we suggested integrating two submodels by incorporating pretest and shrinkage estimation strategies in high dimensional sparse models. Our suggested post-selection estimators are constructed by integration with OFM, which may be either Lasso or Enet variable selection methods with a UFM, which may based on aLasso, SCAD, or MCP variable selection methods. Monte Carlo simulation studies suggest that post-selection listed estimators perform better than usual penalty estimators for both variable selection and prediction, in many instances. The results of two HDD are consistent with the simulation study showing the superior performance of suggested post-selection estimators. However, we fall short in providing the theoretical justifications in this paper, which is an ongoing work and will be communicated in a separate paper.

Further, for future work, one may consider the combining all the estimators produced by overfitted and underfittted into a single estimator to improve the overall prediction error. In another study it would be interesting to include penalty estimators that correspond to Bayes procedures based on priors with polynomial tails.

References

1. Ahmed, S.E.: Shrinkage preliminary test estimation in multivariate normal distributions. J. Stat. Comput. Simul. **43**, 177–195 (1992)
2. Ahmed, S.E.: Penalty, Shrinkage and Pretest Strategies: Variable Selection and Estimation. Springer, New York (2014)
3. Ahmed, S.E., Yüzbaşı, B.: Big data analytics: integrating penalty strategies. Int. J. Manage. Sci. Eng. Manage. **11**(2), 105–115 (2016)
4. Ahmed, S.E., Hossain, S., Doksum, K.A.: Lasso and shrinkage estimation in Weibull censored regression models. J. Stat. Plann. Inference **142**(6), 1273–1284 (2012)
5. Armagan, A., Dunson, D.B., Lee, J.: Generalized double Pareto shrinkage. Stat. Sin. **23**(1), 119 (2013)
6. Beer, D.G., Kardia, S.L., Huang, C.C., Giordano, T.J., Levin, A.M., Misek, D.E., Lin, L., Chen, G., Gharib, T.G., Thomas, D.G., Lizyness, M.L., Kuick, R., Hayasaka, S., Taylor, J.M., Iannettoni, M.D., Orringer, M.B., Hanash, S.: Gene-expression profiles predict survival of patients with lung adenocarcinoma. Nat. Med. **8**(8), 816–824 (2002)

7. Belloni, A., Chernozhukov, V.: Least squares after model selection in high dimensional sparse models. Bernoulli **19**, 521–547 (2009)
8. Bhattacharya, A., Pati, D., Pillai, N.S., Dunson, D.B.: Bayesian shrinkage (2012). arXiv preprint arXiv:1212.6088
9. Bickel, P.J., Ritov, Y., Tsybakov, A.B.: Simultaneous analysis of Lasso and dantzig selector. Ann. Stat. **37**, 1705–1732 (2009)
10. Bullinger, L., Döhner, K., Bair, E., Fröhling, S., Schlenk, R.F., Tibshirani, R., Döhner, H., Pollack, J.R.: Use of gene-expression profiling to identify prognostic subclasses in adult acute myeloid leukemia. New Engl. J. Med. **350**(16), 1605–1616 (2004)
11. Carvalho, C.M., Polson, N.G., Scott, J.G.: The horseshoe estimator for sparse signals, Biometrika **97**, 465–480 (2010)
12. Efron, B., Hastie, T., Johnstone, I., Tibshirani, R.: Least angle regression. Ann. Stat. **32**(2), 407–499 (2004)
13. Fan, J., Li, R.: Variable selection via nonconcave penalized likelihood and its oracle properties. J. Am. Stat. Assoc. **96**(456), 1348–1360 (2001)
14. Hansen, B.E.: The risk of james-stein and Lasso shrinkage (2013). http://www.ssc.wisc.edu/bhansen/papers/Lasso.pdf
15. Huang, J., Ma, S., Zhang, C.H.: Adaptive Lasso for sparse high dimensional regression models. Stat. Sin. **18**(4), 1603–1618 (2008)
16. Kim, Y., Choi, H., Oh, H.S.: Smoothly clipped absolute deviation on high dimensions. J. Am. Stat. Assoc. **103**(484), 1665–1673 (2008)
17. Leng, C., Lin, Y., Wahba, G.: A note on the Lasso and related procedures in model selection. Stat. Sin. **16**(4), 1273–1284 (2006)
18. Liu, H., Yu, B.: Asymptotic properties of Lasso+mLS and Lasso+Ridge in sparse high dimensional linear regression. Electron. J. Stat. **7**, 3124–3169 (2013)
19. Schelldorfer, J., Bühlmann, P., van de Geer, S.: Estimation for high dimensional linear mixed effects models using L_1-penalization. Scand. J. Stat. **38**(2), 197–214 (2011)
20. Tibshirani, R.: Regression shrinkage and selection via the Lasso. J. R. Stat. Soc. Ser. B (Methodological), **58**(1), 267–288 (1996)
21. Tibshirani, R., Saunders, M., Rosset, S., Zhu, J., Knight, K.: Sparsity and smoothness via the fused Lasso. J. Roy. Stat. Soc. Ser. B (Stat. Methodol.) **67**(1), 91–108 (2005)
22. Tran, M.N.: The loss rank criterion for variable selection in linear regression analysis. Scand. J. Stat. **38**(3), 466–479 (2011)
23. Wang, H., Leng, C.: Unified Lasso estimation by least squares approximation. J. Am. Stat. Assoc. **102**(479), 1039–1048 (2012)
24. Yuan, M., Lin, Y.: Model selection and estimation in regression with grouped variables. J. R. Stat. Soc. Ser. B (Stat. Methodol.) **68**(1), 49–67 (2006)
25. Zhang, C.H.: Nearly unbiased variable selection under minimax concave penalty. Ann. Stat. **38**, 894–942 (2010)
26. Zhang, C.H., Zhang, S.S.: Confidence intervals for low-dimensional parameters in high dimensional linear models. Ann. Stat. **76**, 217–242 (2014)
27. Zhao, P., Yu, B.: On model selection consistency of Lasso. J. Mach. Learn. Res. **7**, 2541–2563 (2006)
28. Zou, H.: The adaptive Lasso and its oracle properties. J. Am. Stat. Assoc. **101**(476), 1418–1429 (2006)
29. Zou, H., Hastie, T.: Regularization and variable selection via the elastic net. J. R. Stat. Soc. B **67**, 301–320 (2005)

High-Dimensional Classification for Brain Decoding

Nicole Croteau, Farouk S. Nathoo, Jiguo Cao, and Ryan Budney

Abstract Brain decoding involves the determination of a subject's cognitive state or an associated stimulus from functional neuroimaging data measuring brain activity. In this setting the cognitive state is typically characterized by an element of a finite set, and the neuroimaging data comprise voluminous amounts of spatiotemporal data measuring some aspect of the neural signal. The associated statistical problem is one of the classifications from high-dimensional data. We explore the use of functional principal component analysis, mutual information networks, and persistent homology for examining the data through exploratory analysis and for constructing features characterizing the neural signal for brain decoding. We review each approach from this perspective, and we incorporate the features into a classifier based on symmetric multinomial logistic regression with elastic net regularization. The approaches are illustrated in an application where the task is to infer, from brain activity measured with magnetoencephalography (MEG), the type of video stimulus shown to a subject.

1 Introduction

Recent advances in techniques for measuring brain activity through neuroimaging modalities such as functional magnetic resonance imaging (fMRI), electroencephalography (EEG), and magnetoencephalography (MEG) have demonstrated the possibility of decoding a person's conscious experience based only on non-invasive measurements of their brain signals [11]. Doing so involves uncovering the relationship between the recorded signals and the conscious experience that may then provide insight into the underlying mental process. Such decoding tasks arise in a number of areas, for example, the area of brain–computer interfaces, where humans can be trained to use their brain activity to control artificial devices. At the heart of this task is a classification problem where the neuroimaging data comprise voluminous amounts of spatiotemporal observations measuring some aspect of the neural signal across an array of sensors outside the head (EEG, MEG) or voxels

N. Croteau • F.S. Nathoo (✉) • J. Cao • R. Budney
Department of Mathematics and Statistics, University of Victoria, Victoria, BC, Canada
e-mail: nathoo@uvic.ca

© Springer International Publishing AG 2017

S.E. Ahmed (ed.), *Big and Complex Data Analysis*, Contributions to Statistics,
DOI 10.1007/978-3-319-41573-4_15

within the brain (fMRI). With neuroimaging data the classification problem can be challenging as the recorded brain signals have a low signal-to-noise ratio and the size of the data leads to a high-dimensional problem where it is easy to overfit models to data when training a classifier. Overfitting will impact negatively on the degree of generalization to new data and thus must be avoided in order for solutions to be useful for practical application.

Neuroimaging classification problems have been studied extensively in recent years primarily in efforts to develop biomarkers for neurodegenerative diseases and other brain disorders. A variety of techniques have been applied in this context, including support vector machines [4], Gaussian process classification [22], regularized logistic regression [29], and neural networks [20, 23]. Decoding of brain images using Bayesian approaches is discussed by Friston et al. [10]. While a variety of individual classifiers or an ensemble of classifiers may be applied in any given application, the development of general approaches to constructing features that successfully characterize the signal in functional neuroimaging data is a key open problem. In this article we explore the use of some recent approaches developed in statistics and computational topology as potential solutions to this problem. More specifically, we consider how the combination of functional principal component analysis [27], persistent homology [3], and network measures of brain connectivity [24] can be used to (1) explore large datasets of recorded brain activity and (2) construct features for the brain decoding problem.

The objectives of this article are threefold. First, we wish to introduce the brain decoding problem to researchers working in the area of high-dimensional data analysis. This challenging problem serves as a rich arena for applying recent advances in methodology. Moreover, the specific challenges associated with the brain decoding problem (e.g., low signal-to-noise ratio; spatiotemporal data) can help to further motivate the development of new methods. Our second objective is to describe how functional principal component analysis (FPCA), persistent homology, and network measures of brain connectivity can be used to explore such data and construct features. To our knowledge, FPCA and persistent homology have not been previously considered as approaches for constructing features for brain decoding.

Our third and final objective is to illustrate these methods in a real application involving MEG data, where the goal is to explore variability in the brain data and to use the data to infer the type of video stimulus shown to a subject from a 1-s recording obtained from 204 MEG sensors with the signal at each channel sampled at a frequency of 200 Hz. Each sample thus yields $204 \times 200 = 40,800$ observations of magnetic field measurements outside the head. The goal is to decode which of the five possible video stimuli was shown to the subject during the recording from these measurements. The data arising from a single sample are shown in Fig. 1, where panel (a) depicts the brain signals recorded across all sensors during the 1-s recording, and panel (b) depicts the variance of the signal at each location. From panel (b) we see that in this particular sample the stimulus evoked activity in the regions associated with the temporal and occipital lobes of the brain. The entire dataset for the application includes a total of 1380 such samples (727 training; 653

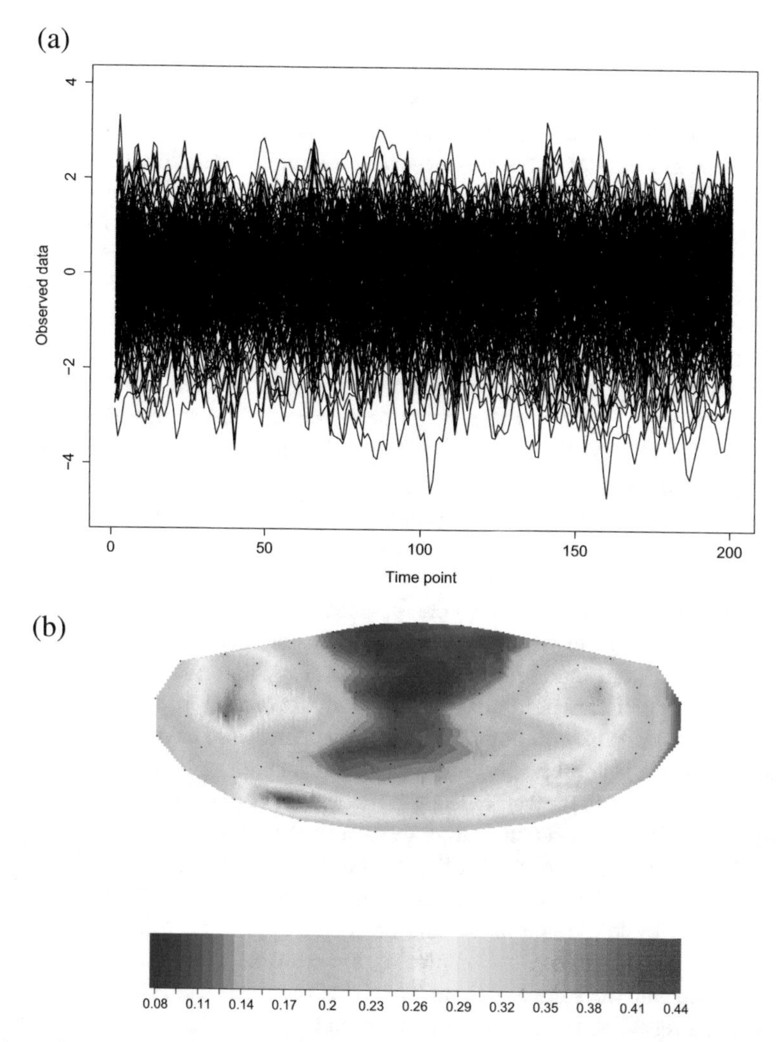

Fig. 1 A single sample from the training data: panel (**a**)—depicts the MEG (magnetic field) signals $Y_{li}(t)$ representing the evoked response collected at $n = 204$ sensors; panel (**b**)—depicts the variance of the signal (after removal of linear trend) at 102 locations. The map is a two-dimensional projection of the sensor array with the *black dots* representing the sensor locations. There are two sensors at each location (each oriented differently) and the variance computed from each of the sensors is averaged to obtain a single value (for the purpose of visual summary only)

test) obtained from the same subject which together yield a dataset of roughly 6 GB in compressed format.

Functional principal component analysis (FPCA) is the extension of standard finite-dimensional PCA to the setting where the response variables are functions, a setting referred to as functional data. For clarity, we note here that the use of the word "functional" in this context refers to functional data as just described, and is not to be confused with functional neuroimaging data which refers to imaging data measuring the function of the brain. Given a sample of functional observations (e.g., brain signals) with each signal assumed a realization of a square-integrable stochastic process over a finite interval, FPCA involves the estimation of a set of eigenvalue-eigenfunction pairs that describe the major vibrational components in the data. These components can be used to define features for classification through the projection of each signal onto a set of estimated eigenfunctions characterizing most of the variability in the data. This approach has been used recently for the classification of genetic data by Leng and Müller [17] who use FPCA in combination with logistic regression to develop a classifier for temporal gene expression data.

An alternative approach for exploring the patterns in brain signals is based on viewing each signal obtained at a voxel or sensor as a point in high-dimensional Euclidean space. The collection of signals across the brain then forms a point cloud in this space, and the shape of this point cloud can be described using tools from topological data analysis [3]. In this setting the data are assumed clustered around a familiar object like a manifold, algebraic variety or cell complex and the objective is to describe (estimate some aspect of) the topology of this object from the data. The subject of persistent homology can be seen as a concrete manifestation of this idea, and provides a novel method to discover nonlinear features in data. With the same advances in modern computing technology that allow for the storage of large datasets, persistent homology and its variants can be implemented. Features derived from persistent homology have recently been found useful for classification of hepatic lesions [1] and persistent homology has been applied for the analysis of structural brain images [6, 21]. Outside the arena of medical applications, Sethares and Budney [25] use persistent homology to study topological structures in musical data. Recent work in Heo et al. [12] connects computational topology with the traditional analysis of variance and combines these approaches for the analysis of multivariate orthodontic landmark data derived from the maxillary complex. The use of persistent homology for exploring structure of spatiotemporal functional neuroimaging data does not appear to have been considered previously.

Another alternative for exploring patterns in the data is based on estimating and summarizing the topology of an underlying network. Networks are commonly used to explore patterns in both functional and structural neuroimaging data. With the former, the nodes of the network correspond to the locations of sensors/voxels and the links between nodes reflect some measure of dependence between the time series collected at pairs of locations. To characterize dependence between time series, the mutual information, a measure of shared information between two time series is a useful quantity as it measures both linear and nonlinear dependence [30], the latter being potentially important when characterizing dependence between brain signals [28]. Given such a network, the corresponding topology can be summarized with a small number of meaningful measures such as those representing the degree of small-world organization [24]. These measures can then be explored to detect differences in the network structure of brain activity across differing stimuli and can be further used as features for brain decoding.

The remainder of the paper is structured as follows. Section 2 describes the classifier and discusses important considerations for defining features. Section 3 provides a review of FPCA from the perspective of exploring functional neuroimaging data. Sections 4 and 5 discuss persistent homology and mutual information networks, respectively, as approaches for characterizing the interaction of brain signals and defining nonlinear features for classification. Section 6 presents an application to the decoding of visual stimuli from MEG data, and Sect. 7 concludes with a brief discussion.

2 Decoding Cognitive States from Neuroimaging Data

Let us assume we have observed functional neuroimaging data $\boldsymbol{Y} = \{y_i(t), i = 1, \ldots, n;\ t = 1, \ldots, T\}$ where $y_i(t)$ denotes the signal of brain activity measured at the ith sensor or voxel. We assume that there is a well-defined but unknown cognitive state corresponding to these data that can be represented by the label $C \in \{1, \ldots, K\}$. The decoding problem is that of recovering C from $\boldsymbol{Y}$. A solution to this problem involves first summarizing $\boldsymbol{Y}$ through an m-dimensional vector of features $\boldsymbol{Y}_f = (Y_{f_1}, \ldots, Y_{f_m})'$ and then applying a classification rule $R^m \rightarrow \{1, \ldots, K\}$ to obtain the predicted state. A solution must specify how to construct the features and define the classification rule, and we assume there exists a set of training samples $\boldsymbol{Y}_l = \{y_{li}(t), i = 1, \ldots, n;\ t = 1, \ldots, T\},\ l = 1, \ldots, L$ with *known* labels $C_l,\ l = 1, \ldots, L$ for doing this.

To define the classification rule we model the training labels with a multinomial distribution where the class probabilities are related to features through a symmetric multinomial logistic regression [9] having form

$$Pr(C = j) = \frac{\exp(\beta_{0j} + \boldsymbol{\beta}_j'\boldsymbol{Y}_f)}{\sum_{k=1}^{K} \exp(\beta_{0k} + \boldsymbol{\beta}_k'\boldsymbol{Y}_f)}, \quad j = 1, \ldots, K \tag{1}$$

with parameters $\boldsymbol{\theta} = (\beta_{01}, \boldsymbol{\beta}_1', \ldots, \beta_{0K}, \boldsymbol{\beta}_K')'$. As the dimension of the feature vector will be large relative to the number of training samples we estimate $\boldsymbol{\theta}$ from the training data using regularized maximum likelihood. This involves maximizing a penalized log-likelihood where the likelihood is defined by the symmetric multinomial logistic regression and we incorporate an elastic net penalty [32]. Optimization is carried using cyclical coordinate descent as implemented in the *glmnet* package [9] in R. The two tuning parameters weighting the l_1 and l_2 components of the elastic net penalty are chosen using cross-validation over a grid of possible values. Given $\hat{\boldsymbol{\theta}}$ the classification of a new sample with unknown label is based on computing the estimated class probabilities from (1) and choosing the state with the highest estimated value.

To define the feature vector $\boldsymbol{Y}_f$ from $\boldsymbol{Y}$ we consider two aspects of the neural signal that are likely important for discriminating cognitive states. The first aspect involves the shape and power of the signal at each location. These are local features computed at each voxel or sensor irrespective of the signal observed at other locations. The variance of the signal computed over all time points is one such feature that will often be useful for discriminating states, as different states may correspond to different locations of activation, and these locations will have higher variability in the signal. The second aspect is the functional connectivity representing how signals at different locations interact. Rather than being location specific, such features are global and may help to resolve the cognitive state in the case where states correspond to differing patterns of interdependence among the signals across the brain. From this perspective we next briefly describe FPCA, persistent homology, and mutual information networks as approaches for exploring these aspects of functional neuroimaging data, and further how these approaches can be used to define features for classification.

3 Functional Principal Component Analysis

Let us fix a particular location i of the brain or sensor array. At this specific location we observe a sample of curves $y_{li}(t)$, $l = 1, \ldots, L$ where the size of the sample corresponds to that of the training set. We assume that each curve is an independent realization of a square-integrable stochastic process $Y_i(t)$ on $[0, T]$ with mean $E[Y_i(t)] = \mu_i(t)$ and covariance $\mathrm{Cov}[Y_i(t), Y_i(s)] = G_i(s, t)$. Mercer's Theorem states that the covariance function $G_i(s, t)$ can be represented as a linear combination of orthonormal basis functions as follows:

$$G_i(s, t) = \sum_{m=1}^{\infty} \lambda_{mi} \rho_{mi}(s) \rho_{mi}(t),$$

where $\{\rho_{mi}(t)\}$ is a set of orthogonal eigenfunctions and $\{\lambda_{mi}\}$ is the corresponding set of eigenvalues with the order $\lambda_{1i} \geq \lambda_{2i} \geq \cdots$ and $\sum_m \lambda_{mi} < \infty$.

Then the stochastic process $Y_i(t)$ can be written in terms of the Karhunen-Loève representation [17]

$$Y_i(t) = \mu_i(t) + \sum_{m=1}^{\infty} \epsilon_{mi} \rho_{mi}(t) \tag{2}$$

where $\{\rho_{mi}(t)\}$ is referred to as the functional principal components (FPCs) with corresponding coefficients

$$\epsilon_{mi} = \int_0^T (Y_i(t) - \mu_i(t)) \rho_{mi}(t) dt \tag{3}$$

with $E[\epsilon_{mi}] = 0$, $Var[\epsilon_{mi}] = \lambda_{mi}$. The coefficients ϵ_{mi} are called the FPC scores. The total variability of process realizations about $\mu_i(t)$ is governed by the FPC scores ϵ_{mi} and in particular by the corresponding variance λ_{mi}, with relatively higher values corresponding to FPCs that contribute more to this total variability.

Given the L sample realizations, the estimates of $\mu_i(t)$ and of the first few FPCs can be used to explore the dominant modes of variability in the observed brain signals at location i. The mean curve is estimated simply as $\hat{\mu}_i(t) = \frac{1}{L}\sum_{l=1}^{L} y_{li}(t)$ and from this the covariance function $G_i(s,t)$ is estimated $\hat{G}_i = \hat{Cov}[Y_i(s_k), Y_i(s_l)]$ using the empirical covariance over a grid of points $s_1, \ldots, s_S \in [0, T]$. The FPCs are then estimated through the spectral decomposition of $\hat{G}_i$ (see, e.g., [27]) with the eigenvectors yielding the estimated FPCs evaluated at the grid points, $\hat{\boldsymbol{\rho}}_{mi} = (\hat{\boldsymbol{\rho}}_{mi}(s_1), \ldots, \hat{\boldsymbol{\rho}}_{mi}(s_S))'$, and the corresponding eigenvalues being the estimated variances $\hat{\lambda}_{mi}$ for the coefficients ϵ_{mi} in (2). The fraction of the sample variability explained by the first M estimated FPCs can then be expressed as $FVE(M) = \sum_{m=1}^{M} \hat{\lambda}_{mi} / \sum_m \hat{\lambda}_{mi}$ and this can be used to choose a nonnegative integer M_i so that the predicted curves

$$\hat{y}_{li}(t) = \hat{\mu}_i(t) + \sum_{m=1}^{M_i} \hat{\epsilon}_{lmi} \hat{\rho}_{mi}(t)$$

explain a specified fraction of the total sample variability. We note that in producing the predicted curve a separate realization of the coefficients ϵ_{mi} from (2) is estimated from each observed signal using (3) and, for a given m, the estimated coefficients $\hat{\boldsymbol{\epsilon}}_{mi} = \{\hat{\epsilon}_{lmi}, l = 1, \ldots, L\}$ are referred to as the order-m FPC scores which represent between subject variability in the particular mode of variation represented by $\hat{\rho}_{mi}(t)$. The scores are thus potentially useful as features for classification.

We compute the FPC scores $\hat{\boldsymbol{\epsilon}}_{mi}$, $m = 1, \ldots, M_i$ separately at each location $i = 1, \ldots, n$. For a given location the number of FPCs, M_i, is chosen to be the smallest integer such that the $FVE(M_i) \geq 0.9$. Thus the number of FPCs, M_i, will vary across locations but typically only a small number will be required. Locations requiring a relatively greater number of FPCs will likely correspond to locations where the signal is more complex. The total number of features introduced by our application of FPCA for brain decoding is then $\sum_{i=1}^{n} M_i$. The FPCs and the associated FPC scores are computed using the *fda* package in R [27].

4 Persistent Homology

Let us now fix a particular sample l from the training set and consider the collection of brain signals, $y_{li}(t)$, observed over all locations $i = 1, \ldots, n$ for that sample. Each signal is observed over the same set of T equally spaced time points $\boldsymbol{Y}_{li} = (y_{li}(1), \ldots, y_{li}(T))'$ and is thus a point in R^T. The sample of signals across the brain/sensors then forms a point cloud in R^T. For example, the single sample depicted in Fig. 1, panel (a), represents a cloud of $n = 204$ points in R^{200}. Using tools from topological data analysis we aim to identify topological structures associated with this point cloud and to use these structures as features for brain decoding.

Persistent homology is an algebraic method for discerning topological features such as clusters, loops, and voids from data. We provide here only an informal description of persistent homology that emphasizes basic concepts and intuition for the construction of features for brain decoding. A more formal introduction to persistent homology including the required definitions and some results from simplicial homology theory and group theory is provided by Zhu [31]. The data in this context consist of a discrete set of points with a metric that gives distances between pairs of points. In our application where each point is a sensor signal we require a metric that is a measure of statistical dependence that will collate both correlated and anti-correlated signals. We therefore employ the absolute Pearson correlation distance metric $D(\boldsymbol{Y}_{li}, \boldsymbol{Y}_{lj}) = 1 - \rho(\boldsymbol{Y}_{li}, \boldsymbol{Y}_{lj})^2$ where $\rho(\boldsymbol{Y}_{li}, \boldsymbol{Y}_{lj})$ is the sample correlation between signals at locations i and j.

While the topology of a discrete set of n points in R^T is trivial, we consider the points as being sampled from or clustered around a subspace with nontrivial topology, and our interest lies in the topology of this subspace. We can create such a space by connecting nearby points. More specifically, we consider a particular distance scale $\epsilon > 0$, and we use the notion of a simplex to connect nearby points and form a type of topological space known as a simplicial complex. The components of a simplicial complex are simplices of differing dimensions, where a p-simplex is the convex hull of $p + 1$ affinely independent points. For example, a 0-simplex is a point, a 1-simplex is an edge, a 2-simplex is a triangle, and a 3-simplex is a solid tetrahedron. A simplicial complex F_ϵ is a collection of simplices of differing dimensions obeying certain rules for inclusion as well as for how the individual simplices it contains should be glued together. For a given p-simplex contained in F_ϵ, all of its lower dimensional faces should be contained in F_ϵ. Further, the intersection of any two simplices in F_ϵ should be either the empty set or a shared face of both simplices. For a given set of n data points and scale ϵ we are able to construct a simplicial complex from the data and determine what is known as the *homology* of this simplicial complex.

Homology is a concept from algebraic topology that informally can be thought of as a construction on a topological space that counts the number of connected components, loops, voids, and higher-dimensional holes of that space. To construct a simplicial complex from the data at a particular scale ϵ, we surround each point in the dataset with a ball of radius $\epsilon/2$ and connect pairs of points with an edge whenever the intersection is non-empty, which occurs precisely when points are separated by no more than distance ϵ. The result is a graph with datapoints as vertices. In addition to edges (1-simplices) between points, higher dimensional simplices are added. A p-dimensional simplex is added whenever a subset of $p + 1$ points is pairwise connected. For example, if three points are connected to form a triangle, the triangle is filled in and the corresponding 2-simplex added to the simplicial complex. Similarly, any four points that are pairwise connected are filled in with a solid tetrahedron. The resulting simplicial complex is called the Vietoris-Rips complex. The homology of such a complex can be computed using linear algebra involving specially defined matrices (known as boundary matrices) and their normal forms.

For a given scale ϵ the homology of the corresponding simplicial complex F_ϵ can be computed and is associated with the data *at that particular scale*. An important quantity associated with F_ϵ is the pth Betti number, Betti_p. Formally, Betti_p is the rank of a particular quotient group known as the pth homology group, the elements of which represent classes of "interesting cycles" in the space, that is, those that surround a hole in the space. Informally it can be thought of as representing the number of p-dimensional holes, which for $p = 0, 1, 2$ corresponds to the *number of connected components*, *loops*, and *voids*, respectively. If the dimension of the topological space is d, then $\text{Betti}_p = 0$ for $p > d$.

For values of ϵ sufficiently small the homology is simply that of n connected components with no higher dimensional holes. For ϵ sufficiently large any two points will be connected and the homology is simply that of a single connected component with no higher dimensional holes. Rather than considering a single scale based on a specific value of ϵ, persistent homology uses a multi-scale construction that tracks the homology of the simplicial complex F_ϵ as $\epsilon \geq 0$ varies between the two extremes. As $F_{\epsilon_1} \subseteq F_{\epsilon_2}$ whenever $\epsilon_1 < \epsilon_2$, varying ϵ creates a nested sequence of simplicial complexes, and this nested sequence is related to an algebraic structure known as a persistence module. The varying homology can be computed and tracked using specially designed computing algorithms. In this case, any given hole (homology class) will be born at a particular scale $\epsilon_1 \geq 0$ where it appears in F_{ϵ_1}, and will die at another scale $\epsilon_2 > \epsilon_1$ where it disappears in F_{ϵ_2}. The persistence of this homology class is then represented by the interval (ϵ_1, ϵ_2). Persistent features remain over a relatively long range of ϵ values and are thus considered as intrinsic the data. Features with short persistence are thought of as arising from noise. A statistically rigorous division of homology classes into those that have long persistence (signal) and short persistence (noise) is not trivial and this issue seems to be mostly ignored in practice. Recent exceptions are the work of Fasy et al. [7] where confidence sets for persistence diagrams are developed, and Bobrowski et al. [2] where the authors study the persistent homology of random simplicial complexes.

For our application the growing scale ϵ corresponds to allowing signals with smaller values of the squared-correlation to be linked together to form simplices in the Vietoris-Rips complex. The nature of change in homology with respect to each dimension p can be depicted graphically using a barcode plot, a plot that tracks the birth and death of holes in each dimension as ϵ varies. Features in the barcode that are born and then quickly die are associated with noise, while features that persist are considered indicative of topological signal in the data. If the barcode plot of dimension $p = 0$ reveals signal and the higher-dimensional barcodes do not, the data are clustered around a metric tree. If both the $p = 0$ and $p = 1$ barcodes reveal signal and the $p = 2$ barcode plot does not, the data are clustered around a metric

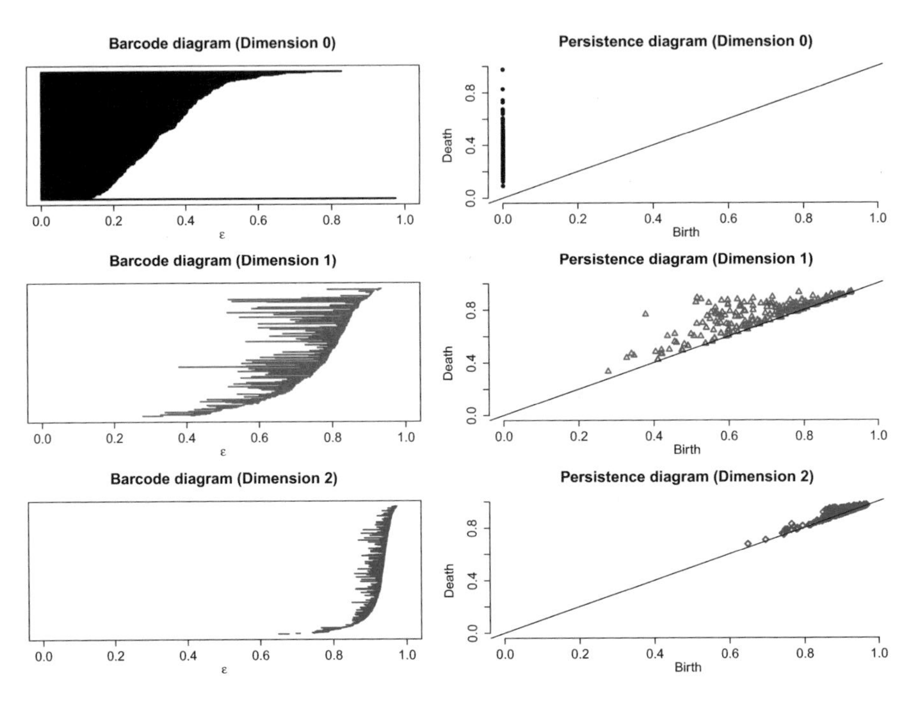

Fig. 2 Persistent homology computed for the single training sample depicted in Fig. 1. The first column displays the barcodes for dimension $p = 0, 1, 2$ in each of the three rows, respectively, and the second column displays the corresponding persistence diagrams

graph. A metric graph is indicative of multiple pathways for signals to get between two sensors/voxels.

For the sample considered in Fig. 1, panel (a), the barcodes for each dimension $p = 0, 1, 2$ are depicted in the first column of Fig. 2. For a given barcode plot, the Betti number for fixed ϵ, corresponding to the simplicial complex F_ϵ, is computed as the number of bars above it. For $p = 0$ (Fig. 2, first row and first column), $\text{Betti}_0 = 204$ connected components are born at $\epsilon = 0$ corresponding to each of the MEG sensors. Betti_0 decreases rapidly as ϵ increases and it appears that between two to four connected components persist over a wide range of ϵ values. The barcode plot for dimension $p = 1$ (Fig. 2, second row and first column) also appears to have features that are somewhat significant, but the $p = 2$ barcodes are relatively short, likely indicating noise. Taken together this can be interpreted as there being many loops in the point cloud. The data resemble a metric graph with some noise added. An equivalent way to depict the persistence of features is through a persistence diagram, which is a scatter plot comparing the birth and death ϵ values for each hole. The persistence diagrams corresponding to each barcode are depicted in the second column of Fig. 2 and have the same interpretation as the barcodes. It is interesting to note that the space of persistence diagrams can be endowed with a metric, and while we will not make use of this fact here, in Sect. 7 we describe an alternative approach for constructing features that makes use of the distance between persistence diagrams.

As for interpretation in the context of functional neuroimaging data, the number of connected components (Betti_0) represents a measure of the overall connectivity or synchronization between sensors, with smaller values of Betti_0 corresponding to a greater degree of overall synchrony. We suspect that the number of loops (Betti_1) corresponds to the density of "information pathways" with higher values corresponding to more complex structure having more pathways. The number of voids (Betti_2) may be related to the degree of segregation of the connections. If a void was to persist through many values of ϵ, then we may have a collection of locations/sensors that are not communicating. Thus the larger the value of Betti_2, the more of these non-communicative spaces there may be.

For each value of p, $p = 0, 1, 2$, we construct features for classification by extracting information from the corresponding barcode by considering the persistence of each homology class appearing at some point in the barcode. This is defined as the difference between the corresponding death and birth ϵ values. This yields a sample of persistence values for each barcode. Summary statistics computed from this sample are then used as features. In particular, we compute the total persistence, PM_p, which is defined as one-half of the sum of all persistence values, and we also compute the variance, skewness, and kurtosis of the sample leading to additional features denoted as PV_p, PS_p, PK_p, respectively. In total we obtain 12 global features from persistent homology.

5 Mutual Information Networks

Let us again fix a particular sample l from the training set and consider the collection of signals, $y_{li}(t)$, observed over all locations $i = 1, \ldots, n$ for the given sample. For the moment we will suppress dependence on training sample l and let $\boldsymbol{Y}_i = (Y_i(1), \ldots, Y_i(T))'$ denote the time series recorded at location i. We next consider a graph theoretic approach that aims to characterize the global connectivity in the brain with a small number of neurobiologically meaningful measures. This is achieved by estimating a weighted network from the time series where the sensors/voxels correspond to the nodes of the network and the links $\hat{\boldsymbol{w}} = (\hat{w}_{ij})$ represent the connectivity, where $\hat{w}_{ij}$ is a measure of statistical dependence estimated from $\boldsymbol{Y}_i$ and $\boldsymbol{Y}_j$.

As a measure of dependence we consider the mutual information which quantifies the shared information between two time series and measures both linear and nonlinear dependence. The coherence between $\boldsymbol{Y}_i$ and $\boldsymbol{Y}_j$ at frequency λ is a measure of correlation in frequency and is defined as $\text{coh}_{ij}(\lambda) = |f_{ij}(\lambda)|^2/(f_i(\lambda) * f_j(\lambda))$ where $f_{ij}(\lambda)$ is the cross-spectral density between $\boldsymbol{Y}_i$ and $\boldsymbol{Y}_j$ and $f_i(\lambda), f_j(\lambda)$ are the corresponding spectral densities for each process (see, e.g., Shumway and Stoffer

[26]). The mutual information within frequency band $[\lambda_1, \lambda_2]$ is then

$$\delta_{ij} = -\frac{1}{2\pi} \int_{\lambda_1}^{\lambda_2} \log(1 - \text{coh}_{ij}(\lambda)) d\lambda$$

and the network weights are defined as $w_{ij} = \sqrt{1 - \exp(-2\delta_{ij})}$ which gives a measure of dependence lying in the unit interval [14]. The estimates $\hat{\boldsymbol{w}}$ are based on values $\lambda_1 = 0$, $\lambda_2 = 0.5$, and computed using the MATLAB toolbox for functional connectivity [30]). After computing the estimates of the network matrices we retained only the top 20 % strongest connections and set the remaining weights to $\hat{w}_{ij} = 0$.

We summarize the topology of the network obtained from each sample with seven graph-theoretic measures, each of which can be expressed explicitly as a function of $\hat{\boldsymbol{w}}$ (see, e.g., Rubinov and Sporns [24]). In computing the measures, the distance between any two nodes is taken as $\hat{w}_{ij}^{-1}$:

1. Characteristic path length: the average shortest path between all pairs of nodes.
2. Global efficiency: the average inverse shortest path length between all pairs of nodes.
3. Local efficiency: global efficiency computed over node neighborhoods.
4. Clustering coefficient: an average measure of the prevalence of clustered connectivity around individual nodes.
5. Transitivity: a robust variant of the clustering coefficient.
6. Modularity: degree to which the network may be subdivided into clearly delineated and non-overlapping groups.
7. Assortativity coefficient: correlation coefficient between the degrees of all nodes on two opposite ends of a link.

The seven measures are computed for each training sample and used as global features for brain decoding.

6 Example Application: Brain Decoding from MEG

In 2011 the International Conference on Artificial Neural Networks (ICANN) held an MEG mind reading contest sponsored by the PASCAL2 Challenge Programme. The challenge task was to infer from brain activity, measured with MEG, the type of a video stimulus shown to a subject. The experimental paradigm involved one male subject who watched alternating video clips from five video types while MEG signals were recorded at $n = 204$ sensor channels covering the scalp. The different video types are:

1. Artificial: screen savers showing animated shapes or text.
2. Nature: clips from nature documentaries, showing natural scenery like mountains or oceans.

3. Football: clips taken from (European) football matches of Spanish La Liga.
4. Mr. Bean: clips from the episode *Mind the Baby, Mr. Bean* of the Mr. Bean television series.
5. Chaplin: clips from the *Modern Times* feature film, starring Charlie Chaplin.

The experiment involved two separate recording sessions that took place on consecutive days. The organizers released a series of 1-s MEG recordings in random order which were downsampled to 200 Hz. A single recording is depicted in Fig. 1, and the data comprise a total of 1380 such recordings. Of these, 677 recordings are labelled training samples from the first day of the experiment and 653 are unlabelled test samples from the second day of the experiment. Thus aside from the challenge of decoding the stimulus associated with test samples an additional challenge arises in that the training and test sets are from different days, leading to a potential domain shift problem. To aid contestants with this problem the organizers released a small additional set of 50 labelled training samples from day 2. The objective was to use the 727 labelled training samples to build a classifier, and the submissions were judged based on the overall accuracy rate for decoding the stimulus of the test samples. The overall winning team obtained an accuracy rate of 68.0 %, which was followed by 63.2 % for the second place entry, and the remaining scores ranged from 62.8–24.2 %. Full details of the competition and results are available in Klami et al. [15]. Following the competition, the labels for the 653 test samples were also released. Our objective is to apply the techniques described in this article to the ICANN MEG dataset and to compare the resulting decoding accuracy rates to those obtained in the actual competition. All rules of the competition were followed and the test data were only used to evaluate our approach, as in the competition.

Examination of the training data reveals the detrended variance of the signal at each sensor to be an important feature for discriminating the stimuli. This is as expected (see discussion in Sect. 2) and so all classifiers we consider include this feature. Experimentation (using only the training data) with classifiers excluding the detrended variance indicated that this is by far the most important feature and the predicted accuracy rates we obtain from cross-validation drop significantly when this feature is excluded. In Fig. 3 we illustrate the average spatial variation of this feature for each of the five stimuli. Differing patterns are seen for each class. For example, in the "Chaplin" class, the signal exhibits greatest power in sensors representing the occipital and parietal lobes whereas, for the "Football" class we see the greatest power in sensors representing the left and right frontal lobes. Including the detrended variance at each sensor yields 204 features to be added to the classifier.

To derive additional features we applied FPCA to all of the training samples separately at each sensor. Figure 4 shows the first three functional principal components. The first FPC, depicted in panel (a), seems to capture the overall level of the signal. The second FPC, depicted in panel (b), appears to represent an overall trend and the third FPC, depicted in panel (c), is a mode of variation having a "U" or an inverted "U" shape. At each sensor, we included as features the minimum number of FPC scores required to explain 90 % of the variability at that sensor across the training samples. The distribution of the number of scores used at each sensor is

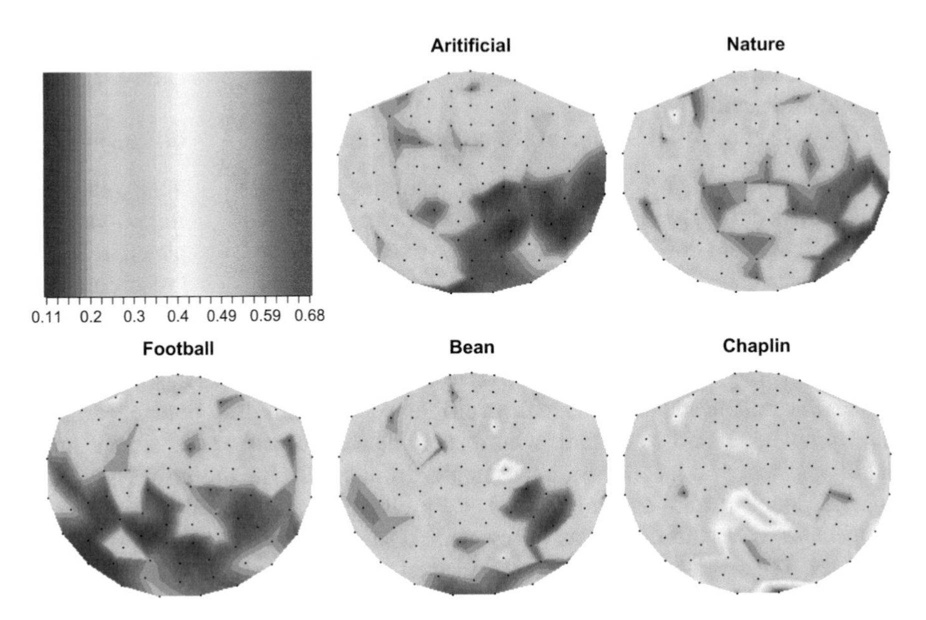

Fig. 3 Spatial variation of the detrended variance by stimulus class. Each map is a two-dimensional projection of the sensor array with the *black dots* representing the sensors. At each sensor we fit a linear regression on time point and compute the variance of the residuals as the feature. There are two sensors (each oriented differently) at each of 102 locations. For the purpose of visual summary, we average the two variance measures for each location and then further average across all training samples within a given stimulus class. We then map the resulting averaged measures across the scalp

depicted in Fig. 4, panel (d). At most sensors either $M_i = 2$ or $M_i = 3$ FPC scores are used as features, and overall, FPCA introduces 452 features. Our cutoff of 90 % was based on an examination of the FPCs for the training data, where it seemed that the fifth and higher FPCs did not represent anything meaningful. It should be noted that this exploratory approach for choosing the cutoff is by no means optimal, and alternative choices could be considered. The spatial variability of the first FPC score is depicted in Fig. 5. Differing spatial patterns across all of the stimuli are visible, in particular for the "Chaplin" class, which tends to have elevated first FPC scores at many sensors.

Persistent homology barcodes of dimension $p = 0, 1, 2$ were computed using the *TDA* package in R [8] for all training samples and the 12 summary features PM_p, PV_p, PS_p, PK_p, $p = 0, 1, 2$ were extracted from the barcodes. To determine the potential usefulness for classification we compared the mean of each of these features across the five stimuli classes using one-way analysis of variance. In most cases the p-value corresponding to the null hypothesis of equality of the mean across all groups was less than 0.05, with the exception of PK_0 (p-value = 0.36) and PM_1 (p-value = 0.34). Mutual information weighted networks were also computed for each training sample and the seven graph theory measures discussed in Sect. 5 were

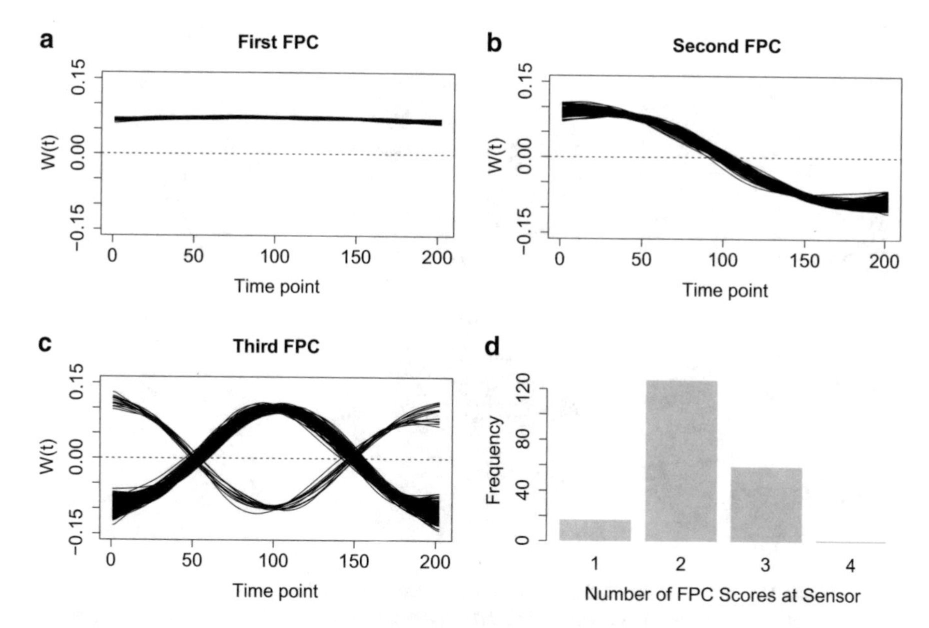

Fig. 4 FPCA applied to the training data: panel (**a**)—the first FPC at each sensor; panel (**b**)—the second FPC at each sensor; panel (**c**)—the third FPC at each sensor; (**d**)—the distribution of the smallest number of FPCs required to explain at least 90 % of the variance at each sensor

calculated. Analysis of variance comparing the mean of each graph measure across stimuli classes resulted in p-values less than 0.001 for all seven features. This initial analysis indicates that both types of features, particularly the network features, may be useful for discriminating the stimuli for these data.

We considered a total of seven classifiers based on the setup described in Sect. 2 each differing with respect to the features included. The features included in each of the classifiers are indicated in Table 1. The simplest classifier included only the detrended variance (204 features) and the most complex classifier included the detrended variance, FPCA scores, persistent homology statistics, and graph theory measures (675 features). As discussed in Sect. 2, the regression parameters $\boldsymbol{\theta}$ are estimated by maximizing the log-likelihood of the symmetric multinomial logistic regression subject to an elastic net penalty. The elastic net penalty is a mixture of ridge and lasso penalties and has two tuning parameters, $\lambda \geq 0$ a complexity parameter, and $0 \leq \alpha \leq 1$ a parameter balancing the ridge ($\alpha = 0$) and lasso ($\alpha = 1$) components. We choose values for these tuning parameters using cross-validation based on a nested cross-validation scheme similar to that proposed in Huttunen et al. [13] that emphasizes the 50 labelled day 2 samples for obtaining error estimates. We consider a sequence of possible values for α lying in the set $\{0, 0.1, 0.2, \ldots, 1.0\}$ and fix α at one such value. With the given value of α fixed, we perform a 200-fold cross-validation. In each fold, the training data consists of all 677 samples from day 1 and a random sample of 25 of the 50 labelled day 2 samples.

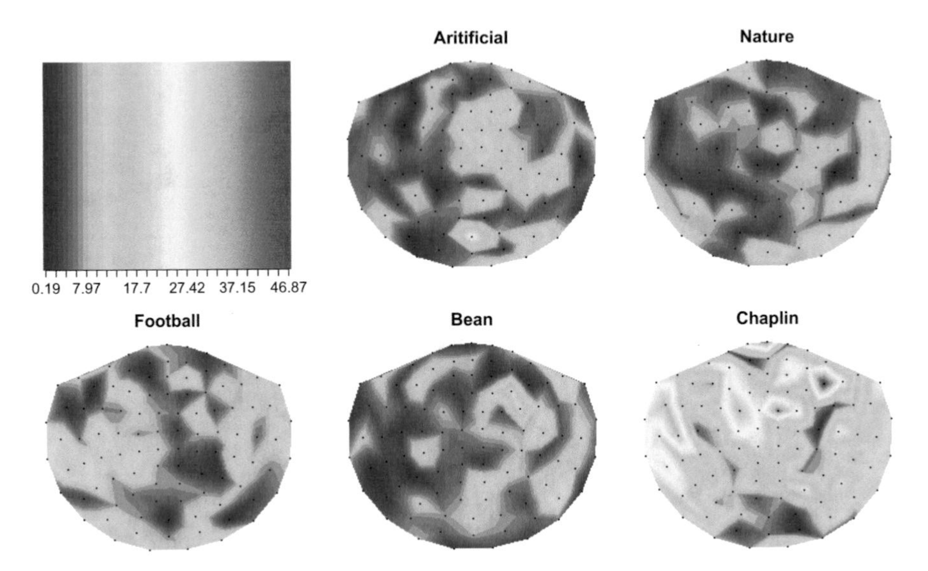

Fig. 5 Spatial variation of the first FPC score by stimulus class. Each map is a two-dimensional projection of the sensor array with the *black dots* representing the sensor locations. There are two sensors (each oriented differently) at each of 102 locations. For the purpose of visual summary, we average the absolute value of the two scores at each location and then further average across all training samples within a given stimulus class. We then map the resulting averaged measures across the scalp

The remaining labelled day 2 samples are set aside as a validation set for the given fold. Within this fold, the $677 + 25 = 702$ samples in the current training set are subjected to another five-fold cross-validation over a sequence of λ values to obtain an optimal λ value for the given α *and* training set. The resulting model is then used to classify the 25 validation samples resulting in a performance estimate $\epsilon_{\alpha,j}$ corresponding to the jth fold, $j = 1, \ldots, 200$. The overall performance estimate for a given α is then obtained as the mean over the 200 folds $\epsilon_\alpha = \frac{1}{200}\sum_{j=1}^{200} \epsilon_{\alpha,j}$. This procedure is repeated for all α in $\{0, 0.1, \ldots, 1.0\}$. The optimal value for the tuning parameter α is that which corresponds to the smallest error ϵ_α. Once the optimal α value has been determined, the optimal value for λ is again chosen by five-fold cross-validation as done previously, but now using all of the 727 training samples from both days.

Table 1 lists the cross-validation predicted accuracy rates for each of the seven classifiers along with the test accuracy obtained from the 653 day 2 test samples. Had we participated in the competition, our choice of classifier would have been based on the cross-validation predicted accuracy rates. While all fairly close, the classifier incorporating detrended variance, FPC scores, and network features would have been chosen as our final model as this is one of two classifiers having the highest predicted accuracy rate 61.68 % and the fewest number of features of the two. The test accuracy from this classifier is 66.46 %, which is just short of 68.0 %

Table 1 Results from the brain decoding competition dataset

Classifier	CV predicted accuracy (%)	Test accuracy (%)
Detrended variance	60.90	61.26
Detrended variance + FPCA	60.90	65.54
Detrended variance + Network features	60.46	61.41
Detrended variance + PH	60.44	61.10
Detrended variance + FPCA + Network features	**61.68**	**66.46**
Detrended variance + FPCA + PH	60.72	64.01
Detrended variance + FPCA + Network features + PH	61.68	65.24

Baseline test accuracy is 23.0 % (chance level); competition winners achieved 68.0 % and second place was 63.2 %. Note that "PH" refers to the 12 features derived using persistent homology
The bold values indicate the classifier with the highest test accuracy

Table 2 Confusion matrix summarizing the performance on the test data for the classifier incorporating detrended variance, FPCA, and network features

	True stimulus				
Predicted stimulus	Artificial	Nature	Football	Mr. Bean	Chaplin
Artificial	90	27	28	6	3
Nature	39	98	16	6	0
Football	14	12	54	12	4
Mr. Bean	5	11	4	76	2
Chaplin	2	3	0	25	116

obtained by the competition winners, but higher than 63.2 % accuracy rate obtained by the first runner-up. *Thus with our entry we would have finished in second place.* The confusion matrix for our classifier is presented in Table 2. Our classifier has highest accuracy for predicting the "Chaplin" (92.8 %) video clips from the MEG data, and lowest accuracy for predicting the "Football" (52.9 %) video clip.

With respect to interpretation of the results, the most important feature appears to be the detrended variance. Figure 3 depicts maps showing the spatial variability of this feature averaged across training samples within a particular stimuli class. The maps depict regions of the scalp, which can be loosely associated with regions of the brain, where the power of the signal is strongest for the different stimuli classes. For example, for the "football" class the signals appear to have higher power in the frontal regions, both left and right whereas, for the "artificial" class the power is strongest in the right frontal and left temporal and occipital regions. The map for the "Chaplin" class is interesting and seems rather different from the others in that the value of the feature seems relatively more distributed across the scalp, though with highest values in the parietal and occipital regions. Interestingly, this is the only black and white clip. This is also the clip for which our classifier had the highest accuracy.

7 Discussion

We have reviewed the brain decoding problem in neuroscience and have discussed approaches from statistics, computational topology, and graph theory for constructing features for this high-dimensional classification problem. We have developed classifiers combining FPCA, persistent homology, and graph theoretic measures derived from mutual information networks. We have considered incorporating the features within a classifier based on symmetric multinomial logistic regression incorporating elastic net regularization and have applied our approach to a real brain decoding competition dataset illustrating good performance.

Overall, examining the results in Table 1 we see that those classifiers incorporating FPC scores all perform quite well, with test accuracy scores being higher than predicted accuracy scores. It is not clear to us what aspect of the FPC scores allows for this increase and we are currently investigating this. This issue may be related to the domain shift problem where all of the test samples were collected on day 2 of the experiment, and all but 50 of the training samples were collected on day 1. The test samples may thus reflect a learning mechanism. We have approached this issue by emphasizing the 50 day 2 training samples when training our classifier. This approach is by no means optimal and alternative techniques for handling domain adaptation in brain decoding problems is of both practical and theoretical interest. Given the positive results we have observed with the classifiers incorporating FPCA, we are exploring the use of more general approaches based on nonlinear manifold representations for functional data such as those recently proposed by Chen and Müller [5]. Another aspect of FPCA we intend to explore is the incorporation of spatial dependence. This is relevant for brain decoding as there will typically be a high level of spatial dependence across sensors/voxels. In fact, very little research has been conducted on this topic with the exception of the recent work of Liu et al. [18].

Regarding the global features, there seems to be a small advantage gained in incorporating the network features but nothing gained by incorporating persistent homology based on our current implementation. We emphasize that this is only for a single dataset and experimental paradigm. Performance on other brain decoding datasets may yield different results in particular as the samples considered in our application were based on fairly short 1-s recordings. When constructing functional connectivity networks we chose to keep the edges having the 20 % strongest connections. Other choices for the cutoff could be considered. An alternative approach that was considered in exploratory work was the use of weighted graphs with all edges between nodes included. Our investigation of this approach did not reveal any advantage in separating the groups relative to the networks based on the hard threshold of 20 %. An alternative approach to choosing this threshold could be based on stability selection for structure estimation [19] and we plan to investigate this.

We are currently exploring an alternative implementation of persistent homology based on the recent work of Kramer et al. [16] where persistent homology is used to analyze spatiotemporal data of flow field patterns from numerical simulations of fluid dynamics. In the setup of Kramer et al. [16], the data consist of a time series of two-dimensional images, and persistent homology is used to characterize the geometric features of each image. Letting $f_t : D \to \mathbb{R}$ denote the image (a spatial field) at time t, $t = 1, \ldots, T$, and D a topological space over which the image is defined, persistent homology is applied to study the structure of the sub-level sets $C(f_t, \theta) = \{x \in D | f_t(x) \leq \theta\}$ as θ varies from $-\infty$ to ∞. The persistence diagrams $\mathrm{PD}_0(f_t)$ and $\mathrm{PD}_1(f_t)$ capture, respectively, the number of connected components and loops of $C(f_t, \theta)$ as θ varies. Computing the persistence diagram $\mathrm{PD}_k(f_t)$ is a mapping taking the image f_t to a point in the space of persistence diagrams of dimension k, Per_k. This mapping is applied to each image in the time series $f_t, t = 1, \ldots, T$, resulting in a point cloud $X_k = \{\mathrm{PD}_k(f_t), t = 1, \ldots, T\} \in \mathrm{Per}_k$. Kramer et al. [16] then use the fact that Per_k is a metric space to summarize features of this point cloud, for example, by computing the distance between consecutive persistence diagrams. The latter summary produces a scalar time series that captures the rate at which the geometry of images is changing over time. For application to brain decoding, we have been investigating this approach where the image at each time point is obtained by interpolating the MEG recordings between sensors. Preliminary results based on this implementation of persistent homology are encouraging and we hope to report on this in a future paper.

Acknowledgements This article is based on work from Nicole Croteau's MSc thesis. F.S. Nathoo is supported by an NSERC discovery grant and holds a Tier II Canada Research Chair in Biostatistics for Spatial and High-Dimensional Data. The authors thank Rachel Levanger for useful discussions on the implementation of persistent homology for space-time data.

References

1. Adcock, A., Rubin, D., Carlsson, G.: Classification of hepatic lesions using the matching metric. Comput. Vis. Image Underst. **121**, 36–42 (2014)
2. Bobrowski, O., Kahle, M., Skraba, P.: Maximally persistent cycles in random geometric complexes. arXiv preprint arXiv:1509.04347 (2015)
3. Carlsson, G. Topology and data. Bull. Am. Math. Soc. **46**, 255–308 (2009)
4. Chapelle, O., Haffner, P., Vapnik, V.N.: Support vector machines for histogram-based image classification. IEEE Trans. Neural Netw. **10**, 1055–1064 (1999)
5. Chen, D., Müller, H.-G.: Nonlinear manifold representations for functional data. Ann. Stat. **40**, 1–29 (2012)
6. Chung, M.K., Bubenik, P., Kim, P.T.: Persistence diagrams of cortical surface data. In: Information Processing in Medical Imaging, pp. 386–397. Springer, Berlin/Heidelberg (2009)
7. Fasy, B.T., Kim, J., Lecci, F., Maria, C.: Introduction to the R package TDA. arXiv preprint arXiv:1411.1830 (2014)
8. Fasy, B.T., Lecci, F., Rinaldo, A., Wasserman, L., Balakrishnan, S., Singh, A.: Confidence sets for persistence diagrams. Ann. Stat. **42**(6), 2301–2339 (2014)
9. Friedman, J., Hastie, T., Tibshirani, R.: Regularization paths for generalized linear models via coordinate descent. J. Stat. Softw. **33**, 1–22 (2010)

10. Friston, K., Chu, C., Mourao-Miranda, J., Hulme, O., Rees, G., Penny, W., Ashburner, J.: Bayesian decoding of brain images. Neuroimage **39**, 181–205 (2008)
11. Haynes, J.-D., Rees, G.: Decoding mental states from brain activity in humans. Nat. Rev. Neurosci. **7**, 523–534 (2006)
12. Heo, G., Gamble, J., Kim, P.T.: Topological analysis of variance and the maxillary complex. J. Am. Stat. Assoc. **107**, 477–492 (2012)
13. Huttunen, H., Manninen, T., Kauppi, J.P., Tohka, J.: Mind reading with regularized multinomial logistic regression. Mach. Vis. Appl. **24**, 1311–1325 (2013)
14. Joe, H.: Relative entropy measures of multivariate dependence. J. Am. Stat. Assoc. **84**, 157–164 (1989)
15. Klami, A., Ramkumar, P., Virtanen, S., Parkkonen, L., Hari, R., Kaski, S.: ICANN/PASCAL2 challenge: MEG mind reading—overview and results. In: Proceedings of ICANN/PASCAL2 Challenge: MEG Mind Reading (2011)
16. Kramar, M., Levanger, R., Tithof, J., Suri, B., Xu, M., Paul, M., Schatz, M., Mischaikow, K.: Analysis of Kolmogorov flow and Rayleigh-Bénard convection using persistent homology. arXiv preprint arXiv:1505.06168 (2015)
17. Leng, X., Muller, H.G.: Classification using functional data analysis for temporal gene expression data. Bioinformatics **22**, 68–76 (2006)
18. Liu, C., Ray, S., Hooker, G.: Functional principal components analysis of spatially correlated data. arXiv:1411.4681 (2014)
19. Meinshausen, N., Buhlmann, P.: Stability selection. J. R. Stat. Soc. Ser. B **72**(4), 417–473 (2010)
20. Neal, R.M., Zhang, J.: High dimensional classification with Bayesian neural networks and Dirichlet diffusion trees. In: Feature Extraction. Springer, Berlin/Heidelberg, pp. 265–296 (2006)
21. Pachauri, D., Hinrichs, C., Chung, M.K., Johnson, S.C., Singh, V.: Topology-based kernels with application to inference problems in Alzheimer's disease. IEEE Trans. Med. Imaging **30**, 1760–1770 (2011)
22. Rasmussen, C.E.: Gaussian processes in machine learning. In: Advanced Lectures on Machine Learning, pp. 63–71. Springer, Berlin/Heidelberg (2004)
23. Ripley, B.D.: Neural networks and related methods for classification. J. R. Stat. Soc. Ser. B Methodol. **56**, 409–456 (1994)
24. Rubinov, M., Sporns, O.: Complex network measures of brain connectivity: uses and interpretations. Neuroimage **52**, 1059–1069 (2010)
25. Sethares, W.A., Budney, R.: Topology of musical data. J. Math. Music **8**, 73–92 (2014)
26. Shumway, R.H., Stoffer, D.S.: Spectral analysis and filtering. In: Time Series Analysis and Its Applications. Springer, New York (2011)
27. Silverman, B.W., Ramsay, J.O.: Functional Data Analysis. Springer, New York (2005)
28. Stam, C.J., Breakspear, M., van Walsum, A.M.V.C., van Dijk, B.W.: Nonlinear synchronization in EEG and whole-head MEG recordings of healthy subjects. Hum. Brain Mapp. **19**, 63–78 (2003)
29. Tomioka, R., Aihara, K., Muller, K.-R.: Logistic regression for single trial EEG classification. Adv. Neural Inf. Process. Syst. **19**, 1377–1384 (2007)
30. Zhou, D., Thompson, W.K., Siegle, G.: MATLAB toolbox for functional connectivity. Neuroimage **47**, 1590–1607 (2009)
31. Zhu, X.: Persistent homology: an introduction and a new text representation for natural language processing. In: Proceedings of the Twenty-Third International Joint Conference on Artificial Intelligence. AAAI Press, Beijing (2013)
32. Zou, H., Hastie, T.: Regularization and variable selection via the elastic net. J. R. Stat. Soc. Ser. B Stat. Methodol. **67**, 301–320 (2005)

Unsupervised Bump Hunting Using Principal Components

Daniel A. Díaz-Pachón, Jean-Eudes Dazard, and J. Sunil Rao

Abstract Principal Components Analysis is a widely used technique for dimension reduction and characterization of variability in multivariate populations. Our interest lies in studying when and why the rotation to principal components can be used effectively within a response-predictor set relationship in the context of mode hunting. Specifically focusing on the Patient Rule Induction Method (PRIM), we first develop a fast version of this algorithm (fastPRIM) under normality which facilitates the theoretical studies to follow. Using basic geometrical arguments, we then demonstrate how the Principal Components rotation of the predictor space alone can in fact generate improved mode estimators. Simulation results are used to illustrate our findings.

1 Introduction

The PRIM algorithm for bump hunting was first developed by Friedman and Fisher [5]. It is an intuitively useful computational algorithm for the detection of local maxima (or minima) on target functions. Roughly speaking, PRIM *peels* the (conditional) distribution of a response from the outside in, leaving at the end rectangular boxes which are supposed to contain a bump (see the formal description in Algorithm 1) at page 328. However, some shortcomings against this procedure have also appeared in the literature when several dimensions are under consideration. For instance, as Polonik and Wang [10] explained it, the method could fail when there are two or more modes in high-dimensional settings. Hirose and Koga [7] also found some instances of superiority of the tree structure of a genetic algorithm over PRIM.

D.A. Díaz-Pachón • J.S. Rao (✉)
Division of Biostatistics, University of Miami, 1120 NW 14 ST 1057, Miami, FL 33136, USA
e-mail: Ddiaz3@miami.edu; jxd101@case.edu

J.-E. Dazard
Center for Proteomics and Bioinformatics, Case Western Reserve University, 10900 Euclid Av., Cleveland, OH 44106, USA
e-mail: jean-eudes.dazard@case.edu

© Springer International Publishing AG 2017

S.E. Ahmed (ed.), *Big and Complex Data Analysis*, Contributions to Statistics,
DOI 10.1007/978-3-319-41573-4_16

Almost at the same time, Dazard and Rao [2] proposed a supervised bump hunting strategy, given that the use of PRIM is still "challenged in the context of high-dimensional data." The strategy, called Local Sparse Bump Hunting (LSBH) is outlined in Algorithm 2 at page 327. Summarizing the algorithm, it uses a recursive partitioning algorithm (CART) to identify subregions the whole space where at most one mode is estimated to be present; then, a Sparse Principal Component Analysis (SPCA) is performed separately on each local partition; and finally, the location of the bump is determined via PRIM in the local, rotated and projected subspace induced by the sparse principal components.

As an example, we show in Fig. 1 simulation results representing a multivariate bimodal situation in the presence of noise, similarly to the simulation design used by Dazard and Rao [2]. We simulated in a three-dimensional input space ($p = 3$) for visualization purposes. The data consists of a mixture of two trivariate normal distributions, taking on discrete binary response values ($Z \in \{1, 2\}$), noised by a trivariate uniform distribution with a null response ($Z = 0$), so that the the data can be written by $X \sim w \cdot N_p(0, \Sigma) + (1 - w) \cdot B_p$, where $B_p \sim U_p[a, b]$, $w \in [0, 1]$ is the mixing weight, and $(a, b) \in \mathbb{R}^2$.

Notice how the data in the PC spaces determined by Partition #1 and #2 do align with the PC coordinate axes Y_{11} and Y_{21}, respectively (Fig. 1).

Our goal in this paper is to provide some theoretical basis for the use of PCs in mode hunting using PRIM and a modified version of this algorithm that we called "fastPRIM." Although the original LSBH algorithm accepts more than one mode by partition, we will restrict ourselves to the case in which there is at most one on each partition, in order to get more workable developments and more understandable results in this work.

In Sect. 2 we define the algorithms we are working with and set some useful notation. Section 3 proposes a modification of PRIM (called fastPRIM) for the particular case in which the bumps are modes in a setting of normal variables that allows to compare the boxes in the original space and in the rotation induced by principal components. The approach goes beyond normality and can be shown to be true for every symmetric distributions with finite second moment, and it is also an important reduction on the computational complexity since it is also useful for samples when $n \gg 0$, via the central limit theorem (Sect. 3.3). In this section we also present simulations which display the differences between considering the original space or the PC rotation for PRIM and fastPRIM. Finally, Sect. 4 proves Theorem 1, a result explaining why the (volume-standardized) output box mode is higher in the PC rotation than in the original input space, a situation observed computationally by Dazard and Rao [2] for which we give here a formal explanation. Theorem 2 shows that in terms of bias and variance, fastPRIM does better than PRIM. Finally, in Sect. 5 we show additional simulations relevant to the results found in Sect. 4.

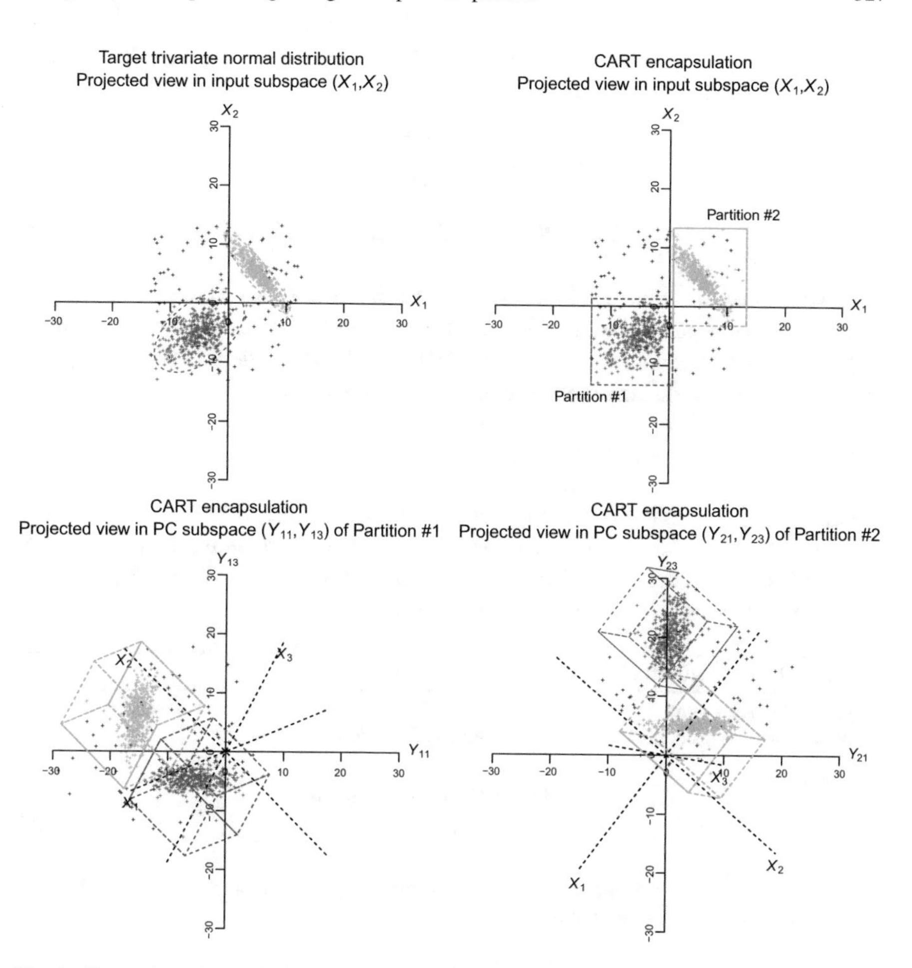

Fig. 1 Illustration of the efficiency of the encapsulation process by LSBH of two target normal distributions (*red and green dots*), in the presence of 10 % ($w = 0.9$) noise distribution (*black dots*) in a three-dimensional input space ($p = 3$). We let the total sample size be $n = 10^3$. *Top row*: each plot represents a projected view of the data in input subspace (X_1, X_2) with 95 % confidence ellipses (*dotted red and green contours—top left panel*) and partitions vertices (*top right panel*). Only those partitions encapsulating the target distributions are drawn. *Bottom row*: each plot represents a projected view of the data in the PC subspace (Y_{11}, Y_{13}) of Partition #1 (*bottom left*), and (Y_{21}, Y_{23}) of Partition #2 (*bottom right*)

2 Notation and Basic Concepts

We set here the concepts that will be useful throughout the paper to define the algorithms and its modifications. Our notation on PRIM follows as a guideline the one used by Polonik and Wang [10].

Let X be a p-dimensional real-valued random vector with distribution F. Let Z be an integrable random variable. Let $m(x) := \mathbf{E}[Z|X = x]$, $x \in \mathbb{R}^p$. Assume without loss of generality that $m(x) \geq 0$.

Define $I(A) := \int_A m(x)dF(x)$, for $A \subset \mathbb{R}^p$. So when $A = \mathbb{R}^p$, then $I(A) = \mathbf{E}Z$. We are interested in a region C such that

$$ave(C) := \frac{I(C)}{F(C)} > \rho, \tag{1}$$

where $\rho = ave(\mathbb{R}^p)$. Note then that $ave(C)$ is just a notational convenience for the average of Z given $X \in C$.

Given a box B whose sides are parallel to the coordinate axes of $\mathbb{R}^p$, we peel small pieces of B parallel to its sides and we stop peeling when what remains of the box B becomes too small. Let the class of all these boxes be denoted by $\mathscr{B}$. Given a subset $S(X) = S \subseteq \mathbb{R}^p$ and a parameter $\beta \in (0, 1)$, we define

$$B^*_\beta = \arg\max_{B \in \mathscr{B}} \{ave(B|S) : F(B|S) = \beta\}, \tag{2}$$

where $ave(B|S) = I(B|S)/F(B|S)$. In words, B^*_β is the box with maximum average of Z among all the boxes whose F-measure, conditioned to the points in the box S, is β. The former definitions set the stage to define Algorithm 1 at page 328 below.

Some remarks are in order given Algorithm 1:

Algorithm 1: Patient Rule Induction Method

- (Peeling) Begin with $B_1 = S$. For $l = 1, \ldots, L-1$, where $(1-\alpha)^L = \beta$, and $\alpha \in (0, 1)$, remove a subbox contained in B_l, chosen among $2p$ candidates given by:

$$\begin{aligned} b_{j1} &:= \{x \in B : x_j < x_{j(\alpha)}\}, \\ b_{j2} &:= \{x \in B : x_j > x_{j(1-\alpha)}\}, \end{aligned} \tag{3}$$

  where $j = 1, \ldots, p$. The subbox b^*_l chosen for removal gives the largest expected value of Z conditional on $B_l \setminus b^*_l(X)$. That is,

$$b^*_l = \arg\min \left\{ I\left(b_{jv}|B_l\right) : j = 1, \ldots, p \text{ and } v = 1, 2 \right\}. \tag{4}$$

  Then B_l is replaced by $B_{l+1} = B_l \setminus b^*_l$ and the process is iterated as long as the current box B_l be such that $F(B_l|S) \geq \beta + \alpha$.
- (Pasting) Alongside the $2p$ boundaries of the resulting box B on the peeling part of the algorithm we look for a box $b^+ \subset S \setminus B$ such that $F(b^+|S) = \alpha F(B|S)$ and $ave((B \cup b^+) \cap S) > ave(B \cap S)$. If there exists such a box b^+, we replace B by $(B \cup b^+)$. If there exists more than one box satisfying that condition, we replace B by the one that maximizes the average $ave((B \cup b^+) \cap S)$. In words, pasting is an enlargement on the Lebesgue measure of the box which is also an enlargement on the average $ave((B \cup b^+) \cap S)$.
- (Covering) After the first application of the peeling-pasting process, we update S by $S \setminus B_1$, where B_1 is the box found after pasting, and iterate the peeling-pasting process replacing $S = S^{(1)}$ by $S^{(2)} = S^{(1)} \setminus B_1$, and so on, removing at each step $k = 1, \ldots, t$ the optimal box of the previous step: $S^{(k)} = S^{(k-1)} \setminus B_{k-1}$, so that $S^{(k)} = S^{(1)} \setminus \cup_{1 \leq b \leq k-1} B_b$. At the end of the PRIM algorithm we are left with a region, shaped as a rectangular box:

$$R_\rho(p, k) = \bigcup_{ave\left(B_k|S^{(k)}\right) \geq \rho} \left\{B_k|S^{(k)}\right\}. \tag{5}$$

Remark 1 The value α is the second tuning parameter and $x_{j(\alpha)}$ is the α-quantile of $F_j(\cdot|B_l)$, the marginal conditional distribution function of X_j given the occurrence of B_l. Thus, by construction,

$$\alpha = F_j\left(b_{jv}|B_l\right) = F\left(b_{jv}|B_l\right). \tag{6}$$

Remark 2 Conditioning on an event, say $\tilde{A}$, is equivalent to conditioning on the random variable $\mathbf{1}\{x \in \tilde{A}\}$; i.e., when this occurs, as in (2), we are conditioning on a Bernoulli random variable.

Remark 3 When dealing with a sample, we define analogs of the terms used previously and replace those terms in Algorithm 1 with:

$$I_n(C) = \frac{1}{n}\sum_{i=1}^{n} Z_i\mathbf{1}\{X_i \in C\},$$

$$F_n(C) = \frac{1}{n}\sum_{i=1}^{n} \mathbf{1}\{X_i \in C\},$$

$$ave_n(C) = \frac{I_n(C)}{F_n(C)},$$

where F_n is the empirical cumulative distribution of $X_1, \ldots, X_n$.

Remark 4 Ignore the pasting stage, considering only peeling and covering. Let us call β_T the probability of the final region. Then

$$\begin{aligned}\beta_T = \mathbf{P}[x \in R_\rho(p)] &= \sum_{k=1}^{t} \beta(1-\beta)^{k-1} \\ &= 1-(1-\beta)^t.\end{aligned}$$

2.1 Principal Components

The theory about PCA is widely known, however we will outline it here for the sake of completeness and to define notation. Among others, Mardia [9] presents a thorough analysis.

If $\mathbf{x}$ is a random centered vector with covariance matrix Σ, we can define a linear transformation $\mathbf{T}$ such that

$$\mathbf{T}\mathbf{x} = \mathbf{y} = \Gamma'\mathbf{x}, \tag{7}$$

Algorithm 2: Local Sparse Bump Hunting

- Partition the input space into R partitions $P_1, \ldots, P_R$, using a tree-based algorithm like CART, in such a way that there is at most one mode in each of the partitions.
- For r from 1 to $\tilde{r}$
  - If P_r is elected for bump hunting (i.e.; if G_r, the number of class labels in P_r, is greater than 1)
    - Run a local SPCA in the partition P_r, rotating and reducing the space to p' ($\leq p$) dimensions, and if possible, decorrelating the sparse principal components (SPC). Call this resulting space $\mathcal{T}(P_r)$.
    - Estimate PRIM meta-parameters α and β in $\mathcal{T}(P_r)$.
    - Run a local and tuned PRIM-based bump hunting within $\mathcal{T}(P_r)$ to get descriptive rules of the bumps in the SPC space of the form $R_\rho^{(r)}(p')$, as in (5), where r indicates the partition being considered.
    - Rotate the local rules $R^{(r)}$ back into the input space to get rules in terms of the sparse linear combinations.
  - Actualize r to $r + 1$.
- Collect the rules from all partitions to get a global rule $\mathcal{R} = \bigcup_{r=1}^{R} R_\rho^{(r)}$ giving a full description of the estimated bumps in the entire input space.

where Γ is a matrix such that its columns are the standardized eigenvectors of $\Sigma := \Gamma \Lambda \Gamma'$; Λ is a diagonal matrix with $\lambda_1 \geq \cdots \lambda_p \geq 0$; and $\lambda_j, j = 1, \ldots, p$, are the eigenvalues of Σ. Then $\mathbf{T}$ is called the principal components transformation.

Let $p' \leq p$. We call $\mathfrak{X}(p)$ the original p-dimensional space where $\mathbf{x}$ lives, $\mathfrak{X}'(p)$ the rotated p-dimensional space where $\mathbf{y}$ lives, and $\mathfrak{X}'(p')$ the rotated and projected space on the p' first PC's.

As we will explain later, we are not advising on the reduction of dimensionality in the context of regression or other learning settings. However, since it is relevant to some features of our simulations, we consider the case $\mathfrak{X}'(p')$ with $p' \leq p$.

3 fastPRIM: A More Efficient Approach to Mode Hunting

Despite successful applications in many fields, PRIM presents some shortcomings. For instance, Friedman and Fisher [5], the proponents of the algorithm, show that in the presence of high collinearity or high correlation PRIM is likely to behave poorly. This is also true when there is significant background noise. Further, PRIM becomes computationally expensive in simulations and real data sets in large dimensions. In this section we propose a modified version of PRIM, called "fastPRIM," aimed to solve these two problems when we are hunting the mode. The high collinearity problem can be solved via principal components. The computational problems can be solved via the CLT and the geometric properties of the normal distribution, if we can warrant $n \gg 0$.

The following situations are variations from simple to complex of the input X and the response Z being normally distributed $N(\mathbf{0}, \Sigma)$ and $N(0, \sigma)$, respectively. We are interested on maximizing the density of Z given X. But there are several ways to define the mode of a continuum distribution. So for simplicity, let us define the mode of Z as the region $C \subset \mathbb{R}^p$ with $P_X[x \in C] = \beta$ that maximizes

$$M(C) := \int_C f_Z(x)dF(x) \tag{8}$$

(note the similarity of $M(C)$ with $I(C)$ in Eq. (1)). In terms of PRIM, we are interested in the box B^*_β defined on Eq. (2). That is, B^*_β is a box such that $\mathbf{P}_X[x \in B^*_\beta] = \beta$, and inside it the mean density of the response Z is maximized. Then, since the mean and the mode of the normal distribution coincide, finding a box of size β centered around the mean of X is equivalent to finding a box that maximizes the mode of Z (since X and Z are both centered around the origin).

Although it is good to have explicit knowledge of our final region of interest, on what follows most of the results—with the exception of Theorem 1 below—can be stated without direct reference to the mode of Z, taking into account that the mode of Z is centered around the mean of X.

3.1 *fastPRIM for Standard Normality*

Let $X \sim N(\mathbf{0}, \mathbf{I})$ with X living in the space $S(X)$. Let $Z \sim N(0, 1)$. Since the whole input space is defined by symmetric uncorrelated variables, PRIM can be modified in a very efficient way. (See below Algorithm 3.)

Algorithm 3: fastPRIM with Standard Normal Predictors

- (Peeling) Instead of peeling just one side of probability α, make $2p$ peels corresponding to each side of the box, giving to each one a probability $\alpha(2p)^{-1}$. Then, after L steps, the remaining box has the same β measure, it is still centered at the origin and its marginals will have probability measure $\beta^{1/p}$.
- (Covering) Call $B_M(k)$ the box found after the k-th step, $k = 1, \ldots, t$ of this modified peeling stage. Setting $S(X) = S^{(1)}(X)$, take the space $S^{(k)}(X) := S^{(1)}(X) \setminus \bigcup_{1 \leq b \leq k-1} B_M(b)$ and repeat on it the peeling stage.

Several comments are worthy to mention related to this modification.

1. Given that the standard normal is spherical, the final box at the end of the peeling algorithm is centered. It is also squared in that all its marginals have the same Lebesgue measure and the same probability measure $\beta^{1/p}$. Then, instead of doing the whole peeling stage, we can reduce it to select the central box whose vertices are located at the coordinates corresponding to the quantiles $\frac{1}{2}\beta^{1/p}$ and $1 - \frac{1}{2}\beta^{1/p}$ of each marginal.
2. Say we want to apply t steps of covering. Since the boxes chosen are centered at the end of the t-th covering step, the final box will have probability measure $\beta_T := 1 - (1 - \beta)^t$ (which, by Remark 4, produces the same probability than PRIM), each marginal has measure $(\beta_T)^{1/p}$, and the vertices of each marginal are located at the coordinates corresponding to the quantiles $\frac{1}{2}(\beta_T)^{1/p}$ and $1 - \frac{1}{2}(\beta_T)^{1/p}$. It means that the whole fastPRIM is reduced to calculating this central box of probability measure $t\beta$.
3. The only non-zero values outside the diagonal in the covariance matrix of $(Z\ X)^T$ of size $(p+1) \times (p+1)$ are possibly the non-diagonal terms in the first row and the first column. Let us call them $\sigma_{ZX_1}, \ldots, \sigma_{ZX_p}$. From this we get that $\mathbf{E}[Z|X] = \sum_{j=1}^{p} \sigma_{ZX_j} X_i$ and $\mathbf{V}[Z|X] = 1 - \sum_{j=1}^{p} \sigma_{ZX_j}^2$.
4. It does not make too much sense to have a pasting stage, since we will be adding the same α we just peeled in portions of $\alpha/(2p)$ at each side. However, a possible way to add this whole stage is to look for the dimension that maximizes the conditional mean, once a portion of probability $\alpha/2$ have been added to each side of the selected dimension. All this, of course, provided that this maximal conditional mean be higher than the one already found during the peeling stage. If this stage is applied as described, the final region will be a rectangular centered box.

Points 1, 2 and 3 can be stated as follows:

Lemma 1 *Assume $Z \sim N(0, 1)$ and $X \sim N(\mathbf{0}, \mathbf{I})$. Let us iterate t times Algorithm 3. Then the whole algorithm can be reduced to a single stage of finding a centralized box with vertices located at the coordinates corresponding to the quantiles $\frac{1}{2}(\beta_T)^{1/p}$ and $1 - \frac{1}{2}(\beta_T)^{1/p}$ of each of the p variables.*

3.2 fastPRIM and Principal Components

Note that if $Z \sim N(\mu, \sigma^2)$ and $X \sim N(\mathbf{0}, \Sigma)$, the same algorithm as in Sect. 3 can be used. The only difference is that the final box will be a rectangular Lebesgue set, not necessarily a square as before (although it continues being a square in probability). Some comments are in order.

First, with each of the variables having possible different variances, we are also peeling the random variables with lower variance. That is, we are peeling precisely the variables that we do not want to touch. The whole idea behind PRIM, however, is to peel from the variables with high variance, leaving the ones with lower variance as untouched as possible. The obvious solution is to use a PCA to project on the variables with higher variance, peel on those variables, and after the box is obtained to add the whole set of variables we chose not to touch. Adding to the notation developed in Sect. 2.1 for PCA, call Y' the projection of Y to its first p' principal components, where $0 < p' \leq p$. Algorithm 4 below makes this explicit.

Algorithm 4: fastPRIM with Principal Components

- (PCA) Apply PCA to X to obtain the space $\mathfrak{X}'(p')$.
- (Peeling) Make $2p'$ peels corresponding to each side of the box, each one with probability $\alpha(2p')^{-1}$. After L steps, the centered box has β measure, and its marginals will have probability $\beta^{1/p'}$ each.
- (Covering) Call $B_M(k)$ the box found after the k-th step, $k = 1, \ldots, t$, of this modified peeling stage. Setting $S(Y') = S^{(1)}(Y')$, take the space $S^{(k)}(Y') := S^{(1)}(Y') \setminus \bigcup_{1 \leq b \leq k-1} B_M(b)$ and repeat on it the peeling stage.
- (Completing) The final box will be given by $[\mathfrak{X}'(p) \setminus \mathfrak{X}'(p')] \cup S^{(t)}(Y')$. That is, to the final box we are adding the whole subspace which we chose not to peel.

In this way, we avoid to select for peeling the variables with lower variance. Concededly, we are still peeling the same amount (we are getting squares, not rectangles, in probability), but we are also getting an important simplification in algorithmic complexity cost. Besides this fact, most of the comments in Sect. 3.1 are still valid but one clarification has to be made: The covariance matrix of $(Z\ Y')$ has size $(p' + 1) \times (p' + 1)$; as before, all the non-diagonal elements are zero, except possibly the ones in the first row and the first column. Call $\sigma_{ZY'_1}, \ldots, \sigma_{ZY'_p}$. Then $\mathbf{E}[Z|Y'] = \sum_{j=1}^{p'} \sigma_{ZY'_j} \lambda_j^{-1} Y'_j$ and $\mathbf{Var}[Z|Y'] = \sigma_Z^2 - \sum_{j=1}^{p'} \lambda_j^{-1} \sigma_{ZY'_j}^2$, where Y'_j is the j-th component of the random vector Y'.

As before, we can state the following lemma:

Lemma 2 *Assume $Z \sim N(\mu, \sigma^2)$ and $X \sim N(\mathbf{0}, \Sigma)$. Iterate t times the covering stage of Algorithm 4. Then the whole algorithm can be reduced to a two-stage setting: First, to find a centralized box with vertices located at the coordinates corresponding to the quantiles $\frac{1}{2}(\beta_T)^{1/p'}$ and $1 - \frac{1}{2}(\beta_T)^{1/p'}$ of each of the p' variables. Second, add the $p - p'$ dimensions left untouched to the final box.*

Remark 5 Even though we have developed the algorithm with $p' \leq p$, it is not wise to try to reduce the dimensions of the input. To be sure, the rotation of the input in the direction of the principal components is a useful thing to do in learning settings, as Díaz-Pachón et al. [4] have showed. However, Cox [1], Hadi and Ling [6], and Joliffe [8], have warned against the reduction of dimensionality.

3.3 *fastPRIM and Data*

The usefulness of the previous result can be more easily seen when, for relatively large n, we consider the iid vectors $X_1, \ldots, X_n$ with finite second moment, since in this way we can approximate to a normal distribution by the Multivariate Central Limit Theorem:

Call $X = [X_1 \cdots X_n]$ and let us assume that $n \gg 0$. By the multivariate central limit theorem, if the vectors of observations are iid, such that their distribution has mean μ_X and variance Σ_X, we can approximate $X^* := n^{1/2}\left(\overline{X} - \mu_X\right)$ to a p-variate normal distribution with parameters $\mathbf{0}$ and Σ_X. That is, $\overline{X}$ can be approximated to a distribution $N(\mu, (1/n)\Sigma_X)$. Now, $Y^* = X^* G$ is the PC transformation of X^*, where G is the matrix of eigenvectors of S, the sample covariance matrix of X^*; i.e., $S = GLG^T$, and L is the diagonal matrix of eigenvalues of S, with $l_{j'} \geq l_j$ for all $j' < j$.

As before, call Y' the projection of Y to its firsts p' principal components. Apply Algorithm 4.

Note that the use of the CLT is indeed well justified: since the asymptotic mean of X^* is $\mathbf{0}$, its asymptotic mode is also at $\mathbf{0}$ (or around $\mathbf{0}$).

3.4 *Graphical Illustrations*

In the following simulations, we first test PRIM and fastPRIM and illustrate graphically how fastPRIM compares to PRIM either in the input space $\mathfrak{X}(p)$ or in the PC space $\mathfrak{X}'(p)$. We generated a synthetic dataset derived from a simulation setup similar to the one used in Sect. 1, although with a single target distribution and a continuous normal response, without noise. Thus, the data X was simulated as $X \sim N_p(0, \Sigma)$ with response $Z \sim N(\mu, \sigma^2)$. To control the amount of variance for each input variable and their correlations, the sample covariance matrix Σ was constructed from a specified sample correlation matrix R and sample variance matrix V such that $\Sigma := V^{1/2} R V^{1/2}$, after ensuring that the resulting matrix Σ is symmetric positive definite.

Simulations were carried out with a continuous normal response with parameters $\mu = 1$ and $\sigma = 0.2$, a fixed sample size $n = 10^3$, and no added noise (i.e., mixing weight $w = 1$). Here, we limited ourselves to a low dimensional space ($p = p' = 2$) for graphical visualization purposes. Simulations were for a fixed peeling quantile α, a fixed minimal box support β, a fixed maximal coverage parameter t, and no pasting for PRIM. Empirical results presented in Fig. 2 show the marked computational efficiency of fastPRIM compared to PRIM. CPU times are plotted against PRIM and fastPRIM coverage parameters $k \in \{1, \ldots, t\}$ and $t \in \{1, \ldots, 20\}$, respectively, in the original input space $\mathfrak{X}(2)$ and PC space $\mathfrak{X}'(2)$.

Further, empirical results presented in Fig. 3 show PRIM and fastPRIM box coverage sequences as a function of PRIM and fastPRIM coverage parameters

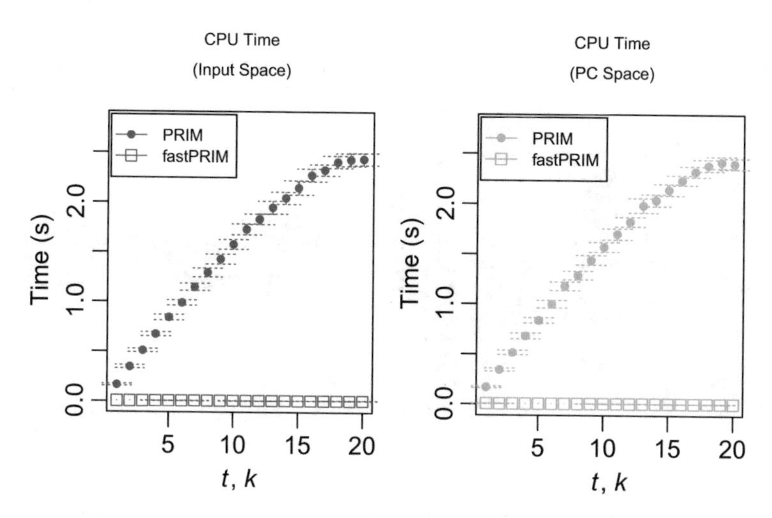

Fig. 2 Total CPU time as a function of coverage. For all plots, comparison of speed metrics are reported against coverage parameter $k \in \{1, \ldots, t\}$ for PRIM and coverage parameter $t \in \{1, \ldots, 20\}$ for fastPRIM, in the original input space $\mathfrak{X}(2)$ (*left*), and the PC space $\mathfrak{X}'(2)$ (*right*) for each algorithm. Total CPU time in seconds (s). Mean estimates and standard errors of the means are reported after generating 128 Monte-Carlo replicates

$k \in \{1, \ldots, t\}$ and $t \in \{1, \ldots, 20\}$, respectively. Notice the centering and nesting of the series of fastPRIM boxes in contrast to the sequence of boxes induced by PRIM (Fig. 3).

4 Comparison of the Algorithms in the Input and PC Spaces

The greatest theoretical advantage of fastPRIM is that, because of the centrality of the boxes, it gives us a framework to compare the output mean in the original input space and in the PC space, something that cannot be attained with the original PRIM algorithm in which the behavior of the final region is unknown (see Fig. 2). Polonik and Wang [10] explain how PRIM tries to approximate regression level curves, an objective that the algorithm does not accomplish in general. With the idea of level curves in mind, it is clear that the bump of a multivariate normal distribution can be seen as the data inside the ellipsoids of concentration. This concept is the key to prove the optimality of the box found on the PC space. By optimality here we mean the box with minimal Lebesgue measure among all possible central boxes found by fastPRIM with probability measure β.

Lemma 3 *Let E be a p-dimensional ellipsoid. The rectangular box that is circumscribing E (i.e., centered at the center of E, with sides parallel to the axes of E, such that each of its edges is of length equal to the axis length of E in the*

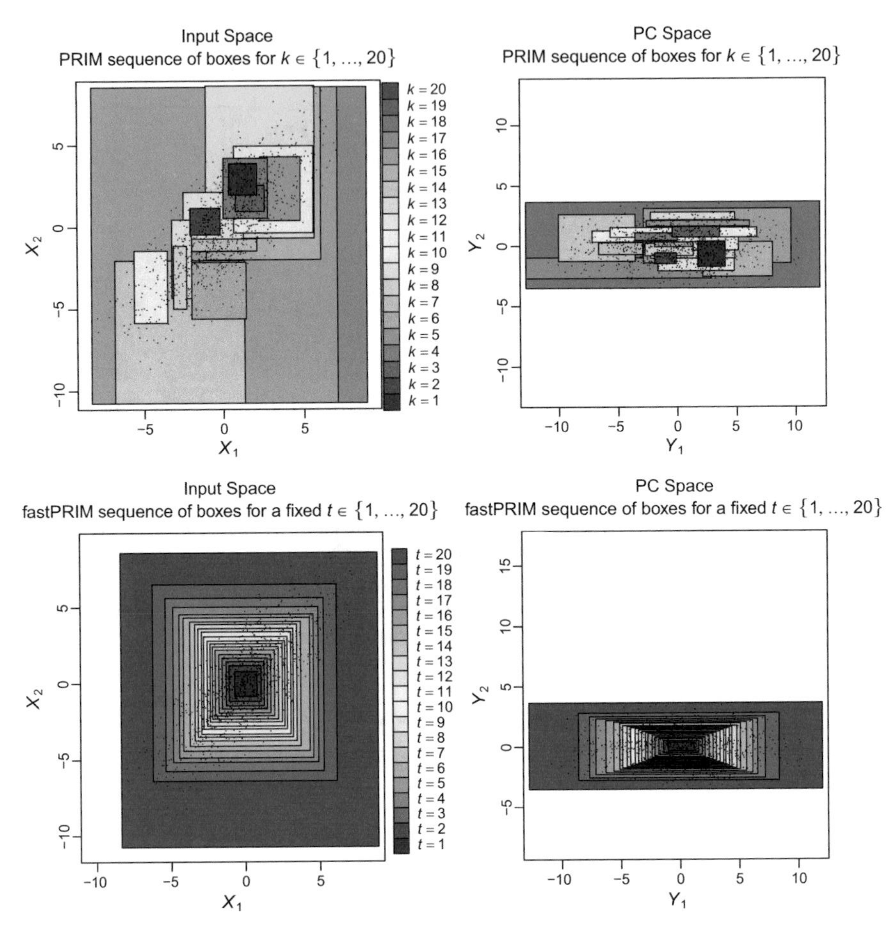

Fig. 3 PRIM and fastPRIM box coverage sequences. *Top row*: PRIM complete sequence of coverage boxes, each corresponding to a coverage step $k \in \{1, \ldots, t\}$ with a fixed peeling quantile $\alpha = 0.05$, and a fixed maximal coverage parameter $t = 20$, corresponding to a fixed minimal box support $\beta = 0.05$. *Bottom row*: fastPRIM complete sequence of coverage boxes, each corresponding to a fixed coverage parameter $t \in \{1, \ldots, 20\}$, with a fixed $\beta = 0.05$. Results are given in the input space $\mathfrak{X}(2)$ (*left*) and in the PC space $\mathfrak{X}'(2)$ (*right*). The *red to blue palette* corresponds to a range of box output means from the largest to the smallest, respectively

corresponding dimension) is the box with the minimal volume of all the rectangular boxes containing E.

The proof of Lemma 3 is well known and is omitted here.

Proposition 1 *Let $X \sim N(\mathbf{0}, \Sigma)$. Assume that the true bump E of X has probability measure $\beta' > 0$. Then, it is possible to find a rectangular box R by fastPRIM that circumscribes E under the PC rotation with minimal Lebesgue measure over all rectangular boxes containing E and the set of all possible rotations.*

Proof The true bump satisfies that $\mathbf{P}[x \in E] = \beta'$. This bump, by definition of normality, lives inside an ellipsoid of concentration E, of volume $\text{Vol}(E) = \pi_p \prod_{1 \leq j \leq p} r_j$, where r_j is the length of the semi axis of the dimension j and π_p is a constant that only depends on the dimension p. By Lemma 3 above, the box R with sides parallel to the axes of E, and circumscribing E, has minimal volume over all the boxes containing E and its volume is $2^p \prod_{1 \leq j \leq p} r_j$, and $2^p > \pi_p$. Let us assume that $\mathbf{P}[x \in R] = \beta$ (thus $\beta' < \beta$).

Note now that R is parallel to the axes in the space of principal components $\mathfrak{X}'(p)$ and it is centered at its origin. Therefore, provided an appropriate small α (it is possible that we need to adjust proportionally α on each direction of the principal components to obtain the box that circumscribes E), the minimal rectangular box R containing the bump E can be approximated through fastPRIM and is in the direction of the principal components. As such, then the box R has smaller Lebesgue measure than any other approximation in every other rotation. □

Remark 6 The box of size β circumscribing the ellipsoid of concentration E is identical to B^*_β in Eq. (2).

Proposition 1 allows us to compare box estimates in the PC space of PRIM (Fig. 2, top-right) versus fastPRIM (Fig. 2, down-right). Remember from Eq. (5) that $R_\rho(p, 1)$ is the box obtained with PRIM after a single stage of coverage. We now restrict ourselves to the case of $R_\rho(p, 1)$ in the direction of the principal components (i.e., its sides are parallel to the axes of $\mathfrak{X}'(p)$). We establish the following result:

Theorem 1 *Assume $X \sim N(0, \Sigma)$ and $Z \sim N(0, \sigma^2)$. Call R the final fastPRIM box resulting from Algorithm 4 and assume $p' = p$. As in (5), call also $\hat{R}_\rho(p, 1)$ the final box from Algorithm 1 after one stage of coverage. Assume that R and $R_\rho(p, 1)$ contain the true bump. Then*

$$\frac{M(R)}{Vol(R)} > \frac{M(R_\rho(p, 1))}{Vol(R_\rho(p, 1))}, \tag{9}$$

that is, the volume-adjusted box output mean of the mode of Z given R is bigger than the volume-adjusted box output mean of the mode of Z given $R_\rho(p)$.

Proof Note that by definition, the two boxes have sides parallel to the axes of $\mathfrak{X}'(p)$. The proof is direct because of the assumptions. By Proposition 1, R is the minimal box of measure β that contains the true bump. Therefore, any other box R' with parallel sides to R that contains the bump also contains R. Since R is centered around the mean of Z, every point z in the support of Z such that $z \in R' \setminus R$ have less density than $\arg\min_z f_Z(z)$. Therefore $M(R) > M(R')$. From Proposition 1 we also get that $Vol(R) < Vol(R')$.

Since $R_\rho(p, 1)$ is but a particular case of a box R', the result follows. □

Not only R has better volume-adjusted output mean than $R_\rho(p, 1)$. We conclude showing the optimality of the latter over the former in terms of bias and variance.

Theorem 2 *Assume $Z \sim N(\mu, \sigma^2)$ and $X \sim N(\mathbf{0}, \Sigma)$. Define E as the true bump, and let us assume that both R and $R_\rho(p)$ cover E. Then $\mathbf{Var}(Z|Y \in R) < \mathbf{Var}(Z|Y \in R_\rho(p))$, and R is unbiased while $R_\rho(p)$ is not.*

Proof Note that R and $R_\rho(p, 1)$ are estimators of B^*_β, as defined in Eq. (2). Algorithm 4 is producing unbiased boxes since by construction it is centered around the mean. In fact, R would be unbiased even if not taken in the direction of the PC. On the other hand, $\hat{R}_\rho(p)$ is almost surely biased, even in the direction of the principal components, since it is producing boxes that are not centered around the mean.

Now, the inequality $\mathbf{Var}(Z|Y \in R) < \mathbf{Var}(Z|Y \in R_\rho(p))$ stems from the fact that R is the box with minimal volume containing E. Since R is in the direction of the principal components, every other box that contains E in the same direction also contains R, in particular $R \subseteq R_\rho(p)$. □

5 Simulations

Next, we illustrate how the optimality of the box encapsulating the true bump is improved in the PC space $\mathfrak{X}'(p)$ as compared to the input space $\mathfrak{X}(p)$. Empirical results presented in Fig. 4 are for the same simulation design and the same fastPRIM and PRIM parameters as described in Sect. 3.4, except that we now allow for higher dimensionality since no graphical visualization is desired here ($p = 100$).

Some of the theoretical results between the original input space and the PC space are borne out based on the empirical conclusions plotted in Fig. 4. In sum, for situations with no added noise, one observes for both algorithms that: (1) the effect of PCA rotation dramatically decreases the box geometric volume; (2) the box output (response) means are almost identical in the PC space and in the original input space; and (3) the volume-adjusted box output (response) means are markedly larger in the PC space than in the original input space—indicating a much more concentrated determination of the true bump structure (Fig. 4).

Some additional comments:

1. As each algorithm covers the space (up to step $k = t$), the box support and the box geometric volume are expected to increase monotonically (up to sampling variability) for both algorithms.
2. The boxes are equivalent for the mean of Z and the mode of Z because Z is normal, we expect the fastPRIM box being centered around the mean and therefore the conditional mean of Z should be 1 (because in this simulation the mean of Z is 1). While, the box for Z given PRIM must have a different conditional expectation. This justifies the fact of looking at the mode of Z inside the boxes, and not directly the mode of Z.
3. Since the the box output (response) mean is almost perfectly constant at 1 for fastPRIM and close to 1 for PRIM, it is expected that the box volume-adjusted

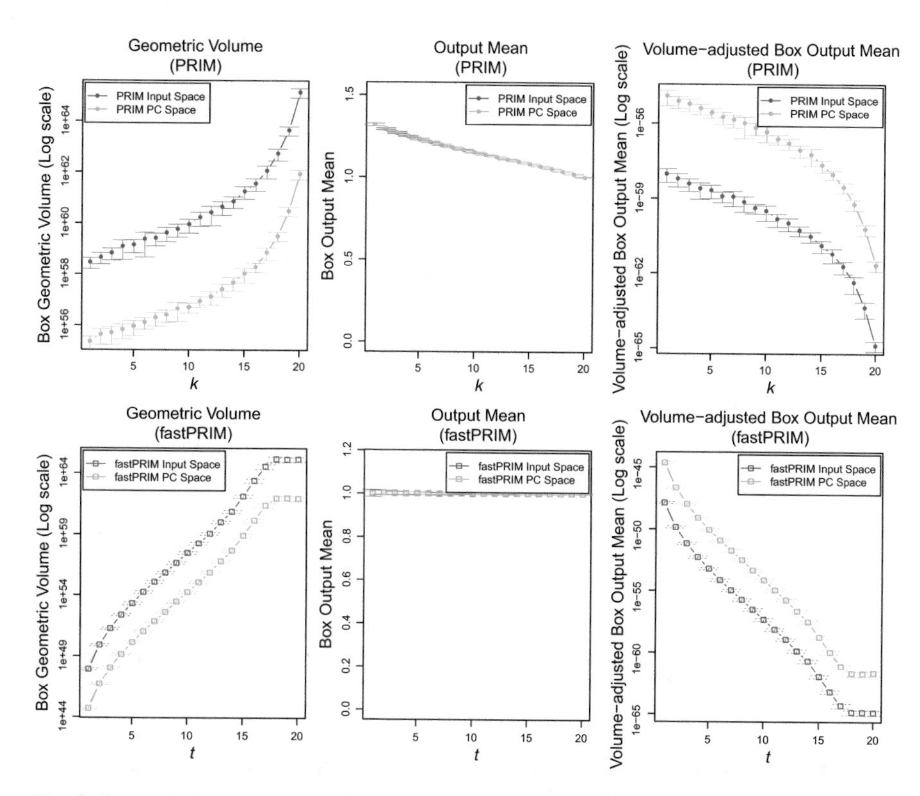

Fig. 4 Box statistics and performance metrics as a function of coverage. For all plots, results are plotted against PRIM coverage parameter $k \in \{1, \ldots, t\}$ and fastPRIM coverage parameter $t \in \{1, \ldots, 20\}$ in the original input space $\mathfrak{X}(100)$ (*red*) vs. the PC space $\mathfrak{X}'(100)$ (*green*), that is for $p = p' = 100$, for each algorithm: PRIM (*top row*) vs. fastPRIM (*bottom row*). *First column*: box geometric volume (Log scale); *second column*: box output (response) mean; *third column*: volume-adjusted box output (response) mean (Log scale). See simulation design for details and metrics definitions. Mean estimates and standard errors of the means are reported after generating 128 Monte-Carlo replicates

output mean decreases monotonically at the rate of the box geometric volume for both algorithms.

4. Also, as coverage k, t increases, the two boxes R and $R_\rho(p)$ of each algorithm converge to each other (covering most of the space), so it is expected that the output (response) means inside the final boxes converge to each other as well (i.e., towards the whole space mean response 1).

To illustrate the effect of increasing dimensionality, we plot in Fig. 5 the profiles of gains in volume-adjusted box output (response) mean as a function of increasing dimensionality $p \in \{2, 3, \ldots, 8, 9, 10, 20, 30, \ldots, 180, 190, 200\}$. Here, the gain is measured in terms of a ratio of the quantity of interest in the PC space $\mathfrak{X}'(p')$ over that in the original input space $\mathfrak{X}(p)$. Empirical results presented are for the same simulation design and the same fastPRIM and PRIM parameters as described

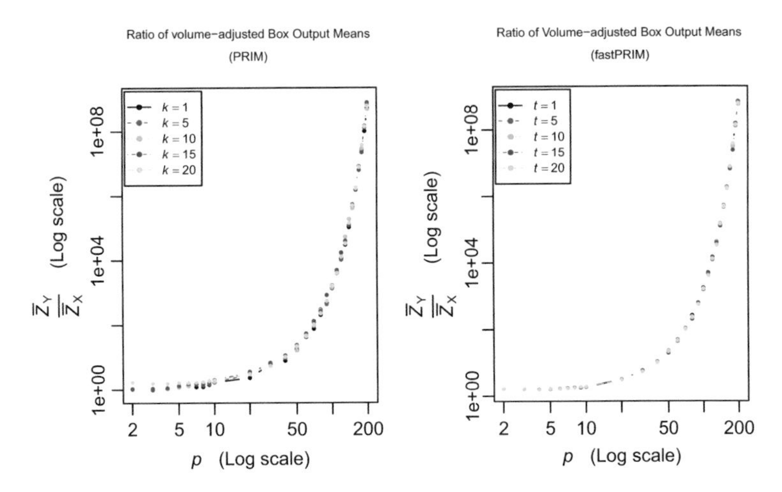

Fig. 5 Gains profiles in volume-adjusted box output (response) mean as a function of dimensionality p. For all plots, comparison of box statistics and performance metrics profiles are reported as a ratio of the values obtained in the PC space $\mathcal{X}'(p')$ (denoted Y) over the original input space $\mathcal{X}(p)$ (denoted X). We show empirical results for varying dimensionality $p \in \{2, 3, \ldots, 8, 9, 10, 20, 30, \ldots, 180, 190, 200\}$, a range of PRIM and fastPRIM coverage parameters ($k, t \in \{1, 5, 10, 15, 20\}$), and for both algorithms: PRIM (*left*) vs. fastPRIM (*right*). Both coordinate axes are on the log scale

in Sect. 3.4. Notice the extremely fast increase in volume-adjusted box output (response) mean ratio as a function of dimensionality p, that is, the marked larger value of volume-adjusted box output (response) mean in the PC space as compared to the one in the input space for both algorithms. Notice also the weak dependency with respect to the coverage parameters (k, t).

Further, using the same simulation design and the same fastPRIM and PRIM parameters as described in Sect. 3.4, we compared the efficiency of box estimates generated by both algorithms in the PC space $\mathcal{X}'(p')$ as a function of dimension p' and coverage parameters k, t for PRIM or fastPRIM, respectively. Notice, the reduced box geometric volume (Fig. 6) and increased box volume-adjusted output (response) mean (Fig. 7) of fastPRIM as compared to PRIM.

Finally, in Figs. 8 and 9 below we compare variances of fastPRIM and PRIM volume-adjusted box output (response) means in the PC space $\mathcal{X}'(p')$ as a function of dimension p' and coverage parameters k, t for PRIM or fastPRIM, respectively. Empirical results are presented for the same simulation design and the same fastPRIM and PRIM parameters as described in Sect. 3.4. Results show that the variance of fastPRIM box geometric volume (Fig. 8) is reduced than its PRIM counterparts for coverage t not too large ($\leq 10 - 15$), which is matched to a reduced variance of fastPRIM *volume-adjusted* box output (response) mean for coverage t not too small ($\leq 10 - 15$).

Of note, the results in Figs. 6 and 7 below, and similarly in Figs. 8 and 9, are for the sample size $n = 1000$ of this simulation design. In particular, efficiency

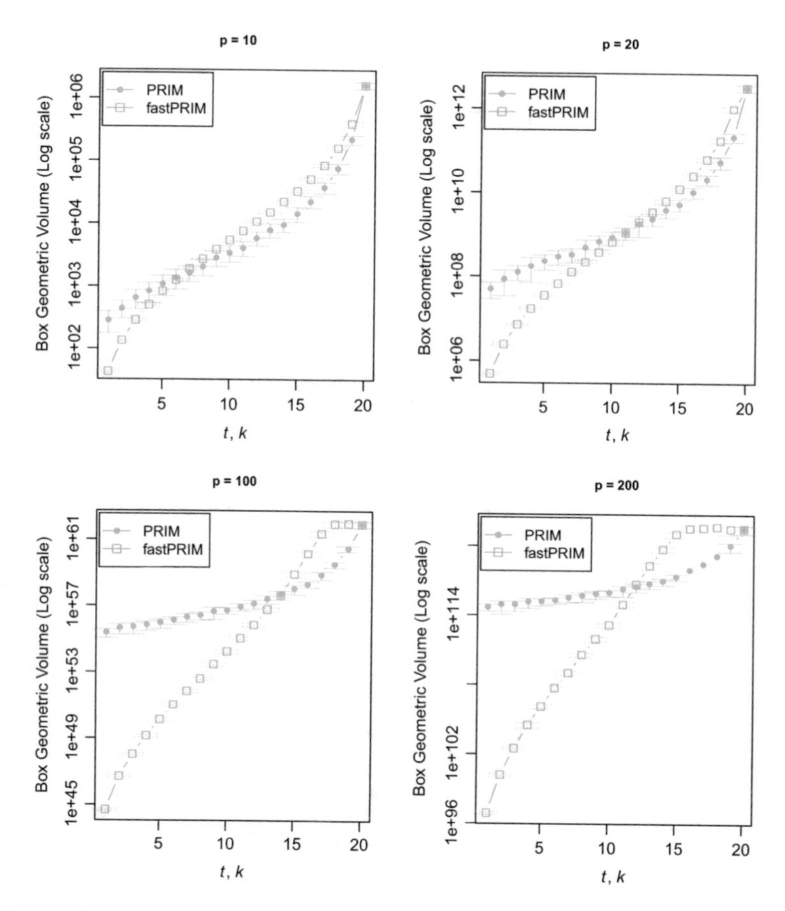

Fig. 6 Comparative profiles of box geometric volumes in the PC space $\mathfrak{X}'(p')$ as a function of dimension p' and coverage parameters $k \in \{1, \ldots, t\}$ or $t \in \{1, \ldots, 20\}$ for PRIM or fastPRIM, respectively. We show results for a range of dimension $p' \in \{10, 20, 100, 200\}$ and a range of PRIM and fastPRIM coverage parameters $k \in \{1, \ldots, t\}$ or $t \in \{1, \ldots, 20\}$. The 'y' axes are on the Log scale

results of fastPRIM versus PRIM box estimates show some dependency with respect to coverage parameters k, t for large coverages and increasing dimensionality. As discussed above, this reflects a finite sample-effect favoring PRIM box estimates in these coverages and dimensionality.

Notice finally in Figs. 6 and 7 how the curves approach each other for the largest coverage step $k = t = 20$, and similarly in Figs. 8 and 9 how the curves approach the identity line. This is in line with the aforementioned convergence point of the two boxes R and $R_\rho(p)$ as coverage increases.

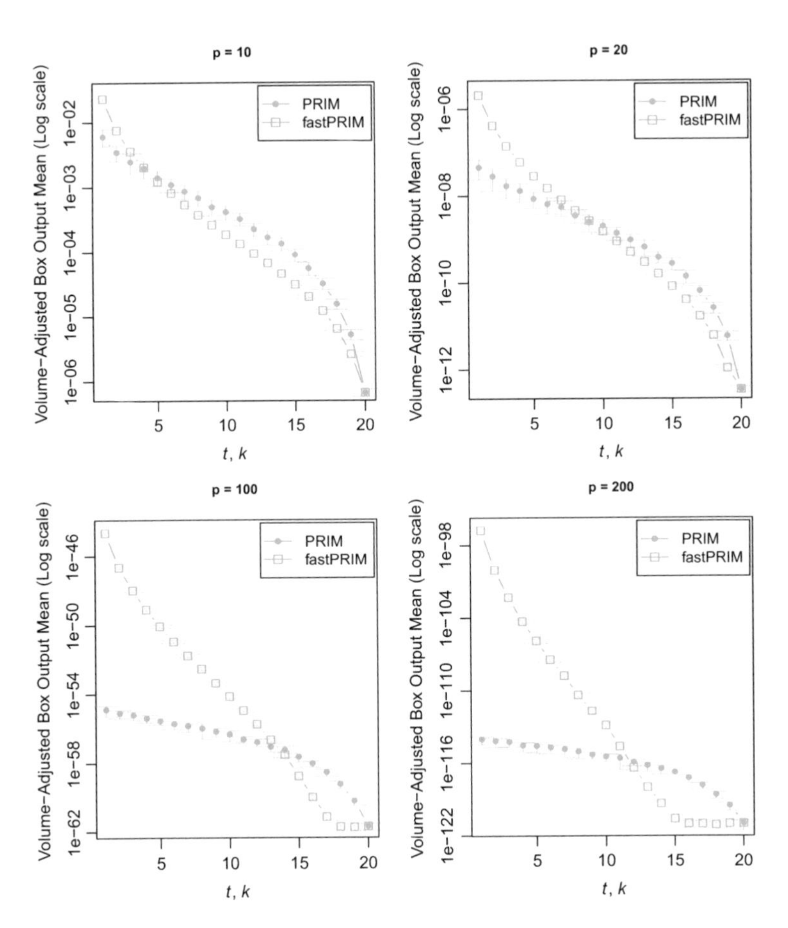

Fig. 7 Comparative profiles of box volume-adjusted output (response) means in the PC space $\mathfrak{X}'(p')$ as a function of dimension p' and coverage parameters $k \in \{1, \ldots, t\}$ or $t \in \{1, \ldots, 20\}$ for PRIM or fastPRIM for PRIM and fastPRIM, respectively. We show results for a range of dimension $p' \in \{10, 20, 100, 200\}$ and a range of PRIM and fastPRIM coverage parameters $k \in \{1, \ldots, t\}$ or $t \in \{1, \ldots, 20\}$. The 'y' axes are on the Log scale

6 Discussion

Our analysis here corroborates what Díaz-Pachón et al. [4] have showed on how the rotation of the input space to one of the principal components is a reasonable thing to do when modeling a response-predictor relationship. In fact, Dazard and Rao [2] use a *sparse* PC rotation for improving bump hunting in the context of high dimensional genomic predictors. And Dazard et al. [3] also show how this technique can be applied to find additional heterogeneity in terms of survival outcomes for colon cancer patients. The geometrical analysis we present here shows that as long as the principal components are not being selected prior to modeling the response,

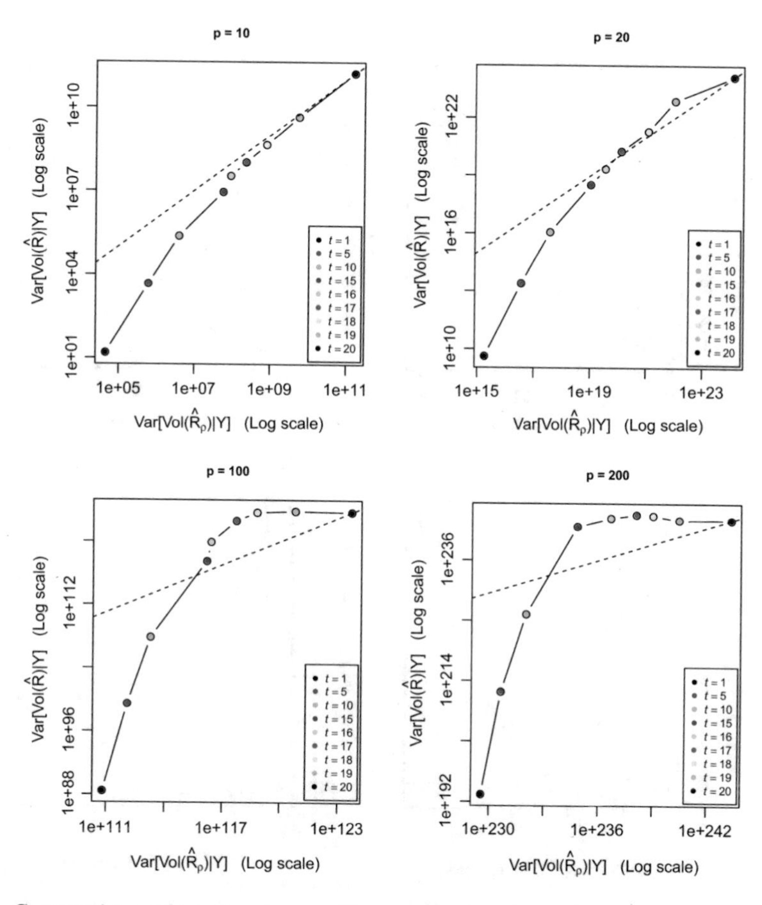

Fig. 8 Comparative profiles of variances of box geometric volumes in the PC space $\mathfrak{X}'(p')$ as a function of dimensionality p' and coverage parameters $k \in \{1, \ldots, t\}$ or $t \in \{1, \ldots, 20\}$ for PRIM or fastPRIM, respectively. In all subplots, we show the variances of box geometric volumes of both algorithms against each other for a range of PRIM and fastPRIM coverage parameters $(k, t \in \{1, 5, 10, 15, 16, 17, 18, 1920\})$ in four dimensions $p' \in \{10, 20, 100, 200\}$. The identity (*doted*) *line* is plotted. All axes are on the Log scale

then these improved variables can produce more accurate mode characterizations. In order to elucidate this effect, we introduced the fastPRIM algorithm, starting with a supervised learner and ending up with an unsupervised one. This analysis opens the question on whether it is possible to go from supervised to unsupervised settings in more general bump hunting situations, not only modes; and more generally, whether is possible to go from unsupervised to supervised in other learning contexts beyond bump hunting.

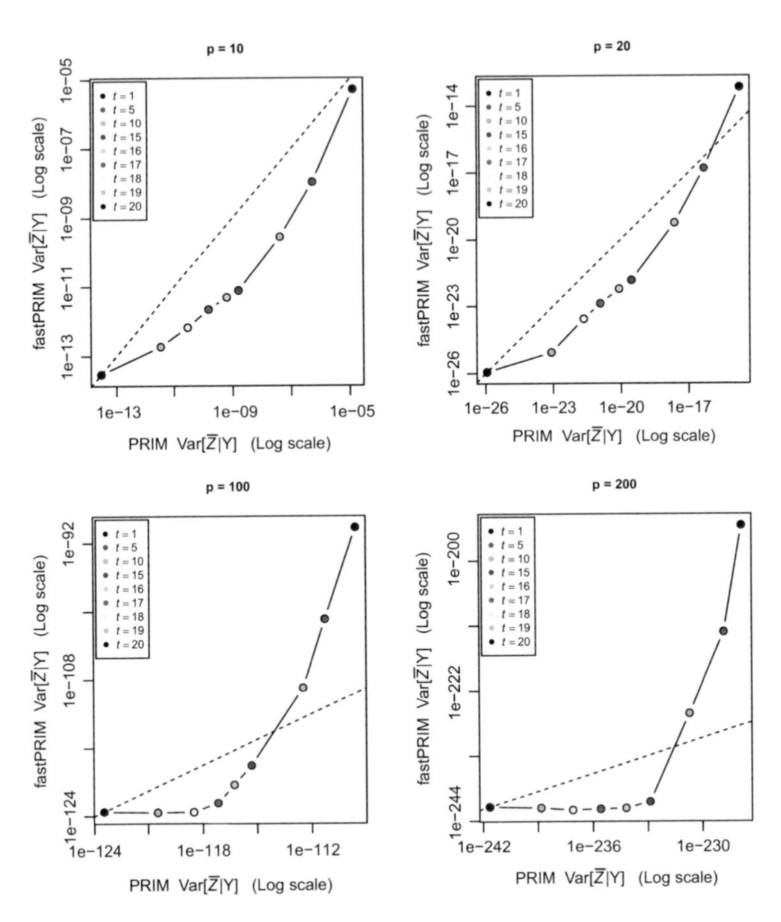

Fig. 9 Comparative profiles of variances of box volume-adjusted output (response) means in the PC space $\mathfrak{X}'(p')$ as a function of dimensionality p' and coverage parameters $k \in \{1, \ldots, t\}$ or $t \in \{1, \ldots, 20\}$ for PRIM or fastPRIM, respectively. In all subplots, we show the variances of the volume-adjusted box output (response) means of both algorithms against each other for a range of PRIM and fastPRIM coverage parameters ($k, t \in \{1, 5, 10, 15, 16, 17, 18, 1920\}$) in four dimensions $p' \in \{10, 20, 100, 200\}$. The identity *(doted) line* is plotted. All axes are on the Log scale

Acknowledgements All authors supported in part by NIH grant NCI R01-CA160593A1. We would like to thank Rob Tibshirani, Steve Marron, and Hemant Ishwaran for helpful discussions of the work. This work made use of the High Performance Computing Resource in the Core Facility for Advanced Research Computing at Case Western Reserve University.

References

1. Cox, D.: Notes on some aspects of regression analysis. J. R. Stat. Soc. Ser. A. **131**, 265/279 (1968)
2. Dazard, J.-E., Rao, J.S.: Local sparse bump hunting. J. Comput. Graph. Stat. **19**(4), 900–929 (2010)
3. Dazard, J.-E., Rao, J., Markowitz, S.: Local sparse bump hunting reveals molecular heterogeneity of colon tumors. Stat. Med. **31**(11–12), 1203–1220 (2012)
4. Díaz-Pachón, D., Rao, J., Dazard, J.-E.: On the explanatory power of principal components (2014). arXiv:1404.4917v1
5. Friedman, J., Fisher, N.: Bump hunting in high-dimensional data. Stat. Comput. **9**, 123–143 (1999)
6. Hadi, S., Ling, R.: Some cautionary notes on the use of principal components regression. Am. Stat. **52**(1), 15–19 (1998)
7. Hirose, H., Koga, G.: A comparative study in the bump hunting between the tree-ga and the prim. Stud. Comp. Int. Dev. **443**, 13–25 (2012)
8. Joliffe, I.: A note on the use of principal components in regression. J. R. Stat. Soc. Ser. C. Appl. Stat. **31**(3), 300–303 (1982)
9. Mardia, K.: Multivariate Analysis. Academic Press, New York (1976)
10. Polonik, W., Wang, Z.: Prim analysis. J. Multivar. Anal., **101**(3), 525–540 (2010)

Identifying Gene–Environment Interactions Associated with Prognosis Using Penalized Quantile Regression

Guohua Wang, Yinjun Zhao, Qingzhao Zhang, Yangguang Zang, Sanguo Zang, and Shuangge Ma

Abstract In the omics era, it has been well recognized that for complex traits and outcomes, the interactions between genetic and environmental factors (i.e., the G$\times$E interactions) have important implications beyond the main effects. Most of the existing interaction analyses have been focused on continuous and categorical traits. Prognosis is of essential importance for complex diseases. However with significantly more complexity, prognosis outcomes have been less studied. In the existing interaction analysis on prognosis outcomes, the most common practice is to fit marginal (semi)parametric models (for example, Cox) using likelihood-based estimation and then identify important interactions based on significance level. Such an approach has limitations. First data contamination is not uncommon. With likelihood-based estimation, even a single contaminated observation can result in severely biased estimation and misleading conclusions. Second, when sample size is not large, the significance-based approach may not be reliable. To overcome these limitations, in this study, we adopt the quantile-based estimation which is robust to data contamination. Two techniques are adopted to accommodate right censoring. For identifying important interactions, we adopt penalization as an alternative to significance level. An efficient computational algorithm is developed. Simulation shows that the proposed method can significantly outperform the alternative. We analyze a lung cancer prognosis study with gene expression measurements.

G. Wang • Y. Zang • S. Zhang
School of Mathematical Sciences, University of Chinese Academy of Sciences, Beijing, China

Key Laboratory of Big Data Mining and Knowledge Management, Chinese Academy of Sciences, Beijing, China
e-mail: wangguohua11@mails.ucas.ac.cn; zangyangguang@mails.ucas.ac.cn; sgzhang@ucas.ac.cn

Y. Zhao • Q. Zhang • S. Ma (✉)
Department of Biostatistics, Yale University, New Haven, CT, USA

VA Cooperative Studies Program Coordinating Center, West Haven, CT, USA
e-mail: yinjun.zhao@yale.edu; zhangqingzhao@amss.ac.cn; shuangge.ma@yale.edu

© Springer International Publishing AG 2017

S.E. Ahmed (ed.), *Big and Complex Data Analysis*, Contributions to Statistics,
DOI 10.1007/978-3-319-41573-4_17

1 Introduction

In the omics era, significant effort has been devoted to searching for genetic markers for disease traits and outcomes. It has been well recognized that, beyond the main effects of genetic (G) and environmental (E) factors, their G×E interactions also play an important role. Extensive data collection and analyses have been conducted. There are multiple families of existing approaches. For comprehensive reviews, we refer to [3, 4, 7, 16, 18] and others. In this study, we adopt the statistical modeling approach, where the interactions are represented with product terms in statistical models. Under this approach, there are two possibilities. The first is to conduct *marginal analysis* and analyze one or a small number of G factors at a time [7, 18]. The second is to conduct *joint analysis* and describe the joint effects of a large number of G factors in a single model [13]. Joint analysis, although may better describe the underlying biology, often suffers high computational cost and lack of stability. Thus, as of today, marginal analysis is still dominatingly popular and will be considered in this study.

Most of the existing G×E studies have been focused on continuous and categorical traits. For complex human diseases such as cancer and diabetes, prognosis is of essential importance. Prognosis outcomes are often subject to censoring, making the analysis significantly more complicated.

Denote T as the survival time of interest, $Z = (Z_1, \ldots, Z_p)^\top \in R^{p\times 1}$ as the p genes, and $X = (X_1, \ldots, X_q)^\top \in R^{q\times 1}$ as the q clinical/environmental risk factors. In the literature, the most common practice proceeds as follows: (a) For gene k, consider the regression model $T \sim \phi(\Sigma_{l=1}^{q}\alpha_{kl}X_l + \gamma_k Z_k + \Sigma_{l=1}^{q}\beta_{kl}X_l Z_k)$, where ϕ is the known function, α_{kl}'s, γ_k, and β_{kl}'s are the unknown regression coefficients. Likelihood-based estimation is applied. The p-value of the estimate of β_{kl}, denoted by p_{kl}, can be computed. (b) With the $p \times q$ p-values $\{p_{kl}\}$, apply a multiple-comparison-adjustment approach such as the FDR (false discovery rate), and identify important interactions. For more detailed discussions and applications, see [7, 18].

Despite considerable successes, the approach described above has limitations. The first is that data contamination is not uncommon, and under likelihood-based estimation, even a single contaminated observation can lead to severely biased estimation and false marker identification. In practice, contamination may happen for multiple reasons. Take cancer studies as an example. Cancer is highly heterogeneous, and different subtypes can have different prognosis patterns. Such heterogeneity introduces contamination. For some patients, the cause of death may be mis-classified, leading to contamination in cancer-specific survival. In addition, the survival times extracted from death records are not always reliable. The second limitation is that when sample size is not large, the significance level based marker identification may not be reliable, as demonstrated in recent studies [17].

To accommodate possible data contamination, in this study, we adopt quantile regression (QR) based estimation. QR is pioneered by Koenker [11] and has been a popular tool in regression analysis. Under low-dimensional settings, the robustness properties of QR have been well studied [10]. Under high-dimensional settings, QR has also been adopted. We refer to a recent review [20] for more discussions. Two techniques, namely the weighted quantile regression and inverse probability weighted quantile regression, have been adopted to accommodate right censoring. Our literature review suggests that the application of QR to prognosis data and interaction analysis is still very limited.

This study may differ from the existing literature in multiple aspects. First it differs from most of the existing interaction analysis studies by adopting robust estimation to better accommodate data heterogeneity. Second it adopts penalization for identifying important interactions, which provides an alternative to the significance-based approach and may lead to better numerical results. Third, it extends the existing QR studies to high-dimensional prognosis data and interaction analysis. The proposed approach can be effectively realized using existing software, and this computational simplicity can be especially valuable for high-dimensional data and interaction analysis. The rest of the article is organized as follows. The proposed method is described in Sect. 2. Numerical study, including simulation in Sect. 3 and data analysis in Sect. 4, demonstrates the effectiveness of proposed method. The article concludes with discussions in Sect. 5.

2 Methods

2.1 Quantile Regression Based Estimation

The τth conditional quantile of T given X, Z for $0 < \tau < 1$ is defined as $Q_\tau(T) = \inf\{t : P(T \le t|X, Z) = \tau\}$. For gene $k(= 1, \ldots, p)$, consider the model:

$$Q_\tau(T) = a_k + \Sigma_{l=1}^q \alpha_{kl} X_l + \gamma_k Z_k + \Sigma_{l=1}^q \beta_{kl} X_l Z_k := \theta_k^\top U_k, \quad (1)$$

where a_k is the intercept term, $\alpha_k = (\alpha_{k1}, \ldots, \alpha_{kq})^\top$ represents the main effects of E factors, γ_k represents the main effect of gene k, $\beta_k = (\beta_{k1}, \ldots, \beta_{kq})^\top$ represents the G×E interactions, and

$$\theta_k = (a_k, \alpha_k^\top, \gamma_k, \beta_k^\top)^\top \in R^{(2q+2)\times 1}, U_k = (1, X^\top, Z_k, Z_k X^\top)^\top \in R^{(2q+2)\times 1}.$$

First ignore censoring. Assume n observations $\{T_i, X_{(i)}, Z_{(i)}\}_{i=1}^n$, where $X_{(i)} = (X_{(i)1}, \ldots, X_{(i)q})^\top$ and $Z_{(i)} = (Z_{(i)1}, \ldots, Z_{(i)p})^\top$. Write $U_{(i)k} = (1, X_{(i)}^\top, Z_{(i)k}, Z_{(i)k} X_{(i)}^\top)^\top$. The unknown regression coefficients can be estimated as

$$\hat{\theta}_k = \arg\min \sum_{i=1}^n \rho_\tau (T_i - \theta_k^\top U_{(i)k}),$$

where $\rho_\tau(u) = u\{\tau - I(u < 0)\}$ is the check loss function. Note that $\hat{\theta}_k$ is also a solution to the following estimating equation:

$$D_n(\theta_k) = n^{-1} \sum_{i=1}^{n} U_{(i)k}\{\tau - 1(T_i - \theta_k^\top U_{(i)k} \leq 0)\} = o_p(a_n) \tag{2}$$

where $a_n \to 0$ as $n \to \infty$.

Practically encountered prognosis data are usually right censored. For the ith observation, let C_i be the censoring time. Then we observe $Y_i = \min(T_i, C_i)$ and $\delta_i = 1(T_i \leq C_i)$. We make the assumption of random censoring. Below we consider two ways of accommodating right censoring in QR, which have been partly motivated by existing studies [1, 19].

2.1.1 Weighted Quantile Regression

First consider the simplified scenario where $F_0(t|U_{(i)k})$, the conditional cumulative distribution function of the survival time T_i given $U_{(i)k}$, is known. Then for gene $k(= 1, \ldots, p)$ under model (1), the QR based objective function is

$$L_n(\theta_k; F_0) = \sum_{i=1}^{n} \left\{w_i(F_0)\rho_\tau(Y_i - \theta_k^\top U_{(i)k}) + (1 - w_i(F_0))\rho_\tau(Y^{+\infty} - \theta_k^\top U_{(i)k})\right\}. \tag{3}$$

$Y^{+\infty}$ is a value sufficiently large and exceeds all $\theta_k^\top U_{(i)k}$, and

$$w_i(F_0) = \begin{cases} 1, & F_0(C_i|U_{(i)k}) > \tau \text{ or } T_i \leq C_i; \\ \frac{\tau - F_0(C_i|U_{(i)k})}{1 - F_0(C_i|U_{(i)k})}, & F_0(C_i|U_{(i)k}) < \tau \text{ and } T_i > C_i. \end{cases}$$

The intuition behind (3) is that the contribution of each observation to (2) only depends on the sign of the residual $T_i - \theta_k^\top U_{(i)k}$. If $C_i > \theta_k^\top U_{(i)k}$ or $T_i \leq C_i$, we immediately know that $T_i - \theta_k^\top U_{(i)k} \leq 0$ and assign weight $w_i(F_0) = 1$. For $T_i > C_i$ and $\theta_k^\top U_{(i)k} > C_i$, we have

$$E\left\{1(T_i < \theta_k^\top U_{(i)k})|T_i > C_i\right\} = \frac{P(C_i < T_i < \theta_k^\top U_{(i)k})}{P(T_i > C_i)} = \frac{\tau - F_0(C_i|U_{(i)k})}{1 - F_0(C_i|U_{(i)k})}.$$

Therefore, we assign weight $w_i(F_0) = \frac{\tau - F_0(C_i|U_{(i)k})}{1 - F_0(C_i|U_{(i)k})}$ to the "pseudo observation" at $(U_{(i)k}, C_i)$ and redistribute the complimentary weight $1 - w_i(F_0)$ at $(U_{(i)k}, Y^{+\infty})$ without altering the quantile fit. For related discussions, see Remark 1 in [19].

Now consider the more flexible scenario where $F_0(t|U_{(i)k})$ is unknown. The strategy is to mimic the above development with assistance of the nonparametric Kaplan-Meier estimate, which is

$$\hat{F}(t) = 1 - \prod_{i=1}^{n} \left\{ 1 - \frac{1}{\sum_{l=1}^{n} 1(Y_l \geq Y_i)} \right\}^{\eta_i(t)} \tag{4}$$

where $\eta_i(t) = I(Y_i \leq t, \delta_i = 1)$. With the KM estimate $\hat{F}(t)$, we are able to estimate the weight function $w_i(\hat{F})$. Then plugging $w_i(\hat{F})$ into (3), we propose the following objective function

$$L_n(\theta_k; \hat{F}) = \sum_{i=1}^{n} \left\{ w_i(\hat{F}) \rho_\tau (Y_i - \theta_k^\top U_{(i)k}) + (1 - w_i(\hat{F})) \rho_\tau (Y^{+\infty} - \theta_k^\top U_{(i)k}) \right\}. \tag{5}$$

Remark 1 A similar approach has been considered in [19] for censored linear quantile regression. Here we extend it to high-dimensional G×E interaction analysis. Different from [19], we use the classic KM estimate as opposed to the local KM estimate. The classic KM estimate is computationally very simple, whereas the local KM estimate may encounter difficulty when the number of E factors is not small. The classic KM estimate can be sufficient in this study as our goal is mainly on the identification of G × E interactions.

2.1.2 Inverse Probability Weighted Quantile Regression

For gene $k(= 1, \ldots, p)$, the objective function is

$$L_n(\theta_k; \hat{G}) = \sum_{i=1}^{n} \frac{\delta_i}{\hat{G}(T_i)} \rho_\tau (Y_i - \theta_k^\top U_{(i)k}), \tag{6}$$

where $\hat{G}(\cdot)$ is the Kaplan-Meier estimate of the cumulative distribution function of the censoring time [14] defined as

$$\hat{G}(t) = \prod_{i=1}^{n} \left\{ 1 - \frac{1}{\sum_{l=1}^{n} 1(Y_l \geq Y_i)} \right\}^{I(Y_i \leq t, \delta_i = 0)}.$$

The inverse probability weighted approach is a classic technique in survival analysis. It uses uncensored data only and assigns different weights depending on the event times. Advancing from the published studies, here we apply it to high-dimensional quantile regression and interaction analysis.

2.2 Penalized Identification of Interactions

With a slight abuse of notation, we use $L_n(\theta_k)$ to denote the objective function in (5) and (6). One way to identify important interactions is to couple the QR objective functions with the "classic" significance-based approach described in Sect. 1. However the concern is that in most of the existing studies, significance level is obtained based on asymptotic distributions. When the sample sizes are small to moderate, the significance level so generated may not be reliable. This gets especially problematic when a huge number of p-values are generated and simultaneously compared.

Motivated by recent studies [17], we consider identifying interactions using penalization. Specifically, for gene k, consider the penalized estimate

$$\hat{\theta}_k = \text{argmin}\left\{L_n(\theta_k) + \sum_{j=1}^{2q+2} \varphi(\theta_{kj}),\right\} \tag{7}$$

where φ is the penalty function. *Interactions with nonzero estimated coefficients are identified as associated with prognosis.*

In the literature, a large number of penalties have been developed and are potentially applicable. Here we adopt the minimax concave penalty (MCP) [22]. Under simpler settings, this penalty has been shown to have satisfactory statistical and numerical properties. Specifically, it enjoys the oracle consistency properties under mild conditions. Compared to other penalties which are also consistent, it can be preferred with its computational simplicity [15]. With MCP, $\varphi(u; \lambda, \gamma) = \lambda \int_0^{|u|}(1 - \frac{x}{\lambda\gamma})_+ dx$, where λ and γ control the degrees of regularization and concavity, respectively. In principle, we can have different tunings for different main/interaction effects. To reduce computational cost, we apply the same tuning to all effects.

With computational concerns, we apply the simple MCP penalty, which may not respect the "main effects, interactions" hierarchy. That is, it is possible that a main effect has a zero coefficient but its interactions have nonzero coefficients. As our main interest lies in identifying interactions, this may not pose a serious problem.

2.3 Computation

The computational aspect is challenging as $\rho_\tau(\cdot)$ is not differentiable and MCP is not convex. Here we resort to the majorize-minimization (MM) approach [6]. Below we provide details for the weighted QR method. The inverse probability weighted QR method can be solved in a similar manner.

Rearrange data such that the first n_0 observations are censored. For gene $k(= 1, \ldots, p)$, the proposed computational algorithm proceeds as follows:

Step 1. Take $Y^{+\infty} = 100 \max\{Y_1, \ldots, Y_n\}$. Appending n_0 pseudo paired observations $(U_{(1)k}, Y^{+\infty}), \ldots, (U_{(n_0)k}, Y^{+\infty})$ to the original data $(U_{(i)k}, Y_i)_{i=1}^n$, we obtain an augmented data set $(U_{(i)k}, Y_i), i = 1, \ldots, n + n_0$. Initialize $\theta_k^{(1)}$. In our numerical study, the unpenalized estimate is used as the initial value.

Step 2. In the sth iteration, establish an approximation function $S_n(\theta|\theta_k^{(s)})$ of the penalized objective function. Minimize or simply find a value that leads to a smaller value of $S_n(\theta|\theta_k^{(s)})$. Denote this estimate as $\theta_k^{(s+1)}$ and move to iteration $s + 1$.

Step 3. Repeat Step 2 until convergence. In our numerical study, we use the L_2-norm of the difference between two consecutive estimates less than 10^{-3} as the convergence criterion. In data analysis, it is observed that the absolute values of some estimated coefficients keep shrinking towards zero. If they fall below a certain threshold (say, 10^{-4}), the estimates are then set as zero.

The key is Step 2. For the weighted QR method, this step can be realized as follows. Let $r_{(i)k} = Y_i - \theta_k^\top U_{(i)k}$, $i = 1, \ldots, n$ and $r_{(n+i)k} = Y^{+\infty} - \theta_k^\top U_{(i)k}$, $i = 1, \ldots, n_0$ be the residual terms, and $v_i(\hat{F}) = w_i(\hat{F})$, $i = 1, \ldots, n$ and $v_{i+n}(\hat{F}) = 1 - w_i(\hat{F})$, $i = 1, \ldots, n_0$ be the weights. Then (5) can be rewritten as

$$L_n(\theta_k; \hat{F}) = \sum_{i=1}^{n+n_0} v_i(\hat{F}) \rho_\tau(r_{(i)k}). \tag{8}$$

Inspired by the majorize-minimization (MM) algorithm [8], at the sth iteration, we introduce a quadratic function $\zeta_\varepsilon(r_{(i)k}|r_{(i)k}^{(s)})$ to approximate the quantile function $\rho_\tau(r_{(i)k})$. Specifically,

$$\zeta_\varepsilon(r_{(i)k}|r_{(i)k}^{(s)}) = \frac{1}{4}\left[\frac{r_{(i)k}^2}{\varepsilon + |r_{(i)k}^{(s)}|} + (4\tau - 2) r_{(i)k} + c\right], \tag{9}$$

where $r_{(i)k}^{(s)} = Y_i - \theta_k^{(s)\top} U_{(i)k}$, c is a constant to ensure that $\zeta_\varepsilon(r_{(i)k}|r_{(i)k}^{(s)})$ is equal to $\rho_\tau(r_{(i)k})$ at $r_{(i)k}^{(s)}$. A small $\varepsilon = 10^{-3}$ is added to the denominator of the approximated expression above to avoid dividing by zero.

As for the MCP, following the local quadratic approximation (LQA) approach [5], we use a quadratic function to approximate it at the sth iteration. Specifically,

$$\varphi(\theta_{kj}; \lambda, \gamma) \approx \varphi(\theta_{kj}^{(s)}; \lambda, \gamma) + \frac{1}{2}\frac{\varphi'(|\theta_{kj}^{(s)}|; \lambda, \gamma)}{\varepsilon + |\theta_{kj}^{(s)}|}(\theta_{kj}^2 - \theta_{kj}^{(s)2}), \tag{10}$$

where $\varphi'(|t|; \lambda, \gamma) = \lambda\{1 - |t|/(\lambda\gamma)\}_+$ is the derivative of $\varphi(t; \lambda, \gamma)$.

Combining (8), (9), with (10), in the sth iteration after removing the irrelevant terms, we approximate the penalized objective function with

$$S_n(\theta_k|\theta_k^{(s)}) = \sum_{i=1}^{n+n_0} \left\{ \frac{v_i(\hat{F})}{2} \left[\frac{r_{(i)k}^2}{\varepsilon + |r_{(i)k}^{(s)}|} + (4\tau - 2) r_{(i)k} \right] \right\} + \sum_{j=1}^{2q+2} \frac{\varphi'(|\theta_{kj}^{(s)}|; \lambda, \gamma)}{\varepsilon + |\theta_{kj}^{(s)}|} \theta_{kj}^2.$$

Note that $S_n(\theta_k|\theta_k^{(s)})$ is a quadratic function, so it is easy to minimize. It is easy to see that $S_n(\theta_k^{(s+1)}|\theta_k^{(s)}) \leq S_n(\theta_k^{(s)}|\theta_k^{(s)})$. In our numerical study, we observe that the proposed algorithm always converges. Our proposed MM approximation is built on those developed in the literature. More specifically, in [8, 9], the convergence properties have been established under mild regularity conditions. That is, the limiting point of the minimizer sequence as $\varepsilon \downarrow 0$ obtained by the MM algorithm is a minimizer of the primal nondifferentiable objective function. Thus, it is reasonable to expect that our MM algorithm also possesses the convergence property. For more details on the approximations, see [8, 9].

The proposed estimate depends on the values of γ and λ. For γ, published studies [2, 22] suggest examining a small number of values or fixing its values. In our experiments, the estimator is not too sensitive to γ, and after some trials we set $\gamma = 6$, which has been adopted in published studies. There are multiple ways of choosing λ. One possibility is to choose its value in a way such that a pre-determined number of effects are selected. In practical genetic studies, usually the investigators have limited experimental resources and hence can only validate a fixed number of (main or interaction) effects. Thus, tuning λ to select a fixed number of effects is practical. Another possibility is to use data-dependent approaches such as cross validation.

3 Simulation

We conduct simulation to evaluate performance of the proposed method. We are interested in comparing performance of the two proposed methods (referred to as M1 and M2 in the tables). As the performance of penalized interaction identification has been partly compared against that of significance-based elsewhere [17], here we are more interested in the comparison against an unrobust objective function. In particular, we consider the least squares (LS) objective function, which has the form

$$\sum_{i=1}^{n} \frac{\delta_i}{\hat{G}(T_i)} (Y_i - \theta_k^\top U_{(i)k})^2 + \sum_{j=1}^{2q+2} \varphi(\theta_{kj}; \lambda, \gamma),$$

where notations have similar implications as under the inverse probability weighted method.

The value of λ affects the performance of different methods, in possibly different ways. To better see the difference of different methods, we take a sequence of λ values, evaluate the interaction identification accuracy at each value, and compute the AUC (area under the ROC curve) as the overall accuracy measure. This approach has been adopted in multiple publications.

SIMULATION I For $n = 200$ samples, consider the linear regression model

$$T_i = X_i^\top \alpha + Z_i^\top \beta + (X_i \otimes Z_i)^\top \eta + \varepsilon_i, \quad i = 1, \ldots, n, \tag{11}$$

where X_i, Z_i, and $X_i \otimes Z_i$ represent the q environmental risk factors, p genes, and $p \times q$ G × E interactions. α, β, and η are the regression coefficients. The p genes have a multivariate normal distribution with marginal means 0 and marginal variances 1, which mimics gene expression data. Consider two types of correlation structures for Z_i. The first is the banded correlation. Further consider two scenarios. Under the first scenario (Band 1), $\rho_{jk} = 0.33$ if $|j-k| = 1$ and $\rho_{jk} = 0$ otherwise. Under the second scenario (Band 2), $\rho_{jk} = 0.6$ if $|j-k| = 1$, $\rho_{jk} = 0.33$ if $|j-k| = 2$, and $\rho_{jk} = 0$ otherwise. The second correlation structure is the auto-regressive (AR) correlation with $\rho_{jk} = \rho^{|j-k|}$. Consider two scenarios with $\rho = 0.2$ (AR(0.2)) and 0.8 (AR(0.8)). The environmental factors also have a multivariate normal distribution. Set $q = 5$ and $p = 500$ and 1000. There are a total of 27 nonzero effects: 3 main effects of the E factors, 4 main effects of the G factors, and 20 interactions. Their coefficients are generated from *Unif*[0.2, 0.8]. Besides, consider three scenarios for the errors: (a) Error 1 has a standard normal distribution, which represents the "standard" scenario with no contamination. (b) Error 2 has a $0.7N(0, 1) + 0.3Cauchy(0, 1)$ distribution, which is partly contaminated. (c) Error 3 has a t-distribution with one degree of freedom, which is heavy-tailed. The censoring times C_i's are generated from two uniform distributions:(1) *Unif*[0, 14], which results in about 10 % censoring. (b) *Unif*[0,1.25], which results in about 40 % censoring.

Summary statistics on AUC based on 100 replicates are shown in Table 1. The following observations can be made. The first is that under all simulation scenarios, the proposed robust methods outperform the unrobust one. For example with Error 3, $p = 1000$, and 10 % censoring, the mean AUCs are 0.783 (M1), 0.764 (M2), and 0.599 (LS), respectively. When the error distribution is contaminated or heavy-tailed, this is "as expected." It is interesting to observe superior performance of the robust methods under the normal error. With high-dimensional covariates and a moderate sample size, the unrobust method may lead to unreliable estimates when one or a small number of observations deviate from the center by chance. The second observation is that the weighted QR method outperforms the inverse probability weighted QR method. The difference can be large under some scenarios. For example under Error 3, $p = 1000$, and 40 % censoring, the mean AUCs are 0.738 (M1) and 0.598 (M2), respectively. This is intuitively reasonable, as the first method can potentially extracts more information from data, whereas the latter uses records with events only. In this study, we have focused on methodological development. It will be interesting to rigorously examine the efficiency of different

Table 1 Simulation I with continuous G measurements

	Band 1			Band 2			AR(0.2)			AR(0.8)		
	M1	M2	LS	M1	M2	LS	M1	M2	LS	M1	M2	LS
$p = 500$, 10 % censoring												
Error 1	0.919	0.891	0.806	0.951	0.938	0.845	0.897	0.874	0.792	0.996	0.951	0.880
	0.043	0.047	0.060	0.030	0.035	0.066	0.044	0.045	0.061	0.020	0.022	0.054
Error 2	0.875	0.859	0.727	0.922	0.907	0.765	0.855	0.837	0.700	0.940	0.941	0.828
	0.047	0.063	0.092	0.031	0.052	0.107	0.058	0.062	0.103	0.034	0.033	0.081
Error 3	0.785	0.757	0.606	0.862	0.813	0.647	0.763	0.736	0.603	0.907	0.877	0.697
	0.054	0.070	0.090	0.046	0.066	0.116	0.062	0.070	0.077	0.045	0.058	0.139
$p = 1000$, 10 % censoring												
Error 1	0.914	0.899	0.796	0.941	0.935	0.847	0.897	0.878	0.791	0.957	0.956	0.879
	0.037	0.040	0.061	0.034	0.036	0.066	0.045	0.050	0.067	0.026	0.024	0.066
Error 2	0.873	0.857	0.724	0.913	0.903	0.754	0.848	0.847	0.698	0.094	0.942	0.818
	0.049	0.068	0.088	0.037	0.049	0.117	0.055	0.056	0.094	0.034	0.031	0.095
Error 3	0.783	0.764	0.599	0.866	0.828	0.550	0.776	0.740	0.612	0.908	0.872	0.710
	0.059	0.070	0.075	0.050	0.069	0.106	0.059	0.064	0.089	0.048	0.067	0.129
$p = 500$, 40 % censoring												
Error 1	0.837	0.772	0.700	0.890	0.874	0.807	0.805	0.725	0.690	0.938	0.940	0.860
	0.056	0.079	0.071	0.040	0.058	0.067	0.045	0.071	0.069	0.028	0.034	0.080
Error 2	0.792	0.687	0.605	0.885	0.809	0.657	0.794	0.654	0.592	0.931	0.089	0.765
	0.059	0.081	0.081	0.044	0.075	0.122	0.052	0.078	0.090	0.033	0.078	0.123
Error 3	0.735	0.601	0.548	0.814	0.662	0.547	0.713	0.580	0.539	0.880	0.775	0.616
	0.066	0.060	0.092	0.067	0.089	0.105	0.053	0.070	0.077	0.054	0.087	0.156

$p = 1000$, 40 % censoring												
Error 1	0.811	0.762	0.708	0.897	0.871	0.816	0.780	0.740	0.687	0.934	0.940	0.865
	0.056	0.072	0.064	0.035	0.058	0.067	0.049	0.081	0.076	0.029	0.038	0.071
Error 2	0.800	0.682	0.583	0.885	0.780	0.654	0.789	0.780	0.585	0.923	0.886	0.784
	0.049	0.077	0.085	0.049	0.100	0.127	0.055	0.081	0.079	0.034	0.070	0.130
Error 3	0.738	0.598	0.548	0.821	0.670	0.547	0.724	0.579	0.539	0.875	0.775	0.620
	0.055	0.070	0.092	0.059	0.093	0.105	0.067	0.058	0.077	0.057	0.087	0.120

In each cell, the first/second row is the mean value/stand deviation of AUC based on 100 replicates

methods in future studies. In addition, performance of all methods depends on the correlation structure and censoring rate. Similar observations have been made in the literature.

Next we mimic SNP and other G measurements that have discrete distributions. Specifically, for the Z values generated above, we dichotomize at -1 and 0.5 to create three levels, mimicking SNP data. The other settings are the same as described above. Summary statistics based on 100 replicates are provided in Table 2. We again observe that under data contamination and heavy-tailed errors, the robust methods can significantly outperform the unrobust one. In addition, the weighted QR method is superior to the inverse probability weighted QR method. We note

Table 2 Simulation I with discrete G measurements

	Band1			Band2			AR(0.2)			AR(0.8)		
	M1	M2	LS	M1	M2	LS	M1	M2	LS	M1	M2	LS
$p = 500$, 10 % censoring												
Error 1	0.909	0.849	0.803	0.927	0.851	0.709	0.868	0.859	0.684	0.968	0.959	0.797
	0.028	0.059	0.065	0.049	0.142	0.074	0.063	0.027	0.020	0.014	0.018	0.108
Error 2	0.856	0.827	0.601	0.939	0.937	0.748	0.885	0.832	0.664	0.902	0.897	0.826
	0.038	0.019	0.136	0.028	0.020	0.078	0.026	0.012	0.077	0.013	0.030	0.039
Error 3	0.774	0.751	0.503	0.856	0.841	0.687	0.797	0.737	0.590	0.882	0.871	0.723
	0.056	0.065	0.045	0.043	0.079	0.096	0.069	0.036	0.083	0.027	0.038	0.103
$p = 1000$, 10 % censoring												
Error 1	0.904	0.843	0.812	0.921	0.854	0.698	0.872	0.851	0.691	0.971	0.955	0.787
	0.030	0.061	0.063	0.051	0.132	0.073	0.067	0.032	0.022	0.012	0.021	0.095
Error 2	0.854	0.819	0.602	0.937	0.934	0.739	0.882	0.840	0.665	0.905	0.899	0.817
	0.041	0.023	0.138	0.031	0.022	0.082	0.027	0.015	0.074	0.015	0.032	0.036
Error 3	0.773	0.753	0.501	0.853	0.837	0.683	0.794	0.742	0.588	0.881	0.867	0.718
$p = 500$, 40 % censoring												
Error 1	0.861	0.653	0.703	0.856	0.697	0.723	0.751	0.667	0.592	0.909	0.822	0.713
	0.070	0.062	0.051	0.048	0.011	0.046	0.048	0.126	0.089	0.014	0.015	0.079
Error 2	0.798	0.631	0.557	0.854	0.730	0.629	0.715	0.607	0.523	0.931	0.871	0.634
	0.022	0.057	0.114	0.054	0.087	0.127	0.081	0.018	0.038	0.012	0.029	0.099
Error 3	0.654	0.652	0.497	0.796	0.669	0.507	0.694	0.575	0.506	0.884	0.728	0.598
	0.069	0.076	0.012	0.022	0.088	0.026	0.057	0.069	0.080	0.036	0.070	0.074
$p = 1000$, 40 % censoring												
Error 1	0.858	0.649	0.695	0.853	0.692	0.714	0.748	0.662	0.588	0.919	0.878	0.809
	0.065	0.043	0.048	0.059	0.025	0.041	0.046	0.087	0.075	0.022	0.025	0.033
Error 2	0.786	0.628	0.556	0.852	0.726	0.615	0.709	0.609	0.519	0.897	0.727	0.657
	0.035	0.052	0.089	0.061	0.081	0.096	0.077	0.023	0.041	0.049	0.125	0.161
Error 3	0.632	0.628	0.476	0.772	0.659	0.503	0.688	0.565	0.501	0.871	0.701	0.674
	0.071	0.074	0.013	0.052	0.079	0.032	0.053	0.071	0.083	0.043	0.011	0.107

In each cell, the first/second row is the mean value/stand deviation of AUC based on 100 replicates

Table 3 Simulation I with continuous G measurements, Error 1, 40 % censoring, and different sample size

	Band1			Band2			AR(0.2)			AR(0.8)		
	M1	M2	LS	M1	M2	LS	M1	M2	LS	M1	M2	LS
$p = 500$												
$n = 50$	0.812	0.692	0.603	0.733	0.728	0.602	0.693	0.624	0.571	0.826	0.828	0.701
	0.043	0.057	0.073	0.036	0.076	0.032	0.052	0.059	0.039	0.073	0.058	0.064
$n = 100$	0.835	0.768	0.692	0.885	0.871	0.801	0.798	0.720	0.682	0.937	0.938	0.851
	0.055	0.034	0.057	0.044	0.063	0.057	0.071	0.068	0.061	0.025	0.033	0.066
$n = 200$	0.837	0.772	0.700	0.890	0.874	0.807	0.805	0.725	0.690	0.938	0.940	0.860
	0.056	0.079	0.071	0.040	0.058	0.067	0.045	0.071	0.069	0.028	0.034	0.080
$n = 500$	0.868	0.781	0.746	0.906	0.882	0.831	0.833	0.738	0.719	0.946	0.944	0.882
	0.042	0.049	0.059	0.062	0.051	0.038	0.031	0.058	0.071	0.041	0.043	0.091
$n = 800$	0.881	0.792	0.767	0.913	0.894	0.853	0.847	0.746	0.751	0.953	0.952	0.909
	0.074	0.063	0.089	0.057	0.088	0.056	0.043	0.082	0.075	0.038	0.042	0.063
$p = 1000$												
$n = 50$	0.759	0.687	0.611	0.731	0.722	0.603	0.691	0.619	0.561	0.819	0.816	0.702
	0.048	0.032	0.085	0.074	0.055	0.049	0.052	0.071	0.060	0.031	0.063	0.052
$n = 100$	0.808	0.757	0.703	0.893	0.865	0.808	0.777	0.735	0.683	0.928	0.933	0.859
	0.035	0.048	0.067	0.032	0.069	0.069	0.053	0.055	0.066	0.057	0.083	0.072
$n = 200$	0.811	0.762	0.708	0.897	0.871	0.816	0.780	0.740	0.687	0.934	0.940	0.865
	0.056	0.072	0.064	0.035	0.058	0.067	0.049	0.081	0.076	0.029	0.038	0.071
$n = 500$	0.832	0.783	0.731	0.913	0.885	0.836	0.793	0.751	0.712	0.948	0.951	0.892
	0.059	0.082	0.041	0.054	0.047	0.082	0.027	0.064	0.043	0.029	0.037	0.051
$n = 800$	0.843	0.792	0.757	0.924	0.893	0.857	0.804	0.763	0.735	0.956	0.959	0.910
	0.074	0.027	0.032	0.051	0.084	0.069	0.052	0.093	0.088	0.056	0.049	0.035

In each cell, the first/second row is the mean value/stand deviation of AUC based on 100 replicates

that in Table 2 under Error 2, performance of the inverse probability weighted QR method can be slightly inferior to the unrobust method.

Moreover, we also take the scenario with continuous G measurements, Error 1, and 40 % censoring as an example and examine performance with different sample sizes. The results with $n = 50, 100, 200, 500$, and 800 are shown in Table 3. The proposed robust approach has advantages with both large and small sample sizes.

SIMULATION II Under the first simulation setting, the random error and covariate effects are independent. Here we consider the more complicated scenario where they are correlated. Specifically, consider the model

$$T_i = W_i\theta + W_i\mu\varepsilon_i, \quad i = 1, \ldots, n, \tag{12}$$

where $W_i = (X_i^\top, Z_i^\top, (X_i \otimes Z_i)^\top)$, $\theta = (\alpha^\top, \beta^\top, \eta^\top)^\top$, and μ is a $(p+q+pq) \times 1$ vector. X_i, Z_i, and $X_i \otimes Z_i$ have the same meanings as under Simulation I, and ε_i has a standard normal distribution. Some components of μ are set to be nonzero:

one corresponds to an important E effect, four correspond to important G effects, and twenty correspond to unimportant G×E interactions. That is, the errors are correlated with five important effects and twenty unimportant effects. An advantage of the QR-based methods is that we can examine different quantiles. For this specific simulation setting, we consider $\tau = 0.1,\ 0.25,\ 0.5,\ 0.75$, and 0.9, under which the nonzero elements of μ equal to 0.5, 0.5, 0.5, −0.5, and −0.5, respectively. The censoring rates are set as 20 % and 40 %. The rest of the settings are similar to those under Simulation I.

Summary statistics are shown in Table 4. The observed patterns are similar to those in Tables 1 and 2. A new observation is that the numerical results also depend on the value of τ. The proposed methods are built on quantile regression, which has the appealing feature of being able to accommodate data heterogeneity, for example, caused by heteroscedastic variance. For example, when the censoring rate is 40 % and the correlation structure is AR(0.2), when $\tau = 0.1$, the mean AUCs are 0.752, 0.685, and 0.673, respectively. When $\tau = 0.75$, the mean AUCs are 0.861, 0.774, and 0.639, respectively.

Table 4 Simulation II

	Band1			Band2			AR(0.2)			AR(0.8)		
τ	M1	M2	LS	M1	M2	LS	M1	M2	LS	M1	M2	LS
$p = 1000$, 20 % censoring												
0.1	0.840	0.832	0.761	0.941	0.895	0.762	0.888	0.837	0.713	0.931	0.911	0.772
	0.025	0.031	0.046	0.026	0.048	0.087	0.040	0.059	0.087	0.012	0.029	0.064
0.25	0.865	0.859	0.731	0.936	0.888	0.763	0.882	0.828	0.709	0.927	0.906	0.762
	0.116	0.092	0.081	0.028	0.048	0.074	0.045	0.060	0.086	0.031	0.042	0.071
0.5	0.886	0.887	0.769	0.933	0.892	0.747	0.897	0.832	0.704	0.969	0.942	0.778
	0.010	0.027	0.056	0.033	0.050	0.082	0.042	0.058	0.077	0.011	0.021	0.073
0.75	0.812	0.805	0.704	0.929	0.897	0.756	0.873	0.825	0.708	0.933	0.932	0.765
	0.120	0.093	0.086	0.030	0.049	0.075	0.038	0.055	0.071	0.021	0.029	0.069
0.9	0.697	0.671	0.513	0.950	0.896	0.758	0.894	0.838	0.706	0.724	0.691	0.526
	0.071	0.072	0.063	0.029	0.044	0.085	0.040	0.050	0.075	0.018	0.029	0.067
$p = 1000$, 40 % censoring												
0.1	0.774	0.723	0.702	0.734	0.716	0.706	0.752	0.685	0.673	0.896	0.812	0.827
	0.038	0.071	0.091	0.049	0.042	0.054	0.033	0.066	0.015	0.031	0.146	0.016
0.25	0.809	0.753	0.751	0.839	0.765	0.768	0.815	0.637	0.620	0.928	0.923	0.806
	0.081	0.047	0.074	0.052	0.049	0.013	0.020	0.026	0.137	0.037	0.019	0.033
0.5	0.803	0.727	0.634	0.899	0.855	0.741	0.774	0.635	0.633	0.876	0.733	0.756
	0.009	0.018	0.015	0.036	0.038	0.107	0.053	0.052	0.012	0.012	0.025	0.065
0.75	0.862	0.731	0.627	0.835	0.747	0.669	0.861	0.774	0.639	0.926	0.746	0.838
	0.029	0.029	0.091	0.064	0.022	0.017	0.016	0.041	0.026	0.028	0.019	0.071
0.9	0.733	0.629	0.632	0.789	0.775	0.782	0.718	0.683	0.696	0.897	0.842	0.841
	0.112	0.053	0.169	0.039	0.091	0.038	0.044	0.019	0.051	0.083	0.015	0.034

In each cell, the first/second row is the mean value/stand deviation of AUC based on 100 replicates

Table 5 Simulation III

Correlation	$\gamma = 1.8$	$\gamma = 3$	$\gamma = 6$	$\gamma = \infty$
M1				
Band1	0.910 (0.045)	0.914 (0.039)	0.919 (0.043)	0.843 (0.051)
Band2	0.946 (0.042)	0.948 (0.057)	0.951 (0.030)	0.881 (0.078)
AR(0.2)	0.889 (0.037)	0.894 (0.068)	0.897 (0.044)	0.832 (0.042)
AR(0.8)	0.985 (0.049)	0.988 (0.067)	0.996 (0.020)	0.924 (0.049)
M2				
Band1	0.885 (0.037)	0.887 (0.053)	0.891 (0.047)	0.833 (0.055)
Band2	0.933 (0.046)	0.935 (0.069)	0.938 (0.035)	0.884 (0.082)
AR(0.2)	0.870 (0.058)	0.872 (0.061)	0.874 (0.045)	0.825 (0.057)
AR(0.8)	0.946 (0.045)	0.948 (0.053)	0.951 (0.022)	0.903(0.056)
LS				
Band1	0.799 (0.035)	0.803 (0.074)	0.806 (0.060)	0.744 (0.053)
Band2	0.841 (0.063)	0.843 (0.047)	0.845 (0.066)	0.792 (0.036)
AR(0.2)	0.787 (0.076)	0.789 (0.046)	0.792 (0.061)	0.746 (0.049)
AR(0.8)	0.874 (0.047)	0.877 (0.061)	0.880 (0.054)	0.827 (0.052)

In each cell, mean AUC (standard deviation) based on 100 replicates. When $\gamma = \infty$, MCP simplifies to Lasso

SIMULATION III We conduct sensitivity analysis and examine the impact of γ value on results. Specifically, consider the scenario with $p = 500$, 10 % censoring, and Error 1. The other settings are the same as in Simulation I. Consider $\gamma = 1.8, 3, 6$ and ∞, following [2, 12, 22]. Note that when $\gamma = \infty$, MCP simplifies to Lasso. The summary results are shown in Table 5. We observe that although the value of γ has an impact, overall the results are not sensitive to this value. In addition, MCP is observed to outperform Lasso, as expected.

4 Analysis of Lung Cancer Prognosis Data

Lung cancer poses a serious public health concern. Gene profiling studies have been widely conducted, searching for genetic markers associated with lung cancer prognosis. Most of the existing studies have been focused on the main effects. In this section, we search for potentially important interactions. We follow [21] and analyze data from four independent studies. The DFCI (Dana-Farber Cancer Institute) study has a total of 78 patients, among whom 35 died during follow-up. The median follow-up time was 51 months. The HLM (Moffitt Cancer Center) study has a total of 76 patients, among whom 59 died during follow-up. The median follow-up time was 39 months. The MI (University of Michigan Cancer Center) study has a total of 92 patients, among whom 48 died during follow-up. The median follow-up time was 55 months. The MSKCC (Memorial Sloan-Kettering Cancer Center) study has a total of 102 patients, among whom 38 died during follow-up. The median follow-up time was 43.5 months. Data on 22,283 probe sets are available for analysis. Gene expression normalization is conducted by a robust method. We refer to [21] for more detailed experimental information.

Although the proposed methods can be straightforwardly applied, we conduct the prescreening of genes to improve stability, following [23]. A total of 2605 genes are analyzed. There are five E factors: age, gender, smoke (smoking status), chemotherapy treatment (denoted as "chemo"), and stage. Age is continuous; Gender, smoke, and chemo are binary; Stage has three levels and is represented using two binary variables.

Simulation suggests that the weighted QR method has dominatingly better performance. Thus we only apply this method. For the tuning parameter λ, we select its value so that the main effects of twenty genes are identified. As shown in Simulation II, results also depend on the value of τ. First we consider $\tau = 0.5$, which is the "default." To achieve better comparability across genes, we also rescale the estimates for different genes in a way that "Age" always has estimated coefficient -1. The detailed results are shown in Table 6. The numbers of identified interactions are 7 (with age), 7 (gender), 10 (smoking), 15 (chemo), and 22 (stage), respectively.

We also apply this method under $\tau = 0.25$ and 0.75. The same λ value as obtained above is applied. The results are shown in Tables 7 and 8, respectively. A total of 25 and 27 genes are identified, respectively. We note that, for the main effects, the three quantile values lead to large overlaps. However, the overlaps in interactions are only moderate. Such an observation is not surprising and has also been made under simpler settings.

5 Discussion

For complex diseases, prognosis is of essential importance. In this article, we have focused on detecting important G×E interactions for prognosis, which has not been extensively studied in the literature. Significantly advancing from the existing studies, two quantile regression-based objective functions are adopted, which are robust to contamination in the prognosis outcome. In addition, penalization is adopted as an alternative way of marker selection. Simulation study under diverse settings shows the superior performance of the weighted QR method. The analysis of lung cancer prognosis data with gene expression measurements demonstrates the practical applicability of proposed method.

Robust methods have been shown to be powerful under low-dimensional settings. The development under high-dimensional settings is still relatively limited. Although several high-dimensional QR methods have been developed, the analysis of interactions is still limited. It will be of interest to more broadly extend low-dimensional robust methods to high-dimensional interaction analysis. The proposed methods are robust to data contamination. In the literature, there are also methods that are robust to model mis-specification [17]. However, some other aspects of

Table 6 Analysis of the lung cancer data using the penalized weighted QR method with $\tau = 0.5$: identified main effects and interactions

	Main effects							Interactions					
Probe	Age	Gender	Smoke	Chemo	Stage II	Stage III	Gene	Age	Gender	Smoke	Chemo	Stage II	Stage III
X202291_s_at	−1.00	1.12	0.07	0.02	−0.03	−1.22	1.24		−0.51		−0.29		−2.20
X205883_at	−1.00	1.19	0.02	1.23	0.02	−0.98	1.20		0.63		1.01		−3.11
X206414_s_at	−1.00	1.04	0.03	0.01	0.05	−0.95	1.01	−0.31	−0.92	0.98	−0.92		2.01
X205258_at	−1.00	1.03	−0.72	0.03	0.03	−0.01	1.22	−0.22			−0.81		−1.71
X218952_at	−1.00	2.11	−1.21	0.50	0.06	−4.02	1.02	−0.43	−2.21	2.11		−0.91	−3.49
X203131_at	−1.00	1.06	0.12	0.02	0.02	−0.92	2.21					−0.33	−1.15
X218701_at	−1.00	0.65	−0.08	0.55	−0.02	−1.13	0.98	−0.77		−1.31	−0.65	−0.93	
X214927_at	−1.00	1.03	0.21	0.72	−0.06	−0.06	0.97				−0.41		
X208763_s_at	−1.00	1.12	0.15	0.03	−0.06	−0.02	1.31			−1.82		0.72	−1.62
X218718_at	−1.00	1.05	−0.06	0.01	−0.02	0.01	0.97					−1.80	−1.06
X201427_s_at	−1.00	0.91	1.03	0.05	0.03	−3.42	1.82			0.51	−0.51		−3.05
X208920_at	−1.00	2.03	0.16	0.92	0.07	−3.71	1.81				−0.67	−0.74	−2.26
X214696_at	−1.00	0.81	−0.08	0.16	0.04	−3.52	2.14		−1.31	0.72	−0.74		−2.41
X205694_at	−1.00	1.22	−0.23	0.12	−0.45	−0.49	1.67			−0.92	−1.89		
X201312_s_at	−1.00	1.14	0.18	0.11	−0.01	−0.52	1.31	−0.35		1.43	−0.61	−0.44	
X201739_at	−1.00	0.76	−0.05	0.19	0.02	−2.10	1.02		−1.25	−0.82	−0.46		−1.72
X205609_at	−1.00	1.32	−0.11	0.21	−0.02	−5.21	1.13				0.91		−3.13
X219572_at	−1.00	1.07	0.22	0.10	0.01	−1.37	1.01	−0.29		1.17	0.21		
X212070_at	−1.00	1.15	−0.14	0.08	0.02	−1.33	2.03	−0.11	−2.10		0.52	−0.81	−1.71
X208718_at	−1.00	1.19	0.81	0.03	0.01	−0.51	0.99						

Table 7 Analysis of the lung cancer data using the penalized weighted QR method with $\tau = 0.25$: identified main effects and interactions

Probe	Main effects							Interactions					
	Age	Gender	Smoke	Chemo	Stage II	Stage III	Gene	Age	Gender	Smoke	Chemo	Stage II	Stage III
X206754_s_at	-1.00	8.32	0.09	0.06	−0.02	−0.01	9.87			−10.23			
X205422_s_at	-1.00	7.22	0.08	0.02	−0.08	−0.01	1.03						
X209335_at	-1.00	1.02	0.01	0.03	−0.02	−0.01	0.09						−3.28
X205883_at	-1.00	7.13	0.06	0.05	−0.05	−0.02	7.62						−10.21
X206414_s_at	-1.00	6.53	0.06	0.09	−0.04	−0.01	8.12						
X205258_at	-1.00	2.12	0.07	0.02	−0.01	−0.01	0.34						−1.05
X218952_at	-1.00	5.11	0.06	0.06	−0.01	−5.36	9.64		−3.42				−9.47
X204072_s_at	-1.00	4.31	0.03	0.05	−0.01	−2.63	10.45						−9.42
X221748_s_at	-1.00	1.16	0.01	0.02	−0.01	−0.01	1.73		−1.12				−1.93
X214927_at	-1.00	1.12	0.03	0.02	−0.02	−1.76	0.79						−1.52
X208763_s_at	-1.00	2.51	0.01	0.04	−0.01	−0.01	0.05						−8.33
X218718_at	-1.00	0.02	0.02	0.05	−0.01	−2.26	1.23					−1.13	−2.71
X201427_s_at	-1.00	0.01	0.05	0.01	−0.06	−8.33	0.25						−9.16
X201328_at	-1.00	1.02	0.01	0.01	−0.01	−0.01	0.07						
X208920_at	-1.00	0.01	0.01	0.01	−0.02	−5.69	9.77						−10.32
X214696_at	-1.00	7.25	0.01	0.01	−0.02	−9.31	11.23						−10.25
X205694_at	-1.00	8.96	0.01	0.03	−0.03	−0.01	10.45				−8.33		
X201312_s_at	-1.00	8.53	0.02	0.03	−0.01	−0.01	8.42						
X217234_s_at	-1.00	8.36	0.05	0.01	−0.02	−0.02	10.63		−4.77				
X201739_at	-1.00	2.03	0.01	0.01	−0.01	−1.91	2.68		−2.51				−5.31
X201916_s_at	-1.00	3.24	0.02	0.07	−0.02	−0.01	10.22						
X205609_at	-1.00	5.33	0.01	−0.03	−0.02	−9.14	11.24						−9.12
X219572_at	-1.00	0.01	0.01	0.01	−0.03	−0.02	1.86				−1.07		
X212070_at	-1.00	6.89	0.01	0.01	−0.02	−9.63	11.31		−7.12				−9.25
X208718_at	-1.00	0.05	0.02	0.01	−0.03	−0.01	0.03						

Table 8 Analysis of the lung cancer data using the penalized weighted QR method with $\tau = 0.75$: identified main effects and interactions

	Main effects							Interactions					
Gene name	Age	Gender	Smoke	Chemo	Stage II	Stage III	Gene	Age	Gender	Smoke	Chemo	Stage II	Stage III
X212599_at	−1.00	10.32	0.01	0.01	0.07	−0.01	13.56						−7.14
X202291_s_at	−1.00	1.51	0.01	0.07	0.04	−0.03	1.03						−1.03
X205422_s_at	−1.00	1.42	0.01	0.02	0.01	0.01	0.11						
X209335_at	−1.00	0.87	0.02	0.05	0.05	−0.01	0.87						−3.41
X201540_at	−1.00	9.32	−0.02	0.02	0.02	−0.01	16.35		−10.31		9.11		−8.25
X205883_at	−1.00	1.55	0.03	0.01	0.01	−1.55	0.42		−0.41		1.52		−5.05
X206414_s_at	−1.00	8.97	0.01	0.01	0.01	0.01	0.41						
X205258_at	−1.00	1.88	−0.01	0.02	0.01	−0.01	1.19						−2.88
X218952_at	−1.00	11.23	−0.02	−0.01	0.02	−5.12	10.68		−9.78				−7.91
X203131_at	−1.00	1.01	0.03	0.01	0.01	0.02	0.98						−1.02
X204072_s_at	−1.00	9.52	0.05	0.01	0.01	−1.98	10.69						−8.27
X218701_at	−1.00	10.51	0.08	0.02	0.02	0.02	11.87				−8.32		
X214927_at	−1.00	1.88	0.02	0.02	0.03	−0.01	1.15						
X208763_s_at	−1.00	1.26	0.04	0.01	0.04	0.01	0.32			−1.21			
X218718_at	−1.00	10.69	−0.01	0.01	0.02	0.03	15.96						−8.12
X205316_at	−1.00	1.95	0.01	0.01	0.04	0.01	0.09						−1.81
X201427_s_at	−1.00	1.47	0.01	0.03	0.01	−2.36	1.21						−4.14
X208920_at	−1.00	9.64	0.01	0.02	0.01	−2.75	13.96						−8.46
X214696_at	−1.00	11.25	−0.02	0.02	0.03	−10.63	15.41		−11.25				−9.25
X205694_at	−1.00	1.30	0.03	0.01	0.04	0.01	0.71				−1.25		
X201312_s_at	−1.00	9.63	−0.05	−0.04	0.02	0.02	7.98			10.53			
X201739_at	−1.00	10.56	0.01	0.01	0.02	−0.11	18.25		−9.14				−9.47
X205609_at	−1.00	8.77	0.01	0.02	0.01	−9.66	15.26				−8.32		−10.11
X219572_at	−1.00	9.30	0.02	0.01	0.01	−10.77	18.66				−9.14		
X212070_at	−1.00	1.33	0.01	0.01	0.03	−0.02	1.32		−1.42				
X214719_at	−1.00	0.02	0.01	0.05	0.01	−0.01	1.06				−1.33		−1.56

robustness, for example to contamination in covariates, remain to be more carefully studied. In addition, it is also of interest to explore "combining" multiple aspects of robustness. In this study, we have focused on methodological development. The establishment of statistical properties will be postponed to future studies. Specifically, it will be of interest to identify sufficient conditions under which the proposed approach has the consistency properties. The relative efficiency of the two quantile methods is also potentially interesting.

Acknowledgements We thank the organizers and participants of "The Fourth International Workshop on the Perspectives on High-dimensional Data Analysis." The authors were supported by the China Postdoctoral Science Foundation (2014M550799), National Science Foundation of China (11401561), National Social Science Foundation of China (13CTJ001, 13&ZD148), National Institutes of Health (CA165923, CA191383, CA016359), and U.S. VA Cooperative Studies Program of the Department of Veterans Affairs, Office of Research and Development.

References

1. Bang, H., Tsiatis, A.A.: Median regression with censored cost data. Biometrics **58**(3), 643–649 (2002)
2. Breheny, P., Huang, J.: Coordinate descent algorithms for nonconvex penalized regression, with applications to biological feature selection. Ann. Appl. Stat. **5**(1), 232 (2011)
3. Caspi, A., Moffitt, T.E.: Gene-environment interactions in psychiatry: joining forces with neuroscience. Nat. Rev. Neurosci. **7**(7), 583–590 (2006)
4. Cordell, H.J.: Detecting gene–gene interactions that underlie human diseases. Nat. Rev. Genet. **10**(6), 392–404 (2009)
5. Fan, J., Li, R.: Variable selection via nonconcave penalized likelihood and its oracle properties. J. Am. Stat. Assoc. **96**(456), 1348–1360 (2001)
6. Hunter, D.R.: MM algorithms for generalized Bradley-Terry models. Ann. Stat. **32**, 384–406 (2004)
7. Hunter, D.J.: Gene-environment interactions in human diseases. Nat. Rev. Genet. **6**(4), 287–298 (2005)
8. Hunter, D.R., Lange, K.: Quantile regression via an MM algorithm. J. Comput. Graph. Stat. **9**(1), 60–77 (2000)
9. Hunter, D.R., Li, R.: Variable selection using MM algorithms. Ann. Stat. **33**(4), 1617 (2005)
10. Koenker, R.: Quantile Regression, vol. 38. Cambridge University Press, Cambridge (2005)
11. Koenker, R., Bassett Jr, G.: Regression quantiles. Econometrica: J. Econom. Soc. 33–50 (1978)
12. Liu, J., Huang, J., Xie, Y., Ma, S.: Sparse group penalized integrative analysis of multiple cancer prognosis datasets. Genet. Res. **95**(2–3), 68–77 (2013)
13. Liu, J., Huang, J., Zhang, Y., Lan, Q., Rothman, N., Zheng, T., Ma, S.: Identification of gene-environment interactions in cancer studies using penalization. Genomics **102**(4), 189–194 (2013)
14. Lopez, O., Patilea, V.: Nonparametric lack-of-fit tests for parametric mean-regression models with censored data. J. Multivar. Anal. **100**(1), 210–230 (2009)
15. Mazumder, R., Friedman, J.H., Hastie, T.: Sparsenet: Coordinate descent with nonconvex penalties. J. Am. Stat. Assoc. **106**(495), 1125–1138 (2011)
16. North, K.E., Martin, L.J.: The importance of gene-environment interaction implications for social scientists. Sociol. Methods Res. **37**(2), 164–200 (2008)
17. Shi, X., Liu, J., Huang, J., Zhou, Y., Xie, Y., Ma, S.: A penalized robust method for identifying gene-environment interactions. Genet. Epidemiol. **38**(3), 220–230 (2014)

18. Thomas, D.: Methods for investigating gene-environment interactions in candidate pathway and genome-wide association studies. Ann. Rev. Public Health **31**, 21 (2010)
19. Wang, H.J., Wang, L.: Locally weighted censored quantile regression. J. Am. Stat. Assoc. **104**(487), 1117–1128 (2009)
20. Wu, C., Ma, S.: A selective review of robust variable selection with applications in bioinformatics. Brief. Bioinform. **16**(5), 873–883 (2015)
21. Xie, Y., Xiao, G., Coombes, K.R., Behrens, C., Solis, L.M., Raso, G., Girard, L., Erickson, H.S., Roth, J., Heymach, J.V., et al.: Robust gene expression signature from formalin-fixed paraffin-embedded samples predicts prognosis of non-small-cell lung cancer patients. Clin. Cancer Res. **17**(17), 5705–5714 (2011)
22. Zhang, C.H.: Nearly unbiased variable selection under minimax concave penalty. Ann. Stat. **38**, 894–942 (2010)
23. Zhu, R., Zhao, H., Ma, S.: Identifying gene-environment and gene–gene interactions using a progressive penalization approach. Genet. Epidemiol. **38**(4), 353–368 (2014)

A Mixture of Variance-Gamma Factor Analyzers

Sharon M. McNicholas, Paul D. McNicholas, and Ryan P. Browne

Abstract The mixture of factor analyzers model is extended to variance-gamma mixtures to facilitate flexible clustering of high-dimensional data. The formation of the variance-gamma distribution utilized is a special and limiting case of the generalized hyperbolic distribution. Parameter estimation for these mixtures is carried out via an alternating expectation-conditional maximization algorithm, and relies on convenient expressions for expected values for the generalized inverse Gaussian distribution. The Bayesian information criterion is used to select the number of latent factors. The mixture of variance-gamma factor analyzers model is illustrated on a well-known breast cancer data set. Finally, the place of variance-gamma mixtures within the growing body of literature on non-Gaussian mixtures is considered.

Keywords Clustering • Factor analysis • High-dimensional data • Mixture models • MVGFA • Variance-gamma distribution • Variance-gamma factor analyzers

1 Introduction

Finite mixture models treat a population as a convex combination of a finite number of probability densities. Therefore, they represent a natural framework for classification and clustering applications. A random vector $\mathbf{X}$ arises from a

---

S.M. McNicholas
Department of Mathematics and Statistics, McMaster University, Hamilton, ON, Canada
e-mail: sharonmc@mcmaster.ca

P.D. McNicholas (✉)
Department of Mathematics and Statistics, McMaster University, Hamilton, ON, Canada
e-mail: mcnicholas@math.mcmaster.ca

R.P. Browne
Department of Statistics and Actuarial Science, University of Waterloo, Waterloo, ON, Canada
e-mail: rpbrowne@uwaterloo.ca

© Springer International Publishing AG 2017
S.E. Ahmed (ed.), *Big and Complex Data Analysis*, Contributions to Statistics,
DOI 10.1007/978-3-319-41573-4_18

(parametric) finite mixture distribution if, for all $\boldsymbol{x} \subset \mathbf{X}$, its density can be written

$$f(\boldsymbol{x} \mid \boldsymbol{\vartheta}) = \sum_{g=1}^{G} \pi_g f_g(\boldsymbol{x} \mid \boldsymbol{\theta}_g),$$

where $\pi_g > 0$ such that $\sum_{g=1}^{G} \pi_g = 1$ are the mixing proportions, $f_g(\boldsymbol{x} \mid \boldsymbol{\theta}_g)$ is the gth component density, and $\boldsymbol{\vartheta} = (\boldsymbol{\pi}, \boldsymbol{\theta}_1, \ldots, \boldsymbol{\theta}_G)$ denotes the vector of parameters with $\boldsymbol{\pi} = (\pi_1, \ldots, \pi_G)$. The component densities $f_1(\boldsymbol{x} \mid \boldsymbol{\theta}_1), \ldots, f_G(\boldsymbol{x} \mid \boldsymbol{\theta}_G)$ are typically taken to be of the same type, most commonly multivariate Gaussian.

Multivariate Gaussian mixtures have become increasingly popular in clustering and classification since they were first considered in this context over 60 years ago (cf. [42, Sect. 2.1]). The Gaussian mixture density is

$$f(\boldsymbol{x} \mid \boldsymbol{\vartheta}) = \sum_{g=1}^{G} \pi_g \phi(\boldsymbol{x} \mid \boldsymbol{\mu}_g, \boldsymbol{\Sigma}_g), \tag{1}$$

where $\phi(\boldsymbol{x} \mid \boldsymbol{\mu}_g, \boldsymbol{\Sigma}_g)$ is the multivariate Gaussian density with mean $\boldsymbol{\mu}_g$ and covariance matrix $\boldsymbol{\Sigma}_g$. Suppose p-dimensional data $\boldsymbol{x}_1, \ldots, \boldsymbol{x}_n$ are observed and no component memberships are known, i.e., a clustering scenario. The likelihood for the Gaussian mixture model in this case can be written

$$\mathscr{L}(\boldsymbol{\vartheta} \mid \boldsymbol{x}) = \prod_{i=1}^{n} \sum_{g=1}^{G} \pi_g \phi(\boldsymbol{x}_i \mid \boldsymbol{\mu}_g, \boldsymbol{\Sigma}_g).$$

The term "model-based clustering" is usually taken to mean the application of mixture models for clustering. The term "model-based classification" is used similarly (e.g., [16, 41]) and is synonymous with "partial classification" (cf. [38, Sect. 2.7])—both terms refer to a semi-supervised version of model-based clustering—while model-based discriminant analysis is completely supervised (cf. [23]).

Over the past few years, there has been a marked increase in work on non-Gaussian mixtures for clustering and classification. Initially, this work focused on mixtures of multivariate t-distributions [2–5, 35, 49, 53], which represent a straightforward departure from normality. More recently, work on the skew-normal distribution [33] and the skew-t distribution [31, 34, 46, 47, 56, 57] has been predominant, as well as work on other approaches (e.g., [13, 14, 26, 48]). Browne and McNicholas [12] add to the richness of this pallet by introducing a mixture of generalized hyperbolic distributions; many other approaches that have been tried are special cases of this "superclass." Herein, we consider an approach that extends the mixture of factor analyzers model to a mixture of variance-gamma factor analyzers.

2 A Mixture of Variance Gamma Distributions

2.1 *Generalized Inverse Gaussian Distribution*

The generalized inverse Gaussian (GIG) distribution was introduced by Good [21] and further developed by Barndorff-Nielsen and Halgreen [6], Blæsild [9], Halgreen [22], and Jørgensen [25]. Write $Y \backsim \text{GIG}(\psi, \chi, \lambda)$ to indicate that a random variable Y follows a generalized inverse Gaussian (GIG) distribution with parameters (ψ, χ, λ) and density

$$p(y \mid \psi, \chi, \lambda) = \frac{(\psi/\chi)^{\lambda/2} y^{\lambda-1}}{2K_\lambda\left(\sqrt{\psi\chi}\right)} \exp\left\{-\frac{\psi y + \chi/y}{2}\right\}, \tag{2}$$

for $y > 0$, where $\psi, \chi \in \mathbb{R}^+$, $\lambda \in \mathbb{R}$, and $K_\lambda(\cdot)$ is the modified Bessel function of the third kind with index λ.

2.2 *Generalized Hyperbolic Distribution*

McNeil et al. [40] give the density of a random variable $\boldsymbol{X}$ following the generalized hyperbolic distribution,

$$\begin{aligned} f(\boldsymbol{x} \mid \boldsymbol{\theta}) &= \left[\frac{\chi + \delta(\boldsymbol{x}, \boldsymbol{\mu} \mid \boldsymbol{\Sigma})}{\psi + \boldsymbol{\alpha}'\boldsymbol{\Sigma}^{-1}\boldsymbol{\alpha}}\right]^{\frac{\lambda - p/2}{2}} \\ &\times \frac{[\psi/\chi]^{\lambda/2} K_{\lambda-p/2}\left(\sqrt{[\psi + \boldsymbol{\alpha}'\boldsymbol{\Sigma}^{-1}\boldsymbol{\alpha}][\chi + \delta(\boldsymbol{x}, \boldsymbol{\mu} \mid \boldsymbol{\Sigma})]}\right)}{(2\pi)^{p/2} |\boldsymbol{\Sigma}|^{1/2} K_\lambda\left(\sqrt{\chi\psi}\right) \exp\left\{(\boldsymbol{\mu} - \boldsymbol{x})' \boldsymbol{\Sigma}^{-1}\boldsymbol{\alpha}\right\}}, \end{aligned} \tag{3}$$

where $\boldsymbol{\mu}$ is a location parameter, $\boldsymbol{\alpha}$ is a skewness parameter, $\boldsymbol{\Sigma}$ is a scale matrix, χ and ψ are concentration parameters, λ is an index parameter, $\delta(\boldsymbol{x}, \boldsymbol{\mu} \mid \boldsymbol{\Sigma}) = (\boldsymbol{x} - \boldsymbol{\mu})' \boldsymbol{\Sigma}^{-1} (\boldsymbol{x} - \boldsymbol{\mu})$ is the squared Mahalanobis distance between $\boldsymbol{x}$ and $\boldsymbol{\mu}$, and $\boldsymbol{\theta} = (\lambda, \chi, \psi, \boldsymbol{\mu}, \boldsymbol{\Delta}, \boldsymbol{\alpha})$ is the vector of parameters. Herein, we use the notation $\boldsymbol{X} \backsim \mathcal{G}_p(\lambda, \chi, \psi, \boldsymbol{\mu}, \boldsymbol{\Sigma}, \boldsymbol{\alpha})$ to indicate that a p-dimensional random variable $\boldsymbol{X}$ has the generalized hyperbolic density in (3). Note that some constraint needs to be imposed on (3) to ensure identifiability; see [12] for details.

A generalized hyperbolic random variable $\boldsymbol{X}$ can be generated by combining a random variable $Y \backsim \text{GIG}(\psi, \chi, \lambda)$ and a multivariate Gaussian random variable $\boldsymbol{V} \backsim \mathcal{N}(\boldsymbol{0}, \boldsymbol{\Sigma})$ via the relationship

$$\boldsymbol{X} = \boldsymbol{\mu} + Y\boldsymbol{\alpha} + \sqrt{Y}\boldsymbol{V}, \tag{4}$$

and it follows that $\boldsymbol{X} \mid y \backsim \mathcal{N}(\boldsymbol{\mu} + y\boldsymbol{\alpha}, y\boldsymbol{\Sigma})$. From Bayes' theorem, we obtain $Y \mid \boldsymbol{x} \backsim \text{GIG}(\psi + \boldsymbol{\alpha}'\boldsymbol{\Sigma}^{-1}\boldsymbol{\alpha}, \chi + \delta(\boldsymbol{x}, \boldsymbol{\mu} \mid \boldsymbol{\Sigma}), \lambda - p/2)$. See [12] for details.

2.3 A Mixture of Variance-Gamma Distributions

The variance-gamma distribution arises as a special, limiting case of the generalized hyperbolic distribution (3) by setting $\lambda > 0$ and $\chi \to 0$. Note that the variance-gamma distribution is also known as the generalized or Bessel function distribution. To obtain this representation of the variance-gamma distribution, we need to note that for small, positive b:

$$K_a(b) \approx \begin{cases} -\log\left(\frac{b}{2}\right) - \varepsilon & \text{if } a = 0, \\ \frac{\Gamma(a)}{2}\left(\frac{2}{b}\right)^a & \text{if } a > 0, \end{cases}$$

where $K_a(b)$ is the modified Bessel function of the third kind with index a and ε is the Euler-Mascheroni constant. Noting that $\lambda > 0$, we have

$$\left(\frac{\psi}{\chi}\right)^{\lambda/2} \frac{1}{K_\lambda(\sqrt{\chi\psi})} \approx \frac{2^{1-\lambda}}{\Gamma(\lambda)}\psi^\lambda \tag{5}$$

for small, positive χ. Using the result in (5), we obtain the following variance-gamma density as a special, limiting case of (3):

$$v(\boldsymbol{x} \mid \boldsymbol{\mu}, \boldsymbol{\Sigma}, \boldsymbol{\alpha}, \lambda, \psi) = \left[\frac{\delta(\boldsymbol{x}, \boldsymbol{\mu} \mid \boldsymbol{\Sigma})}{\psi + \boldsymbol{\alpha}'\boldsymbol{\Sigma}^{-1}\boldsymbol{\alpha}}\right]^{\frac{\lambda - p/2}{2}} \frac{2^{1-\lambda}\psi^\lambda K_{\lambda-p/2}\left(\sqrt{(\psi + \boldsymbol{\alpha}'\boldsymbol{\Sigma}^{-1}\boldsymbol{\alpha})\delta(\boldsymbol{x}, \boldsymbol{\mu} \mid \boldsymbol{\Sigma})}\right)}{\Gamma(\lambda)\,(2\pi)^{p/2}\,|\boldsymbol{\Sigma}|^{1/2}\exp\left\{(\boldsymbol{\mu} - \boldsymbol{x})'\,\boldsymbol{\Sigma}^{-1}\boldsymbol{\alpha}\right\}}, \tag{6}$$

for $\lambda > 0$ and with the same notation as before. The notation $\boldsymbol{X} \backsim \mathcal{V}_p(\boldsymbol{\mu}, \boldsymbol{\Sigma}, \boldsymbol{\alpha}, \lambda, \psi)$ is used to indicate that a p-dimensional random variable $\boldsymbol{X}$ has the variance-gamma density in (6). By analogy with the generalized hyperbolic case, a random variable $\boldsymbol{X} \backsim \mathcal{V}_p(\boldsymbol{\mu}, \boldsymbol{\Sigma}, \boldsymbol{\alpha}, \lambda, \psi)$ can be generated by combining a random variable $Y \backsim \text{gamma}(\lambda, \psi/2)$ and a multivariate Gaussian random variable $\boldsymbol{V} \backsim \mathcal{N}(\boldsymbol{0}, \boldsymbol{\Sigma})$ using the relationship

$$\boldsymbol{X} = \boldsymbol{\mu} + Y\boldsymbol{\alpha} + \sqrt{Y}\boldsymbol{V}. \tag{7}$$

Note that $Y \backsim \text{gamma}(\lambda, \psi/2)$ denotes a gamma random variable Y with the shape-rate parameterization, i.e., with density

$$g(y \mid a, b) = \frac{b^a}{\Gamma(a)} y^{a-1} \exp\{-by\}, \tag{8}$$

for $y > 0$ and $a, b \in \mathbb{R}^+$.

From (7), we have $\boldsymbol{X} \mid y \backsim \mathcal{N}(\boldsymbol{\mu} + y\boldsymbol{\alpha}, y\boldsymbol{\Delta})$. Therefore, noting that

$$\begin{aligned}
&\delta(\boldsymbol{x}, \boldsymbol{\mu} + y\boldsymbol{\alpha} \mid y\boldsymbol{\Sigma}) \\
&\quad = \boldsymbol{\alpha}'\boldsymbol{\Sigma}^{-1}\boldsymbol{\alpha}y - (\boldsymbol{x} - \boldsymbol{\mu})'\boldsymbol{\Sigma}^{-1}\boldsymbol{\alpha} - \boldsymbol{\alpha}'\boldsymbol{\Sigma}^{-1}(\boldsymbol{x} - \boldsymbol{\mu}) + \delta(\boldsymbol{x}, \boldsymbol{\mu} \mid \boldsymbol{\Sigma})/y,
\end{aligned}$$

Bayes' theorem gives

$$\begin{aligned}
f(y \mid \boldsymbol{x}) &= \frac{\phi(\boldsymbol{x} \mid y) g(y)}{v(\boldsymbol{x})} \\
&= \left[\frac{\psi + \boldsymbol{\alpha}'\boldsymbol{\Sigma}^{-1}\boldsymbol{\alpha}}{\delta(\boldsymbol{x}, \boldsymbol{\mu} \mid \boldsymbol{\Sigma})}\right]^{\frac{\lambda - p/2}{2}} \frac{y^{\lambda - p/2 - 1} \exp\left\{-\left[y\left(\psi + \boldsymbol{\alpha}'\boldsymbol{\Sigma}^{-1}\boldsymbol{\alpha}\right) + y^{-1}\delta(\boldsymbol{x}, \boldsymbol{\mu} \mid \boldsymbol{\Sigma})\right]/2\right\}}{2K_{\lambda - p/2}\left(\sqrt{\left(\psi + \boldsymbol{\alpha}'\boldsymbol{\Sigma}^{-1}\boldsymbol{\alpha}\right)\delta(\boldsymbol{x}, \boldsymbol{\mu} \mid \boldsymbol{\Sigma})}\right)},
\end{aligned}$$

and so $Y \mid \boldsymbol{x} \backsim \text{GIG}(\psi + \boldsymbol{\alpha}'\boldsymbol{\Sigma}^{-1}\boldsymbol{\alpha}, \delta(\boldsymbol{x}, \boldsymbol{\mu} \mid \boldsymbol{\Sigma}), \lambda - p/2)$.

There are several limiting and special cases of the variance-gamma distribution. Most relevant to clustering applications is the special case called the asymmetric Laplace distribution (cf. [29]), which arises upon setting $\lambda = 1$ and $\psi = 2$. With the addition of a location parameter, the (shifted) asymmetric Laplace distribution was used for mixture model-based clustering and classification by Franczak et al. [18].

Unfortunately, an identifiability issue will arise if we proceed with (6) as is. To see why this is so, consider that (6) can be written

$$\begin{aligned}
&v(\boldsymbol{x} \mid \boldsymbol{\mu}, \boldsymbol{\Sigma}, \boldsymbol{\alpha}, \lambda, \psi) \\
&= \left[\left(\frac{1}{\psi^2}\right)\frac{\psi\delta(\boldsymbol{x}, \boldsymbol{\mu} \mid \boldsymbol{\Sigma})}{1 + \frac{1}{\psi}\boldsymbol{\alpha}'\boldsymbol{\Sigma}^{-1}\boldsymbol{\alpha}}\right]^{\frac{\lambda - p/2}{2}} \\
&\quad \times \frac{2^{1-\lambda}\psi^{\lambda}K_{\lambda - p/2}\left(\sqrt{(1 + \frac{1}{\psi}\boldsymbol{\alpha}'\boldsymbol{\Sigma}^{-1}\boldsymbol{\alpha})\psi\delta(\boldsymbol{x}, \boldsymbol{\mu} \mid \boldsymbol{\Sigma})}\right)}{\Gamma(\lambda)(2\pi)^{p/2}|\boldsymbol{\Sigma}|^{1/2}\exp\left\{(\boldsymbol{\mu} - \boldsymbol{x})'\boldsymbol{\Sigma}^{-1}\boldsymbol{\alpha}\right\}}, \\
&= \left[\frac{\delta(\boldsymbol{x}, \boldsymbol{\mu} \mid \boldsymbol{\Sigma}_*)}{1 + \boldsymbol{\alpha}_*'\boldsymbol{\Sigma}_*^{-1}\boldsymbol{\alpha}_*}\right]^{\frac{\lambda - p/2}{2}} \frac{2^{1-\lambda}K_{\lambda - p/2}\left(\sqrt{(1 + \boldsymbol{\alpha}_*'\boldsymbol{\Sigma}_*^{-1}\boldsymbol{\alpha}_*)\delta(\boldsymbol{x}, \boldsymbol{\mu} \mid \boldsymbol{\Sigma}_*)}\right)}{\Gamma(\lambda)(2\pi)^{p/2}|\boldsymbol{\Sigma}_*|^{1/2}\exp\left\{(\boldsymbol{\mu} - \boldsymbol{x})'\boldsymbol{\Sigma}_*^{-1}\boldsymbol{\alpha}_*\right\}},
\end{aligned}$$

where

$$\boldsymbol{\alpha}_* = \frac{1}{\psi}\boldsymbol{\alpha} \qquad \text{and} \qquad \boldsymbol{\Sigma}_*^{-1} = \psi\boldsymbol{\Sigma}^{-1}.$$

To overcome this problem, set $\mathbb{E}[Y] = 1$ in (7), i.e., impose the restriction $\lambda = \psi/2$. For notational clarity, define $\gamma := \lambda = \psi/2$. Then, our variance-gamma density can be written

$$v_*(\boldsymbol{x} \mid \boldsymbol{\mu}, \boldsymbol{\Sigma}, \boldsymbol{\alpha}, \gamma) = \left[\frac{\delta(\boldsymbol{x}, \boldsymbol{\mu} \mid \boldsymbol{\Sigma})}{2\gamma + \boldsymbol{\alpha}'\boldsymbol{\Sigma}^{-1}\boldsymbol{\alpha}}\right]^{\frac{\gamma - p/2}{2}} \times \frac{2\gamma^{\gamma} K_{\gamma - p/2}\left(\sqrt{(2\gamma + \boldsymbol{\alpha}'\boldsymbol{\Sigma}^{-1}\boldsymbol{\alpha})\delta(\boldsymbol{x}, \boldsymbol{\mu} \mid \boldsymbol{\Sigma})}\right)}{\Gamma(\gamma)\,(2\pi)^{p/2}\,|\boldsymbol{\Sigma}|^{1/2}\exp\left\{(\boldsymbol{\mu} - \boldsymbol{x})'\,\boldsymbol{\Sigma}^{-1}\boldsymbol{\alpha}\right\}}, \tag{9}$$

and $Y \mid \boldsymbol{x} \backsim \text{GIG}(2\gamma + \boldsymbol{\alpha}'\boldsymbol{\Sigma}^{-1}\boldsymbol{\alpha}, \delta(\boldsymbol{x}, \boldsymbol{\mu} \mid \boldsymbol{\Sigma}), \gamma - p/2)$. Our mixture of variance-gamma distributions has density

$$v_{\text{mix}}(\boldsymbol{x} \mid \boldsymbol{\vartheta}) = \sum_{g=1}^{G} \pi_g v_*(\boldsymbol{x} \mid \boldsymbol{\mu}_g, \boldsymbol{\Sigma}_g, \boldsymbol{\alpha}_g, \gamma_g),$$

with the same notation as before.

3 A Mixture of Variance Gamma Factor Analyzers

3.1 Background

The number of free parameters in a p-dimensional, G-component mixture of variance-gamma distributions can be prohibitively large for even relatively small values of p. The scale matrices $\boldsymbol{\Sigma}_1, \ldots, \boldsymbol{\Sigma}_G$ contain $Gp(p+1)/2$ free parameters, i.e., a number that is quadratic in p. There are $2G(1+p) - 1$ further free parameters, i.e., a number that is linear in p. Accordingly, it is natural to first look to the component scale matrices as a means of introducing parsimony. One approach is to introduce lower dimensional latent variables.

Given p-dimensional data $\boldsymbol{x}_1, \ldots, \boldsymbol{x}_n$, factor analysis finds q-dimensional latent factors $\boldsymbol{u}_1, \ldots, \boldsymbol{u}_n$, with $q < p$, that explain a great deal of the variability in the data. The factor analysis model can be written

$$\boldsymbol{X}_i = \boldsymbol{\mu} + \boldsymbol{\Lambda}\boldsymbol{U}_i + \boldsymbol{e}_i, \tag{10}$$

for $i = 1, \dots, n$, where $\boldsymbol{U}_i \sim \mathcal{N}(\boldsymbol{0}, \boldsymbol{I}_q)$, with $q < p$, and $\boldsymbol{e}_i \sim \mathcal{N}(\boldsymbol{0}, \boldsymbol{\Psi})$. Note that $\boldsymbol{U}_1, \dots, \boldsymbol{U}_n$ are distributed independently, and independently of the errors $\boldsymbol{e}_1, \dots, \boldsymbol{e}_n$, which are also distributed independently. The matrix $\boldsymbol{\Lambda}$ is a $p \times q$ matrix of factor loadings, and $\boldsymbol{\Psi}$ is a $p \times p$ diagonal matrix with strictly positive entries. The marginal distribution of $\boldsymbol{X}_i$ from model (10) is $\mathcal{N}(\boldsymbol{\mu}, \boldsymbol{\Lambda}\boldsymbol{\Lambda}' + \boldsymbol{\Psi})$.

Ghahramani and Hinton [20] and McLachlan and Peel [39] consider a mixture of factor analyzers model, where

$$\boldsymbol{X}_i = \boldsymbol{\mu}_g + \boldsymbol{\Lambda}_g \boldsymbol{U}_{ig} + \boldsymbol{e}_{ig} \tag{11}$$

with probability π_g, for $i = 1, \dots, n$ and $g = 1, \dots, G$.

3.2 The Model

This model can be extended to the variance-gamma distribution by first noting that $\boldsymbol{V}$ in (7) can be decomposed using a factor analysis model, i.e.,

$$\boldsymbol{V} = \boldsymbol{\Lambda}\boldsymbol{U} + \boldsymbol{e},$$

where $\boldsymbol{U} \sim \mathcal{N}(\boldsymbol{0}, \mathbf{I}_q)$ and $\boldsymbol{e} \sim \mathcal{N}(\boldsymbol{0}, \boldsymbol{\Psi})$. Then, we can write

$$\boldsymbol{X} = \boldsymbol{\mu} + Y\boldsymbol{\alpha} + \sqrt{Y}(\boldsymbol{\Lambda}\boldsymbol{U} + \boldsymbol{e}), \tag{12}$$

where $Y \backsim \text{gamma}(\gamma, \gamma)$, and it follows that $\boldsymbol{X} \mid y \sim \mathcal{N}(\boldsymbol{\mu} + y\boldsymbol{\alpha}, y(\boldsymbol{\Lambda}\boldsymbol{\Lambda}' + \boldsymbol{\Psi}))$. Then, similar to the mixture of skew-t factor analyzers (MSTFA) model of Murray et al. [46] and the mixture of generalized hyperbolic factor analyzers (MGHFA) model of Tortora et al. [55], we have a mixture of variance-gamma factor analyzers (MVGFA) model with density

$$v_{\text{mixfac}}(\boldsymbol{x} \mid \boldsymbol{\vartheta}) = \sum_{g=1}^{G} \pi_g v_*(\boldsymbol{x} \mid \boldsymbol{\mu}_g, \boldsymbol{\Lambda}_g\boldsymbol{\Lambda}_g' + \boldsymbol{\Psi}_g, \boldsymbol{\alpha}_g, \gamma_g). \tag{13}$$

3.3 Parameter Estimation

Let z_{ig} denote component membership, where $z_{ig} = 1$ if $\boldsymbol{x}_i$ is in component g and $z_{ig} = 0$ otherwise, for $i = 1, \dots, n$ and $g = 1, \dots, G$. The alternating expectation-conditional maximization (AECM) algorithm [45] can be useful when there are multiple sources of unobserved data (missing data and/or latent variables) and one wishes to find maximum likelihood estimates. The AECM algorithm is a variant of the expectation-maximization (EM) algorithm [17] and, similar to the

EM algorithm, is based on the complete-data log-likelihood. Note that the complete-data likelihood is the likelihood of the observed data together with the unobserved data. In our mixture of variance-gamma factor analyzers model, the complete-data consist of the observed $\boldsymbol{x}_i$ as well as the missing labels z_{ig}, the latent y_{ig}, and the latent factors $\boldsymbol{u}_{ig}$, for $i = 1, \ldots, n$ and $g = 1, \ldots, G$. The AECM algorithm allows specification of different complete-data at each stage of the algorithm.

In each E-step, the expected value of the complete-data log-likelihood is computed. The conditional expected value of Z_{ig} is given by

$$\mathbb{E}[Z_{ig} \mid \boldsymbol{x}_i] = \frac{\pi_g v_{\text{mixfac}}(\boldsymbol{x}_i \mid \boldsymbol{\vartheta}_g)}{\sum_{h=1}^{G} \pi_h v_{\text{mixfac}}(\boldsymbol{x}_i \mid \boldsymbol{\vartheta}_h)} =: \hat{z}_{ig}.$$

Note that $Y_{ig} \mid \boldsymbol{x}_i, z_{ig} = 1 \backsim \text{GIG}(2\gamma_g + \boldsymbol{\alpha}'_g \boldsymbol{\Sigma}_g^{-1} \boldsymbol{\alpha}_g, \delta\left(\boldsymbol{x}_i, \boldsymbol{\mu}_g \mid \boldsymbol{\Sigma}_g\right), \gamma_g - p/2)$ and so we have convenient forms for the following expected values:

$$\mathbb{E}[Y_{ig} \mid \boldsymbol{x}_i, z_{ig} = 1] = \sqrt{\frac{\delta(\boldsymbol{x}_i, \boldsymbol{\mu}_g | \boldsymbol{\Sigma}_g)}{2\gamma_g + \boldsymbol{\alpha}_g' \boldsymbol{\Sigma}_g^{-1} \boldsymbol{\alpha}_g}}$$

$$\times \frac{K_{\gamma_g - \frac{p}{2} + 1}\left(\sqrt{[2\gamma_g + \boldsymbol{\alpha}_g' \boldsymbol{\Sigma}_g^{-1} \boldsymbol{\alpha}_g] \delta(\boldsymbol{x}_i, \boldsymbol{\mu}_g | \boldsymbol{\Sigma}_g)}\right)}{K_{\gamma_g - \frac{p}{2}}\left(\sqrt{[2\gamma_g + \boldsymbol{\alpha}_g' \boldsymbol{\Sigma}_g^{-1} \boldsymbol{\alpha}_g] \delta(\boldsymbol{x}_i, \boldsymbol{\mu}_g | \boldsymbol{\Sigma}_g)}\right)} =: a_{ig},$$

$$\mathbb{E}[1/Y_{ig} \mid \boldsymbol{x}_i, z_{ig} = 1] = -\frac{2\lambda_g - p}{\delta(\boldsymbol{x}_i, \boldsymbol{\mu}_g | \boldsymbol{\Sigma}_g)}$$

$$+ \sqrt{\frac{2\gamma_g + \boldsymbol{\alpha}_g' \boldsymbol{\Sigma}_g^{-1} \boldsymbol{\alpha}_g}{\delta(\boldsymbol{x}_i, \boldsymbol{\mu}_g | \boldsymbol{\Sigma}_g)}} \frac{K_{\gamma_g - \frac{p}{2} + 1}\left(\sqrt{[2\gamma_g + \boldsymbol{\alpha}_g' \boldsymbol{\Sigma}_g^{-1} \boldsymbol{\alpha}_g] \delta(\boldsymbol{x}_i, \boldsymbol{\mu}_g | \boldsymbol{\Sigma}_g)}\right)}{K_{\gamma_g - \frac{p}{2}}\left(\sqrt{[2\gamma_g + \boldsymbol{\alpha}_g' \boldsymbol{\Sigma}_g^{-1} \boldsymbol{\alpha}_g] \delta(\boldsymbol{x}_i, \boldsymbol{\mu}_g | \boldsymbol{\Sigma}_g)}\right)} =: b_{ig},$$

$$\mathbb{E}[\log Y_{ig} \mid \boldsymbol{x}_i, z_{ig} = 1] = \log \sqrt{\frac{\delta(\boldsymbol{x}_i, \boldsymbol{\mu}_g | \boldsymbol{\Sigma}_g)}{2\gamma_g + \boldsymbol{\alpha}_g' \boldsymbol{\Sigma}_g^{-1} \boldsymbol{\alpha}_g}}$$

$$+ \frac{\partial}{\partial t} \log \left\{ K_t \left(\sqrt{[2\gamma_g + \boldsymbol{\alpha}_g' \boldsymbol{\Sigma}_g^{-1} \boldsymbol{\alpha}_g] \delta(\boldsymbol{x}_i, \boldsymbol{\mu}_g | \boldsymbol{\Sigma}_g)} \right) \right\} \Bigg|_{t = \gamma_g - \frac{p}{2}} =: c_{ig}.$$

When the latent factors $\boldsymbol{U}_{ig}$ are part of the complete-data, the following expectations are also needed,

$$\mathbb{E}[\boldsymbol{U}_{ig} \mid \boldsymbol{x}_i, z_{ig} = 1] = \boldsymbol{\beta}_g(\boldsymbol{x}_i - \boldsymbol{\mu}_g - a_{ig}\boldsymbol{\alpha}_g) =: \boldsymbol{E}_{1ig},$$

$$\mathbb{E}[(1/Y_{ig})\boldsymbol{U}_{ig} \mid \boldsymbol{x}_i, z_{ig} = 1] = \boldsymbol{\beta}_g[b_{ig}(\boldsymbol{x}_i - \boldsymbol{\mu}_g) - \boldsymbol{\alpha}_g] =: \boldsymbol{E}_{2ig},$$

$$\mathbb{E}[(1/Y_{ig})\boldsymbol{U}_{ig}\boldsymbol{U}_{ig}' \mid \boldsymbol{x}_i, z_{ig} = 1] = b_{ig}[\boldsymbol{I}_q - \boldsymbol{\beta}_g\boldsymbol{\Lambda}_g + \boldsymbol{\beta}_g(\boldsymbol{x}_i - \boldsymbol{\mu}_g)(\boldsymbol{x}_i - \boldsymbol{\mu}_g)'\boldsymbol{\beta}_g']$$

$$- \boldsymbol{\beta}_g[(\boldsymbol{x}_i - \boldsymbol{\mu}_g)\boldsymbol{\alpha}_g' + \boldsymbol{\alpha}_g(\boldsymbol{x}_i - \boldsymbol{\mu}_g)']\boldsymbol{\beta}_g' + a_{ig}\boldsymbol{\beta}_g\boldsymbol{\alpha}_g\boldsymbol{\alpha}_g'\boldsymbol{\beta}_g' =: \boldsymbol{E}_{3ig},$$

where $\boldsymbol{\beta}_g = \boldsymbol{\Lambda}'_g(\boldsymbol{\Lambda}_g\boldsymbol{\Lambda}'_g + \boldsymbol{\Psi}_g)^{-1}$. As usual, all expectations are conditional on the current parameter estimates.

At the first stage of the AECM algorithm, the complete-data comprise the observed $\mathbf{x}_i$, the missing labels z_{ig}, and the latent y_{ig}, and we update the mixing proportions π_g, the component means $\boldsymbol{\mu}_g$, the skewness $\boldsymbol{\alpha}_g$, and the concentration parameter γ_g. The complete-data log-likelihood is

$$l_1 = \sum_{i=1}^{n}\sum_{g=1}^{G} z_{ig}\big[\log \pi_g + \log \phi(\mathbf{x}_i \mid \boldsymbol{\mu}_g + y_{ig}\boldsymbol{\alpha}_g, y_{ig}(\boldsymbol{\Lambda}_g\boldsymbol{\Lambda}'_g + \boldsymbol{\Psi}_g)) + \log g(y_{ig} \mid \gamma_g, \gamma_g)\big].$$

After forming the (conditional) expected value of l_1, updates for π_g, $\boldsymbol{\mu}_g$, and $\boldsymbol{\alpha}_g$ are:

$$\hat{\pi}_g = \frac{n_g}{n}, \quad \hat{\boldsymbol{\mu}}_g = \frac{\sum_{i=1}^n \hat{z}_{ig}\mathbf{x}_i(\bar{a}_g b_{ig} - 1)}{\sum_{i=1}^n \hat{z}_{ig}(\bar{a}_g b_{ig} - 1)}, \quad \text{and} \quad \hat{\boldsymbol{\alpha}}_g = \frac{\sum_{i=1}^n \hat{z}_{ig}\mathbf{x}_i(b_{ig} - \bar{b}_g)}{\sum_{i=1}^n \hat{z}_{ig}(\bar{a}_g b_{ig} - 1)},$$

respectively, where $n_g = \sum_{i=1}^n \hat{z}_{ig}$, $\bar{a}_g = (1/n_g)\sum_{i=1}^n \hat{z}_{ig}a_{ig}$, and $\bar{b}_g = (1/n_g)\sum_{i=1}^n \hat{z}_{ig}b_{ig}$. The update for γ_g arises as the solution to the equation

$$\varphi(\gamma_g) - \hat{z}_{ig}\log\gamma_g = \bar{c}_g - \bar{a}_g + 1,$$

where $\varphi(\cdot)$ is the digamma function and $\bar{c}_g = (1/n_g)\sum_{i=1}^n \hat{z}_{ig}c_{ig}$.

At the second stage, the complete-data comprise the observed $\mathbf{x}_i$, the missing z_{ig}, the latent y_{ig}, and the latent $\mathbf{u}_{ig}$. At this stage, $\boldsymbol{\Lambda}_g$ and $\boldsymbol{\Psi}_g$ are updated, and the complete-data log-likelihood can be written

$$l_2 = \sum_{i=1}^{n}\sum_{g=1}^{G} z_{ig}\big[\log \pi_g + \log \phi(\mathbf{x}_i \mid \boldsymbol{\mu}_g + y_{ig}\boldsymbol{\alpha}_g + \boldsymbol{\Lambda}_g\mathbf{u}_{ig}, y_{ig}\boldsymbol{\Psi}_g) + \log \phi(\mathbf{u}_{ig} \mid \mathbf{0}, y_{ig}\mathbf{I}_q) + \log g(y_{ig} \mid \gamma_g, \gamma_g)\big].$$

That is,

$$\begin{aligned} l_2 = C - \frac{1}{2}\sum_{i=1}^{n}\sum_{g=1}^{G} z_{ig}\Bigg[& \log|\boldsymbol{\Psi}_g| + \frac{1}{y_{ig}}\operatorname{tr}\{(\mathbf{x}_i - \boldsymbol{\mu}_g)(\mathbf{x}_i - \boldsymbol{\mu}_g)'\boldsymbol{\Psi}_g^{-1}\} \\ & - 2\operatorname{tr}\{(\mathbf{x}_i - \boldsymbol{\mu}_g)\boldsymbol{\alpha}'_g\boldsymbol{\Psi}_g^{-1}\} + y_{ig}\operatorname{tr}\{\boldsymbol{\alpha}_g\boldsymbol{\alpha}'_g\boldsymbol{\Psi}_g^{-1}\} - \frac{2}{y_{ig}}\operatorname{tr}\{(\mathbf{x}_i - \boldsymbol{\mu}_g)'\boldsymbol{\Psi}_g^{-1}\boldsymbol{\Lambda}_g\mathbf{u}_{ig}\} \\ & + 2\operatorname{tr}\{\boldsymbol{\alpha}'_g\boldsymbol{\Psi}_g^{-1}\boldsymbol{\Lambda}_g\mathbf{u}_{ig}\} + \frac{1}{y_{ig}}\operatorname{tr}\{\boldsymbol{\Lambda}_g\mathbf{u}_{ig}\mathbf{u}'_{ig}\boldsymbol{\Lambda}'_g\boldsymbol{\Psi}_g^{-1}\}\Bigg], \end{aligned}$$

where C is constant with respect to $\boldsymbol{\Lambda}_g$ and $\boldsymbol{\Psi}_g$. Taking the (conditional) expected value of l_2 gives

$$Q_2 = C - \frac{1}{2}\sum_{i=1}^{n}\sum_{g=1}^{G}\hat{z}_{ig}\Big[\log|\boldsymbol{\Psi}_g| + b_{ig}\,\mathrm{tr}\{(\boldsymbol{x}_i - \hat{\boldsymbol{\mu}}_g)(\boldsymbol{x}_i - \hat{\boldsymbol{\mu}}_g)'\boldsymbol{\Psi}_g^{-1}\}$$
$$- 2\,\mathrm{tr}\{(\boldsymbol{x}_i - \hat{\boldsymbol{\mu}}_g)\hat{\boldsymbol{\alpha}}_g'\boldsymbol{\Psi}_g^{-1}\} + a_{ig}\,\mathrm{tr}\{\hat{\boldsymbol{\alpha}}_g\hat{\boldsymbol{\alpha}}_g'\boldsymbol{\Psi}_g^{-1}\} - 2\,\mathrm{tr}\{(\boldsymbol{x}_i - \hat{\boldsymbol{\mu}}_g)'\boldsymbol{\Psi}_g^{-1}\boldsymbol{\Lambda}_g\boldsymbol{E}_{2ig}\}$$
$$+ 2\,\mathrm{tr}\{\hat{\boldsymbol{\alpha}}_g'\boldsymbol{\Psi}_g^{-1}\boldsymbol{\Lambda}_g\boldsymbol{E}_{1ig}\} + \mathrm{tr}\{\boldsymbol{\Lambda}_g\boldsymbol{E}_{3ig}\boldsymbol{\Lambda}_g'\boldsymbol{\Psi}_g^{-1}\}\Big].$$

Differentiating Q_2 with respect to $\boldsymbol{\Lambda}_g$ gives

$$S_1(\boldsymbol{\Lambda}_g, \boldsymbol{\Psi}_g) = \frac{\partial Q_2}{\partial \boldsymbol{\Lambda}_g}$$
$$= -\frac{1}{2}\sum_{i=1}^{n}\hat{z}_{ig}\left[-2\boldsymbol{\Psi}_g^{-1}(\boldsymbol{x}_i - \hat{\boldsymbol{\mu}}_g)\boldsymbol{E}_{2ig}' + 2\boldsymbol{\Psi}_g^{-1}\hat{\boldsymbol{\alpha}}_g\boldsymbol{E}_{1ig}' + \boldsymbol{\Psi}_g^{-1}\boldsymbol{\Lambda}_g(\boldsymbol{E}_{3ig}' + \boldsymbol{E}_{3ig})\right],$$

and solving $S_1(\hat{\boldsymbol{\Lambda}}_g, \hat{\boldsymbol{\Psi}}_g) = \boldsymbol{0}$ gives the update

$$\hat{\boldsymbol{\Lambda}}_g = \left\{\sum_{i=1}^{n}\hat{z}_{ig}\left[(\boldsymbol{x}_i - \hat{\boldsymbol{\mu}}_g)\boldsymbol{E}_{2ig}' - \hat{\boldsymbol{\alpha}}_g\boldsymbol{E}_{1ig}'\right]\right\}\left\{\sum_{i=1}^{n}\hat{z}_{ig}\boldsymbol{E}_{3ig}\right\}^{-1}.$$

Differentiating Q_2 with respect to $\boldsymbol{\Psi}_g^{-1}$ gives

$$S_2(\boldsymbol{\Lambda}_g, \boldsymbol{\Psi}_g) = \frac{\partial Q_2}{\partial \boldsymbol{\Psi}_g^{-1}} = \frac{1}{2}\sum_{i=1}^{n}\hat{z}_{ig}\boldsymbol{\Psi}_g - \frac{1}{2}\sum_{i=1}^{n}\hat{z}_{ig}\Big[b_{ig}(\boldsymbol{x}_i - \hat{\boldsymbol{\mu}}_g)(\boldsymbol{x}_i - \hat{\boldsymbol{\mu}}_g)'$$
$$- 2\hat{\boldsymbol{\alpha}}_g(\boldsymbol{x}_i - \hat{\boldsymbol{\mu}}_g)' + a_{ig}\hat{\boldsymbol{\alpha}}_g\hat{\boldsymbol{\alpha}}_g' - 2(\boldsymbol{x}_i - \hat{\boldsymbol{\mu}}_g)\boldsymbol{E}_{2ig}'\boldsymbol{\Lambda}_g' + 2\hat{\boldsymbol{\alpha}}_g\boldsymbol{E}_{1ig}'\boldsymbol{\Lambda}_g' + \boldsymbol{\Lambda}_g\boldsymbol{E}_{3ig}\boldsymbol{\Lambda}_g'\Big],$$

and solving $\mathrm{diag}\{S_2(\hat{\boldsymbol{\Lambda}}_g, \hat{\boldsymbol{\Psi}}_g)\} = \boldsymbol{0}$ we obtain

$$\hat{\boldsymbol{\Psi}}_g = \frac{1}{n_g}\mathrm{diag}\Big\{\sum_{i=1}^{n}\hat{z}_{ig}\Big[b_{ig}(\boldsymbol{x}_i - \hat{\boldsymbol{\mu}}_g)(\boldsymbol{x}_i - \hat{\boldsymbol{\mu}}_g)' - 2\hat{\boldsymbol{\alpha}}_g(\boldsymbol{x}_i - \hat{\boldsymbol{\mu}}_g)' + a_{ig}\hat{\boldsymbol{\alpha}}_g\hat{\boldsymbol{\alpha}}_g'$$
$$- 2(\boldsymbol{x}_i - \hat{\boldsymbol{\mu}}_g)\boldsymbol{E}_{2ig}'\hat{\boldsymbol{\Lambda}}_g' + 2\hat{\boldsymbol{\alpha}}_g\boldsymbol{E}_{1ig}'\hat{\boldsymbol{\Lambda}}_g' + \hat{\boldsymbol{\Lambda}}_g\boldsymbol{E}_{3ig}\hat{\boldsymbol{\Lambda}}_g'\Big]\Big\}.$$

Note that the direct inversion of the matrix $\boldsymbol{\Lambda}_g\boldsymbol{\Lambda}_g' + \boldsymbol{\Psi}_g$ requires inversion of a $p \times p$ matrix, which can be very slow for larger values of p. From the Woodbury identity [59], we have the formula

$$(\boldsymbol{\Lambda}_g\boldsymbol{\Lambda}_g' + \boldsymbol{\Psi}_g)^{-1} = \boldsymbol{\Psi}_g^{-1} - \boldsymbol{\Psi}_g^{-1}\boldsymbol{\Lambda}_g(\boldsymbol{I}_q + \boldsymbol{\Lambda}_g'\boldsymbol{\Psi}_g^{-1}\boldsymbol{\Lambda}_g)^{-1}\boldsymbol{\Lambda}_g'\boldsymbol{\Psi}_g^{-1}, \tag{14}$$

which requires inversion of diagonal $p \times p$ matrices—which is trivial—and a $q \times q$ matrix, resulting in a significant speed-up for $q \ll p$.

We determine convergence of our EM algorithms via the Aitken acceleration [1]. Specifically, the Aitken acceleration is used to estimate the asymptotic maximum of the log-likelihood at each iteration and we consider the algorithm converged if this estimate is sufficiently close to the current log-likelihood. The Aitken acceleration at iteration k is

$$a^{(k)} = \frac{l^{(k+1)} - l^{(k)}}{l^{(k)} - l^{(k-1)}},$$

where $l^{(k)}$ is the log-likelihood at iteration k. Böhning et al. [10] and Lindsay [36] use an asymptotic estimate of the log-likelihood at iteration $k+1$, i.e.,

$$l_{\infty}^{(k+1)} = l^{(k)} + \frac{1}{1 - a^{(k)}}(l^{(k+1)} - l^{(k)}),$$

and the algorithm can be considered to have converged when

$$l_{\infty}^{(k+1)} - l^{(k)} < e, \tag{15}$$

for small e, provided this difference is positive (cf. [44]). The criterion in (15) is used in the analyses in Sect. 4, with $e = 0.1$.

3.4 Model Selection

In model-based clustering applications, the Bayesian information criterion [BIC; 52] is often used to determine the number of components G (if unknown) as well as the number of latent factors, if applicable. The BIC can be written

$$\text{BIC} = 2l(\hat{\boldsymbol{\theta}}) - \rho \log n,$$

where $l(\hat{\boldsymbol{\theta}})$ is the maximized log-likelihood, $\hat{\boldsymbol{\theta}}$ is the maximum likelihood estimate of the model parameters $\boldsymbol{\theta}$, ρ is the number of free parameters in the model, and n is the number of observations. The BIC has long been used for mixture model selection and its use was motivated through Bayes factors [15, 27, 28]. While many alternatives have been suggested (e.g., [8]) none have yet proved superior in general. Lopes and West [37] illustrate that the BIC can be effective for choosing the number of factors in a factor analysis model.

It is worth noting, however, that the BIC can be unreliable for model selection for larger values of p. In such cases, one approach is to fix G a priori, e.g., in their MGHFA analysis of a 27-dimensional data set, Tortora et al. [55] fix $G = 2$ and use the BIC to select the number of latent factors—an analogous approach is taken in the analyses in Sect. 4. Other approaches are possible and include using a LASSO-penalized approach (e.g., [7]), which will be discussed further in Sect. 5.

4 The Wisconsin Breast Cancer Data

The purpose of this illustration is to show that the MVGFA model is a useful addition to the model-based clustering toolkit, i.e., that even though it is a special and limiting case, the MVGFA is useful in addition to the MGHFA model. The Wisconsin breast cancer data are available from the UCI Machine Learning Repository [32] and comprise 30 quantitative features computed from digitized images of 569 fine needle aspirates of breast masses, where 357 are benign and 212 are malignant. Bouveyron and Brunet-Saumard [11] use these data to illustrate the performance of two Gaussian mixture approaches to clustering high-dimensional data. Similarly, we fix $G = 2$ components in this analysis. The MVGFA model is fitted to these data for $q = 1, \ldots, 22$ latent factors, k-means starting values are used, and the best model (i.e., the number of latent factors) is selected using the BIC. For comparison, the same procedure is taken for the MGHFA model. All code is written in R [50].

Because we know whether each mass is benign or malignant, we can assess the respective performance of the selected MVGFA and MGHFA models in terms of classification accuracy, which can be measured using the adjusted Rand index [ARI; 24, 51]. The ARI has expected value 0 under random classification and takes the value 1 for perfect class agreement. Negative values of the ARI are also possible, and indicate classification that is worse than one would expect under random classification. The selected MVGFA model has $q = 20$ latent factors and the associated predicted classifications misclassify just 47 of the 569 breast masses (ARI $= 0.695$; Table 1). The selected MGHFA model has $q = 19$ latent factors and gives slightly inferior classification performance, misclassifying 51 of the 569 masses (ARI $= 0.672$; Table 1).

Table 1 Cross-tabulation of the classifications (A, B) associated with the selected MVGFA and MGHFA models, respectively, for the Wisconsin breast cancer data

	MVGFA		MGHFA	
	A	*B*	*A*	*B*
Benign	326	31	319	38
Malignant	16	195	13	198

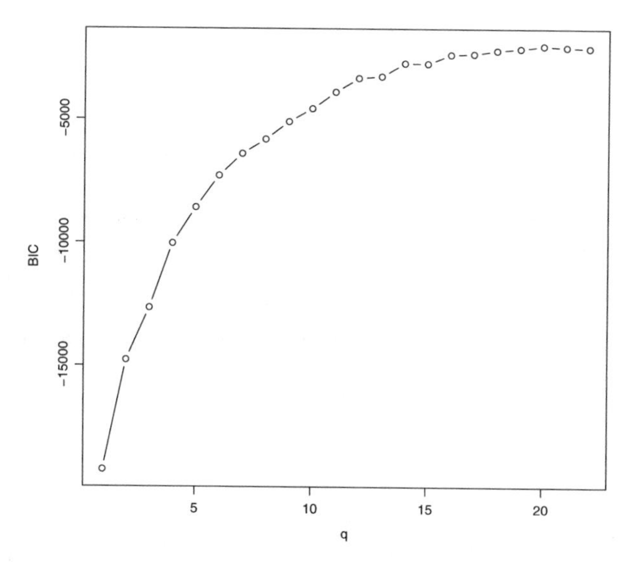

Fig. 1 Plot of BIC value versus number of latent factors q for the MVGFA model fitted to the Wisconsin breast cancer data

Considering a plot of the log-likelihood versus the number of factors for the MVGFA model (Fig. 1), it is clear that the BIC prefers larger values of q for these data—a plot focused on the region where $q \in [16, 20]$ is given in the Appendix (Fig. 3). The analogous plots for the MGHFA model are very similar. The superior performance of the MVGFA model for these data is not intended to suggest that the MVGFA model is better, in general, than the MGHFA model but rather to show that it can outperform the MGHFA model in some cases. Accordingly, the MVGFA model is a useful addition to the suite of non-Gaussian extensions of the mixture of factor analyzers model.

Note that the number of latent factors is run from $q = 1, \ldots, 22$ latent factors because $q = 22$ is the largest number of latent factors that leads to a reduction in the number of free scale parameters. That is, $q = 22$ is the largest number of latent factors such that

$$(30 - q)^2 > 30 + q.$$

This criterion follows from recalling that the reduction in free covariance parameters under the factor analysis model is given by

$$\frac{1}{2}p(p+1) - \left[pq + p - \frac{1}{2}q(q-1)\right] = \frac{1}{2}\left[(p-q)^2 - (p+q)\right]$$

(cf. [30]) and noting that $p = 30$ for the Wisconsin breast cancer data.

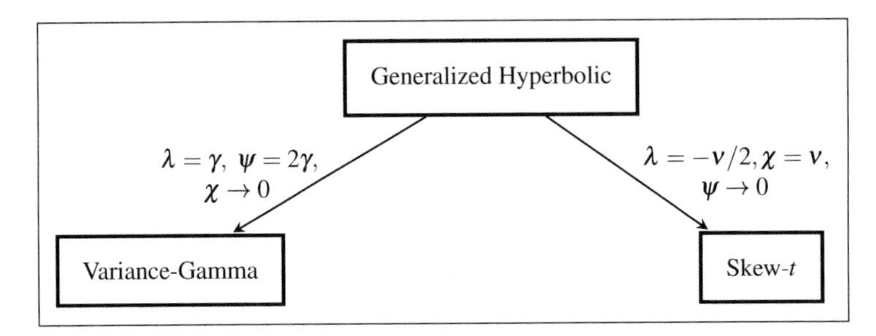

Fig. 2 Two distributions available as special and limiting cases of the generalized hyperbolic distribution

5 Discussion

The mixture of factor analyzers model has been extended to variance-gamma mixtures using a formulation of the variance-gamma distribution that arises as a special ($\lambda = \gamma, \psi = 2\gamma$), limiting ($\chi \to 0$), case of the generalized hyperbolic distribution. Updates are derived for parameter estimation within the AECM algorithm framework, which is made feasible by exploitation of the relationship with the GIG distribution. As illustrated in Fig. 2, there is a clear analogy between our formulation of the variance-gamma distribution and the formulation of the skew-*t* distribution used by Murray et al. [46, 47]. Future work will see an extensive comparison of the MSTFA, MVGFA, and MGHFA models as well as other approaches that can be viewed as extensions of the mixture of factor analyzers model.

Bhattacharya and McNicholas [7] illustrate that the BIC does not perform well for selecting the number of components and the number of latent factors for the mixture of factor analyzers model, and parsimonious versions thereof [43], when p is large. To help circumvent this problem, Bhattacharya and McNicholas [7] develop a LASSO-penalized BIC, and pursuing a similar approach for the MVGFA model will be a topic of future work. Future work will also include consideration of alternatives to the BIC for selecting the number of latent factors q, investigation of alternatives to the AECM algorithm for parameter estimation, e.g., variational Bayes approximations (cf. [54]), as well as the use of a mixture of variance-gamma distributions and the MVGFA model within the fractionally supervised classification framework [58]. Multiple scaled mixtures of variance-gamma distributions will also be considered and can be viewed as an extension of the work of Franczak et al. [19].

Acknowledgements The authors are grateful to an anonymous reviewer for providing helpful comments. This work is supported by an Alexander Graham Bell Scholarship (CGS-D) from the Natural Sciences and Engineering Research Council of Canada (S.M. McNicholas).

Appendix

See Fig. 3.

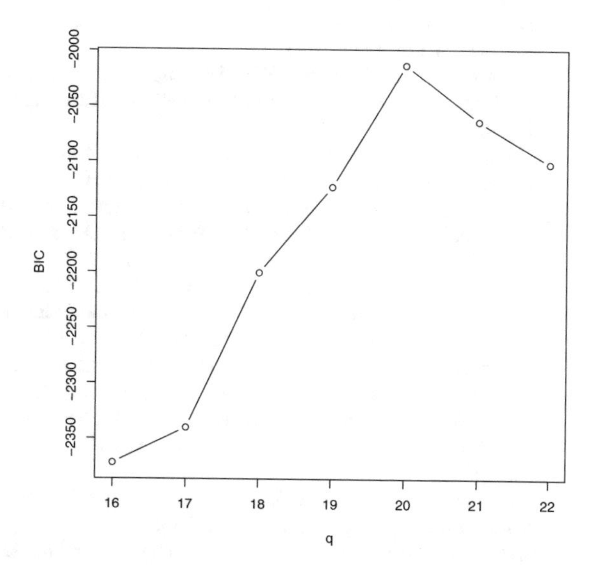

Fig. 3 Plot of BIC value versus number of latent factors q for the MVGFA model fitted to the Wisconsin breast cancer data, focusing on $q \in [16, 22]$

References

1. Aitken, A.C.: A series formula for the roots of algebraic and transcendental equations. Proc. R. Soc. Edinb. **45**, 14–22 (1926)
2. Andrews, J.L., McNicholas, P.D.: Extending mixtures of multivariate t-factor analyzers. Stat. Comput. **21**(3), 361–373 (2011)
3. Andrews, J.L., McNicholas, P.D.: Mixtures of modified t-factor analyzers for model-based clustering, classification, and discriminant analysis. J. Stat. Plann. Inf. **141**(4), 1479–1486 (2011)
4. Andrews, J.L., McNicholas, P.D.: Model-based clustering, classification, and discriminant analysis via mixtures of multivariate *t*-distributions: the *t*EIGEN family. Stat. Comput. **22**(5), 1021–1029 (2012)
5. Andrews, J.L., McNicholas, P.D., Subedi, S.: Model-based classification via mixtures of multivariate t-distributions. Comput. Stat. Data Anal. **55**(1), 520–529 (2011)
6. Barndorff-Nielsen, O., Halgreen, C.: Infinite divisibility of the hyperbolic and generalized inverse Gaussian distributions. Zeitschrift für Wahrscheinlichkeitstheorie und Verwandte Gebiete **38**, 309–311 (1977)
7. Bhattacharya, S., McNicholas, P.D.: A LASSO-penalized BIC for mixture model selection. Adv. Data Anal. Classif. **8**(1), 45–61 (2014)
8. Biernacki, C., Celeux, G., Govaert, G.: Assessing a mixture model for clustering with the integrated completed likelihood. IEEE Trans. Pattern Anal. Mach. Intell. **22**(7), 719–725 (2000)
9. Blæsild, P.: The shape of the generalized inverse Gaussian and hyperbolic distributions. Research Report 37, Department of Theoretical Statistics, Aarhus University, Denmark (1978)

10. Böhning, D., Dietz, E., Schaub, R., Schlattmann, P., Lindsay, B.: The distribution of the likelihood ratio for mixtures of densities from the one-parameter exponential family. Ann. Inst. Stat. Math. **46**, 373–388 (1994)
11. Bouveyron, C., Brunet-Saumard, C.: Model-based clustering of high-dimensional data: a review. Comput. Stat. Data Anal. **71**, 52–78 (2014)
12. Browne, R.P., McNicholas, P.D.: A mixture of generalized hyperbolic distributions. Can. J. Stat. **43**(2), 176–198 (2015)
13. Browne, R.P., McNicholas, P.D., Sparling, M.D.: Model-based learning using a mixture of mixtures of Gaussian and uniform distributions. IEEE Trans. Pattern Anal. Mach. Intell. **34**(4), 814–817 (2012)
14. Dang, U.J., Browne, R.P., McNicholas, P.D.: Mixtures of multivariate power exponential distributions. Biometrics **71**(4), 1081–1089 (2015)
15. Dasgupta, A., Raftery, A.E.: Detecting features in spatial point processes with clutter via model-based clustering. J. Am. Stat. Assoc. **93**, 294–302 (1998)
16. Dean, N., Murphy, T.B., Downey, G.: Using unlabelled data to update classification rules with applications in food authenticity studies. J. R. Stat. Soc. Ser. C **55**(1), 1–14 (2006)
17. Dempster, A.P., Laird, N.M., Rubin, D.B.: Maximum likelihood from incomplete data via the EM algorithm. J. R. Stat. Soc. Ser. B **39**(1) 1–38 (1977)
18. Franczak, B.C., Browne, R.P., McNicholas, P.D.: Mixtures of shifted asymmetric Laplace distributions. IEEE Trans. Pattern Anal. Mach. Intell. **36**(6), 1149–1157 (2014)
19. Franczak, B.C., Tortora, C., Browne, R.P., McNicholas, P.D.: Unsupervised learning via mixtures of skewed distributions with hypercube contours. Pattern Recogn. Lett. **58**(1), 69–76 (2015)
20. Ghahramani, Z., Hinton, G.E.: The EM algorithm for factor analyzers. Tech. Rep. CRG-TR-96-1, University Of Toronto, Toronto (1997)
21. Good, J.I.: The population frequencies of species and the estimation of population parameters. Biometrika **40**, 237–260 (1953)
22. Halgreen, C.: Self-decomposability of the generalized inverse Gaussian and hyperbolic distributions. Zeitschrift für Wahrscheinlichkeitstheorie und Verwandte Gebiete **47**, 13–18 (1979)
23. Hastie, T., Tibshirani, R.: Discriminant analysis by Gaussian mixtures. J. R. Stat. Soc. Ser. B **58**(1), 155–176 (1996)
24. Hubert, L., Arabie, P.: Comparing partitions. J. Classif. **2**(1), 193–218 (1985)
25. Jørgensen, B.: Statistical Properties of the Generalized Inverse Gaussian Distribution. Springer, New York (1982)
26. Karlis, D., Meligkotsidou, L.: Finite mixtures of multivariate Poisson distributions with application. J. Stat. Plan. Inf. **137**(6), 1942–1960 (2007)
27. Kass, R.E., Raftery, A.E.: Bayes factors. J. Am. Stat. Assoc. **90**(430), 773–795 (1995)
28. Kass, R.E., Wasserman, L.: A reference Bayesian test for nested hypotheses and its relationship to the Schwarz criterion. J. Am. Stat. Assoc. **90**(431), 928–934 (1995)
29. Kotz, S., Kozubowski, T.J., Podgorski, K.: The Laplace Distribution and Generalizations: A Revisit with Applications to Communications, Economics, Engineering, and Finance. Birkhauser, Boston (2001)
30. Lawley, D.N., Maxwell, A.E.: Factor analysis as a statistical method. J. R. Stat. Soc. Ser. D **12**(3), 209–229 (1962)
31. Lee, S.X., McLachlan, G.J.: On mixtures of skew normal and skew t-distributions. Adv. Data Anal. Classif. **7**(3), 241–266 (2013)
32. Lichman, M.: UCI machine learning repository. University of California, Irvine, School of Information and Computer Sciences. http://archive.ics.uci.edu/ml (2013)
33. Lin, T.I.: Maximum likelihood estimation for multivariate skew normal mixture models. J. Multivar. Anal. **100**, 257–265 (2009)
34. Lin, T.I.: Robust mixture modeling using multivariate skew t distributions. Stat. Comput. **20**(3), 343–356 (2010)

35. Lin, T.I., McNicholas, P.D., Hsiu, J.H.: Capturing patterns via parsimonious t mixture models. Stat. Probab. Lett. **88**, 80–87 (2014)
36. Lindsay, B.G.: Mixture models: Theory, geometry and applications. In: NSF-CBMS Regional Conference Series in Probability and Statistics, vol. 5, Institute of Mathematical Statistics, Hayward, CA (1995)
37. Lopes, H.F., West, M.: Bayesian model assessment in factor analysis. Stat. Sin. **14**, 41–67 (2004)
38. McLachlan, G.J.: Discriminant Analysis and Statistical Pattern Recognition. Wiley, New York (1992)
39. McLachlan, G.J., Peel, D.: Mixtures of factor analyzers. In: Proceedings of the Seventh International Conference on Machine Learning, Morgan Kaufmann, SF, pp. 599–606 (2000)
40. McNeil, A.J., Frey, R., Embrechts, P.: Quantitative Risk Management: Concepts, Techniques and Tools. Princeton University Press, Princeton (2005)
41. McNicholas, P.D.: Model-based classification using latent Gaussian mixture models. J. Stat. Plan. Inf. **140**(5), 1175–1181 (2010)
42. McNicholas, P.D.: Mixture Model-Based Classification. Chapman & Hall/CRC Press, Boca Raton (2016)
43. McNicholas, P.D., Murphy, T.B.: Parsimonious Gaussian mixture models. Stat. Comput. **18**(3), 285–296 (2008)
44. McNicholas, P.D., Murphy, T.B., McDaid, A.F., Frost, D.: Serial and parallel implementations of model-based clustering via parsimonious Gaussian mixture models. Comput. Stat. Data Anal. **54**(3), 711–723 (2010)
45. Meng, X.L., van Dyk, D.: The EM algorithm—an old folk song sung to a fast new tune (with discussion). J. R. Stat. Soc. Ser. B **59**(3), 511–567 (1997)
46. Murray, P.M., Browne, R.B., McNicholas, P.D.: Mixtures of skew-t factor analyzers. Comput. Stat. Data Anal. **77**, 326–335 (2014)
47. Murray, P.M., McNicholas, P.D., Browne, R.B.: A mixture of common skew-*t* factor analyzers. Stat **3**(1), 68–82 (2014)
48. O'Hagan, A., Murphy, T.B., Gormley, I.C., McNicholas, P.D., Karlis, D.: Clustering with the multivariate normal inverse Gaussian distribution. Comput. Stat. Data Anal. **93**, 18–30 (2016)
49. Peel, D., McLachlan, G.J.: Robust mixture modelling using the t distribution. Stat. Comput. **10**(4), 339–348 (2000)
50. R Core Team: R: A Language and Environment for Statistical Computing. R Foundation for Statistical Computing, Vienna, Austria (2015)
51. Rand, W.M.: Objective criteria for the evaluation of clustering methods. J. Am. Stat. Assoc. **66**(336), 846–850 (1971)
52. Schwarz, G.: Estimating the dimension of a model. Ann. Stat. **6**, 461–464 (1978)
53. Steane, M.A., McNicholas, P.D., Yada, R.: Model-based classification via mixtures of multivariate t-factor analyzers. Commun. Stat. Simul. Comput. **41**(4), 510–523 (2012)
54. Subedi, S., McNicholas, P.D.: Variational Bayes approximations for clustering via mixtures of normal inverse Gaussian distributions. Adv. Data Anal. Classif. **8**(2), 167–193 (2014)
55. Tortora, C., McNicholas, P.D., Browne, R.P.: A mixture of generalized hyperbolic factor analyzers. Adv. Data Anal. Classif. (2015, to appear). doi: 10.1007/s11634-015-0204-z
56. Vrbik, I., McNicholas, P.D.: Analytic calculations for the EM algorithm for multivariate skew-mixture models. Stat. Probab. Lett. **82**(6), 1169–1174 (2012)
57. Vrbik, I., McNicholas, P.D.: Parsimonious skew mixture models for model-based clustering and classification. Comput. Stat. Data Anal. **71**, 196–210 (2014)
58. Vrbik, I., McNicholas, P.D.: Fractionally-supervised classification. J. Classif. **32**(3), 359–381 (2015)
59. Woodbury, M.A.: Inverting modified matrices. Statistical Research Group, Memorandum Report 42. Princeton University, Princeton, NJ (1950)

Printed in the United States
By Bookmasters